W9-APU-883

# PHARMACOLOGY, BIOLOGY, AND CLINICAL APPLICATIONS OF ANDROGENS

## Current Status and Future Prospects

Proceedings of the Second International Androgen Workshop, Long Beach, California, February 17–20, 1995

### EDITORS

**SHALENDER BHASIN**
Charles R. Drew University of Medicine and Science
Los Angeles, California

**HENRY L. GABELNICK**
Contraceptive Research and Development Program
Arlington, Virginia

**JEFFREY M. SPIELER**
Agency for International Development
Washington, D.C.

**RONALD S. SWERDLOFF**
Harbor-UCLA Medical Center
Torrance, California

**CHRISTINA WANG**
Harbor-UCLA Medical Center
Torrance, California

**CHUCK KELLY**
Technical Editor
Long Beach, California

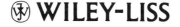

A JOHN WILEY & SONS, INC., PUBLICATION
New York • Chichester • Brisbane • Toronto • Singapore

**Address All Inquiries to the Publisher**
**Wiley-Liss, Inc., 605 Third Avenue, New York, NY 10158-0012**

**Library of Congress Cataloging-in-Publication Data**

International Androgen Workshop (2nd : 1995 : Long Beach, Calif.)
    Biology, pharmacology, and clinical applications of androgens :
current status and future prospects / editors, Shalender Bhasin ..
[et al.].
      p.  cm.
    Includes index.
    ISBN 0-471-13320-5 (cloth : alk. paper)
    1. Androgens—Therapeutic use—Congresses. I. Bhasin, Shalender,
1953–  . II. Title.
    [DNLM: 1. Androgens—therapeutic use—congresses. 2. Androgens-
-physiology—congresses. WJ 875 I606b 1995]
RM296.I58  1995
615'.366—dc20
DNLM/DLC
for Library of Congress                  95-46146
                                            CIP

**The text of this book is printed on acid-free paper.**

10  9  8  7  6  5  4  3  2  1

# CONTENTS

**PART III: ANDROGEN: EFFECTS ON THE BRAIN: COGNITIVE,
SEXUAL, AND AGGRESSIVE BEHAVIOR**

**PART IV: EFFECTS ON METABOLISM**

## PART V: ANDROGEN THERAPY

## PART VI: ANDROGENS AND MALE CONTRACEPTION

## PART VII: ANDROGEN DELIVERY SYSTEMS

### PART VIII: WORKSHOP PARTICIPANTS

# PREFACE

The First International Androgen Workshop was held in Marco Island, Florida in the spring of 1990. That Workshop was a great success. It generated a number of new ideas and provided the impetus for a number of new clinical trials. In fact, the subsequent 4-1/2 years turned out to be the most exciting in the androgen field. This period witnessed the cloning of the 5-alpha reductase gene and the characterization of the molecular biology of the androgen receptor. Following the clinical trials with the 5-alpha reductase inhibitor finesteride, the Food and Drug Administration approved this drug for use in benign prostatic hyperplasia. A number of other landmark studies were completed during this period, including the demonstration that androgen-induced azoospermia and/or severe oligozoospermia provides effective and reversible contraception. It was demonstrated that combined administration of a GnRH antagonist or a gestagen and androgen can induce consistent azoospermia in normal men. There was significant progress in the development of several new testosterone formulations. These studies resolved some issues, but many areas of uncertainty persisted. Therefore, many investigators in the field felt that it was time to bring back the experts under one roof in order to review the state of the art; to identify areas of disagreement, and/or uncertainty; and, to outline critical areas for future research. This led to the formation of a steering committee which guided the selection of topics and speakers.

The Second International Androgen Workshop was truly the result of a collaborative effort of many investigators and federal and non-federal funding agencies. Primary funding for the Workshop was provided by the Contraceptive Research and Development Program (CONRAD) with support from US AID. The Workshop also received significant support from the Food and Drug Administration, National Institute of Child Health and Human Development, World Health Organization, the ALZA Corporation, Biotechnology General Corporation, the Theratech Corporation, Stolle Research and Development, Roerig Pfizer, the Upjohn Company, Merck and Company, and Eli Lilly and Company.

The Workshop was attended by over 200 investigators from six continents and representatives from several federal and international regulatory agencies and pharmaceutical companies. The Workshop provided a forum for investigators from around the world to review up-to-date information, challenge the dogma, and thus help delineate the areas of agreement and uncertainty. This publication represents the proceedings of the Workshop.

This book is not intended to be an encyclopedic reference. Instead, the authors were encouraged to present their opinions on areas of controversy and highlight the cutting edge. The debates and the point-counterpoint sessions provided an effective venue for crystallizing areas of agreement and disagreement in the field. Therefore, these proceedings present the state-of-the-art in androgen biology and the range of expert opinions, and ideas for future research.

We are greatly indebted to Chuck Kelly for his tireless efforts in putting this book together.

Shalender Bhasin
Henry Gabelnick
Jeff Spieler
Ronald Swerdloff
Christina Wang

# CONTRIBUTORS

**A. Adimoejla,** *Airlangga University* [**375**]

**Gerianne M. Alexander, PhD,** *Assistant Professor, Department of Psychology, University of New Orleans, New Orleans, Louisiana* [**169**]

**K.M. Arsyad, MD,** *Faculty of Medicine, Sriwidjajaj University, Palembang, Indonesia* [**375**]

**Stefan Arver,** *Karolinska Institute, Stockholm, Sweden* [**449**]

**Linda E. Atkinson,** *ALZA Corporation, Palo Alto, California* [**437**]

**Carrie J. Bagatell,** *Department of Medicine, University of Washington, Medicine Service, Seattle Veterans Affairs Medical Center, Seattle, Washington* [**225**]

**C. Wayne Bardin,** *Center for Biomedical Research, The Population Council, New York, New York* [**493**]

**Elizabeth Barrett-Conner, MD,** *Professor and Chair, Department of Family Medicine and Preventive Medicine, University of California at San Diego, San Diego, California* [**215**]

**David J. Baylink,** *Departments of Medicine and Biochemistry, Loma Linda University and Jerry L. Pettis Medical Center, Loma Linda, California* [**259**]

**Hermann M. Behre, MD,** *Professor, Institute of Reproductive Medicine,* *University of Steinfurter, Strauss, Germany* [**409, 471**]

**Shalender Bhasin, MD,** *Professor of Medicine, Harbor-UCLA Medical Center, Torrance, California* [**199, 283, 355, 481**]

**Gabriel Bialy, PhD,** *Acting Deputy Director, Center for Population Research, National Institute of Child Health and Human Development, Bethesda, Maryland* [**387**]

**William J. Bremner, MD, PhD,** *Professor and Chair, Department of Medicine, Veterans' Administration Medical Center, Seattle, Washington* [**225**]

**Terry Brown, PhD,** *Associate Professor, Department of Population Dynamics, Johns Hopkins University, Baltimore, Maryland* [**45, 503**]

**Carlos Callegari,** *Harbor–UCLA Medical Center, Torrance, California* [**355**]

**Richard Casaburi, PhD, MD,** *Associate Professor of Medicine, Harbor-UCLA Medical Center, Torrance, California* [**283**]

**Don H. Catlin, MD,** *Director of UCLA Analytical Laboratory, UCLA-Olympic Laboratory, Los Angeles, California* [**289**]

**Chawnshang Chang, PhD,** *Associate Professor, Department of Human Oncology, University of Wisconsin, Madison, Wisconsin* [**65**]

**Chen-Tien Chang,** *Department of Human Oncology and Program in Endocrinology–Reproductive Physiology, University of Wisconsin, Madison, Wisconsin* [**65**]

**Glenn R. Cunningham, MD** *Professor and Associate Chief of Staff, Veterans' Administration Medical Center, Houston, Texas* [**79, 437**]

**James M. Dabbs, Jr., PhD,** *Professor of Psychology, Georgia State University, Atlanta, Georgia* [**179**]

**David M. deKretser, MD,** *Professor and Director, Institute of Reproduction and Development, Monash University, Melbourne, Australia* [**3**]

**Adrian S. Dobs,** *Johns Hopkins University, Baltimore, Maryland* [**449**]

**Timothy M.M. Farley,** *UNDP/ UNFPA/WHO/World Bank Special Program of Research, Development, and Research Training in Human Reproduction, World Health Organization, Geneva, Switzerland* [**345**]

**Gary Stephen Ferenchick, MD,** *Associate Professor of Medicine, Michigan State University, Lansing, Michigan* [**201**]

**Joel S. Finkelstein, MD,** *Assistant Professor of Medicine, Harvard Medical School, Boston, Massachusetts* [**265**]

**Jack Geller, MD,** *Adjunct Professor, Program Director, Internal Medicine, Mercy Hospital Medical Center, San Diego, California* [**103**]

**Roger A. Gorski, PhD,** *Professor, Department of Anatomy, UCLA School of Medicine, Los Angeles, California* [**157, 159**]

**James E. Griffin,** *Department of Internal Medicine, The University of Texas, Southwestern Medical Center, Dallas, Texas* [**57**]

**K.M. Grigor,** *Department of Pathology, University of Edinburgh, Edinburgh, Scotland* [**17**]

**Michael D. Griswold, PhD,** *Professor of Biochemistry, Washington State University, Pullman, Washington* [**11**]

**P. Hadiluwih,** *Diponegoro University* [**375**]

**David J. Handelsman, MD, PhD,** *Associate Professor, Director Andrology Unit, University of Sydney, Sydney, Australia* [**395, 459**]

**M.P. Hedger,** *Institute of Reproduction and Development, Monash University, Monash Medical Centre, Clayton, Victoria, Australia* [**3**]

**Richard Horton, MD,** *Professor of Medicine, USC School of Medicine, Los Angeles, California*

**Peiwan Hsaio,** *Department of Human Oncology and Program in Endocrinology–Reproductive Physiology, University of Wisconsin, Madison, Wisconsin* [**65**]

**John T. Isaacs, PhD,** *Professor of Oncology and Urology, Johns Hopkins University, Baltimore, Maryland* [**95**]

**Narender Kumar,** *Center for Biomedical Research, The Population Council, New York, New York* [**493**]

**Tehming Liang, MD, PhD,** *Associate Professor and Chair, Department of Dermatology, Wright State University School of Medicine, Dayton, Ohio* [**247**]

**Din-Lii Lin,** *Department of Human Oncology and Program in Endocri-*

nology–Reproductive Physiology, University of Wisconsin, Madison, Wisconsin [**65**]

**Alvin M. Matsumoto, MD,** Chief of Gerontology, Veterans' Administration Medical Center, Seattle, Washington [**367**]

**Norman A. Mazer,** Pharmaceutics, University of Utah, Salt Lake City, Utah, and TheraTech, Inc., Salt Lake City, Utah [**449**]

**J.F. McFarlane,** Institute of Reproduction and Development, Monash University, Monash Medical Centre, Clayton, Victoria, Australia [**3**]

**C. McKinnell,** MRC Reproductive Biology Unit, Centre for Reproductive Biology, Edinburgh, Scotland [**17**]

**A. Wayne Meikle, MD,** Professor of Medicine, University of Utah Medical School, Salt Lake City, Utah [**449**]

**M. Millar,** MRC Reproductive Biology Unit, Centre for Reproductive Biology, Edinburgh, Scotland [**17**]

**N. Moeloek,** University of Indonesia [**375**]

**Eberhard Nieschlag, MD,** Professor of Medicine, Director, Institute of Reproductive Medicine, University of Steinfurter, Strauss, Germany [**409, 471, 503**]

**Marie-Claire Orgebin-Crist, PhD,** Professor of Obstetrics-Gynecology, Vanderbilt University, Nashville, Tennessee [**27**]

**W. Pangkahila,** Udayna University [**375**]

**C. Alvin Paulsen, MD,** Professor Emeritus of Medicine, University of Washington Medical School, Seattle, Washington [**335**]

**Jon L. Pryor, MD,** Assistant Professor, Urologic Surgery and Cell Biology/Neuroanatomy, University of Minnesota, Minneapolis, Minnesota [**111**]

**Joshua Riebe,** Department of Human Oncology and Program in Endocrinology–Reproductive Physiology, University of Wisconsin, Madison, Wisconsin [**65**]

**G.P. Risbridger,** Institute of Reproduction and Development, Monash University, Monash Medical Centre, Clayton, Victoria, Australia [**3**]

**Ken Roberts,** Department of Urologic Surgery, University of Minnesota Medical School, Minneapolis, Minnesota [**11**]

**Alan D. Rogol, MD,** Professor of Medicine, University of Virginia Health Science Center, Charlottesville, Virginia [**301**]

**David W. Russell,** Department of Molecular Genetics, The University of Texas, Southwestern Medical Center, Dallas, Texas [**57**]

**Steven W. Sanders,** TheraTech, Inc., Salt Lake City, Utah [**449**]

**P.T.K. Saunders,** MRC Reproductive Biology Unit, Centre for Reproductive Biology, Edinburgh, Scotland [**17**]

**Fritz H. Schröder, MD,** Professor and Chairman, Department of Urology, Erasmus Universiteit, Rotterdam, Netherlands [**121, 137**]

**Richard M. Sharpe, PhD,** Center for Reproductive Biology, Edinburgh, Scotland [**17**]

**Barbara B. Sherwin, PhD,** Professor, Department of Psychology and OB-GYN, McGill University, Montreal, Canada [**319**]

**Peter J. Snyder, MD,** *Professor of Medicine, University of Pennsylvania, Philadelphia, Pennsylvania* [**143, 437**]

**Barbara Steiner,** *Harbor–UCLA Medical Center, Torrance, California* [**355**]

**Thomas Storer,** *Laboratory of Exercise Sciences, El Camino College, Torrance, California* [**283**]

**Chingyuan Su,** *Department of Human Oncology and Program in Endocrinology–Reproductive Physiology, University of Wisconsin, Madison, Wisconsin* [**65**]

**Kalyan Sundaram, PhD,** *Senior Scientist, Center for Biomedical Research, The Population Council, New York, New York* [**493**]

**Ronald S. Swerdloff, MD,** *Professor of Medicine, Harbor-UCLA Medical Center, Torrance, California* [**355, 481, 487, 503**]

**J. Lisa Tenover, MD, PhD,** *Medical Director, Internal Medicine/Geriatrics, Emory University, Wesley Woods Health Center, Atlanta, Georgia* [**309**]

**Walter Tribley,** *Department of Biochemistry and Biophysics, Washington State University, Pullman, Washington* [**11**]

**Geoffrey M.H. Waites, ScD, PhD,** *Professor, Department of OB-GYN, University Hospital of Geneva, Geneva, Switzerland* [**345**]

**Christina Wang, MD,** *Professor of Medicine, Director, Clinical Study Center, Harbor-UCLA Medical Center, Torrance, California* [**433, 487**]

**Gerhard F. Weinbauer,** *Institute of Reproductive Medicine, University of Munster, WHO Collaborating Center for Research in Human Reproduction, Munster, Germany* [**409, 471**]

**Jon E. Wergedel, MD,** *Research Chemist, Research Service, Pettis Veterans' Hospital, Loma Linda, California* [**259**]

**Jean D. Wilson, MD,** *Professor and Chair, Department of Medicine, Southwestern Medical School, Dallas, Texas* [**57, 503**]

**F.C.W. Wu, MD,** *Department of Medicine, University of Manchester, Hope Hospital, Manchester, United Kingdom* [**191, 381**]

# PART I: ANDROGEN PHYSIOLOGY

# 1

# THE REGULATION OF LEYDIG CELL FUNCTION

**DM de Kretser, JF McFarlane, MP Hedger, GP Risbridger**

**Institute of Reproduction and Development, Monash University Monash Medical Centre, Clayton, Victoria, 3168, Australia**

## INTRODUCTION

The basic elements in the regulation of Leydig cell function are well established and involve the stimulation by LH secretion from the pituitary induced by gonadotrophin releasing hormone (GnRH). LH, released in a pulsatile manner by this episodic GnRH stimulus, acts via a transmembrane receptor to stimulate a pulse of testosterone release. While the importance of the pulsatile mode of stimulation has been established for pituitary LH secretion, it is still unclear whether an episodic mode of stimulation is important for testosterone secretion since the testis can respond to a continuous stimulus of LH/hCG.

The accumulating data concerning the molecular mechanisms of LH action on testosterone production by the Leydig cell have clarified certain physiological issues, but a number of key areas still require further attention. These issues, rather than the well-established data, are highlighted in this review.

## ONTOGENY AND REPLICATION OF LEYDIG CELLS

It is well accepted that Leydig cells exhibit two generations, fetal and adult, separated by a prepubertal phase in which the testis of the postnatal mammal is devoid of Leydig cells (Mendis-Handagama et al., 1987). Unfortunately, in the most widely studied mammal, the rat, this does not occur because of the temporal proximity of sexual maturity to birth. Although Leydig cells develop as a fetal generation, these cells do not regress before the onset of pubertal development, characterized by increased LH levels which initiate differentiation of the adult generation of Leydig cells.

Both generations of Leydig cells arise from mesenchymal precursors that are still poorly characterized. Using enzymatic digestion, several investigators have isolated populations of Leydig cell precursors in the mouse and rat which have the

*Pharmacology, Biology, and Clinical Applications of Androgens*, edited by Shalender Bhasin et al.
ISBN 0-471-13320-5 © 1996 Wiley-Liss, Inc.

capacity to bind LH and produce androgens (Kerr et al., 1985; Hardy et al., 1990; Risbridger and Davies, 1994). Hardy et al. (1990) were the first to report the *in vitro* differentiation of these precursor cells into immature Leydig cells. There is general agreement that LH is an important stimulus to the process of differentiation and that the precursor cells have the capacity for LH binding and indeed express the LH receptor gene (Shan and Hardy, 1992).

There is also agreement that factors other than LH are involved in the differentiation of precursor cells and $IGF_1$, $TGF_\alpha$, $TGF_\beta$, interleukin 1 and bFGF have all been implicated indirectly (see review Teerds et al., 1994). Evidence that factors other than LH are involved can be obtained from observations that in the rat fetus, differentiation of Leydig cells from precursors takes in about 1-3 days, whereas in the adult testis, the regeneration of Leydig cells after treatment with ethane dimethane sulphonate (EDS) takes approximately 21 days (Jackson et al., 1986). Furthermore, regeneration of Leydig cells in the cryptorchid rat testis after EDS treatment takes approximately 10-14 days; again, indicating that factors other than LH are involved (O'Leary et al., 1986).

Some growth factors have been implicated in the proliferation of precursors and immature Leydig cells and in the latter case, IGF1 and $TGF_\alpha$, are stimulatory, while $TGF_\beta$ is inhibitory (Teerds et al., 1994). Teerds and colleagues suggest that the development of Leydig cells involves several phases:

| | |
|---|---|
| I | Proliferation of precursor cells |
| II | Differentiation of precursor cells to form immature Leydig cells, the latter being characterized by the production of 5α-reduced androgens rather than testosterone |
| III | Proliferation of immature Leydig cells |
| IV | Differentiation of immature Leydig cells to form mature Leydig cells. |

This type of model allows formal testing of some hypotheses but an important issue that requires clarification is the specific criteria for recognition and characterization of each cell type in this process. Unless these are clearly enunciated, conflicting results are likely to be published from different laboratories.

## THE ROLE OF THE LH RECEPTOR

The cloning of the LH receptor gene demonstrated that it belonged to a large gene family composed of approximately 100 members that couple through GTP-binding proteins to intracellular second messengers (Themmen et al., 1994). The gene encodes a protein with an extracellular binding domain encoded by the first 10 exons, a hydrophobic domain including seven transmembrane segments and an intracellular G protein-coupling domain (McFarland et al., 1989). Study of LH receptor mRNA's has identified at least four sizes, namely, 6.5, 4.3, 2.6 and 1.2 kb, but up to 13 variations have been identified and some of these variants encode proteins which do not contain part of the transmembrane and intracellular domains

(Themmen et al., 1994). Although the expression of variant mRNA's appear to be low in most states, Remy et al. (1993) showed that co-expression of the extracellular binding domain and the transmembrane-intracellular domain led to reconstitution of a high affinity LH receptor capable of signal transduction. Furthermore, expression of a truncated transcript lacking the intracellular/transmembrane domain led to high affinity hCG binding but no signal transduction (Vu Hai et al., 1992). Co-expression of both the binding domain and the intracellular/transmembrane domain led to enhanced adenyl cyclase production.

It is unclear how these splice variants are generated, but their level of expression may alter physiological responses. Furthermore, significant developmental changes occur in the splice variants of the LH receptor mRNA's found on Leydig cells, since initially, a truncated version lacking a transmembrane-/intracellular domain is expressed with full length receptor mRNA being expressed later in development (Tena-Sempere et al., 1994). Further evidence that transcript size is regulated emerges from experiments in which hypophysectomy caused a decrease in the 7.0kb, 4.2kb, 2.5kb LH receptor mRNA, but an increase in the 1.8kb form (Teerds et al., 1994). Further studies are necessary to understand the physiological relevance of these splice variants of LH receptor mRNA.

## ACTION OF LH

There is increasing evidence to indicate that the initiation of LH action by binding to the LH receptor results in activation of not only the CAMP pathway but also initiates rapid changes in intracellular $Ca^{++}$ (Saez, 1994). The latter, through the activation of phospholipases in the lipoxygenase pathway and via the calcium-/calmodulin protein kinase C pathway, can stimulate androgen production independently of CAMP (Cooke ,1990). Having examined the relevant data, Saez (1994) concluded that, despite evidence of alternative signal transduction pathways, the major effect of LH/hCG on steroidogenesis is mediated through cAMP.

There is considerable data to indicate that in many species a rise in circulating LH results in a rapid (within two hours) rise in circulating testosterone levels which peak at 24 hours and decline (Hodgson and de Kretser, 1984). Furthermore, episodic LH secretory pulses cause pulsatile testosterone secretion in many species (Lincoln, 1976). However, in man, even very large doses of hCG cause only a small acute rise in testosterone secretion (Padron et al., 1980). The reasons for this differing pattern of testosterone secretion between species is unknown.

Insufficient attention is paid to sampling times during *in vivo* experiments assessing responses to LH/hCG injections. In the adult rat, a biphasic pattern of testosterone secretion to a single injection of hCG is evident, but in the cryptorchid rat, the second phase at 48-72 hours is attenuated (Hodgson and de Kretser, 1985). Conversely, in hypophysectomized and immature rats , the initial phase is attenuated but the second peak is normal, probably reflecting the cellular differentiation induced by the injection of hCG (Hodgson and de Kretser, 1984). The latter effects are dramatic and lead to doubling in size of the Leydig cells in the hypophysectomized rat.

## ACUTE STEROID RESPONSE TO LH

Recently, several investigators have evaluated the mechanisms involved in the acute response of the Leydig cell to LH stimulation. There is increasing evidence that the rate limiting step in steroidogenesis is the delivery of the cholesterol to the inner mitochondrial membrane, which is the site of the cholesterol side-chain cleavage complex (SCC) (Stocco and Clark, 1994). A steroid carrier protein (SCP-2) has been shown to transfer cholesterol from lipid droplets to mitochondria and is located primarily in peroxisomes (Mendis-Handagama et al., 1990). While LH stimulation causes a redistribution of SCP-2 in Leydig cells, SCP-2 levels do not change significantly in response to acute stimulation or to treatment with cycloheximide.

Another protein, termed steroidogenesis activator peptide (SAP), which is located only in steroidogenic tissues, is acutely regulated by trophic hormone stimulation and can increase cholesterol transport into mitochondria (Pederson and Brownie, 1987). SAP has been shown to be nearly identical to the carboxy terminus of a heat shock protein known as glucose-regulated protein 78 (Mertz and Pederson, 1989). Its specific role in the acute regulation of steroidogenesis requires further study.

The peripheral benzodiazepine receptor (PBR) has been implicated in the acute control of Leydig cell function by its high concentration in the outer mitochondrial membrane and by the observation that stimulation of steroid secretory cells by PBR agonists resulted in increases in steroid secretion (Papadopolous, 1993). Further support for this concept emerged from data which demonstrated that the endogenous ligand for PBR, known as the diazepam binding inhibitor (DBI), and an 8.2kDa peptide, were identical and capable of stimulating an acute rise in steroid secretion (Besman et al., 1989). Some inconsistencies in the temporal responses of PBR and DBI to the steroid response in hypophysectomized rats have questioned the role of these proteins in the acute response (Cavallaro et al., 1993), but the demonstration that an antisense oligonucleotide to DB1 blocked the effects of hCG on steroidogenesis in MA10 Leydig cells supports its role (Boujrad et al., 1993).

A further group of proteins, termed 30kDa mitochondrial proteins, have also been implicated in the acute response, particularly by their localization to steroid producing tissues; their stimulation in a dose and time dependent manner, their sensitivity to cycloheximide treatment, and the total inhibition of steroidogenesis by agents blocking the conversion of a 37kDa precursor to the 30kDa protein (Stocco and Clark, 1994). The purification of this protein has been accomplished and its structural characteristics are awaited with interest.

Clearly, further studies are necessary to determine which of the above mentioned molecules are essential to the acute steroid response by Leydig cells.

## LOCAL REGULATION OF LEYDIG CELL FUNCTION

The concept that the Leydig cells function can be modulated by factors secreted by the seminiferous tubules was first suggested by Aoki and Fawcett (1978).

Subsequently, considerable circumstantial evidence has accumulated to support this concept with data emerging from a variety of experimental paradigms (de Kretser, 1987). Many attempts have been made to characterize the factors produced by the seminiferous tubules which influence Leydig cell function with testicular interstitial fluid and Sertoli cell culture media constituting the major sources (Sharpe and Cooper, 1984; Verhoeven, 1992). Confusing results have been obtained with some studies characterizing stimulators and others providing evidence of inhibitory materials. Part of this confusion arose from the failure of investigators to utilize properly characterized bioassays which utilized dose-response measurements of activity. Using a carefully characterized bioassay system (Hedger et al., 1990) it is evident that both stimulatory and inhibitory activities are present in such sources as testicular interstitial fluid and seminiferous tubule culture media (Hedger et al., 1994). The nature of these molecules requires further characterization although some reports have claimed that these substances have been isolated to homogeneity (Cheng et al., 1993). No sequence information has been published, nor have the cDNAs encoding these molecules been cloned.

Although these molecules remain to be characterized, the testis contains many factors which may exert local regulatory processes, and these have been reviewed recently by Verhoeven (1992). These include, IGF1 and IGF-1 binding proteins, the inhibin, activin and TGF$_\beta$ family of proteins, LHRH, vasopressin, epidermal growth factor and interleukin 1. Other systems include bFGF, which inhibits testosterone production by Leydig cells (Murono and Washburn, 1990), and data are accumulating to suggest that the seminiferous tubules, in particular germ cells, produce bFGF (Han et al., 1993).

One of the major difficulties in this field is the manner in which this data, largely derived from *in vitro* studies, relates to *in vivo* function. Considerable attention needs to be paid to the development of systems which allow the influence of these factors to be explored in an *in vivo* setting. One possibility involves the use of *in vivo* synchronization of spermatogenic stages using the vitamin A deprivation system (Morales and Griswold, 1987). Other longer term prospects involves the knock out of specific gene functions within the testis.

## CONCLUDING REMARKS

It is evident that the secretion of testosterone *in vivo* by the testis involves a heterogeneous group of cells which include Leydig cell precursors, immature Leydig cells, and adult (mature) Leydig cells. The fact that the *in vivo* response arises from this menage of cells is often forgotten and our attempts to mimic these systems *in vitro* can be disrupted by this heterogeneity. The frequent conflicting results of published studies may arise from poor characterization of the cells used, the media conditions employed, and the failure to use dose-responses in evaluating the actions of putative control systems.

As discussed earlier, better markers to identify specific stages of Leydig cell differentiation are required rather than the use of LH binding or 3$\beta$ hydroxysteroid dehydrogenase activity. It is only when such criteria are developed that our understanding of the process of Leydig cell regulation will advance.

# REFERENCES

Aoki A and Fawcett DW (1978): Is there a local feedback from the seminiferous tubules affecting activity of the Leydig cells? Biol Reprod 19:144-158.

Besman MJ, Yanagibashi K, Lee TD, Kawamura M, Hall PF, Shively JE (1989): Identification of des-(Gly-Ile)-endozepine as an effector of corticotropin-dependent adrenal steroidogenesis: stimulation of cholesterol delivery is mediated by the peripheral benzodiazepine receptor. Proc Natl Acad Sci USA. 86:4897-4901.

Boujrad N, Hudson JR, Papadopoulos V (1993): Inhibition of hormone-stimulated steroidogenesis in cultured Leydig cell tumor cells by a cholesterol-linked phosphorothioate oligodeoxynucleotide antisense to diazepam binding inhibitor. Proc Natl Acad Sci USA 90:5728-5731.

Cavallaro S, Pani L, Guidotti A, Costa E. (1993): ACTH-induced mitochondrial DBI receptor (MDR) and diazepam binding inhibitor (DBI) expression in adrenals of hypophysectomized rats is not cause-effect related to its immediate steroidogenic action. Life Sci 53:1137-1147.

Cheng CY, Zwain IH, Li AHY, Grima J. (1993): The roles of Sertoli cell proteins in germ cell-Sertoli cell-Leydig cell interaction in the testis. In Mornex R, Jaffiol C, Leclere J (eds): "Progress in Endocrinology". Parthenon Publishing, Lancashire: pp 619-625.

Cooke BA. (1990): Is cyclic AMP an obligatory second messenger for luteinizing hormone. Mol Cell Endocrinol 69:C11-C15.

de Kretser DM (1987): Local regulation of testicular function. Int Rev Cytol 10: 89-112.

Han IS, Sylvester SR, Kim KH, Schelling ME, Venkateswaran S, Blanckaert VD, McGuiness MP, Griswold MD. (1993): Basic FGF is a testicular germ cell product which may regulate Sertoli cell function. Mol Endocrinol 7:889-897.

Hardy MP, Kelce WR, Klinefelter GR, Ewing LL (1990): Differentiation of Leydig cell precursors *in vitro*: a role for androgen. Endocrinology 127:488-490.

Hedger MP, Robertson DM, de Kretser DM, Risbridger GP (1990): The quantification of steroidogenesis-stimulating activity in testicular interstitial fluid by an *in vitro* bio-assay employing adult rat Leydig cells. Endocrinology 127:1967-1977.

Hedger MP, McFarlane JR, de Kretser DM, Risbridger GP. (1994): Multiple factors with steroidogenic-regulating activity in testicular intertubular fluid from normal and experimentally cryptorchid adult rats. Steroids 59:676-685.

Hodgson YM, de Kretser DM (1984): Acute responses of Leydig cells to hCG: Evidence for early hypertrophy of Leydig cell. Mol Cell Endocr 35:75-82.

Hodgson YM, de Kretser DM (1985): The testosterone response of cryptorchid rats and hypophysectomized rats to human chorionic gonaodotrophin (hCG) stimulation. Aust J Biol Sci. 38: 445-455.

Jackson AE, O'Leary P, Ayers M, de Kretser DM (1986): The effects of ethylene dimethane sulphonate (EDS) on rat Leydig cells: evidence to support a connective tissue origin of Leydig cells. Biol Reprod 35: 425-437.

Kerr JB, Robertson DM, de Kretser DM (1985): Morphological and functional characterization of interstitial cells from mouse testis fractionated on Percoll density gradient. Endocrinology 116:1030-1043.

Lincoln GA. (1976): Seasonal variation in the episodic secretion of luteinizing hormone and testosterone in the ram. J Endocr 69: 213-226.

McFarland KC, Sprengel R, Phillips HS, Kohler M, Rosenblil N, Nikolics K, Segaloff DL, Seeburg PH. (1989): Lutropin choriogonadotropin receptor: an unusual member of the G protein-coupled receptor family. Science 245:494-499.

Mendis-Handagama SMLC, Risbridger GP, de Kretser DM (1987): Morphometric analysis of the components of the neonatal and the adult testis interstitium. Int J Androl 10: 525-534.

Mendis-Handagama SMLC, Zirkin BR, Scallen TJ, Ewing LL. (1990): Studies on peroxisomes of the adult rat Leydig cell. J Androl 11:270-278.

Mertz LM, Pedersen RC (1989): Steroidogenesis activator polypeptide maybe a product of glucose regulated protein 78 (GRP 78). Endocr Res 15:101-115.

Morales G, Griswold MD (1987): Retinol-induced stage synchronization in seminiferous tubules of the rat. Endocrinology 121:432-434.

Murono EP, Washburn AL (1990): Basic fibroblast growth factor inhibits delta 5 3 beta hydroxysteroid dehydrogenase-isomerase activity in cultured immature Leydig cells. Biochem Biophys Res Commun 168:248-253.

O'Leary P, Jackson AE, Averill S, de Kretser DM. (1986): The effects of ethane dimethane sulphonate (EDS) on bilaterally cryptorchid rat testes. Mol Cell Endocrinol 45:183-190.

Padron RS, Wischusen J, Hudson B, Burger HG, de Kretser DM (1980): Prolonged biphasic response of plasma testosterone to single intramuscular injections of human chorionic gonadotrophin. J Clin Endocrinol Metab 50:1100-1104.

Papadopoulos V (1993): Peripheral-type benzodeazepine/diazepam binding inhibitor receptor: biological role in steroidogenic cell function. Endocrine Rev 14: 222-240.

Pedersen RC, Brownie AC (1987): Steroidogenesis-activator polypeptide isolated from a rat Leydig cell tumor. Science 236:188-190.

Remy JJ, Bozon V, Couture L, Goxe B, Salesse R, Garnier J (1993): Reconstitution of a high affinity functional lutropin receptor by coexperession of its extracellular and membrane domains. Biochem Biophys Res Commun. 193:1023-1030.

Risbridger GP, Davies A (1994): Isolation of rat Leydig cell and precursor forms after administration of ethane dimethane sulfonate. Am J Physiol 286:E975-979.

Saez JM (1994) Leydig cells: Endocrine, paracrine and autocrine regulation. Endocrine Rev 15: 574-626.

Shan LX, Hardy MP (1992): Developmental changes in levels of luteinizing hormone receptor and androgen receptor in rat Leydig cells. Endocrinology 131: 1107-1114.

Sharpe RM, Cooper I (1984): Intratesticular secretion of a factor(s) with major stimulatory effects on Leydig cell testosterone secretion in vitro. Mol Cell Endocr 37:159-168.

Stocco DM, Clark BJ (1994): Regulation of the acute production of steroids in steroidogenic cells. Verhoeven G, Habenicht UF (eds): "Molecular and Cellular Endocrinology", Berlin: Springer Verlag, pp 67-98.

Teerds KJ, Veldhuizen-Tsoerkan MB, Rommerts FFG, de Rooij DG, Dorrington JH. (1994): Proliferation and differentiation of testicular interstitial cells: aspects of Leydig cell development in the (pre)pubertal and adult testis. In Verhoeven G,' Habenicht UF (eds), "Molecular and Cellular Endocrinology of the Testis", Berlin, Springer Verlag, pp 37-65.

Tena-Sempere M, Zhang FP, Huhtaniemi I (1994): Persistent expression of a truncated hormone receptor messenger ribonucleic acid in the rat testis after selective Leydig cell destruction by ethylene dimethane sulfonate. Endocrinology 135:1018-1024.

Themmen APN, Kraaij R, Grootengoed AJ (1994): Regulation of gonadotrophin receptor gene expression. Mol Cell Endocrinol 100:15-19.

Verhoeven G (1992): Local control systems within the testis. In de Kretser DM (ed): "The Testes". Bailliere's Clinical Endocrinology and Metabolism 6: 313-333.

Vu Hai MT, Misrahi M, Houllier A, Jolivet A, Milgrom E (1992): Variant forms of the pig lutropin/choriogonadotropin receptor. Biochemistry 31: 8377-8383.

# 2

# ANDROGEN REGULATION OF SERTOLI CELL FUNCTION

Walter Tribley[1], Ken Roberts[2], and
Michael D. Griswold[1]

[1]Department of Biochemistry and Biophysics
Washington State University
Pullman, Washington 99164-4660
[2]Department of Urologic Surgery
University of Minnesota Medical School
Minneapolis, Minnesota 55455

## INTRODUCTION

The important regulatory role of androgens in spermatogenesis is well recognized and accepted. Animal models, primarily rodents, deprived of the consequences of androgen action by hypophysectomy, or by genetic mutations (such as the testicular feminized mutation-Tfm), exhibit arrested spermatogenesis. Following removal of androgens from an adult rat by hypophysectomy, or treatment with ethane dimethane sulfonate, abnormal morphological changes are first observed (3-4 days) in germ cells associated with stages VII-VIII of the cycle of the seminiferous epithelium (Russell and Clermont, 1977). Continued hormone deprivation leads to loss of spermatogenesis in partially regressed rodent testes, but both follicle stimulating hormone (FSH) and testosterone are required to restore the fully regressed testes (Fritz, 1978). Despite the wealth of biological information pertaining to the importance of androgen action in spermatogenesis, there is little reliable information about how testosterone exerts its effects. This remains one of the major enigmas in male reproduction.

## PRESENCE OF ANDROGEN RECEPTORS IN THE TESTIS

The availability of antibodies to the steroid receptors has led to the localization of androgen receptors in Sertoli and peritubular cells (Sar et al., 1993). Recently, putative androgen receptors were detected by immunohistochemistry and Western blots in round and elongating spermatids (Vornberger et al., 1994). These results opened, yet again, the question of direct androgen action on germ cells. In a review in 1978, Fritz summarized the three major lines of genetic evidence that

*Pharmacology, Biology, and Clinical Applications of Androgens,* edited by Shalender Bhasin et al.
ISBN 0-471-13320-5 © 1996 Wiley-Liss, Inc.

support the lack of androgen action on germ cells in the testis (Fritz, 1978). First, germ cell development into primary spermatocytes is evident in Tfm mice that lack functional androgen receptors. The androgen receptor is encoded by the X-chromosome, and some level of XY pair inactivation occurs after the spermatocyte stage in many rodents. Taken together, this evidence argues for the lack of a need for an androgen receptor in spermatogonia and spermatocytes. A second point brought out by Fritz is that the common vole lacks the X-chromosome in all sper-matogonia or advanced germ cells. Therefore, spermatogenesis in the vole can proceed without androgen receptors. The final point made by Fritz was that in 1975, using techniques involving the production of chimeras from Tfm and normal mice, Mary Lyons and colleagues generated chimeric male mice that sired Tfm offspring. The authors of the original article postulated that this outcome was possible only if the germ cells of the chimera were of Tfm origin and the somatic cells came from the normal blastula. Any contention that the recently reported immunodetection of androgen receptors in germ cells is of critical biological impor-tance must explain the contradictory genetic evidence. In addition, the potential biological activity of putative steroid receptors in elongated spermatids must be questioned since these cells are undergoing a progressive deactivation of genome activity and an increase in chromatin condensation.

There appears to be agreement on the presence of androgen receptors in peritubular cells. Work from the laboratory of Skinner has demonstrated that peritubular cells in culture secrete a factor, termed "P-Mod-S" that affects the secretory capability of cultured Sertoli cells (Anthony and Skinner, 1991). It is possible that this mesenchymal factor may prove to be important in the action of androgens on spermatogenesis.

## ANDROGEN ACTION ON SERTOLI CELLS

The evidence against androgen action in germ cells and the absence of data from *in vivo* studies on P-Mod-S leave us with the likelihood that the primary action of androgens in spermatogenesis takes place in Sertoli cells. However, there is little good documentation of the gene products in Sertoli cells that are regulated by testosterone. Most attempts to measure responses of Sertoli cells to androgens have involved the use of primary cell cultures. While these cultures consist almost exclusively of Sertoli cells, most of the published results were obtained from experi-ments that utilized prepubertal rats in which the effect of androgens on spermato-genesis is minimal. Results from these types of experiments have shown little or no effect of testosterone on the synthesis of specific macromolecules. Some experi-ments have clearly shown that there is a long term trophic effect of testosterone on general protein synthesis, or RNA synthesis, in the treated cells in culture (Louis and Fritz, 1979; Lamb, et al., 1981; Roberts and Griswold, 1989).

In an extensive series of experiments using hypophysectomized rats, we examined the androgen response of steady state levels of specific mRNAs in Sertoli cells *in vivo* (Hugly, et al., 1988). Rats of two ages (20 days old and 40 days old) were hypophysectomized and for the next 20 days were either allowed to regress, treated with testosterone alone, FHS alone, or a combination of the two. The end-points measured in this experiment included testis weights and levels of SGP-2 and testicular transferrin mRNA. These two mRNAs are found only in Sertoli cells in the testis. The results showed that testosterone was effective in maintaining testis weight and levels of the specific mRNAs in the rats hypophysectomized at 40 days of age, but FSH was more effective in the younger group. These results demonstrated that some of the actions of FSH in the prepubertal rats are assumed by testosterone in the adult rats.

It has been suggested that testosterone may not be regulating spermatogenesis via androgen receptor mediated pathways (Sharpe, et al., 1994). One of the strongest points in favor of this suggestion is the observation that the level of testosterone required to maintain spermatogenesis is 40-fold higher than is required to saturate the androgen receptors. Roberts and Zirkin have directly addressed this issue experimentally and have concluded that the requirement for high testosterone levels is a result of the inhibition of testosterone action by androgen binding protein (ABP) in the seminiferous tubule fluid (Roberts and Zirkin, 1993).

## SEARCH FOR ANDROGEN RESPONSIVE GENES

The proposed, and generally accepted mechanism of action of steroid hormones, involves the interaction of steroid with receptor, and the subsequent function of the receptor, as a transcriptional activator of very specific gene products. Knowledge of this mechanism has prompted a number of studies designed to determine which gene products are regulated in Sertoli cells. We have used two-dimensional gel electrophoresis to search for proteins induced by testosterone (Roberts and Griswold, 1989). Sertoli cells from 20 day-old rats, 40 day-old and 40 day-old rats that had been hypophysectomized 20 days earlier, were placed in culture and left untreated, or treated with testosterone for 5 days. Each experimental treatment group was incubated with $^{35}$S-methionine for the last 24 hours of culture. The cells were collected, lysed and subjected to two-dimensional gel electrophoresis, followed by fluorography. The resulting fluorograms were scanned at high resolution and subjected to computer analysis of spot location and intensities. While only 235 to 328 proteins, or spots, could be assayed by this technique, a number of proteins changed in radioactive intensity as a result of testosterone treatment. In general, 14-16% of the spots increased in intensity by at least 100% as a result of testosterone treatment, and 13 to 17% of the spots decreased in intensity by at least 50%, as a result of the treatment. The proteins that changed in intensity represented less than 0.2% of the total incorporated radioactivity and could be classed as low abundance proteins. Thus, we concluded from this study of long-term effects that testosterone acted on Sertoli cells in culture to affect the synthesis of a relatively large number of low abundance proteins. It is likely that only the secondary trophic effects of testosterone were examined in this study.

We and others have also used subtractive hybridization procedures in attempts to identify and isolate mRNAs representing androgen responsive genes (Sharpe et al., 1994) and unpublished observations. Subtractive procedures have been used on mRNA from cultured Sertoli cells and from the testes of EDS-treated rats. In general, these procedures have identified mRNAs that proved in further experiments not to be testosterone responsive. We are currently applying the sensitive technique of polymerase chain reaction (PCR) display in attempts to identify mRNAs that are induced as a result of androgen action. This procedure involves the use of random primer sets to generate a profile of the mRNA sequences present in a cell. These profiles are displayed and compared between treatment groups on electrophoretic gels. Bands present in one sample and absent in another can be sequenced and should represent unique mRNA species. Results so far suggest that only a limited subset of mRNAs is induced by testosterone in cultured Sertoli cells.

## CONCLUSIONS

Androgen regulation of spermatogenesis is a result of testosterone action on Sertoli cells. The consequence of long term testosterone action on Sertoli cells includes a general trophic effect and stimulation of RNA and protein synthesis. Many activities of Sertoli cells that are regulated in prepubertal animals by FSH are regulated by androgens in the adult. Despite considerable efforts, attempts to identify the initial androgen responsive genes in Sertoli cells have been unsuccessful. The mechanism by which androgen regulates Sertoli cell functions remains an enigma.

## REFERENCES

Anthony, CT, Skinner MK (1991): Analysis of Peritubular Cell-Sertoli Cell Interaction Mediated by PMODS. XIth North American Testis Workshop, Montreal, Canada.

Fritz I (1978): Sites of actions of androgens and follicle stimulation hormone on cells of the seminiferous tubule. In Litwack G (ed): "Biochemical Actions of Hormones." New York: Academic Press, pp 249-278.

Hugly S, Roberts K, Griswold MD (1988): Transferrin and sulfated glycoprotein-2 messenger ribonucleic acid levels in the testis and isolated Sertoli cells of Hypophysectomized rats. Endocrinology 122:1390-1396.

Lamb DJ, Tsai YH, Steinberger A, Sanborn BM (1981): Sertoli cell nuclear transcriptional activity: stimulation by follicle-stimulating hormone and testosterone *in vitro*. Endocrinology 108:1020-1026.

Louis BG, Fritz IB (1979): Follicle-stimulating hormone and testosterone independently increase the production of androgen-binding protein by Sertoli cells in culture. Endocrinology 104:454-460.

Roberts K, Griswold MD (1989): Testosterone induction of cellular proteins in cultured Sertoli cells from hypophysectomized rats and rats of different ages. Endocrinology 125:1174-1179.

Roberts K, Zirkin B (1993): Androgen binding protein inhibition of androgen-dependent transcription explains the high minimal testosterone concentration required to maintain spermatogenesis. Endocrine J 1:41-47.

Russell LD, Clermont Y (1977): Degeneration of germ cells in normal, hypophysectomized and hormone treated hypophysectomized rats. Anat Rec 187:347-366.

Sar M, Hall SH, Wilson EM, French FS (1993): Androgen Regulation of Sertoli cells. In Russell LD, Griswold MD (eds.): "The Sertoli Cell." Clearwater, FL: Cache River Press, pp 509-516.

Sharpe RM, McKinnell C, McClaren T, Millar M, West TP, Maguire S, Gaughan J, Syed V, Jegou B, Kerr JB, Saunders PTK (1994): Interactions between androgens, Sertoli cells and germ cells in the control of spermatogenesis. In Verhoeven G, Habenicht U-F (eds.): "Molecular and Cellular Endocrinology of the testis." Berlin: Springer-Verlag, pp 115-142.

Vornberger W, Prins G, Musto NA, Suarez-Quian CA (1994): Androgen receptor distribution in rat testis: new implication for androgen regulation of spermatogene sis. Endocrinology 134:2307-2316.

# 3

# TESTOSTERONE AND GERM CELL DEVELOPMENT (SPERMATOGENESIS)

**Richard M. Sharpe[1], C. McKinnell[1], M. Millar[1], W. B. Bremner[2], K.M. Grigor[3], and PTK Saunders[1]**

[1]MRC Reproductive Biology Unit, Centre for Reproductive Biology
37 Chalmers Street
Edinburgh EK3 9EW, Scotland, UK

[2]Department of Medicine and Population Center for Research in Reproduction, VA Medical Center
Seattle, Washington 98108, USA

[3]Department of Pathology,
University of Edinburgh
Edinburgh EH 8 9AG, Scotland, UK

## INTRODUCTION

Testosterone clearly plays an indispensable role in the normal development of germ cells during the process of spermatogenesis and this is known to be the case in most, and probably all, mammals (Sharpe, 1994). Despite our appreciation of the central role that testosterone has to play in these events, we remain in the dark as to how it exerts its effects on spermatogenesis. This ignorance has not only hampered our efforts to diagnose and treat the causes of male infertility, it has also made more difficult the development of new male contraceptive methods, especially those that are centered on the suppression of intratesticular testosterone levels and/or action. It seems fairly certain that if we can understand how testosterone controls spermatogenesis, then we must be far better placed to both unravel the disorders of this process which result in infertility and to design methods which will allow suppression of spermatogenesis for contraceptive purposes. This article reviews in brief how far we have come along this pathway of understanding and identifies some of the mysteries that remain to be solved.

*Pharmacology, Biology, and Clinical Applications of Androgens*, edited by Shalender Bhasin et al.
ISBN 0-471-13320-5 © 1996 Wiley-Liss, Inc.

## SITES OF TESTOSTERONE ACTION IN THE TESTIS

It is logically presumed that testosterone exerts its effects on spermato-genesis by first interacting with the androgen receptor and that the receptor-ligand complex then interacts with specific recognition sites within the promoter region of androgen-responsive genes (Parker, 1991). The sites of expression of the androgen receptor in the rat testis have been well documented and two recent publications (Vornberger et al., 1994; Bremner et al., 1994) have categorized this in detail. There is complete agreement that androgen receptors are present within the nuclei of pertitubular cells, Sertoli cells, some (and perhaps all) Leydig cells, and the endo-thedial cells of small arterioles (Fig. 1). Our own data (Bremner et al., 1994) has shown no evidence for the expression of androgen receptors in any germ cells, whereas the study by Vornberger et al. (1994), which used similar techniques, indicated that step 11 spermatids, might contain androgen receptor protein. The possibility that germ cells might contain androgen receptors has been debated for two decades or more and the weight of evidence, based on binding studies, immu-nohistochemistry, and a variety of molecular approaches, suggest that germ cells do not contain androgen receptors (Sharpe, 1994). However, there is no ready expla-nation for the observations of Vornberger et al. (1994), although in our own immu-nohistochemistry studies we have noted that condensing spermatids are somewhat prone to stain non-specifically, and perhaps this is related to the dramatic reorgani-zation of nuclear chromatin that is occurring in these cells.

Thus, in the absence of persuasive evidence to the contrary, the most widely accepted view is that germ cells do not contain androgen receptors, and therefore all of the supportive effects of testosterone on germ cell development are indirect. These effect are presumed to be mediated via effects on the Sertoli cells, which are in intimate contact with the germ cells (Sharpe, 1994), though some role of pertitu-bular cells is possible (Skinner, 1991). Indeed, in the rat, it is clear that during fetal and prebubertal development, expression of androgen receptors in pertitubular cell nuclei is very intense whereas in Sertoli cell nuclei, it only becomes faintly evident in the postnatal period and then increases progressively in intensity throughout puberty (Bremner et al., 1994; Majdic et al., 1995). The most striking feature regarding expression of the androgen receptor protein in Sertoli cells in the adult rat testis is its marked stage-dependence (Fig 1; Vornberger et al., 1994; Bremner et al., 1994). Sertoli cells in seminiferous tubules at stages IX-XIII show little or no immunostaining for the androgen receptor, but from stages XIV-VII there is a progressive increase in the intensity of immunostaining, with the peak occurring at stages VI-VII (Fig. 1); thereafter, during stage VIII, the intensity of immunostaining declines very rapidly. This stage-dependence fits reasonably well with what is known about the biochemical consequences of testosterone action on the seminifer-ous tubules, as is discussed below. At present, it remains unclear what causes this stage-dependent pattern of immunostaining for the androgen receptor in Sertoli cells; i.e., is the receptor only present at certain stages because of differences in transcription of the androgen receptor gene, or is the stage-dependent pattern just a reflection of subtle changes in the conformation of the receptor protein at the differ-ent stages? There is currently no information which allows us to choose between these, or other, possible explanations.

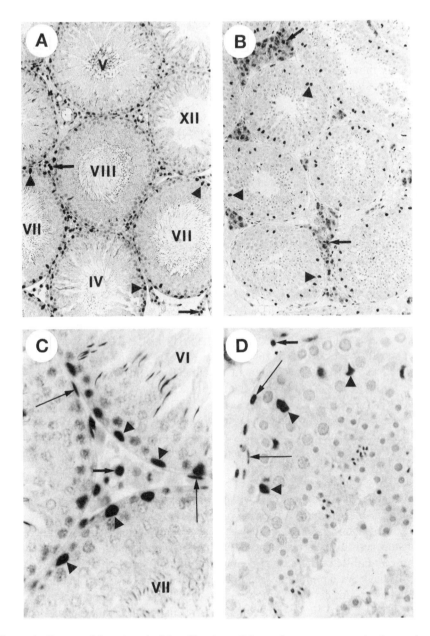

Figure 1. Immunohistochemical localization of the androgen receptor in the testis of a normal adult rat (A, C) or a normal adult man (B,D). There is intense immunostaining of Sertoli cell nuclei (arrowheads), although in the rat, this varies according to the stage of the spermatogenic cycle (Roman numerals). There is also immunostaining of pertitubular cell nuclei (long arrows) of Leydig cells (short arrows), and of the muscle wall of small arterioles (not marked) in both species. Magnification x100 (top x360 (bottom).

Close examination of a number of normal and abnormal human testes has failed to reveal any obvious stage-dependent pattern of immunostaining for the androgen receptor in Sertoli cells, though in all other respects, the pattern of immunostaining is identical to that in the rat (Fig. 1). Until the basis for the stage-dependent immunostaining in rat Sertoli cells is deciphered, it remains difficult to assess the implications and importance of the apparent absence of this phenomenon in the human.

## MECHANISMS OF TESTOSTERONE ACTION

In most androgen-responsive tissues, interaction of an androgen with its nuclear receptor results in altered transcription of a small number of specific genes. So far, no such straightforward mechanism of testosterone action has been identified in the seminiferous tubules, despite long and detailed investigation (Sharpe et al., 1994a). One of the approaches used in these studies was aimed at identifying specific proteins secreted by the seminiferous epithelium which were androgen-regulated. Although this appeared to identify successfully a number of such proteins (Sharpe et al., 1992a), our most recent analyses suggest that it is the **secretion** rather than the **synthesis** of these, and many other proteins, which is controlled somehow by testosterone.

Our initial findings demonstrated that the overall secretion of newiy-synthesized proteins by seminiferous tubules (ST) isolated from normal adult rats was markedly stage-dependent (Sharpe et al., 1992). ST in stages VI-VIII secreted approximately twice as much protein as did ST at earlier or later stages of the spermatogenic cycle, despite there being no detectable change in overall protein synthesis by ST at the different stages (Fig. 2). The increase in protein secretion by ST at stages VI-VIII is completely testosterone-dependent (Fig. 2). However, what makes this effect of testosterone of considerable interest is that it is remarkably prone to disruption; thus, within 24 hours of exposure of rats to testicular toxicants, or to local testicular heating, the normal androgen-dependent increase in protein secretion by ST at stages VI-VIII has been eliminated (McLaren et al., 1994; Sharpe et al., 1994a). This change occurs without any effect on testosterone levels or on the stage-dependent pattern of expression of the androgen receptor (our published data) as described above. Thus, it appears that several agents which disrupt normal spermatogenesis also disrupt events downstream from androgen-receptor interaction, resulting in failure of the normal doubling in protein secretion by ST at stages VI-VIII. Though we do not know the precise mechanisms involved, findings such as this lead us to consider that the testosterone-dependent increase in protein secretion by ST at stages VI-VIII, is somehow of central importance to the process of sper-matogenesis.

In attempting to understand more about the testosterone-driven increase in protein secretion, we have undertaken a detailed quantification of a substantial number of the individual secreted proteins using image analysis and 2-dimensional SDS-PAGE (McKinnell and Sharpe, 1995). For most of these proteins, their iden-tity is unknown, though their cellular source(s) has been determined by comparable analysis of secreted proteins by isolated germ cells and by isolated ST, which have been depleted specifically of one or other of the meiotic, or post-meiotic germ cells

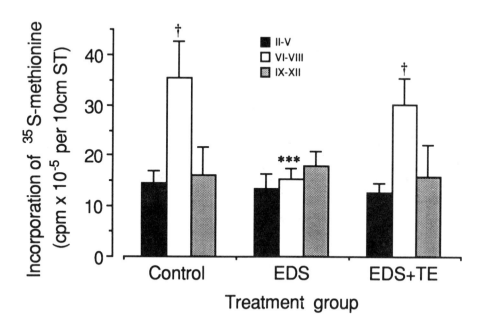

Figure 2. Stage-dependent differences in total protein secretion *in vitro* over 24 hours by seminiferous tubules (ST) isolated from control rats, from rats in which testosterone withdrawal had been induced by treatment with EDS four days earlier or from EDS-treated rats in which intratesticular testosterone levels had been restored by exogenous administration (EDS+TE). Values are means ±SD.[+]p<0.001, compared with ST at stages VI-VIII in the other two treatment groups. Reproduced with permission from Sharpe et al. (1992).

(McKinnell and Sharpe, 1992; Sharpe et al., 1994a).  The findings of this analysis have been surprising.  First, the majority of Sertoli cell-derived proteins (especially the abundant proteins) are secreted constitutively and this secretion is virtually unaffected by testosterone withdrawal or replacement (Fig. 3).  Second, all round spermatid-derived proteins that we have so far analyzed are secreted in a regulated manner and secretion of all of these proteins is testosterone-dependent, i.e., when testosterone is withdrawn by EDS-induced Leydig cell destruction, the proteins are still synthesized in the same amount, but far less is secreted (Fig. 3; McKinnell et al., 1995).

What these findings indicate is that Sertoli cells, which are clearly an androgen target cell, do not appear to respond to testosterone, at least in terms of the

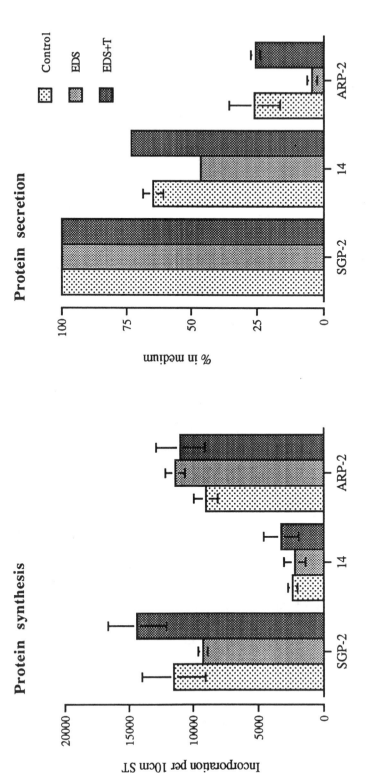

Figure 3. Changes in total synthesis and secretion of three proteins *in vitro* over 24 hours by seminiferous tubules at stages VI-VIII isolated from control rats, from rats in which testosterone withdrawal has been induced by treatment with EDS 4 days earlier or from EDS-treated rats in which intratesticular testosterone levels had been restored by exogenous administration (EDS+T). Values are the mean and range from duplicate experiments. SGP-2=sulphated glycoprotein-2, a know Sertoli cell product. 14= an unidentified protein which also derives from the Sertoli cells. ARP-2= an unidentified protein which derives from round spermatids and which was shown previously to be androgen regulated (Sharpe et al., 1992). Note that only the secretion of ARP-2 is affected markedly by testosterone withdrawal and replacement, whereas synthesis of all 3 protein is unaffected by treatment.

secretion of most major protein products. In contrast, round spermatids, which do not possess androgen receptors as far as we can tell (see above), respond in a major way to testosterone in terms of protein secretion. We do not have a satisfactory explanation for these rather paradoxical observations, though there are a number of possibilities. For example, the changes in germ cell protein secretion may be secondary to a primary change in some unknown function of the Sertoli cells. Alternatively, testosterone could be acting directly on the germ cells, either via membrane effects of the testosterone, or by interacting with androgen-binding protein (ABP), secreted by the Sertoli cells, which then binds to ABP receptors on the germ cells. There is some indirect supporting evidence for the latter possibility (Sharpe, 1994; Sharpe et al., 1994a), but, overall, there is no compelling evidence for or against either of the possibilities mentioned. Future research should tackle this important problem as well as addressing how the secretion of so many (and perhaps all) round spermatid-derived proteins might be regulated in a wholesale manner.

## CONSEQUENCES OF TESTOSTERONE ACTION

Irrespective of precisely how and where testosterone acts in the seminiferous epithelium, the consequences of its actions are to enable germ cells to develop normally into spermatozoa. In the rat, it appears that germ cells pass through a 'testosterone-regulated window' at four times during their development, i.e., as preleptotene spermatocytes, pachytene spermatocytes, round spermatids, and elongate spermatids. This 'window' occurs at stages VII-VIII of the spermatogenic cycle (Sharpe, 1994) and is presumably related somehow to the changes in protein secretion which occur at these stages if testosterone is present (see above). If testosterone is absent or levels are inadequate, then normal germ cell development does not occur as these cells pass through the 'window,' and they will subsequently degenerate; this sequence of events is presumably related to failure of the normal increase in protein secretion during this 'window.' However, perhaps the crucial question that arises from this is whether similar events occur in human seminiferous tubules? The apparent absence of any stage-dependent difference in expression of the androgen receptor (Fig. 1) is perhaps an argument against this possibility, though in reality, we have no hard evidence for or against. What is certain is that in man, as in the rat, spermatogenesis is completely dependent upon exposure to high intratesticular levels of testosterone, and it seems rather unlikely that testosterone would exert its effects in fundamentally different ways in the two species. If this assumption is correct, then it may also be true that in man, as in the rat, interference with normal spermatogenesis may occur commonly through disruption of one or more events in the androgen action pathway, even if the testosterone level itself remains unaffected. With this in mind, it should also be remembered that testosterone has other important effects on the testis, including the regulation of blood flow and vasomotion (Damber et al., 1992; Collin et al., 1993) and the production of both seminiferous tubule fluid (Je'gou et al., 1983; Sharpe et al., 1994b) and interstitial fluid (Maddocks and Sharpe, 1989; Sharpe et al., 1994b), all of which are likely to be of fundamental importance in creating and maintaining an appropriate environment for normal germ cell development.

## UNSOLVED MYSTERIES OF TESTOSTERONE ACTION

From the brief review above, it will be clear to the reader that most aspects of testosterone action on spermatogenesis remain shrouded in mystery. How androgens act on the seminiferous tubules appears to be fundamentally different to how androgens act elsewhere. One remarkable illustration of this difference is that testosterone levels in the testis need to be far higher than elsewhere in the body for effects to occur on spermatogenesis; in the rat, intratesticular levels need to be approximately 40-fold higher than the levels in peripheral blood, whereas in man, this difference is probably even more extreme, being around 200-fold (Sharpe, 1994). Why? If testosterone is acting via androgen receptors, then these would be saturated at around normal blood levels of testosterone; yet, we know that such levels are completely incapable of supporting normal spermatogenesis. This remains a perplexing mystery which we desperately need to solve. Does it indicate that testosterone is acting via non-receptor mechanisms, or does testosterone interact with the Sertoli cell androgen receptor in a different way elsewhere in the body (there is no good evidence that it does)? These are fundamentally important, and very basic questions to which we need answers if we are to unravel the secrets of the control of spermatogenesis. Such discoveries would be bound to have major impact on our ability to develop new contraceptive approaches in man.

## REFERENCES

Bremner WJ, Millar MR, Sharpe RM, Saunders PTK (1994): Immunohistochemical localization of androgen receptors in the rat testis; evidence for stage-dependent expression and regulation by androgens. Endocrinology 135: 1227-1234.

Collin O, Bergh A, Damber JE, Widmark A (1993): Control of testicular vasomotion by testosterone and tubular factors in rats. J Reprod Fertil 97:15-121.

Damber JE, Maddocks S, Widmark A, Bergh A (1992): Testicular blood flow and vasomotion can be maintained by testosterone in Leydig cell-depleted rats. *Int J Androl* 15;385-393.

Maddocks S, Sharpe RM (1989). Interstitial fluid volume in the rat testis-androgen dependent regulation by the seminiferous tubules. *J Endocrinol* 120;215-222.

Majdic G, Millar M, Saunders PTK (1995). Temporal changes in expression of androgen receptor in fetal rat testes and associated ducts detected by immuno histo-chemistry and reverse transcription plus polymerase chain reaction. J Endocrinol (Submitted).

McKinnell C, Sharpe RM (1992): The role of specific germ cell types in modulation of the secretion of androgen-regulated proteins (ARPs) by stage VI-VIII seminiferous tubules from the adult rat. Mol Cell Endocrinol 83: 219-231.

McKinnell C, Sharpe RM (1995). Testosterone and spermatogenesis: evidence that androgens regulate cellular secretory mechanism in stage VI-VIII seminiferous tubules from adult rats. J Androl (Submitted).

McLaren TT, Foster PMD, Sharpe RM (1994): Identification of stage-specific changes in protein secretion by isolated seminiferous tubules from rats following exposure to short-term local testicular heating. J Reprod Fertil 102: 293-300.

Parker MG (Ed) (1991). Nuclear hormone receptors. Academic Press, New York.

Sharpe RM (1994). Regulation of spermatogenesis: In: *The Physiology of Reproduction, second edition* (Eds; E Knobil & JD Neill). pp 1363-1434. Raven Press, New York.

Sharpe RM, Maddocks S, Millar M, Saunders PTK, Kerr JB, McKinnell C (1992). Testosterone and spermatogenesis: Identification of stage- specific, androgen-regulated proteins secreted by adult rat seminiferous tubules. J Androl 13: 172-184.

Sharpe RM, McKinnell C, McLaren TT, Millar M, West AP, Maguire S, Gaughan J, Syed V, Je'gou B, Kerr JB, Saunders PTK (1994a): Interactions between andro gens, Sertoli cells and germ cells in the control of spermatogenesis. In: *Molecular and Cellular Endocrinology of the Testis: Ernst Schering Research Foundation Workshop, Supplement 1* (Eds: G Verhoeven & U-F Habenicht). pp 115-142. Springer-Verlag, Berlin.

Sharpe RM, Kerr JB, McKinnell C, Millar M(1994b). Temporal relationship between androgen-dependent changes in the volume of seminiferous tubule fluid, lumen size and seminiferous tubule protein secretion in rats. J Reprod Fertil 101: 193-198.

Skinner MK (1991). Cell-cell interactions in the testis. Endocrine Rev 12; 45-77.

Vornberger W, Prins G, Musto NA, Suarez-Quian CA (1994): Androgen receptor distribution in rat testis: new implications for androgen regulation of spermatogenesis. *Endocrinology* 134: 2307-2316.

# 4

# ANDROGENS AND EPIDIDYMAL FUNCTION

Marie-Claire Orgebin-Crist

Center for Reproductive Biology Research
Vanderbilt University School of Medicine
Nashville, Tennessee  37232-2633

The fact that the epididymis and its functions are regulated by androgens was recognized early in this century.  The first experimental evidence came from the studies of Benoit (1926), who observed that the ratio of nucleus/cytoplasm in the mouse epididymis decreased after birth as the epididymis differentiated, and increased dramatically after orchiectomy, as the epididymis dedifferentiated.  Benoit could not demonstrate the nature of the testicular factor responsible for the control of epididymal function since the first androgen prepared in chemically pure form was not available until five years later (Butenandt, 1931).  Since then, numerous studies have shown that the administration of testosterone reverses, although not entirely as will be seen below, the effect of castration on the gross morphologic structure of the epididymis, as well as on the ultrastructure of the epididymal epithelium (Orgebin-Crist et al., 1975).

## EPIDIDYMAL PROCESSES UNDER ANDROGEN CONTROL

The metabolic activity of the epididymis is likewise regulated by androgens.  Table 1 lists the epididymal processes which have been demonstrated to be under androgen control.  Androgens regulate not only the growth and differentiation of the epididymis, but also tightly control the microenvironment of the maturing spermatozoa by regulating the transport of ions and small organic molecules across the epididymal epithelium, the synthesis of adhesion proteins (such as E-cadherin, present in junctional complexes between epididymal cells), and the synthesis and secretion into the luminal fluid of proteins, which are in contact with the maturing spermatozoa.  Some of these proteins possess enzymatic activities which have the potential to either modify the plasma membrane of the maturing spermatozoa (glycosyltransferases, glucosidases, proteases), or protect the mature spermatozoa against oxidative damage during storage in the cauda epididymidis (glutathione peroxidase, $\gamma$-glutamyl transpeptidase).  In this highly regulated microenvironment, spermatozoa develop the ability to move forward, to bind to the zona pellucida, and

*Pharmacology, Biology, and Clinical Applications of Androgens,* edited by Shalender Bhasin et al.
ISBN 0-471-13320-5 © 1996 Wiley-Liss, Inc.

TABLE 1. EPIDIDYMAL PROCESSES UNDER ANDROGEN CONTROL

| | |
|---|---|
| 1) Transport of Small Molecules Across Epididymal Epithelium | |
|    - Ions (Na$^+$) | Wong et al., 1977[1] |
|    - Carnitine | Marquis et al., 1965 |
|    - Inositol | Pholpramool et al., 1982 |
|    - Amino acids | Hinton et al., 1982 |
|    - Sugars | Brooks, 1979 |
| 2) Synthesis | |
|    - DNA | Brooks, 1977 |
|    - RNA | Brooks, 1977 |
| 3) Synthesis and Secretion | |
|    - Small organic molecules | Dawson et al., 1959 |
|    - Proteins and glycoproteins | Cameo et al., 1976 |
| 4) Enzyme Activity | |
|    - Glycolytic enzymes | Brooks, 1976 |
|    - Lipid oxidation enzymes | Brooks, 1978 |
|    - Steroid metabolizing enzymes | |
|     . 5α-reductase | Djoseland, 1976 |
|     . 3α-dehydrogenase | Robaire et al., 1981 |
|    - Polyamine Synthesis Enzymes | |
|     . ornithine decarboxylase | de las Heras et al., 1987 |
|     . S-adenosyl-L-methionine decarboxylase | de las Heras et al., 1991 |
|    -Detoxification Enzymes | |
|     . glutathione S. transferase | Robaire et al., 1982 |
|     . glutathione peroxidase | Rigaudiere et al., 1992 |
|     . glutamyl transpeptidase | Agrawal et al., 1989 |
|    -Oxidation-Reduction Enzyme | |
|     aldo-keto reductase | Fabre et al., 1994 |
|    -Hydrolases | |
|     . esterase | Abou-Haila, 1987 |
|     . β-glucuronidase | Conchie et al., 1959 |
|     . α-mannosidase | Conchie et al., 1959 |
|     . β-galactosidase | Conchie et al., 1959 |
|     . N-acetyl-β-D-glucosaminidase | Conchie et al., 1959 |
|     . acid phosphatase | Mayorga et al., 1981 |
|    - Protease | |
|     . cathepsin D | Mayorga et al., 1981 |
|     . angiotensin converting enzyme | Jaiswal et al., 1985 |
| 5) Maturation and Storage of | |
|    Spermatozoa | Orgebin-Crist, 1973 |

[1]In cases of multiple references only what is believed to be the princeps reference is cited.

to penetrate and fertilize the egg. When androgens are withdrawn, either by or-chiectomy or hypophysectomy, they fail to perform these functions unless exogenous androgen is administered (Orgebin-Crist et al., 1975).

## ANDROGEN REGULATION OF EPIDIDYMAL FUNCTION

In recent years the molecular mechanisms of steroid hormone action have been deciphered to a large extent (Truss and Beato, 1993). However, specific information relating to the mechanism of androgen action has not been as extensive because few androgen-regulated genes have been well characterized. It is believed that androgens, like other steroids, exert their functions through an intracellular androgen receptor (AR). The unliganded AR is associated with heat-shock proteins and is inactive. When androgen is available, it binds to the AR and the hormone-AR associates with the nuclear matrix and specific DNA sequences, called androgen response elements (AREs), located in promoter, or enhancer regions of target genes. This binding triggers gene transcription which is further modulated by transcription regulators (Lindzey et al., 1994). The epididymis shares with other androgen-dependent tissues, the same molecular mechanism of androgen action. For example, a functional ARE in the promoter of the gene for an aldose reductase-like protein in the mouse vas deferens, has recently been identified (Fabre et al., 1994). However, there are special, and, in some cases, unique aspects of the androgen regulation of epididymal function which will be considered.

## SOURCE OF ANDROGENS

The initial step in androgenic regulation depends upon the availability of the ligand for the AR. The epididymis receives a dual source of androgens: the blood, where androgens are bound to a sex hormone-binding globulin, and the rete testis fluid, where androgens are bound to an androgen-binding protein secreted by Sertoli cells. Testosterone, the dominant testicular androgen, undergoes enzymatic reduction to $5\alpha$-dihydrotestosterone (DHT), which is the major effector of the androgen-induced response in the epididymis. Luminal androgens and/or other testicular factors present in the rete testis fluid are essential for the normal function of the proximal epididymis. After efferent duct ligation, which interrupts the flow of rete testis fluid into the epididymis, but maintains normal levels of circulating androgens, the initial segment of the epididymis dedifferentiates and some proteins cease to be synthesized and secreted into the lumen. The same phenomenon occurs after castration and androgen treatment, even when testosterone is administered in supra-physiologic doses (Holland et al., 1992). This indicates that, in addition to circulating androgens, a direct contribution of testicular effluents is necessary for the normal functioning of the epididymis.

## TISSUE SPECIFICITY OF GENE EXPRESSION

Another aspect of epididymal androgen regulation is the tissue specificity of androgen regulated gene expression. This is not a unique feature of epididymal androgen regulation. It has been known for some time that "housekeeping" genes with a wide tissue distribution are androgen regulated only in some tissues (Berger and Watson, 1989). For example, $\gamma$-glutamyl transpeptidase mRNA responds to androgen in the proximal epididymis, but not in the kidney. On the other hand, the

TABLE 2. REGULATION OF TISSUE-SPECIFIC mRNA AND/OR PROTEIN EXPRESSION

| | | Decrease after Castration | Restoration with Testosterone | |
|---|---|---|---|---|
| Endogenous[1] Proviral | epididymis | complete | partial | Cornwall et al., 1992c |
| Sequence | kidney | complete | complete | |
| Cytochrome[1] | epididymis | partial | partial | Cornwall et al., 1992a |
| c oxidase | liver | partial | complete | |
| Subunit II | kidney | partial | complete | |
| γ-Glutamyl[1] | epididymis (prox) | complete | complete | Palladino et al., 1994 |
| Transpeptidase Types II & III | kidney | none | none | |
| 5α-Reductase | epididymis (dist) | partial | complete | Viger et al., 1991 |
| Type 1 | liver | increase | none | |
| | prostate (ventral) | none | increase | |
| β-Glucuronidase[2] | epididymis | partial | none | Abou-Haila et al., 1995 |
| | liver | none | none | |
| | kidney | partial | increase | |

[1]mRNA expression.
[2]enzyme activity.

enzyme activity of the β-glucuronidase gene product is induced in the kidney in response to androgens, but not in the epididymis, and remains unaffected in the liver (Table 2).

## REGION-SPECIFICITY OF GENE EXPRESSION

Another feature of androgen regulation, which is quite possibly unique to the epididymis, is its regionalized gene expression. Although the epididymis is a long convoluted duct lined by the same cell type, a polarized columnar principal cell, each region has a specific pattern of protein (Figure 1) and mRNA expression (Figure 2). The expression of some genes is restricted to a narrow region of the epididymis. For example, the mRNA for a cystatin-related protein is expressed only in the initial segment, while 5α-reductase type 2 mRNA is expressed only in the caput, and the leukocyte differentiation antigen CDw52 mRNA is expressed only in the corpus. Other genes are expressed in more than one segment. For example, retinol-binding protein mRNA is expressed predominantly in both the initial segment and the caput, while the carboxypeptidase y-like protein (D/E) mRNA, is expressed from the caput to the cauda.

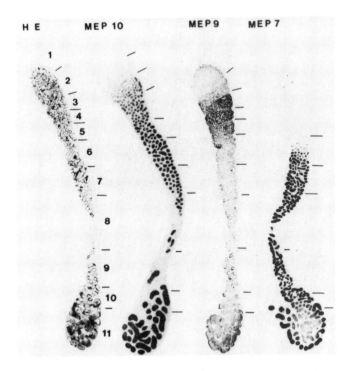

FIGURE 1. The section on the left represents a longitudinal section stained with hematoxylin and eosin (HE). The sections on the right represent the immunolocalization of three secretory proteins (MEP 7, 9, 10) in the epididymis. Reproduced with permission from Rankin et al., 1992.

Not only does the epididymis exhibit a highly regionalized gene expression, but the regulation of gene expression by androgens is also region-specific (Table 3). For example, the expression of some genes present only in the initial segment, such as proenkephalin mRNA, a cystatin-related protein mRNA, or 5α-reductase 1 mRNA, disappears after castration and is not restored when exogenous testosterone is administered. As discussed above, this implies that expression of these genes is dependent upon components of the testicular fluid. In the case of proenkephalin mRNA, the responsible factor appears to be associated with spermatozoa. In the case of the cystatin-related protein and 5α-reductase 1 mRNAs, the factor(s) has not been identified. Other genes which are expressed in several regions of the epididymis display a differential response to androgens depending on the segment. For example, E-cadherin mRNA expression is only partially decreased in the initial segment, but is drastically reduced in the caput and cauda. Androgen replacement maintains normal levels of gene expression even in the initial segment. γ-Glutamyl transpeptidase offers the best example to date of differential androgen response in the epididymis. Although γ-glutamyl transpeptidase types II, III and IV mRNA transcripts disappear from the initial segment after castration, types II and III are reinduced by exogenous testosterone, but type IV is not reinduced. On the other hand, the type II transcript, but not type IV, is responsive to androgens in the cauda.

## REGION-SPECIFIC mRNA EXPRESSION IN THE EPIDIDYMIS[a]

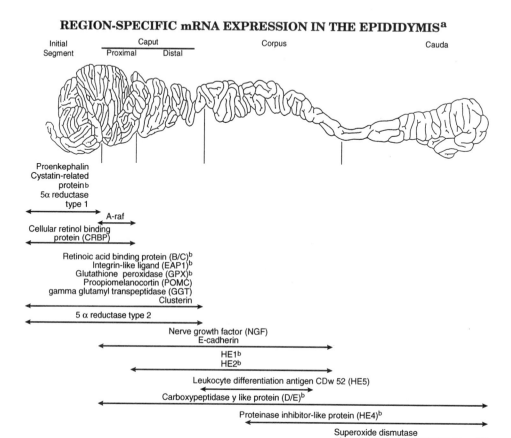

FIGURE 2. Proenkephalin: Garrett et al., 1991; cystatin-related protein: Cornwall et al., 1992b; 5α-reductase types 1 and 2: Viger et al., 1991, Robaire et al., 1995; A-raf: Winer et al., 1993; CRBP: Rajan et al., 1990; B/C and D/E: Walker et al., 1990; EAP1: Perry et al., 1992; GPX: Faure et al., 1991; POMC: Gizang-Ginsberg et al., 1987; GGT: Palladino et al., 1994; Clusterin: Cyr et al., 1992a; NGF: Ayer-LeLievre, 1988; E-cadherin: Cyr et al., 1992b; HE1, HE2 and HE4: Krull et al., 1993; HE5: Kirchhoff et al., 1991; Superoxide dismutase: Perry et al., 1993.

[a]This diagram indicates the region where there is predominant    expression of each gene listed.

[b]Gene expressed predominantly in the epididymis.

TABLE 3. REGION-SPECIFIC REGULATION OF EPIDIDYMAL
mRNA EXPRESSION

| | | Decrease after Castration | Restoration with Testosterone | |
|---|---|---|---|---|
| Predominantly Expressed in Initial Segment | | | | |
| Proenkephalin | | Complete | None | Garrett et al., 1990 |
| Cystatin-related protein | | Complete | None | Cornwall et al., 1992b |
| 5 α-Reductase 1 | | Complete | None | Viger et al., 1991 |
| Expressed in Epididymis | | | | |
| Clusterin | IS | None | None | Cyr et al., 1992a |
| | Caput | None | None | |
| | Cauda | Increase | Complete | |
| γ-Glutamyl Transpeptidase II | IS | Complete | Complete | Palladino et al., 1994 |
| | Caput | Complete | Partial | |
| | Cauda | Partial | Complete | |
| γ-Glutamyl Transpeptidase III | IS | Complete | Complete | |
| | Caput | Complete | Partial | |
| γ-Glutamyl Transpeptidase IV | IS | Complete | None | |
| | Cauda | None | None | |
| E-Cadherin | IS | Partial | Complete | Cyr et al., 1992b |
| | Caput | Complete | Complete | |
| | Cauda | Complete | Complete | |

In some instances, the recovery of mRNA expression, or the reinduction of specific gene products, is not complete following castration and testosterone replacement. For example, γ-glutamyl transpeptidase type II mRNA exhibits only a partial recovery in the caput and a full recovery in the cauda. This implies that for some genes there is a multifactorial regulation of gene expression.

## CELL-SPECIFICITY OF GENE EXPRESSION

The epididymis presents a final level of complexity. Not only is gene expression region-specific but it is also cell-specific. Many mRNAs and/or proteins show a characteristic checkerboard pattern of expression within the same region of the epididymis. That is, some principal cells exhibit strong expression whereas adjacent principal cells display none, or very low levels of expression (Table 4).

TABLE 4. CELL-SPECIFIC EPIDIDYMAL mRNA AND/OR PROTEIN EXPRESSION

| | |
|---|---|
| Proenkephalin[1] | Garrett et al., 1991 |
| Yf Subunit of Glutathione S Transferase[2] | P. Veri et al., 1993 |
| Clusterin[2] | Hermo et al., 1991 |
| Immobilin[2] | Hermo et al., 1992 |
| 5α-Reductase Type I[2] | Viger et al., 1994 |
| Phospholipid Binding Protein (MEP 9)[2] | Rankin et al., 1992 |
| Carboxypeptidase Y-Like Protein (MEP 7)[2] | Rankin et al., 1992 |
| Retinoic Acid Binding Protein (MEP 10)[2] | Rankin et al., 1992 |

[1]mRNA; [2]protein

## CONCLUSION

From the above, it is quite clear that tissues within the same animal, or in the case of the epididymis, different regions of the same tissue, containing the same genome and expressing the same AR, respond differentially to androgens. The diversity and specificity of the control of gene expression may be regulated at different levels: (1) ligand specificity and availability, (2) cell-specific receptor expression, (3) differences in nuclear matrix composition which can expose or shelter DNA sequences to transcription factors, (4) differences in binding affinity between chromatin and AR, or requirement for multiple receptor binding sites creating dissimilar thresholds of response, (5) different tissue-specific transcription regulators binding to DNA sequences located in the promoter or enhancer region, which can regulate the expression of target genes, or (6) differences in mRNA stability (Truss and Beato, 1993). Any of these mechanisms, alone or in combination, could modulate tissue-, region-, and cell-specific gene expression in the epididymis, as well as differential androgen regulation.

In summary, androgens, in concert with unidentified testicular factors, regulate the cell- and region-specific expression, transport, secretion, and absorption of luminal fluid components. As a result, an optimal milieu is created where spermatozoa develop and maintain their ability to fertilize. Much of what we know concerning the specificity of androgenic regulation of gene expression has been learned from non-reproductive tissue, such as the kidney or reproductive tissues, such as the prostate and the seminal vesicle. Yet, as we have seen, the epididymis presents another level of complexity: the specificity of gene expression within the same tissue. Analysis of the mechanisms regulating this region- and cell-specific gene expression will provide a better understanding of the molecular mechanisms which control the microenvironment of the maturing spermatozoa.

## REFERENCES

Abou-Haila A, Fain-Maurel MA (1987): Postnatal differentiation and endocrine control of esterase isoenzymes in the mouse epididymis. J Reprod Fertil 79:437-446.

Abou-Haila A, Tulsiani DRP, Skudlarek M, Orgebin-Crist M-C (1995): Differential androgen regulation of the molecular forms of ß-D-glucuronidase in the mouse epididymis, liver and kidney. Submitted.

Agrawal YP, Vanha-Perttula T (1989): Y-Glutamyl transpeptidase in rat epididymis: effects of castration, hemicastration and efferent duct ligation. Int J Androl 12:321-328.

Ayer-LeLievre C, Olson L, Ebendal T, Hallbook F, Persson H (1988): Nerve growth factor mRNA and protein in the testis and epididymis of mouse and rat. Proc Natl Acad Sci USA 85:2628-2632.

Benoit MJ (1926): Recherches anatomiques, cytologiques et histophysiologiques sur les voies excretrices du testicule, chez les mammiferes. Arch Anat Histol Embryol 5:173-412.

Berger FG, Watson G (1989): Androgen-regulated gene expression. Annu Rev Physiol 51:51-65.

Brooks DE (1976): Activity and androgenic control of glycolytic enzymes in the epididymis and epididymal spermatozoa of the rat. Biochem J 156:527-537.

Brooks DE (1977): The androgenic control of the composition of the rat epididymis determined by efferent duct ligation or castration. J Reprod Fert 49:383-385.

Brooks DE (1978): Activity and androgenic control of enzymes associated with the tricarboxylic acid cycle, lipid oxidation and mitochondrial shuttles in the epididymis and epididymal spermatozoa of the rat. Biochem J 174:741-752.

Brooks DE (1979): Carbohydrate metabolism in the rat epididymis: evidence that glucose is taken up by tissue slices and isolated cells by a process of facilitated transport. Biol Reprod 21:19-26.

Butenandt A (1931): Uber die chemisch untersuchung der sexualhormone. Z Angew Chem 44:905-908.

Cameo MS, Blaquier JA (1976): Androgen-controlled specific proteins in rat epididymis. J Endocrin 69:47-55.

Conchie J, Findlay J (1959): Influence of gonadectomy, sex hormones and other factors, on the activity of certain glycosidases in the rat and mouse. J Endocrin 18:132-146.

Cornwall GA, Orgebin-Crist M-C, Hann S (1992a): Differential expression of the mouse mitochondrial genes and the mitochondrial RNA-processing endoribonuclease RNA by androgens. Mol Endocrin 6:1032-1042.

Cornwall GA, Orgebin-Crist M-C, Hann SR (1992b): The CRES gene: a unique testis-regulated gene related to the cystatin family is highly restricted in its expression to the proximal region of the mouse epididymis. Mol Endocrin 6:1653-1664.

Cornwall GA, Orgebin-Crist M-C, Hann SR (1992c): Expression of an endogenous murine leukemia virus-related proviral sequence is androgen-regulated and primarily restricted to the epididymis/vas deferens and oviduct/uterus. Biol Reprod 47:665-675.

Cyr DG, Robaire B (1992a): Regulation of sulfated glycoprotein-2 (clusterin) messenger ribonucleic acid in the rat epididymis. Endocrin 130:2160-2166.

Cyr DG, Hermo L, Blaschuk OW, Robaire B (1992b): Distribution and regulation of epithelial cadherin messenger ribonucleic acid and immunocytochemical localization of epithelial cadherin in the rat epididymis. Endocrin 130:353-363.

Dawson RMC, Rowlands IW (1959): Glycerylphosphorylcholine in the male reproductive organs of rats and guinea-pigs. Quart J Exp Physiol 44:26-34.

de las Heras MA, Calandra RS (1987): Androgen-dependence of ornithine decarboxylase in the rat epididymis. J Reprod Fert 79:9-14.

de las Heras MA, Calandra RS (1991): S-adenosyl-L-methionine decarboxylase activity in the rat epididymis: ontogeny and androgenic control. J Androl 12:209-213.

Djoseland O (1976): Androgen metabolism by rat epididymis. Effect of castration and anti-androgens. Steroids 27:47-64.

Fabre S, Manin M, Pailhoux E, Veyssiere G, Jean C (1994): Identification of a functional androgen response element in the promoter of the gene for the androgen-regulated aldose reductase-like protein specific to the mouse vas deferens. J Biol Chem 269:5857-5864.

Faure J, Ghyselinck NB, Jimenez C, Dufaure J-P (1991): Specific distribution of messenger ribonucleic acids for 24-kilodalton proteins in the mouse epididymis as revealed by in situ hybridization: developmental expression and regulation in the adult. Biol Reprod 44:13-22.

Garrett JE, Garrett SH, Douglas J (1990): A spermatozoa-associated factor regulated proenkephalin gene expression in the rat epididymis. Mol Endocrin 4:108-118.

Garrett SH, Garrett JE, Douglas J (1991): In situ histochemical analysis of region-specific gene expression in the adult rat epididymis. Molec Reprod Dev 30:1-17.

Gizang-Ginsberg E, Wolgemuth DJ (1987): Expression of the proopiomelanocortin gene is developmentally regulated and affected by germ cells in the male mouse reproductive system. Develop Biol 84:1600-1604.

Hermo L, Wright J, Oko R, Morales CR (1991): Role of epithelial cells of the male excurrent duct system of the rat in the endocytosis secretion of sulfated glycoprotein-2 (clusterin). Biol Reprod 44:1113-1131.

Hermo L, Oko R, Robaire B (1992): Epithelial cells of the epididymis show regional variations with respect to the secretion of endocytosis of immobilin as revealed by light and electron microscope immunocytochemistry. Anat Rec 232:202-220.

Hinton BT, Howards SS (1982): Rat testis and epididymis can transport [$^3$H]3-0-methyl-D-glucose, [$^3$H] aminoisobutyric acid across its epithelia. Biol Reprod 27:1181-1189.

Holland MK, Vreeburg JTM, Orgebin-Crist M-C (1992): Testicular regulation of epididymal protein secretion. J Androl 13:266-273.

Jaiswal AK, Panda JN, Kumar MV and Joshi P (1985): Androgen dependence of testicular and epididymal angiotensin converting enzyme. Andrologia 17:92-97.

Kirchhoff C, Habben I, Ivell R, Krull N (1991): A major human epididymis-specific cDNA encodes a protein with sequence homology to extracellular proteinase inhibitors. Biol Reprod 45:350-357.

Krull N, Ivell R, Osterhoff C, Kirchhoff C (1993): Region-specific variation of gene expression in the human epididymis as revealed by in situ hybridization with tissue-specific cDNAs. Molec Reprod Dev 34:16-24.

Lindzey J, Kumar MV, Grossman M, Young C, Tindall DJ (1994): Molecular mechanisms of androgen action. Vit Horm 49:383-432.

Marquis NR, Fritz IB (1965): Effects of testosterone on the distribution of carnitine and carnitine acetyltransferase in tissues of the reproductive system of the male rat. J Biol Chem 240:2197-2200.

Mayorga LS, Bertini F (1981): Acid hydrolases in the epididymis of normal, castrated vasectomized, cryptorchid and cryptepididymal rats. Int J Androl 4:208-219.

Orgebin-Crist M-C (1973): Maturation of spermatozoa in the rabbit epididymis: Effect of castration and testosterone replacement. J Exp Zool 185:301-310.

Orgebin-Crist M-C, Danzo BJ, Davies J (1975): Endocrine control of the development and maintenance of sperm fertilizing ability in the epididymis. In: Greep R, Hamilton DW (eds.): "Handbook of Physiology-Endocrinology V." Baltimore, MD: Williams & Wilkins, Chapter 15, pp 319-338.

Palladino MA, Hinton BT (1994): Expression of multiple gamma-glutamyl transpeptidase messenger ribonucleic acid transcripts in the adult rat epididymis is differentially regulated by androgens and testicular factors in a region-specific manner. Endocrin 135:1146-1156.

Perry ACF, Jones R, Barker PJ, Hall L (1992): A mammalian epididymal protein with remarkable sequence similarity to snake venom haemorrhagic peptides. Biochem J 286:671-675.

Perry ACF, Jones R, Hall L (1993): Isolation and characterization of a rat cDNA clone encoding a secreted superoxide dismutase reveals the epididymis to be a major site of its expression. Biochem J 293:21-25.

Pholpramool C, White RW, Setchell BP (1982): Influence of androgens on inositol secretion and sperm transport in the epididymis of rats. J Reprod Fert 66:547-553.

Rajan N, Sung WK, Goodman DS (1990): Localization of cellular retinol-binding protein mRNA in rat testis and epididymis and its stage-dependent expression during the cycle of the seminiferous epithelium. Biol Reprod 43:835-842.

Rankin TL, Tsuruta KJ, Holland MK, Griswold MD, Orgebin-Crist M-C (1992): Isolation, immunolocalization, and sperm-association of three proteins of 18, 25, and 29 kilodaltons secreted by the mouse epididymis. Biol Reprod 46:747-766.

Rigaudiere N, Ghyselinck NB, Faure J, Dufaure JP (1992): Regulation of the epididymal gluthathione peroxidase-like protein in the mouse: dependence upon androgens and testicular factors. Molec Cell Endocrin 89:67-77.

Robaire B, Zirkin B.R. (1981): Hypophysectomy and simultaneous testosterone replacement: effects on male rat reproductive tract and epididymal $\nabla^4$-5$\alpha$-reductase and 3$\alpha$-hydroxysteroid dehydrogenase. Endocrin 109:1225-1233.

Robaire B, Hales BF (1982): Regulation of epididymal glutathione S-transferases: effects of orchidectomy and androgen replacement. Biol Reprod 26:559-565.

Robaire B, Viger RS (1995): Regulation of epididymal epithelial cell functions. Biol Reprod 54:226-236.

Truss M, Beato M (1993): Steroid hormone receptors: interaction with deoxyribonucleic acid and transcription factors. Endocrin Rev 14: 459-479.

Veri J-P, Hermo L, Robaire B (1993): Immunocytochemical localization of the Yf subunit of glutathione S-transferase P shows regional variation in the staining of epithelial cells of the testis, efferent ducts, and epididymis of the male rat. J Androl 14:23-44.

Viger RS, Robaire B (1991): Differential regulation of steady state 4-ene steroid 5α-reductase messenger ribonucleic acid levels along the rat epididymis. Endocrin 128:2407-2414.

Viger RS, Robaire B (1994): Immunocytochemical localization of 4-Ene steroid 5α-reductase type 1 along the rat epididymis during postnatal development. Endocrin 134:2298-2306.

Walker JE, Jones R, Moore A, Hamilton DW, Hall L (1990): Analysis of major androgen-regulated        cDNA clones from the rat epididymis. Mol Cell Endocrin 74:61-68.

Winer MA, Wadewitz AG, Wolgemuth DJ (1993): Members of the raf gene family exhibit segment-specific patterns of expression in mouse epididymis. Molec Reprod Dev 35:16-23.

Wong PYD, Yeung CH (1977): Hormonal regulation of fluid reabsorption in isolated rat cauda epididymidis. Endocrin 101:1391.

# DISCUSSION: ANDROGEN PHYSIOLOGY
## Chairpersons: William Bremner, Ilpo Huhtaniemi

**Margaret Wierman:** This question is for Dr. Griswold or Dr. Sharpe. I was fascinated by your reports on the differential expression of genes that are regulated by androgens and through the androgen receptor. Based on the recent work with the estrogen receptor knockout in the mouse and the human homologue recently reported in NEJM, what is your current understanding about the role of estrogen on Sertoli or Leydig cell function?

**Michael Griswold:** The evidence for the presence of the estrogen receptor in Sertoli cells in the rat, is still open to question. The direct effects of the estrogen receptor knockout in the male are still unclear.

**Richard Sharpe:** There is evidence that estrogens might be involved in an intratesticular long loop feedback system, whereby you negatively regulate Leydig cell supply. Estrogens produced within the testis, whether it is by the Leydig cells in the adult or by Sertoli cells in the fetal testes, exert feedback effect on steroidogenic enzymes within the Leydig cells, but also on Leydig precursor cells.

**Margaret Wierman:** In the estrogen receptor knockout animal model there were marked defects in the male with spermatogenesis. In the human male with estrogen receptor defect, a low sperm count was found. The human patient and the knockout mice also have abnormalities in skeletal maturation, suggesting that androgen's effect on bones is through conversion to estrogens. Thus, the question is, what is the role of estrogen and estrogen receptors in the testes?

**Michael Griswold:** There is some information from Gorsky's Lab in Wisconsin that the estrogen receptor appears to be present in Sertoli cells during embryogenesis and then disappears during the prepubertal phase.

**Ilpo Huhtaniemi:** There is another difference in testosterone production, which is the high intratesticular level in the human testes. It is about ten fold higher than in the rodent, and we do not understand why the level has to be so high in man.

**Gail Risbridger:** My question is specifically for Richard Sharpe and concerns the issue of Leydig cell regulation and what locally stimulates testosterone production. There are different types of Leydig cells and they have different developmental phases. They respond to and are regulated differently by LH. One would therefore assume that local factors are also having different actions at those specific stages and we seem to have lost site of that. I think that it is not the approach in the *in vitro* models that is wrong, it is the failure to put those ideas back into the context of the biological process of Leydig cell development. How do you respond to that?

**Richard Sharpe:** I agree Gail. My continuing concern is about the "overuse" of *in vitro* model systems without considering when or how such effects might occur *in vivo*. Many researches never make any attempt (yourself excepted) to check the relevance of their results to the physiological situation, and although this can be difficult to do, it should at least be attempted.

**Gail Risbridger:** The problem is that we are not recognizing there is not just a single type of Leydig cell. Maybe some of those disparate findings that people have will be resolved if they actually looked more carefully and considered the biological process they were studying rather than just considering a phenomena.

**Richard Sharpe:** I agree.

**Wayne Meikle:** My question relates to the multiple substances that the testes make and particularly the Leydig cell and how these may modulate the LH response in producing testosterone. How do you put all of these growth factors, cytokines and displaced releasing hormones that are made in the Leydig cell in perspective, and how do they help us understand Leydig cell physiology? Are they really important there?

**David deKretser:** There are a large number of factors which are produced by Leydig cells and there are a large number of factors which are produced by Sertoli cells, which are reputed to have actions on Leydig cells. I think so far they are in the realm of phenomenology rather than truly established physiology. Equally, I think, there are other substances that are going to be characterized which may have local roles in regulation. Many of these substances have actions in multi-systems, so if one is looking at gene "knockouts" to solve these issues, then they should be cell specific and tissue specific knockouts.

**Richard M. Sharpe -** I have always been unable to make physiological sense of the multiplicity of effects of so many growth factors on Leydig cell function, until the concept of biochemical radar was proposed. This concept proposes that a cell, such as the Leydig cell, continuously monitors its environment. It sends out a signal which could be a peptide or it could be testosterone or even a binding protein but the Leydig cell also has receptors for the same signal. Other cells, and they could be within the testes or they could be far away in the pituitary gland, secrete factors, which either bind the signal, or metabolize it or even add to it. All of these complex interactions ultimately condense down to a single simple signal which the Leydig cell receives back. So, one signal is sent out and one is received back, but in the interim, many factors from any cells have had the possibility to modify this signal and in the process, enable the Leydig cell to live in harmony with both the local environment and that of the body as a whole.

**William Bremner:** There are data for an effect of FSH as well as growth hormone and prolactin on testosterone production. Do either one of you want to comment on that?

**David deKretser:** I think that if FSH does exert an action on Leydig cell function, in view of the absence of FSH receptors on Leydig cells, that the most likely source of this action is in fact via the Sertoli cell. There is some data to suggest that FSH might also have an action on macrophages and there is evidence of influence of macrophages on neighboring Leydig cell testosterone production. I don't think there is any doubt that the FSH effect is real. It is just a question of what the mechanism is by which it is exerted.

**Eberhardt Nieschlag:** I would like to add to the discussion David deKretser had started when pointing out the different responses of Leydig cells in different species and even within the same species. In men, when you give the hCG at 8:00 o'clock in the morning, the response occurs 24 hours later. When you give the same injection at 8:00 o'clock in the evening, the maximum response also occurs the next ˙ing. So the absolute time required is not so much of importance, but a chronobiological phenomenon plays a role here. The blood flow through the testes, which may change during the day, could explain the intraindividual as well as the interspecies phenomenon. We have to take into account chronobiological phenomena when looking at the responses of cells and tissues.

**Stephen Winters:** If we track testosterone and LH secretory episodes in peripheral blood in men, we see robust LH secretory episodes with very small fluctuations of 10 to 15% for testosterone. In old world monkeys, by contrast, there are large LH pulses and large spontaneous testosterone pulses. So between those two species of primates, there is a dramatic difference of LH-testosterone secretions. One of the differences is the frequency of the GnRH pulse generator. The monkey has a slower GnRH pulse generator than human, with 6 to 9 pulses over 24 hours versus humans pulsing at about once per hour. Thus, I propose that the difference you discussed in testosterone secretions relates partly to the pulsable pattern of LH secretion in humans.

**David deKretser:** Actually, I think you have also raised an important issue and that is, do the Leydig cells require a pulsatile LH signal or is that just simply a "hangover" from the pituitary-GnRH pulse generator activity? What you are suggesting is that in view of the high frequency of the human pulse generator, the Leydig cell is exposed almost to a tonic stimulus. I don't think we have a clear picture as to whether a pulsatile signal is absolutely required by the testes.

**Patricia Cuasnicu:** Some of these proteins, e.g., mouse MEP or rat acidic epididymal proteins, that you have considered specific to the epididymis, are present in other tissues, e.g., in the salivary gland.

**Marie-Claire Orgebin-Crist:** Some proteins like protein DE, which is the rat homologue of MEP7, was thought to be specifically expressed in the epididymis and has now been shown to be expressed in other tissues as well. In my talk, I was careful to say, "predominantly expressed" in the epididymis and I think this is still true for protein DE.

**Ronald Swerdloff:** I would like to ask if the cross talk between Sertoli and germ cell may be important in the regional responses to testosterone within the spermatogenic tubules. It seems highly unlikely to me that the testosterone would be able to target the germ cells at one specific stage or at multiple levels of advancement without some kind of a mediator, such as Sertoli cell. Dr. Sinha-Hikim in our laboratories, has shown that stage-specific degeneration of germ cell with hormone deprivation to be directly correlated with the level of apoptosis that occurs in a stage-specific fashion. Perhaps this will serve as a marker for identification of Sertoli cell factors that might be influencing this process.

**Richard Sharpe:** Certainly with regard to FSH, testosterone, and stage-specific action, I paint a picture of testosterone acting at a particular stage. In fact, there are stages where testosterone effects seem to be most prominent. This doesn't necessarily mean that its effects are absent from other stages. FSH is probably interacting in this whole process by acting on different steps or stages from those affected by testosterone. However, I think that there is tremendous overlap, and maybe even redundancy in action, between FSH and testosterone because the processes that are driven by FSH during development largely switch to be controlled by testosterone in adult life. With regard to androgens being unable to affect germ cells just at a particular stage, I see no problem in believing that this can happen - NOT by targeting the testosterone at particular germ cells, but by varying the androgen-responsiveness of the germ cells.

**Robert McLachlan:**  We have found that high dose testosterone treatment to an intact rat or to a GnRH immunized rat, spermatogenesis is substantially restored.  In both of those models FSH is also present.  If you look critically at the testicular weights, or more importantly at the spermatogonial number in such animals, they are still significantly reduced by perhaps 20% to 25% despite the presence of both androgens and FSH.  What comment do you have about that and should we think about a third factor being required?

**Richard Sharpe:**  I think that what constitutes quantitative maintenance of spermatogenesis and what is qualitative is a very thorny question.  Part of the answer might relate to the "redundancy" in action between FSH and testosterone which I referred to a few minutes ago because this may mean that a very similar end result (in terms of maintenance of spermatogenesis) may be achieved with several different hormonal profiles because of the overlap in action between FSH and testosterone. The other problem is that very often testosterone levels do not appear to be as high as in the normal situation.  This is particularly true in studies using hypophysectomized animals and in species other than the rat, and certainly in the human.

**Robert McLachlan:**  It is possible that, in fact, there are thresholds of androgen action on spermatogenesis.  It is important that in restoration studies, that quantitation is performed.  If you look critically at germ cell numbers, there are clearly different androgen thresholds for aspects of spermatogenic restoration.

**Richard Sharpe:**  The duration of experiments is also critical.  For example, if testosterone substitution results in levels which are 80% of normal, then you are going to maintain spermatogenesis fairly effectively, but the longer you carry on that treatment, the more chance there will be that the deficiency in androgen support will become manifest.

**William Bremner:**  It is often stated that the epididymis would be an excellent site to target because the length of time it would take to induce the contraceptive effect would be short and the return to fertility would also be short.  There could be an avoidance of effects on systemic endocrinology.  Do you have mechanism or site to suggest in the epididymis that might be targeted as a potential contraceptive?

**Marie-Claire Orgebin-Crist:**  Yes, specific interference with the maturation or storage of spermatozoa in the epididymis would be an attractive contraceptive approach.

**David Handelsman:**  It has been observed in the rat that DHT, which is not aromatizable, can induce quantitatively complete spermatogenesis, which doesn't seem to leave much role for aromatization and action via estrogen receptor. I would also like to support Richard's comment that there is biological redundancy between FSH and testosterone.  We have recently been able to show that you can actually induce quantitatively complete spermatogenesis in the total absence of FSH in congenitally gonadotropin deficient mice.

**Abraham Morgenthler:**  For Dr. deKretser, I wish to ask you to summarize ᴺᵐe of the biochemical effects of the cryptorchid state on Leydig cells?

**David deKretser:** The disorder in Leydig cell function that takes place with any of the disruptive modes of spermatogenic damage is characterized by Leydig cells that are larger and have greater proportion of organelles that are involved in steroid production, i.e., endoplasmic reticulum, mitochondria, and lipid droplets. The cells, in response to HCG, produce more testosterone, but the sensitivity is reduced which may be related to a 50% reduction in the LH receptor numbers on Leydig cells.

**Glenn Cunningham:** Dr. Sharpe, what regulates the stem cells? Is it possible to suppress, as contraceptive target, the stem cell proliferation?

**Richard Sharpe:** I think there is extremely little known about what regulates stem cell proliferation and all aspects of the early spermatogonial stages and spermatogenesis. Because of this, I think we cannot identify an aspect of spermatogonial development which would be suitable for contraceptive attack. My own personal conviction is that the later in spermatogenesis a contraceptive agent acts, the less chance there is of untoward side effects. Therefore, targeting the epididymis, or very late effects in spermiogenesis, would seem to offer the safest contraceptive options.

# 5

# ANDROGEN RECEPTOR STRUCTURE, FUNCTION, REGULATION, AND DYSFUNCTION

**Terry R. Brown**

**Department of Population Dynamics**
**Division of Reproductive Biology**
**Johns Hopkins University**
**Baltimore, Maryland 21205**

## INTRODUCTION

Androgens promote normal virilization of the male urogenital tract during embryogenesis, masculinization of the male phenotype at puberty, and maintenance of the function of male sex organs during adulthood. The primary androgen secreted by the testis is testosterone, which controls differentiation of the Wolffian ducts (epididymides, vasa deferentia, and seminal vesicles). The more biologically potent $5\alpha$-reduced product of testosterone, namely $5\alpha$-dihydrotestosterone (DHT), regulates differentiation of the prostate and development of the urogenital sinus and external genitalia (scrotum, penis, and penile urethra). The actions of testosterone and DHT are mediated by the intracellular androgen receptor (AR), which belongs to the subfamily of nuclear receptor proteins including the glucocorticoid (GR), progesterone (PR), and mineralocorticoid (MR) receptors, all of which are members of the larger superfamily of ligand-dependent transcription factors.

## ANDROGEN RECEPTOR STRUCTURE/FUNCTION

The AR gene locus spans over 90 kb and has been mapped to the $q_{11-12}$ region of the human X-chromosome (Kuiper et al., 1989). The human AR gene is a single copy gene comprised of 8 exons. Northern blot analysis of RNA revealed the presence of a predominant 10.6-kb AR mRNA, with less abundant, alternatively processed species in the range of 7- and 4.6-kb. The human AR promoter lacks TATA/CCAAT boxes and is characterized by a short GC-box (-59/-32) and a long homopurine stretch (-117/-60) relative to the transcription start site (Faber et al., 1993). Two major transcription initiation sites are located in a 13-bp region located 1127-bp (AR-TIS I) and 1116-bp (AR-TIS II) upstream of the translation initiation

*Pharmacology, Biology, and Clinical Applications of Androgens*, edited by Shalender Bhasin et al.
ISBN 0-471-13320-5 © 1996 Wiley-Liss, Inc.

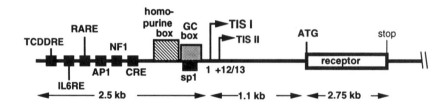

Figure 1. Diagram of androgen receptor (AR) gene promoter. Two transcription start sites (TIS I and II) are located approximately 1.1 kb upstream from the translation initiation methionine codon (ATG) of the 2.75 kb open reading frame. The AR promoter lacks TATA/CAAT elements but has GC-rich (-32 to -59 bp) and homopurine (-60 to -117 bp) boxes immediately 5' to TIS I and II. Consensus sequences for several regulatory protein binding sites are located within the 2.5 kb 5' enhancer region.

site. The GC-box contains a single SP1 binding site and directs initiation from the AR-TIS II site. However, the primary transcript of AR is initiated from the AR-TIS I site in all tissues examined to date. Other potential cis-acting elements within the AR promoter include a nuclear factor (NF)-1 binding motif, an accessory protein (AP)-1 binding motif (with one base mismatch), and response elements for cAMP (CRE), retinoic acid receptors (two), IL-6 (three), and TCDD (one) (Mizokami et al., 1994). Deletion analysis showed that a region between 530 bp and 380 bp upstream of the AR gene transcription initiation site, which includes one potential CRE with a two base mismatch, is responsible for cAMP induction of AR transcription.

The 5'- and 3'-untranslated regions are 1.1- and 6.8-kb in length, respectively. Recently, a portion of the 5'-untranslated region containing a stem-loop secondary structure was discovered to play a role in the induction of AR translation (Mizokami and Chang, 1994). A putative role for the 3'-untranslated region in the stability and/or translation of AR mRNA has also been suggested. The 110-114 kDa receptor protein contains 910-919 amino acids encoded by a 2.75 kb open reading frame (Lubahn et al., 1988). A smaller, 87 kDa form of the AR protein with unknown function and translated from an alternative initiation-methionine codon has been observed at lower concentration (10%) on Western blots. Studies of the steroid receptors, including human AR, have revealed the presence of three conserved functional domains.

## Transcriptional Activation Domain

The amino terminus is the least conserved region with the greatest variation in length among the various receptors, but is essential for transcriptional activation (Jenster et al., 1991). In the human AR, this region is encoded by the first and largest exon of the X-chromosomal gene. A transcriptional activating function

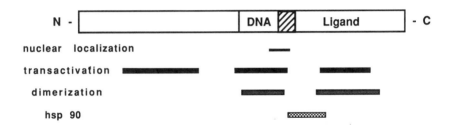

Figure 2. Functional domains common to steroid receptors including the androgen receptor. The central DNA- and carboxy-terminal ligand binding domains are separated by the "hinge" (slashed area) region containing the nuclear localization signal sequence. The relative location of peptide regions important for nuclear localization, transactivation, dimerization, and heat shock protein (hsp 90) binding functions are indicated by the bars.

(TAF) region in AR was localized within the region of amino acids 142-239 in the N-terminal domain and determined to be critical for regulation of target gene transcription (Zhou et al., 1994b). By contrast, deletion of amino acids 199-239 within this region caused a significant increase in transactivation compared to wild-type AR, suggesting that the N-terminus contains both activator and repressor functions. A striking feature of the DNA sequence encoding the N-terminal domain are two polymorphic in-frame trimeric repeats, of GGN and $(CAG)_n(CAA)$ (Trifiro et al., 1994). The polymorphic GGN repeat encodes a glycine stretch which can vary from 16-27 residues. The long GGN repeat is specific to the human AR as a shorter glycine region occurs in the rat and mouse AR, and is not present in the GR, MR, PR and ER. The polyglutamine, $CAG_n$, tract also varies polymorphically from 11 to 31 residues. The polymorphic variation within these two regions accounts for the variation in amino acid number in the human AR protein reported by various research groups. A practical application of these polymorphic tandem triplet repeats is their use in pedigree analysis in families with X-linked diseases, such as androgen insensitivity syndrome (AIS). The function of the polyglutamine stretch is not clear but is postulated to have a role as a transcription activating domain by analogy to other transcription factors containing GC-rich sequences which interact with other regulatory factors, such as SP1.

## DNA-Binding Domain

The most highly conserved region of steroid receptors is the central, cysteine-rich DNA-binding domain (Lubahn et al., 1988). Exons 2 and 3 of the AR gene encode the DNA-binding domain of the receptor which shares approximately 80% homology with GR and PR. By analogy with GR, the DNA-binding domain of AR structurally consists of two zinc-fingers incorporating two perpendicularly oriented alpha-helices. Specific amino acids in the N-terminal alpha-helix directly contact the DNA and define the specificity of the receptor for its hormone response element. The invariant residues, gly[577], ser[578], and val[581] within this proximal (P)-box are present in AR, GR and PR and account for their recognition of the same response element nucleotide sequence (Freedman, 1992). The distal (D)-box, consisting of five amino acids (ASRND) within the second zinc-finger, is thought to play a role in AR dimerization for DNA binding as previously demonstrated for GR. AR and GR differ by a single amino acid within the D-box. Mutations within these regions can be used to study DNA binding and dimerization properties of the AR that impact upon AR transactivation functions. Nucleotide sequence specific DNA binding of receptors to their respective response elements leads to DNA bending and suggests that interactions between various cis-acting factors bound to DNA can occur by drawing them into close proximity within the transcriptional activation complex. In addition, the DNA binding of AR may be influenced by its interaction with other nuclear proteins.

A bipartite nuclear targeting signal sequence, similar to that of the protein, nucleoplasmin, overlaps the DNA binding and "hinge" regions encoded at the junction of exons 3 and 4 (Zhou et al., 1994a). Amino acids 617-633 represent two clusters of basic amino acids separated by 10 amino acids that shuttle the AR through nuclear pores. In the absence of ligand, the AR is distributed within the cytoplasm and nucleus. The presence of androgen induces a rapid migration of AR to the nucleus. Mutation of the basic amino acids in the 617-633 region of AR causes an almost complete cytoplasmic localization of the receptor and absence of its transactivation function. Furthermore, the bipartite nuclear targeting sequence of AR includes flanking sequence and is modulated by interactions between the $NH_2$- and COOH-terminal regions.

## Steroid-Binding Domain

The carboxyl-terminus, encoded by exons 4-8 of the AR gene, specifies the steroid binding properties of the receptor (Jenster et al., 1991). Transcriptional functions of native steroid receptors are repressed by the C-terminal ligand-free steroid-binding domain. Ligand binding releases this repression by mechanisms not fully understood involving a conformational change that may be associated with the release of heat shock proteins, thus allowing the formation of receptor dimers and binding of receptors to steroid response elements to promote transactivation. Intramolecular interactions between the amino-terminal and steroid-binding domains are regulated by the specificity of hormone binding and modulate receptor dimerization and DNA binding (Zhou et al., 1994b). A second putative TAF function has been assigned to the steroid-binding domain of AR by homology with the activating domain of other receptors. In addition, post-translational phosphorylation is common to steroid receptors, including AR. High affinity androgen binding occurs with both the unphosphorylated and phosphorylated forms of AR, however a higher level of phosphorylated AR is observed in the presence of androgen due either to stabilization of the ligand-bound receptor or to a higher degree of protein phosphorylation. Interestingly, a mutant AR with deletion of its steroid-binding domain retains constitutive activity to induce transcription in the absence of hormone binding. These studies suggest that the steroid-binding domain of AR acts to repress target gene transcription in the absence of androgen, perhaps, due to an inhibitory conformation adopted by the ligand-free protein.

AR is localized in the nucleus in the presence of the androgens, testosterone, dihydrotestosterone and methyltrienolone (R1881), and with high concentrations of estradiol and progesterone, as well as with the antiandrogens, hydroxyflutamide and cyproterone acetate (Zhou et al., 1994b). AR is degraded rapidly ($t^{1/2} = 1$ h) except in the presence of androgen ($t^{1/2} = 6$ h). The antiandrogens, flutamide and hydroxyflutamide, lack agonist activity and inhibit R1881-induced activation of transcription and androgen-induced stabilization of AR. Hydroxyflutamide acts as a true antiandrogen since it lacks agonist activity and inhibits androgen-induced transcriptional activation by preventing binding of AR to DNA.

## ANDROGEN RECEPTOR DYSFUNCTION

### Androgen Insensitivity Syndrome

The human androgen insensitivity syndrome (AIS) presents as male pseudohermaphroditism in subjects with a normal 46,XY karyotype despite normal male levels of testosterone secretion by testicular Leydig cells during fetal life (Brown and Migeon, 1987). The external genitalia in affected individuals with AIS ranges from a female phenotype and blind-ending vaginal pouch at birth and breast development at puberty in the complete form, to ambiguous genitalia with hyposapdias at birth

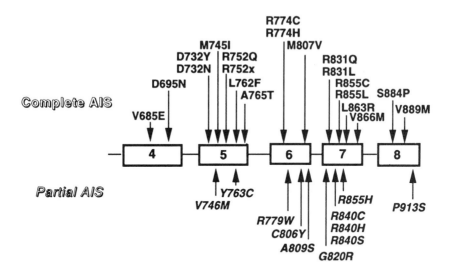

Figure 3. Mutations within exons 4-8 of the androgen receptor gene encode single amino acid substitutions within the steroid-binding domain of subjects with complete (top) and partial (bottom) androgen insensitivity (AIS). The position of the affected amino acid residue is indicated by the number with the normal residue to the left and the substituted residue on the right. The letter x is used to indicate a stop codon.

and gynecomastia at puberty in partial forms, to milder forms with an apparent normal male phenotype and infertility. The androgen-dependent Wolffian duct derivatives remain hypoplastic whereas the Mullerian ducts regress in response to secretion of Mullerian Inhibiting Substance from Sertoli cells. The testes are located in the abdominal or inguinal region and are characterized postpubertally by hyperplastic Leydig cells and seminiferous tubules containing immature Sertoli cells and primitive germ cells that have not progressed beyond the spermatogonia stage. In early infancy and postpubertally, the hallmark endocrine findings in AIS are serum testosterone concentrations within or above the normal male range and elevated LH levels. Estrogenic responses from aromatization of testosterone often prevail in the face of diminished or absent androgen sensitivity.

Our group pioneered studies during the 1970's demonstrating the biochemical and cellular basis of AIS by classifying steroid binding in genital skin fibroblasts from subjects with the clinical diagnosis of AIS into several categories (Brown and Migeon, 1987). Those studies were followed more recently by molecular genetic studies to identify molecular lesions in the AR gene (Brown et al., 1994; McPhaul et al., 1993; Pinsky et al., 1992; Quigley et al., 1994; Trapman and Brinkmann, 1993). Absence of androgen binding (AR-) in genital skin fibroblasts is now known to be associated with complete and partial deletions of the AR gene, and with single base mutations that introduce a premature termination codon, disturb mRNA splicing, or cause substitution of amino acids in the steroid binding domain. Normal androgen binding (AR+) is present in cultured genital skin fibroblasts of some subjects with the clinical phenotype and endocrine profile of AIS. Although the molecular defect was originally believed to occur at some point distal to the AR (i.e. "post-receptor") in the pathway for androgen action, recent molecular analyses of the AR gene have revealed mutations within the DNA-binding domain encoded by exons 2 and 3. These mutations predominantly influence the DNA-binding and dimerization properties of AR that impact upon AR transactivation functions. The majority of AR gene mutations identified in subjects with AIS occur within the steroid-binding domain, however the distribution of mutations leading to partial and complete forms of AIS are similar throughout this domain. These mutations affect the level of androgen binding (AR± or AR-), the steroid binding specificity, and the association/dissociation kinetics of ligand-receptor interaction. Exon 5 harbors the greatest number of point mutations causing AIS, such that substitution of nearly 50% of the amino acid residues encoded by this exon have been documented among subjects with partial or complete AIS. The amino acid sequence encoded by exon 5 is the most highly conserved portion of the steroid-binding domain among members of the AR/GR/PR/MR subfamily of steroid receptors. In addition, five codons within exons 6 and 7 appear as "hot spots" for mutation based upon their relative frequency of mutation and the several alternative amino acid substitutions that occur with each codon (Murono et al., 1995). Four arginine residues at positions 774, 831, 840 and 855, and valine 866 are altered in numerous families with AIS, often involving a single base substitution in a CpG dinucleotide sequence. As reported for other genes with high rates of mutation, these doublets are subject to a high frequency of C-T transition by methylation of cytosine to 5-methylcytosine, followed by spontaneous deamination to thymine. In addition, arginine codons are over represented in approximately 40% of all AR mutations despite their frequency at 4% among all residues within AR. Arg is completely conserved among members of the AG/GR/-AR/GR/PR/MR subfamily of receptors at positions 774, 831 and 855, but is unique to AR at position 840.

Complete AR gene deletion in two families and partial deletions involving multiple exons (4-8, 3-8, and 6-7) and single exons (2, 3, or 5) have been reported for families with complete AIS (Brown et al., 1994). Surprisingly, deletion of exon 4 was reported for a subject with isolated infertility and deletion of the 5' portion of exon 3 caused only hypospadias in another subject. Less than 5% of subjects with AIS have deletion mutations, with the vast majority of affected individuals having single nucleotide substitutions.

## Male Breast Cancer

Breast cancer is very rare in men and the etiology is unknown. Factors such as hypoandrogenism in Klinefelters syndrome, testicular atrophy, orchitis, undescended testes, testicular trauma and infertility have been determined as risk factors for male breast cancer. Recently, two germline mutations in the androgen receptor gene of subjects with breast cancer and partial androgen insensitivity have been reported (Lobaccaro et al., 1993; Wooster et al., 1992). Both of these mutations occurred within exon 3 encoding the second zinc-finger of the DNA-binding domain of the androgen receptor. Each was caused by a point mutation in adjacent codons causing amino acid substitutions of $arg^{607} \Rightarrow glu$ and $arg^{608} \Rightarrow lys$. The me-

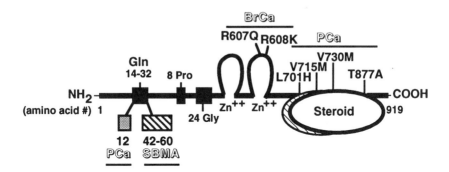

Figure 4. Mutant forms of the androgen receptor (AR) associated with the human diseases of prostate cancer (PCa), spinal bulbar muscular atrophy (SBMA), and male breast cancer (BrCa). The human AR is represented schematically showing the $NH_2$-terminal polymeric amino acid repeats, the central two zinc-fingers, and the steroid-binding domain. Contraction of the polyglutamine region has been reported in PCa whereas expansion of this region occurs in SBMA. Male breast cancer has occurred in subjects with partial androgen insensitivity and amino acid substitutions in the DNA-binding domain. Paradoxical responses of prostate tumors to endocrine therapy have been associated with several different somatic cell mutations in the AR steroid-binding domain.

chanism by which these mutant receptors can lead to breast cancer is unknown as the function of these mutant receptors has not been characterized in a transfection system. One could postulate that these amino acid substitutions within the DNA-binding domain might lead to alternative recognition of hormone response elements such that their respective androgen specificity of transactivation might be altered.

## Prostate Cancer

Cancer of the prostate is one of the most common malignancies in men. The growth of prostatic carcinomas is sensitive to androgen and hormonal manipulation has been used for its treatment. About 75% of prostate cancers initially respond to endocrine therapy. However, more than half of the responders gradually become resistant to this therapy. Changes in tumors from an androgen-responsive to an androgen-resistant state have been explained by adaptation or clonal selection of cancer cells. Thus relapsed tumors consist primarily of androgen-independent cells. These cells contain variable levels of androgen receptor by ligand binding assays and often retain immunocytochemically detectable androgen receptor protein. These findings suggest that structural abnormalities may arise in the androgen receptors of tumor cells to alter their function.

A mutation in the androgen receptor of LNCaP cells, derived from a metastatic lesion in the lymph node of a subject with prostate cancer, provided the first evidence that such mutations might exist in prostate tumor cells (Veldscholte et al., 1992). Subsequently, our laboratory was the first to identify a somatic cell mutation in an organ-confined tumor of a subject with prostatic carcinoma (Newmark et al., 1992). The mutation G$\Rightarrow$A of codon 730 was present in approximately 50% of cells from the tumor specimen, whereas only the normal coding sequence was identified in DNA from peripheral lymphocytes of the same individual. The mutation in LNCaP cells occurs in codon 877 (thr$\Rightarrow$ala) of exon 8 and the mutation in exon 5 of our patient caused substitution of val$^{730}$$\Rightarrow$met. The AR mutation in LnCaP cells causes a paradoxical stimulatory activity in the presence of the anti-androgen, hydroxyflutamide. Recent studies have shown that this same mutation is present in the prostate tumors from other subjects suggesting that this region is hypermutable during the evolution of tumors to the metastatic form and from androgen-responsive to androgen-independent (Gaddipata et al., 1994). One subject with the AR gene mutation, thr$^{877}$$\Rightarrow$ala, in a metastatic tumor also had a second mutation, leu$^{701}$$\Rightarrow$his, in the primary tumor (Suzuki et al., 1994).

In an androgen-unresponsive tumor from another subject, a G$\Rightarrow$A transition occurred in codon 715 of the AR gene causing the substitution of met for val (Culig et al., 1993). In transfection assays, this mutation did not significantly alter transactivation by androgens such as dihydrotestosterone or mibolerone, but increased the relative ability of progesterone and the adrenal androgens, androstenedione and dehydroepiandrosterone, to induce androgen-responsive gene transcription. These findings suggest that the mutant receptor leads to a gain of function, rather than a loss. Another AR gene alteration that contracted the number of glutamine repeats from 24 in some cells to 18 in others, occurred in the tumor from a subject with a paradoxical response to flutamide therapy (Schoenberg et al., 1994).

The functional significance of this example of genetic instability in tumor cells is unknown.

Taken together, these results suggest an involvement of AR mutations in tumor progression rather than in tumor promotion. Functional characterization indicates an increase in receptor activity related to alterations in its ligand-binding properties. Whereas the majority of specimens investigated represent primary lesions of early and intermediate stages, further examination of highly malignant prostatic lesions and tumor metastases is required to determine the full extent of androgen receptor involvement in tumor progression.

## Spinal Bulbar Muscular Atrophy

An intriguing pathognomonic alteration in exon 1 is the abnormal length of the polyglutamine repeat associated with spinal and bulbar muscular atrophy (SBMA; Kennedy syndrome) (LaSpada et al., 1991). This very rare neuromuscular disorder becomes manifest in men between the ages of 30 and 40 years, and is characterized by progressive neuron degeneration and predominant proximal and bulbar muscle weakness. The appearance of gynecomastia, testicular atrophy and infertility are often associated with this syndrome and indicative of a form of mild androgen insensitivity. In all subjects with SBMA, the polyglutamine region is expanded beyond 42 residues, whereas in all other individuals the number of glutamines never exceeds 32. A possible consequence of an increased length of the polyglutamine region could be a change in the structural constraint of the N-terminal domain of AR resulting in modification of transcription initiation complexes on target genes. Conflicting reports of deficient and normal trans-activating properties of the AR protein containing an expanded polyglutamine tract with androgen-responsive reporter genes have been provided to explain the occurrence of SBMA (Trifiro et al., 1994). Resolution of this issue may reside within specific cell types (e.g. neurons) or on specific target gene response element sequences that respond differentially to the polymorphic AR. Similar alterations in GC-rich triplet repeats of the genes associated with myotonic dystrophy, fragile-X syndrome, and Huntington's disease have also been reported (Caskey et al., 1992).

## SUMMARY

Cloning of the androgen receptor gene and expression of the protein by molecular techniques have increased our understanding of its structure and function. Mutations of the receptor in subjects with androgen insensitivity and the association of mutant androgen receptors with human disease has presented additional opportunities to understand androgen-dependent pathophysiology.

## ACKNOWLEDGMENTS

The work performed in my laboratory was supported by NIH grant DK43147.

# REFERENCES

Brown TR, Chang YT, Ghirri P, Migeon CJ, Murono K, Scherer P, Zhou Z (1994): Molecular biology of human androgen insensitivity syndrome. In Bartke A (ed): "Function of Somatic Cells in the Testis." Serono Symposia, Springer-Verlag, New York, pp 411-429.

Brown TR, Migeon CJ (1987): Androgen insensitivity syndromes: paradox of phenotypic feminization with male genotype and normal testicular androgen secretion. In Cohen MP, Foa PP (eds.): "Hormone Resistance and Other Endocrine Paradoxes." New York, Springer-Verlag, pp 157-203.

Caskey CT, Pizzuti A, Fu Y-H, Fenwick RG, Nelson DL (1992): Triplet repeat mutations in human disease. Science 256:784-789.

Culig Z, Hobisch A, Cronauer MV, Cato ACB, Hittmair A, Radmayr C, Eberle J, Bartsch G, Klocker H (1993): Mutant androgen receptor detected in an advanced stage prostatic carcinoma is activated by adrenal androgens and progesterone. Mol Endocrinol 7:1541-1550.

Faber PW, van Rooij HCJ, Schipper HJ, Brinkman AO, Trapman J (1993): Two different, overlapping pathways of transcription initiation are active on the TATA-less human androgen receptor promoter. J Biol Chem 268:9296-9301.

Freedman LP (1992): Anatomy of the steroid receptor zinc finger region. Endocr Rev 13:129-145.

Gaddipati JP, McLeod DG, Heidenberg HB, Sesterhenn IA, Finger MJ, Moul JW, Srivastava S (1994): Frequent detection of codon 877 mutation in the androgen receptor gene in advanced prostate cancers. Cancer Res 54:2861-2864.

Jenster G, van der Korput HAGM, van Vroonhoven C, van der Kwast TH, Trapman J, Brinkman AO (1991): Domains of the human androgen receptor involved in steroid binding, transcriptional activation, and subcellular localization. Mol Endocrinol 5:1396-1404.

Kuiper GGJM, Faber PW, van Rooij HCJ, van der Korput JAGM, Ris-Staplers C, Klassen P, Trapman J, Brinkmann AO (1989): Structural organization of the human androgen receptor gene. J Mol Endocrinol 2:R1-R4.

LaSpada AR, Wilson EM, Lubahn DB, Harding AE, Fischbeck KH (1991): Androgen receptor gene mutations in X-linked spinal and bulbar muscular atrophy. Nature 352:77-79.

Lobaccaro J-M, Lumbroso S, Belon C, Galtier-Dereure F, Bringer J, Lesimple T, Namer M, Cutuli BF, Pujol H, Sultan C (1993): Androgen receptor gene mutation in male breast cancer. Hum Mol Genet 2:1799-1802.

Lubahn DR, Brown TR, Simental JA, Higgs HN, Migeon CJ, Wilson EM, French FS (1989): Sequence of the intron/exon junctions of the coding region of the human androgen receptor gene and identification of a point mutation in a family with complete androgen insensitivity. Proc Natl Acad Sci USA 86:9534-9538.

Lubahn DB, Joseph DR, Sar M, Tan J-A, Higgs HN, Larson RE, French FS, Wilson EM (1988): The human androgen receptor: complementary deoxyribonucleic acid cloning, sequence analysis, and gene expression in prostate. Mol Endocrinol 2:1265-1275.

McPhaul MJ, Marcelli M, Zoppi S, Griffin JE, Wilson JD (1993): Genetic basis of endocrine disease 4. The spectrum of mutations in the androgen receptor gene that causes androgen resistance. J Clin Endocrinol Metab 76:17-23.

Migeon CJ, Berkovitz GD, Brown TR (1994): Sexual differentiation and ambiguity. In Kappy MS, Blizzard RM, Migeon CJ (eds.): "The Diagnosis and Treatment of Endocrine Disorders in Childhood and Adolescence." Charles C Thomas, Springfield, IL, pp 573-715.

Mizokami A, Chang C (1994): Induction of translation by the 5'-untranslated region of human androgen receptor mRNA. J Biol Chem 269:25655-25659.

Mizokami A, Yeh S-Y, Chang C (1994): Identification of 3',5'-cyclic adenosine monophosphate response element and other cis-acting elements in the human androgen receptor gene promoter. Mol Endocrinol 8:77-88.

Murono K, Mendonca BB, Arnhold I, Rigon A, Migeon CJ, Brown TR (1995): Androgen insensitivity due to point mutations encoding amino acid substitutions in the androgen receptor steroid-binding domain. Will appear in vol. 6 of Human Mutation, in press.

Newmark JR, Hardy DO, Tonb DC, Carter BS, Epstein JI, Isaacs WB, Brown TR, Barrack ER (1992): Androgen receptor gene mutations in human prostate cancer. Proc Natl Acad Sci USA 89:6319-6323.

Pinsky L, Trifiro M , Kaufman M, Beitel LK, Mhatre A, Kazemi-Esfarjani P, Sebbaghian M, Lumbroso S, Alvardo C, Vasiliou M, Gottlieb B (1992): Androgen resistance due to mutations of the androgen receptor. Clin Invest Med 15:456-472.

Quigley CA, DeBellis A, Marschke KB, El-Awady MK, Wilson EM, French FS (1995): Androgen receptor defects: historical, clinical and molecular perspectives. Will appear in 1995, vol. 16. Endocr Rev 15: in press.

Schoenberg MP, Hakimi JM, Wang S, Bova GS, Epstein JI, Fischbeck KH, Isaacs WB, Walsh PC, Barrack ER (1994): Microsatellite mutation (CAG24 -->18) in the androgen receptor gene in human prostate cancer. Biochem Biophys Res Commun 198:74-80.

Suzuki H, Sato H, Watabe Y, Masai M, Seino S, Shimazaki J (1994): Androgen receptor gene mutations in human prostate cancer. J Steroid Biochem Molec Biol 46:759-765.

Trapman J, Brinkmann AO (1993): Mutations in the androgen receptor. Ann NY Acad Sci 684:85-93.

Trifiro MA, Kazemi-Esfaranji P, Pinsky L (1994): X-linked muscular atrophy and the androgen receptor. Trends Endocrinol Metab vol. 9:in press.

Veldscholte J, Berrevoets C, Brinkmann AO, Grootegoed JA, Mulder E (1992): Anti-androgens and the mutated androgen receptor of LNCaP cells: differential effects on binding affinity, heat shock protein interaction, and transcription activation. Biochemistry 31:2393-2399.

Wooster R, Mangion J, Eeles R, Smith S, Dowsett M, Averill D, Barrett-Lee P, Easton DF, Ponder BAJ, Stratton MR (1992): A germline mutation in the androgen receptor gene in two brothers with breast cancer and Reifenstein syndrome. Nature Genet 2:132-134.

Zhou Z-X, Sar M, Simental JA, Lane MV, Wilson EM (1994a): A ligand-dependent bipartite nuclear targeting signal in the human androgen receptor. J Biol Chem 269:13115-13123.

Zhou Z-X, Wong C-I, Sar M, Wilson EM (1994b): The androgen receptor: an overview. Rec Prog Horm Res 49:249-274.

# 6

# STEROID 5α-REDUCTASE: ONE DISORDER/TWO ENZYMES/ MANY UNSOLVED PROBLEMS

[1]Jean D. Wilson, [2]James E. Griffin, and [3]David W. Russell

[1,2]Departments of Internal Medicine and [3]Molecular Genetics
The University of Texas
Southwestern Medical Center
Dallas, Texas 75235-8857 USA

## INTRODUCTION

The first androgenic hormone characterized was androsterone, a 5α-reduced 19 carbon steroid isolated by Butenandt in 1931 from the urine of adult men; this androgen is potent in bioassay systems and was assumed to be the male hormone until Laquer and his colleagues demonstrated in 1935 that the testicular androgen is testosterone, a 19 carbon steroid with a 4,5 double-bond (Tausk, 1984). It was generally assumed thereafter that the metabolism of testosterone to androsterone served to inactivate and promote the excretion of the hormone. However, in 1968, studies in two laboratories established that the mediator of most androgen action is an intermediate in this pathway, the 5α-reduced derivative of testosterone, dihydrotestosterone (Griffin et al., 1995). It was subsequently shown that a rare autosomal recessive form of human male pseudohermaphroditism, pseudovaginal perineoscrotal hypospadias, is due to steroid 5α-reductase deficiency (Wilson et al., 1993). The 5α-reductase reaction thus plays a crucial role in male developmental biology, physiology, and pharmacology.

## CHARACTERIZATION OF STEROID 5α-REDUCTASES

5α-reductase enzyme activity in tissue extracts can be detected at two pH optima. In many androgen target tissues, such as prostate, the principal 5α-reductase activity is detected at pH 5, whereas in many nongenital tissues, activity is detected at alkaline pH (8.0). When the cDNAs for the human enzymes were cloned, the cDNA for encoding the pH 8 enzyme was cloned first, and it is now

Table 1. Comparison of Human Steroid 5α-Reductases

|                                      | Enzyme            | Enzyme            |
| ------------------------------------ | ----------------- | ----------------- |
| Chromosome Locus of the Gene         | 5 (p15)           | 2 (p23)           |
| Gene Structure                       | 5 exons, 4 introns | 5 exons, 4 introns |
| Amino Acid Sequence Homology         |                   |                   |
| pH Optima                            | 6-8.5             | 5.0               |
| Apparent Km for Testosterone         | 1-5 μM            | 01.-1 μM          |
| NADPH                                | 3-10 μM           | 3-10 μM           |
| Activity in Subjects with 5α-        |                   |                   |
| Reductase Deficiency                 | Normal            | Impaired          |

termed steroid 5α-reductase 1; the cDNA encoding the pH 5 enzyme was cloned subsequently, and it is now termed steroid 5α-reductase 2 (Russell and Wilson, 1994). The characteristics of the two enzymes are summarized in Table 1. The predicted coding sequence for enzyme 1 was normal in 22 families with steroid 5α-reductase deficiency, and mutations of the steroid 5α-reductase 2 gene are responsible for the disorder (Andersson et al., 1991; Thigpen et al., 1992; Wilson et al., 1993).

Each of the enzymes is a low abundance, hydrophobic protein with a predicted molecular weight of 28,000-29,000. The hydrophobic amino acids are uniformly distributed, suggesting that the proteins are intrinsic membrane proteins. The gene structures for the two enzymes are similar with five coding exons and four introns each. Determinants for steroid hormone binding are located on the carboxyl- and amino-terminal ends of the molecule, and determinants of NADPH binding are present in the carboxyl-terminal half of the molecule. The two enzymes have different pharmacological properties. For example, enzyme 2 is more susceptible to inhibition by the 4-azasteroid finasteride than is enzyme 1.

## STEROID 5α-REDUCTASE 2 DEFICIENCY

The cloning of the 5α-reductase 2 cDNA made it possible to define the mutations responsible for steroid 5α-reductase 2 deficiency. In an early study it was shown that deletion of the entire coding sequence for the steroid 5α-reductase 2 gene is responsible for the disorder in a tribe residing in the New Guinea Highlands (Andersson et al., 1991). In subsequent studies a variety of techniques, including PCR amplification, conformation-dependent DNA polymorphism analysis, and DNA sequencing, have been utilized for analysis of additional families with 5α-reductase deficiency (Thigpen et al., 1992; Wilson et al., 1993).

The families represent more than 20 ethnic groups; the diagnosis is made on the basis of clinical findings, pedigree analysis, endocrine criteria, and in many instances analysis of 5α-reductase activity in cultured skin fibroblasts. Coding sequence abnormalities have been documented in the vast majority of such families, and most are the consequence of point mutations that cause amino acid substitutions, splice-junction alterations, nonsense codons, or small deletions. In most of the families the mutations are homozygous, but about a third are compound heterozygotes (different mutations on the two alleles). No mutations have been detected in one family in whom the diagnosis seems clearcut on clinical and endocrine grounds. Mutations of only one allele were present in three families. We believe that the latter two groups are homozygotes and compound heterozygotes,

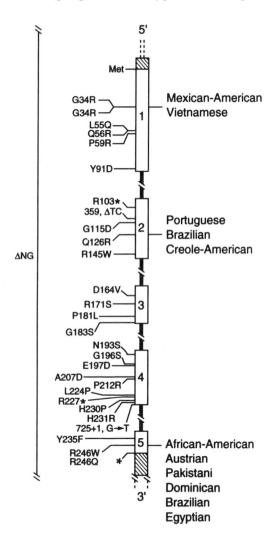

Fig. 1. Mutations of the steroid 5α-reductase 2 gene. A schematic diagram of the five coding exons of the steroid 5α-reductase 2 gene is shown in the middle. On the left are shown the location of 28 different mutations, and the sites of recurring mutations are shown on the right. (Reprinted with permission from Wilson et al., 1993.)

respectively, for mutations that map outside the exons and the immediate flanking intron sequences of the 5α-reductase 2 gene. The mutations are distributed throughout the coding sequence (Fig. 1) and disturb enzyme function by several mechanisms, including impairment of binding of testosterone or NADPH to the enzyme, formation of nonfunctional (deletions, premature termination codons, splice junction abnormalities) or unstable enzymes, and diminished amounts of the gene product [no enzyme protein detected on immunoblot analysis].

Identical mutations have been identified in different ethnic groups (Fig. 1). In some instances, this recurrence is probably due to unrecognized founder effects. In other instances, for example, the sharing of the R246W mutation among families in Egypt, Brazil, and the Dominican Republic, the phenomenon may be due to recurring new mutations.

In addition to the subjects studied in our laboratory, at least 14 additional families have been reported in the literature in whom the diagnosis appears to be clearcut (Wilson et al., 1993). Consanguinity was documented in about 40%, and homozygosity was present in about 60%; the slight discrepancy between these figures is almost certainly due to the fact that several of the homozygotes in whom consanguinity was not documented came from areas with known high coefficients of inbreeding. About 30% of all subjects are compound heterozygotes or presumed compound heterozygotes, and approximately 45% had other affected family members. The fact that the disorder is genetically heterogeneous - at least 35 mutations responsible for the defect in 48 families - is in keeping with findings in other rare autosomal recessive mutations. This feature unfortunately complicates the development of rapid molecular screening procedures for making the diagnosis.

Approximately 55% of patients have a blind-ending vagina (pseudovagina) as originally described (Table 2). However, it was early recognized that in some sibships, one affected sibling had a pseudovagina whereas the other had only a single perineal orifice, a urethra that on closer inspection provided the outlet for a urogenital sinus in which a vaginal pouch or dimple was demonstrable on the side of the urethra, and this finding is present in about a third of subjects. Of greater interest, perhaps, in about 10% of affected subjects the phallus is so large at birth

Table 2. Clinical Features of 5α-Reductase Deficiency

| | |
|---|---|
| Karyotype | 46,XY |
| Inheritance | Autosomal Recessive |
| External Phenotype | Female with some clitoromegaly at birth and variable virilization at puberty; male breasts |
| Urogenital Tract | Testes; epididymides, vasa deferentia, and seminal vesicles empty into vagina; no mullerian duct derivatives |
| Endocrinology | |
|     Testosterone | Normal male production rates and plasma levels |
|     Estradiol | Normal male production rates and plasma levels |
|     Gonadotropins | Normal to slightly elevated plasma LH levels |
| Pathogenesis | Mutation in the gene encoding steroid 5α-reductase 2 |

that affected infants are identified as males with hypospadias and raised as boys. Thus, the anatomical features range from partial to profound impairment of virilization of the external genitalia. The most consistent features in the disorder are underdevelopment of the phallus and absence/hypoplasia of the prostate. The reason for the variability in expression (even within families) is not clear. It is also worth noting that the testes have been extraabdominal - present in the inguinal canals, labia majora, or scrotum - in all subjects. Likewise, spermatogenesis is absent or profoundly impaired in all subjects in whom it has been examined; whether this abnormality is a direct effect of the mutation or the secondary consequence of incomplete testicular descent, is uncertain.

In addition to the variable impairment of virilization at birth, other clinical features are puzzling. First, although plasma dihydrotestosterone levels are low they are never undetectable and may fall within the low normal range. Circulating dihydrotestosterone in this disorder could be synthesized by residual activity of the mutant enzyme, or it could be derived from steroid 5α-reductase 1. Studies of two groups of affected individuals clearly indicate that the latter source must predominate. New Guinea subjects with a deletion of the entire coding sequence for enzyme 2 (Andersson et al., 1991) and who, as a consequence, can make no functional enzyme nevertheless have measurable plasma dihydrotestosterone (Imperato-McGinley et al., 1991). Likewise, one subject from a family with a splice junction abnormality (Thigpen et al., 1992) does not synthesize a functional steroid 5α-reductase 2; nevertheless, basal levels of plasma dihydrotestosterone in this subject were in the low normal range and rose to supraphysiological levels when he was given large amounts of testosterone propionate by injection (Price et al., 1984). These findings demonstrate that steroid 5α-reductase 1 must contribute to plasma dihydrotestosterone, recognizing that in some patients dihydrotestosterone may also be formed in small amounts from the residual activity of mutated steroid 5α-reductase 2.

Imperato-McGinley et al. (1979a, 1979b) reported that 18 of 19 individuals from the Dominican Republic cluster were initially raised as females but subsequently changed gender role behavior to male at the time of expected puberty. A similar phenomenon has been described in additional families in other parts of the world. Recognition of this phenomenon has served to reinvigorate the argument as to the relative roles of biological determinants and psychological factors in the development of gender identity. It is of interest that such behavioral change is not characteristic of mutations of the androgen receptor in which gender behavior usually conforms to the predominant anatomical development, and hence to gender assignment.

## IS TESTOSTERONE A HORMONE?

After more than a quarter of a century of research on the problem, many uncertainties exist as to the true role of dihydrotestosterone in androgen physiology. Dihydrotestosterone binds more tightly to the androgen receptor than does testosterone, largely as the result of a much slower dissociation rate of the hormone-receptor complex (Grino et al,, 1990), but the two hormones have the same Bmax of binding to the receptor. Furthermore, in *in vitro* assays involving the mouse mammary tumor virus (MMTV) promoter, testosterone at high concentration can enhance the transcription of reporter genes maximally (Deslypere et al., 1992). Consequently, it is possible that the function of 5α-reduction is to enhance a weak hormonal signal, an enhancement that is not necessary when intracellular testosterone levels are high (as might be the case in tissues such as the Wolffian ducts).

However, study of this problem is complicated by several compounding factors: (1.) Low levels of steroid 5α-reductase 1 are present in many tissues, and the activity of this enzyme is enhanced at the time of expected puberty (Thigpen et al., 1993); as mentioned above, dihydrotestosterone derived from this enzyme can always be detected in the circulation of subjects with steroid 5α-reductase 2 deficiency. (2.) Even when low levels are present in tissues, dihydrotestosterone, not testosterone, can be the major occupant of the nuclear androgen receptors in the steady state (Grino et al., 1990). (3.) Many uncertainties exist as to the nature and specificity of the androgen regulatory elements in the DNA that mediate the control of gene transcription by the hormone. Consequently, it is possible that some (or all) androgen actions absolutely require the dihydrotestosterone-receptor complex.

Resolution of this dilemma will not be possible until mice are available in which both 5α-reductase genes are knocked out (so-called double knockout mice), assuming that there is no 5α-reductase 3 that has yet to be identified, or until potent pharmacological agents are developed that will completely block both enzymes.

## CONCLUSION

In the quarter century since it was deduced that dihydrotestosterone formation may be important in androgen action, a wealth of information has accumulated about its role in physiology and pathophysiology, culminating in the cloning of cDNAs encoding two 5α-reductase enzymes and documentation that mutations in the steroid 5α-reductase 2 gene are the cause of a rare form of human intersex. Perplexing and difficult problems remain unresolved; for example, it is not clear whether dihydrotestosterone functions only as a nonspecific amplifier of androgen action or whether it exerts a unique role for some actions of the hormone.

## REFERENCES

Andersson S, Berman DM, Jenkins EP, Russell DW (1991): Deletion of steroid 5α-reductase 2 gene in male pseudohermaphroditism. Nature 354:159-161.
Deslypere JP, Young M., Wilson JD, McPhaul MJ (1992): Testosterone and 5α-dihydrotestosterone interact differently with the androgen receptor to enhance transcription of the MMTV-CAT reporter gene. Mol Cell Endocrinol 88:15-22.
Griffin JE, McPhaul MJ, Russell DW, Wilson JD (1995): The androgen resistance syndromes: Steroid 5α-reductase 2 deficiency, testicular feminization and related disorders. In Scriver CR, Beaudet AL, Sly WS, Valle D (ed): "The Metabolic and Molecular Bases of Inherited Disease." 7th ed, New York: McGraw-Hill, pp 2967-2998.

Grino PB, Griffin JE, Wilson JD (1990): Testosterone at high concentrations interacts with the human androgen receptor similarly to dihydrotestosterone. Endocrinology 126:1165-1172.

Imperato-McGinley J, Miller M, Wilson JD, Peterson RE, Shackleton C, Gajdusek DC (1991): A cluster of male pseudohermaphroditism with 5α-reductase deficiency in Papua New Guinea. Clin Endocrinol 34:293-298.

Imperato-McGinley J, Peterson RE, Gautier T, Sturla E (1979): Male pseudohermaphroditism secondary to 5α-reductase deficiency: a model for the role of androgens in both the development of the male phenotype and the evolution of a male gender identify. J Steroid Biochem 11:637-645.

Imperato-McGinley J, Peterson RE, Gautier R, Sturla E (1979): Androgens and the evolution of male-gender identity among male pseudohermaphrodites with 5α-reductase deficiency. N Engl J Med 300:1233-1237.

Price P, Wass JAH, Griffin JE, Leshin M, Savage MO, Large DM, Bu'Lock DE, Anderson DC, Wilson JD, Besser GM (1984): High dose androgen therapy in male pseudohermaphroditism due to 5α-reductase deficiency and disorders of the androgen receptor. J Clin Invest 74:1496-1508.

Russell DW, Wilson JD (1994): Steroid 5α-reductase: two genes/two enzymes. Annu Rev Biochem 63:25-61.

Tausk M (1984): Androgens and anabolic steroids. Discov Pharmacol 2:307-318.

Thigpen AE, Davis DL, Milatovich A, Mendonca BB, Imperato-McGinley J, Griffin JE, Francke U, Wilson JD, Russell DW (1992): Molecular genetics of steroid 5α-reductase 2 deficiency. J Clin Invest 90:799-809.

Thigpen AE, Silver RI, Guileyardo JM, Casey ML, McConnell JD, Russell DW (1993): Tissue distribution and ontogeny of steroid 5α-reductase. J Clin Invest 92:903-910.

Wilson JD (1982): Gonadal hormones and sexual behavior. In Besser GM, Martini L (eds): "Clinical Neuroendocrinology." New York: Academic Press, Vol 2, pp 1-29.

Wilson JD, Griffin JE, Russell DW (1993): Steroid 5α-reductase 2 deficiency. Endocr Rev 14:577-593.

# 7

# ANDROGEN-RESPONSIVE GENES

**Chawnshang Chang, Tien-Min Lin, Peiwen Hsiao,
Chingyuan Su, Joshua Riebe, Chen-Tien Chang,
and Din-Lii Lin**

**Department of Human Oncology
and Program in Endocrinology-
Reproductive Physiology
University of Wisconsin
Madison, Wisconsin 53792**

## INTRODUCTION

The molecular mechanism of the action of androgen (A) has been studied thoroughly in various androgen target organs. For example, in prostate, $5\alpha$-reductase can convert testosterone (T) into a more potent androgen, $5\alpha$-dihydrotestosterone (DHT). The action of both T and DHT are mediated through the same intracellular protein, the androgen receptor (AR) (Chang, 1988a,b), which belongs to the steroid hormone receptor superfamily. The A-AR complex can either induce or suppress the androgen-responsive genes, via binding, to androgen-response elements (ARE) that, in general, are located in the 5' flanking region of androgen target genes. So far more than 30 androgen target genes have been characterized, and many of these genes are induced by androgens. In addition, androgens also repress the expression of several other target genes (Table 1). Among these androgen target genes, we have chosen glutathione-S-transferase (GST), FAR17a, interleukin-4, interleukin-5, $\gamma$-interferon, and sex-limiting protein, for further discussion.

## DIFFERENTIAL REGULATION OF GST Yb1 mRNA LEVELS IN PROSTATE, LIVER AND BRAIN BY ANDROGEN

Northern blot analysis of GST YB1 mRNA levels in various rat tissues has suggested that androgen may differentially regulate the expression of GST Yb1 gene. In the ventral prostate, GST Yb1 mRNA levels increased rapidly after castration, reached a peak of 6-fold as compared to the normal on the third day, and then declined to 50% of the normal on the tenth day after castration. On the other hand, in the liver, GST Yb1 mRNA reached 30% of the normal control one day after castration, but recovered gradually to normal by the fifth day post-castration. No

Table 1. Androgen-Repressed Genes

| Target genes | Function | Tissue distribution | Reference |
|---|---|---|---|
| PAcP | Prostate-specific marker | Prostate | Henttu et al. (1993) |
| AR | Development of male sex accessory organ | Ubiquitous | Grossmann et al. (1994) |
| TR2 | Orphan receptor involved in Vit A & D pathways | Ubiquitous | Chang et al. (1988c) |
| GST Yb1 | Multiple function enzyme, detoxification enzyme | Ubiquitous | Chang et al. (1987) |
| Cytochrome p450 | Cytochrome | Ubiquitous | Henderson et al. (1991) |
| SMP2 | Liver-specific gene | Rat liver | Song et al. (1990) |
| pSvr-1 | Unknown | Rat seminal vesicles | Izawa et al. (1990) |
| TRPM-2 | Apoptosis | Rat ventral prostate | Buttyan et al. (1989) |
| Glycoprotein hormone LH α subunit | Feedback mechanism of androgen | Pituitary gonadotropin | Clay et al. (1993) |
| Interleukin-4 | Cytokine | Anti-CD3 activated T cells | Araneo et al. (1991) |
| Interleukin-5 | Cytokine | Anti-CD3 activated T cells | Araneo et al. (1991) |
| γ-interferon | Cytokine | Anti-CD3 activated T cells | Araneo et al. (1991) |

significant change in the GST Yb1 mRNA levels was observed in the brain (Zhang and Chang, paper in preparation). These results clearly show that androgen can either induce or repress the same gene (GST-Yb1) in different tissues. These observations make the GST-Yb1 gene a very interesting model for studying the details of androgen mechanism and a useful tool for isolating the transcriptional factors which may contribute to these different regulations (Zhang & Chang, paper in preparation).

## SELECTIVE ANDROGEN ACTION (TESTOSTERONE VERSUS DIHYDROTESTOSTERONE)

It has been known for some time that T and its 5α-reduced derivative, DHT, exert different actions in the male during both gestational and post-natal development. Nevertheless, these two androgens bind to the same AR with DHT showing higher binding affinity, and both hormones have the same $B_{max}$ of binding. To investigate different androgen action potential contributing to the preference of AR in binding to DHT, Deslypere *et al.* have demonstrated in transiently transfected Chinese hamster ovary (CHO) cells that DHT can induce the same MMTV-ARE-CAT reporter activity as 10-fold more concentrated T (Deslypere, 1991). The limited 5α-reductase activities found in CHO cells and also the apparent Kd values for the interaction of DHT and T to AR lead the authors to conclude that the different androgen potencies between DHT and T are attributed to their affinity to the AR.

However, the explanation in CHO cells may not be applicable to the case in which DHT, but not T, can reduce the amount of interleukin-4 (IL-4), IL-5 and γ-interferon (γIFN) produced from murine T-cell hybridoma after activation with anti-CD3 antibodies (Araneo et al., 1991). A close interaction between T-cell and local macrophage, which metabolizes T to DHT, is proposed as another mechanism determining how androgen regulates expression of its target gene via peripheral activation. To investigate whether any promoter cis-acting element contributes to this differential effect of DHT, versus T on IL-4 expression, we have obtained serial deletion mutants of human IL-4 promoter upstream with the CAT reporter gene (Li-Weber et al., 1992). Because the pBLCAT3 plasmid contains an unidentified ARE (our unpublished results), all human IL-4 promoter deletion mutants were reconstructed as an ARE-free pBS-CAT expression vectors. Under our experimental conditions, we failed to demonstrate any potential ARE on human IL-4 promoter region when transfected into the same murine T-cell hybridoma cells mentioned above. The species specificity of the IL-4 expression may not explain this phenomena since their promoter region were demonstrated to be highly conserved among animals. The instability of these murine T-cell hybridoma cells, as demonstrated by their inability to express a reverse transcription polymerase chain reaction (RT-PCR) detectable murine IL-4 mRNA, may have contributed to our failure in identifying the potential ARE.

Another androgen target gene, FAR17a, was isolated from golden hamster flank organ subtraction library generated between testosterone propionate-treated and nontreated animals (Seki et al., 1991). This FAR17a has been up-regulated by DHT; while T, in the presence of the 5α-reductase competitor progesterone, fails to stimulate FAR17a expression assessed from Northern dot-blot obtained from 5-day steroid-treated hamsters. To study the molecular mechanism by which DHT, but not T, stimulates this gene expression, a 1.4 kb FAR17a promoter was put in a CAT and/or luciferase reporter gene constructs (Adachi and Chang, paper in preparation).

These reporter plasmids were tested in three different cell lines, CV1, LNCaP-FGC and CHO, with specific characteristics available in each cell line. LNCaP-FGC is an AR-positive cell line, while CV1 and CHO do not express AR. CHO is a cell line without 5α-reductase. pSG5-AR was co-transfected when CV1 and CHO cells were utilized. MMTV-CAT was used as a positive control here. Results obtained from all three cell lines showed significant amounts of promoter activities; however, there was no R1881, a synthetic androgen, responsiveness. To investigate whether T and DHT make a difference in reporter gene expression and considering that R1881 is not a natural androgen, the experiments were repeated with T and DHT. The results failed to show any improvement in androgen influence on promoter activities. A longer promoter region and/or intron sequence may be needed to make the reporter-gene-containing construct become androgen-responsive, or perhaps species and/or tissue specificity in gene expression in other cell lines which better represent hamster flank organ, should be considered. Nevertheless, one may also not expect to see promoter activities regulated by DHT if this regulation is an indirect phenomenon, which is suggested by a required 5-day DHT treatment, to induce a significant increase in FAR17a transcription assessed by Northern blot.

In summary, although IL-4 and FAR17a can be differentially regulated by DHT (but not T) at protein and mRNA levels, respectively, the detailed mechanism at the molecular level remains unclear.

## ANDROGEN RESPONSE ELEMENTS (ARE)

Based on the cloning and sequence analysis of all known androgen-responsive genes, we may be able to summarize two types of ARE (consensus vs. nonconsensus) in Table 2. The detailed molecular mechanism of interaction between AR and these two types of ARE remains unclear.

Table 2. Functional ARE Sequences in Androgen-Regulated Genes.

| Sequences | Genes | References |
|---|---|---|
| *Consensus Sequences:* | | |
| 5'-AGTACGtgaTGTTCT-3' | C3 (first intron) | Claessens et al., 1989 |
| 5'-GAAACAgccTGTTCT-3' | SLP | Adler et al., 1991 |
| 5'-AGCACTtgcTGTTCT-3' | PSA | Riegman et al., 1991 |
| 5'-ATAGCAtctTGTTCT-3' | Probasin (ARE 1) | Rennie et al., 1993 |
| 5'-AGTCCCactTGTTCT-3' | ODC | Crozat et al., 1992 |
| 5'-AGTACTtgtTGTTCT-3' | GUS (intron 9) | Lund et al., 1991 |
| 5'-AGCTCAgctTGTACT-3' | Factor IX | Crossley et al., 1992 |
| 5'-AGAACAaccTGTTGA-3' | MEP 24 | Ghyselinck et al., 1993 |
| 5'-TGAAGTtccTGTTCT-3' | MVDP | Fabre et al., 1994 |
| *Nonconsensus Sequences:* | | |
| 5'-GTAAAGTACTCCAAGAA | Probasin (ARE 2) | Rennie et al., 1993 |
| 5'-GGAACAGCAAGTGCT-3' | KLK2 | Murtha et al., 1993 |

# ANDROGEN VS. GLUCOCORTICOID-SPECIFIC GENE REGULATION

Using the AR DNA-binding domain to search for all potential ARE, Roche et al. (1992) found that all the identified AREs are similar to the consensus GRE. These results suggest that other factors may be needed to distinguish between ARE and GRE.

Sex-limited protein (Slp) is a mouse serum protein encoded by a major histocompatibility complex class III gene (Adler et al., 1991, 1992, 1993). The protein is expressed predominantly in liver and nearly exclusively in sexually mature males or testosterone-treated females. It is encoded by a gene (C4-Slp) whose hormonal dependence has been attributed to an androgen-responsive transcriptional enhancer introduced accidentally, alongside the C4-Slp promoter, in the guise of the 5' long terminal repeat of an ancient retrovirus.

Hemenway et al. (1987) first localized a hormonal regulatory element within 2 kb upstream of the Slp gene. A fragment from this region can function as an androgen-dependent enhancer in CAT transfection assay. This enhancer was found to reside within the 5' long terminal repeat (LTR) of an ancient endogenous provirus, indicating that the hormonal regulation of Slp is a retrotransposon-induced insertional mutation that has been preserved in evolution.

Slp gene can be activated by androgens but not by glucocorticoids or progestins when tested in receptor-deficient CV-1 cells with co-transfection of AR, GR, or PR. Androgen induction requires both a consensus glucocorticoid (hormone) response element and auxiliary elements also present within the 120-base-pair DNA fragment. Co-transfection assays with AR plus wild-type GR or GR-DBD (DNA binding domain), at 1:1 and 1:3 ratio, revealed that GR can bind to DNA to repress AR action by blocking AR binding, but not transactivate from the hormone-response element within the enhancer. The positive effect of androgen and the null effect of glucocorticoid may require the amino-terminal domains of the respective receptors. Furthermore, multiple nonreceptor factors may be involved in androgen specificity, with respect to both the elevation of androgen receptor activity and the inactivity of glucocorticoid receptor, since clustered base changes at any of several sites can reduce or abolish androgen induction and do not increase glucocorticoid response.

A fundamental issue in steroid hormone regulation is the question of how specific transcription can be started *in vivo* when several receptors (e.g., MR, PR, GR, AR) can bind to the same DNA sequence *in vitro*. GR is ubiquitous and abundant relative to AR. Therefore, for the androgen-specific genes, it may be as problematic to remain inactive in the presence of glucocorticoids as to express when androgens increase. Because AR response depends on sequences that can also function as GREs, an efficient specificity mechanism may be simultaneously positive for AR and null for GR, to prevent leaky GR activation, i.e., androgen-specific induction is attained by interaction of AR (directly and/or indirectly) with a variety of accessory transcription factors. When GR binds to the common receptor binding site, it can be prevented from transactivating by some components of the androgen-specific complex. To allow expression, accessory factors need only favor interaction of AR over GR. Therefore, the specific cohorts, and not the receptor binding site, may orchestrate precise hormonal response *in vivo* (Adler et al., 1992, 1993).

## REFERENCES

Adler AJ, Scheller A, Hoffman Y, Robins DM (1991): Multiple components of a complex androgen-dependent enhancer. Mol Endocrinol 5:1587-1596.

Adler AJ, Danielsen M, Robins DM (1992): Androgen-specific gene activation via a consensus glucocorticoid response element is determined by interaction with nonreceptor factors. Proc Natl Acad Sci (USA) 89:11660-11663.

Adler AJ, Scheller A, Robins DM (1993): The stringency and magnitude of androgen-specific gene activation are combinational functions of receptor and nonreceptor binding site sequences. Mole Cell Biol 13:6326-6335.

Araneo BA, Dowell T, Diegel M, Daynes RA (1991): Dihydrotestosterone exerts a depressive influence on the production of interleukin-4 (IL-4), IL-5, and gamma-interferon, but not IL-2 by activated murine T cells. Blood 78:688-699.

Buttyan R, Oljson C, Pintar J, Chang C, Bandykm, Ngp, Sawczwk I, (1988): Induction of the TKPM-2 gene in cells undergoing programmed cell death. Mol Cell Biol 9:3473-3481.

Chang C, Saltzman AG, Sorensen N, Hipakka RA, Liao S (1987): Identification of glutathione S-transferase Yb1 mRNA or the androgen-repressed mRNA by cDNA cloning and sequence analysis. J Biol Chem 262:11901-11903.

Chang C, Kokontis J (1988): Identification of a new member of steroid receptors super-family by cloning and sequence analysis. Biochem Biophys Res Commun 155:971-977.

Chang CS, Kokontis J, Liao ST (1988a): Molecular cloning of human and rat complementary DNA encoding androgen receptors. Science 240:324-326.

Chang CS, Kokontis J, Liao ST (1988b): Structural analysis of complementary DNA and amino acid sequences of human and rat androgen receptors. Proc Natl Acad Sci (USA) 85:7211-7215.

Claessens F, Celis L, Peeters B, Heyns W, Verhoeven G, Rombauts W (1989): Functional characterization of an androgen response element in the first intron of the C3(1) gene of prostatic binding protein. Biochem Biophys Res Comm 164:833-840.

Clay CM, Keri RA, Finicle AB, Heckert LL, Hamernik DL, Marschke KM, Wilson EM, French FS, Nilson JH (1993): Transcriptional repression of the glycoprotein hormone alpha subunit gene by androgen may involve direct binding of androgen receptor to the proximal promoter. J Biol Chem 268:13556-13564.

Crossley M, Ludwig M, Stowell KM, De Vos P, Olek K, Brownlee GG (1992): Recovery from hemophilia B Leyden: an androgen-responsive element in the factor IX promoter. Science 257:377-379.

Crozat A, Palvimo JJ, Julkunen M, Janne OA (1992): Comparison of androgen regulation of ornithine decarboxylase and S-adenosylmethionine decarboxylase gene expression in rodent kidney and accessory sex organs. Endocrinology 130:1131-1144.

Deslypere JP, Young M, Wilson JD, McPhaul MJ (1992): Testosterone and 5 alpha-dihydrotestosterone interact differently with the androgen receptor to enhance transcription of the MMTV-CAT reporter gene. Mol Cell Endocrinol 88:15-22.

Fabre S, Manin M, Pailhoux E, Veyssiere G, Jean C (1994): Identification of a functional androgen response element in the promoter of the gene for the androgen-regulated aldose reductase-like protein specific to the mouse vas deferens. J Biol Chem 269:5857-5864.

Ghyselinck NB, Dufaure I, Lareyre JJ, Rigaudiere N, Mattei MG (1993): Structural organization and regulation of the gene for the androgen-dependent glutathione peroxidase-like protein specific to the mouse epididymis. Mol Endocrinol 7:258-272.

Grossmann ME, Lindzey J, Kumar MV, Tindall DJ (1994): The mouse androgen receptor is suppressed by the 5'-untranslated region of the gene. Mol Endocrinol 8:448-455.

Hemenway C, Robins DM (1987): DNase I-hypersensitive sites associated with expression and hormonal regulation of mouse C4 and Slp genes. Proc Natl Acad Sci USA 84:4816-4820.

Henderson CJ, Wolf CR (1991): Evidence that the androgen receptor mediates sexual differentiation of mouse renal cytochrome P450 Expression. Biochem J 278: 499-503.

Henttu P, Vihko P (1993): Growth factor regulation of gene expression in the human prostatic carcinoma cell line LNCaP. Cancer Res 53:1051-1058.

Izawa M (1990): cDNA cloning of androgen-repressed mRNA in rat seminal vesicles: partial characterization of a cDNA clone, pSvr-1. Endocrinologia Japonica 37:233-238.

Li-Weber M, Eder A, Krafft-Czepa K, Krammer PH (1992): T cell-specific negative regulation of transcription of the human cytokine IL-4. J Immunol 148:1913-1918.

Lund SD, Gallagher PM, Wang B, Porter SC, Ganschow RE (1991): Androgen responsiveness of the murine beta-glucuronidase gene is associated with nuclease hypersensitivity, protein binding, and haplotype-specific sequence diversity within intron 9. Mol Cell Biol 11:5426-5434.

Murtha P, Tindall DJ, Young CY (1993): Androgen induction of a human prostate-specific kallikrein, hKLK2: characterization of an androgen response element in the 5' promoter region of the gene. Biochemistry 32:6459-6464.

Rennie PS, Bruchovsky N, Leco KJ, Sheppard PC, McQueen SA, Cheng H, Hamel A, Bock ME, MacDonald BS, et al., (1993): Characterization of two cis-acting DNA elements involved in the androgen regulation of the probasin gene. Mol Endocrinol 7:23-36.

Riegman PH, Vlietstra RJ, van der Korput JA, Brinkmann AO, Trapman J (1991): The promoter of the prostate-specific antigen gene contains a functional androgen responsive element. Mol Endocrinol 5:1921-1930.

Roche PJ, Hoare SA, Parker MG (1992): A concensus DNA-binding site for the androgen receptor. Mol Endocrinal 6: 2229-2235.

Seki T, Ideta R, Shibuya M, Adachi I (1991): Isolation and characterization of cDNA for an androgen-regulated mRNA in the flank organ of hamsters. J Invest Dermatol 96:926-931.

Song CS, Kim JM, Roy AK, Chatterjee B (1990): Structure and regulation of the senescence marker protein 2 gene promoter. Biochemistry 29:542-551.

## DISCUSSION: ANDROGENS AND DEVELOPMENT OF REPRODUCTIVE TISSUES
### Chairpersons: Jean Wilson, Richard Horton

**Richard Horton**: In the normal male, we have a ratio of T to DHT in plasma of about 10 to 1. If you look at apparent free steroid the ratio would be 20 to 1. My question is, could one conclude that *circulating* DHT plays little or no role on androgen physiology?

**Jean Wilson**: The question as to whether dihydrotestosterone is a hormone is an interesting one. It is not possible to study the question with steroid 5 alpha-reductase inhibitors because they do not totally block the enzyme. The ideal circumstance to study the effects of plasma DHT would be in the double knockout animal. The double knockout animals will have a total absence of steroid 5 alpha-reductase 1 and 2. We will be able to determine whether at low circulating levels DHT can act as a physiological hormone. To my knowledge there is only one circumstance in biology in which DHT is proved to be a hormone and not a local mediator and that is in the Australian phalangen, Tricowris Welpecula, in which the prostate does not contain 5 alpha-reductase, but the hormone that occupies the nuclear receptors is DHT; in that circumstance, the DHT reaches the prostate from the circulation.

**Shalender Bhasin:** In patients with relatively complete mutations of androgen receptor or 5 alpha-Reductase gene, are there differences in spermatogenesis or sperm densities?

**Jean Wilson**: Mutations of the androgen reception caused profound decreases in spermatogenesis. Mutations of 5 alpha-Reductase 2 also caused profound decreases in spermatogenesis; however, the latter subjects also have a high instance of maldescent of the testes so that it is not possible to ascertain whether the effect is primary or secondary.

**Richard Sharpe:** My first question is how important is the conformational structure of the androgen receptor? How do changes in its phosphorylation or changes of its structure alter its function? The second question is in cells which normally express the androgen receptor (not transfected cells), what is known about the role of inactivation of steroid? I ask this question because a few years ago, a student of mine did some studies, which showed that seminiferous tubules from the rat metabolized testosterone to a remarkable degree.

**Jean Wilson:** I agree that the factors that determine steady state androgen levels in tissues are of importance in androgen action. The rate limiting enzyme in many target tissues is not clear; one candidate is 17 beta-hydroxysteroid dehydrogenase 2, the enzyme that converts testosterone to androstenedione in peripheral tissues. That enzyme appears to be critical in determining the steady state level of dihydrotestosterone in some tissues.

**Terry Brown:** In response to the phosphorylation issue, all the receptors are phosphorylated. In the androgen receptor, many of the serine residues that can be phosphorylated reside within the N-terminal region which is thought to be involved in transcriptional activation. The question is whether there is one or more of these sites that are critical in phosphorylation in regulating the activity of the receptor. There is a discrepancy in the literature whether hormone binding to the androgen receptor does or does not change phosphorylation. There is the question of whether the phosphorylation in itself affects the conformation and the ability of the receptor to activate transcription. There was some thought in the past that the receptor could autophosphorylate itself or whether there are, in fact, DNA related kinases that may be involved in phosphorylation in terms of the binding of the receptor to DNA. In many of the receptors, different growth factors operate either through PKA or PKC pathways and can influence phosphorylation and activity of the receptors in the absence of ligand. If the receptors phosphorylate by growth factor, then the necessity for the presence of the ligand in certain cases to activate gene transcription is obviated.

**Robert Lustig:** Dr. Wilson, can you explain the dichotomy between the female phenotype at birth and the genital mass phenolization that occurs at puberty of patients with 5 alpha-reductase deficiency?

**Jean Wilson**: There is no patient with 5 alpha-reductase deficiency yet described who has no detectable circulating DHT. We have studied two families with mutations of 5 alpha-reductase 2 gene who do not make functional enzyme 2, and we know that subjects from those families form DHT from circulating testosterone in considerable amounts. So we deduce that that DHT in those two families has to be coming from enzyme 1. Since enzyme 1 is expressed more at the time of male puberty than during embryogenesis, it functions to form DHT either in tissues or as a source of circulating DHT to allow some virilization at the time of puberty.

**Robert Lustig:** So you would say it is an enzyme ontogeny?

**Jean Wilson:** There may be other aspects involved, but my guess is that it is an issue of the ontogeny of the enzyme.

**Jack Geller:** Dr. Wilson, I wanted to ask you about the issue of the measurement of biological activity of T versus DHT based upon binding affinity to the androgen receptor. From your studies, DHT, based on its binding affinity to the androgen receptor, is about five times as potent as T in the prostate. Is there any other way of verifying this data with a more direct biological test such as measurement of DNA responses or cell number responses in an incubation system?

**Jean Wilson**: I am putting a lot of hope on the double enzyme knockout mouse and that we will be as lucky as Berthold and be able to obtain clear-cut data from it.

**Jack Geller**: Do you think it would be impossible to do an experiment *in vitro* using finasteride as an inhibitor of DHT formation to compare T to DHT; e.g., by incubating androgen sensitive cells with T plus finasteride and DHT plus finasteride and comparing biologic effects?

**Jean Wilson:** It certainly would be possible if we were more successful than we have been to date in identifying *in vitro* systems that respond to androgen. This has been a problem in androgen physiology for 30 years, and we still do not have very good *in vitro* markers of hormone action.

**Ilpo Huhtaniemi:** We know now what effects estrogen receptor knockout has on the male phenotype, but is anything known about the effects of androgen receptor deficiency on the female phenotype?

**Jean Wilson:**  Mary Lyon performed an experiment in which she made $X^{tfm}O$ mice; in that same experiment, she made XO that carried the tfm mutation, and those animals were fertile, almost as fertile, as other XO mice.  So she concluded that the androgen receptor is not necessary for normal female reproduction.

**Wayne Taylor:**  Dr. Chang, regarding differential regulation of the glutathione transferase promoter, does this work through the androgen receptor or androgen response element?  Are the four androgen receptors associated proteins differentially expressed in the prostate and the liver?

**Chawnshang Chang:**  First, all androgen response elements were identified from androgen inducible genes.  Glutathione transferase represents the first identified androgen repressed gene but I cannot answer whether there is such androgen response element in this gene.  In terms of the androgen associated protein, we were able to find six different proteins that can be associated with androgen receptor.  We do not know whether these are tissue specific.

**Blake Neubauer:**  Dr. Wilson, you reported that finasteride is a prototypic type II 5 alpha-reductase inhibitor based upon initial rate velocity.  We have demonstrated in the LNCAP cell line which has exclusively type I 5 alpha-reductase activity, that there is potent inhibition of type I 5 alpha-reductase with finasteride.  Would you comment on the clinical efficacy of finasteride as a type I 5 alpha-reductase inhibitor?

**Jean Wilson:**  It is my belief that in the dosage that was approved by the FDA (5 mg/day), finasteride inhibits both enzymes in most peripheral tissues.  The problem is that in some tissues, in at least experimental animals, it is difficult to demonstrate inhibition of 5 alpha-Reductase type I by finasteride.

**Melissa Hines:**  Can you explain why some patients with 5 alpha-Reductase deficiency change their identity to a male at puberty and others do not?  Are these due to differences in some aspect of the defect, or differences in its expression?

**Jean Wilson:**  5 alpha-reductase deficiency has been described in about 55 families worldwide.  In those families in which individuals were assigned female gender at birth and allowed to reach adulthood without any intervention, a change in apparent gender role behavior has occurred in about 2/3 of the families and has not occurred in the other third.  It is not related to the severity of the mutation because changes in gender male behavior can occur in subjects with mild mutations or severe mutations.  What the determinant is, I do not know.  It may or may not be a coincidence that the majority of changes in gender role behavior have occurred in societies in which males have a dominant role.

**Ronald Swerdloff:**  My first question is whether we now can explain what makes the muscle tissue different from the other tissues.  Is this a differential sensitivity, is it a difference in the 5 alpha-reductase content or alterations in promoter regions or other factors?  The second question is the issue of idiopathic oligospermia and androgen receptor defects which was reported some time ago by Dr. Wilson's colleagues.  The last question deals with the issue of acquired defects in the androgen receptor; do we have an understanding of how often or whether that actually occurs?

**Jean Wilson:** The most likely obvious mechanism for an acquired mutation would either be an autoimmune phenomenon or an expansion with age of a trinucleotide repeat. Some patients with the Kennedy syndrome look in many ways as if they have an acquired androgen receptor abnormality. The issue of the idiopathic oligospermia is not yet settled.

**Terry Brown:** In collaboration with Richard Sherins, we screened about 30 patients from his clinic, with so-called idiopathic infertility. We have not detected any mutations in the androgen receptor coding region in those individuals.

**Jean Wilson:** I still do not understand androgen action in muscle, but the Dominican Republic patients have low normal levels of circulating DHT when their muscle hypertrophy occurs. Although 5 alpha-reductase cannot be demonstrated in skeletal muscles of humans, half or more of the androgen present in muscle nuclei is DHT. So I do not know what the active hormone is in muscle. It could either be T or DHT.

**F.C. Wu:** We heard from Dr. de Kretser this morning that there are different generations of Leydig cells. Immature Leydig cells tend to produce 5 alpha-reduced androgens whereas mature Leydig cells produce testosterone. To what extent could this phenomenon be explained by the ontogeny of either 5 alpha-reductase 1 or 2, and if so, could that be regulated by LH?

**Jean Wilson:** I do not know the answer to that question.

**F.C. Wu** - Which 5 alpha-reductase is expressed predominantly in Leydig cells?

**Jean Wilson:** I do not know. Does anyone here know which enzyme is expressed in Leydig cells?

**Bernard Robaire:** We have examined the presence of mRNAs for type I and type II 5 alpha-reductase throughout development in whole testes and in isolated Leydig cells from rats aged 7 to 90 days. We found that type I in the rat is expressed at a low level very early in life, comes down to a trough by day 21, goes back up and peaks when the enzyme activity peaks. The intensity of the signal is lower but still detectable in the adult. Type II is almost undetectable and we cannot see any changes with age. The primary mRNA for 5 alpha-reductase in the rat testes is type I.

**Erwin Goldberg:** We found a consensus sequence for AR in the promoter region of the human LDHC gene. We made deletion constructs of this region, and when the AR sequence is present, there is repression of promoter activity. There is no androgen receptor on germ cells, and the only place that LDHC gene is expressed is in the germ cells. Dr. Chang, can you comment on these perplexing observations?

**Chawnshang Chang:** I do not know whether this is just a simple *in vitro* data without any physiological significance.

**Erwin Goldberg:** I find it a curious association that this element is functional in a germ cell specific gene but that the androgen receptor may not be present on germ cells.

**Terry Brown:** I do not know that we really resolved the issues of whether androgen receptors are not expressed in germ cells, or have we?

**John Isaacs:** This is a question for Dr. Chang. There are laboratories which have transfected the PC-3 human prostate cancer cell line which does not express

PSA or the androgen receptor with a vector coding for androgen receptor and using a reporter construct driven by the PSA promoter region. When these transfected cells are given androgens they express the PSA driven reporter exogenous construct very nicely, but they do not express the endogenous PSA gene. Even though the androgen receptor is present, ligand is present, and in theory, the same type of promoter is present. You can drive an artificial construct, but you do not drive the endogenous one. This brings up two issues; 1) the artificiality of such transfected reporter constructs as testing response elements, and 2) how to explain such differential expression of endogenous and exogenous genes?

**Chawnshang Chang:** Actually, I do not know whether the genomic structure of PSA-CAT construct is still identical to endogenous PSA gene. A similar situation may also apply to AR. The result for AR expression in different tissue may also be different.

**John Isaacs:** Correct. You are showing that it is the same androgen receptor, so the transfection of that receptor can transactivate an exogenously introduce genetic construct that uses the PSA upstream promoter. There is also the same promoter which is part of the endogenous PSA gene and it does not drive the production of PSA off the endogenous sequences. The receptor and the ligand must not be the whole story.

**Chawnshang Chang:** We tested about 6 different strong promoters that linked to androgen receptors and transfected to the different cells including androgen insensitive PC-3 cells. AR are equally expressive in all cells we tested. But if you replace these stronger promoters with natural AR promoters, you may start to see tissue or cell-specific expression of AR. One possible explanation is AR expression may need some specific CIS-acting elements (in AR promoter) and some transacting factors (transcriptional factors) which may be tissue specific.

**Terry Brown:** Many of these genes have negative regulating sequences within the 5' region that seem to, if they are present, modify the androgen receptor activity. It is only when you isolate the response elements by themselves that you get the androgen induction.

**F. H. Schroder:** I wonder if Dr. Wilson could explain to me why in those families with congenital 5 alpha-reductase 2 deficiency who have relatively high levels of type I derived DHT, that DHT is not capable of maintaining or stimulating normal prostatic growth and function.

**Jean Wilson:** Alfred Jost showed in his studies that you cannot get virilization of the male urogenital tract after a critical window of time during development; e.g., late in embryogenesis exogenous androgens can cause growth of the phallus but not formation of the prostate. I think that the critical window of time is passed in adolescent subjects with 5 alpha-reductase deficiency. Their DHT is turned only at the time of expected puberty but it is too late to cause formation of a prostate.

# PART II:
# ANDROGEN AND
# THE PROSTATE

# 8

# OVERVIEW OF ANDROGENS ON THE NORMAL AND ABNORMAL PROSTATE

**Glenn R. Cunningham**

**Departments of Medicine and Cell Biology**
**Baylor College of Medicine and VA Medical Center**
**Houston, Texas 77030**

## INTRODUCTION

Androgen is required for both normal prostate development and initiation of most benign and malignant prostate neoplasms. The prostate presents the biologist and the clinician with several perplexing findings. Other than man, only the dog spontaneously develops benign prostatic hyperplasia. Malignant prostatic neoplasms rarely have been reported in any species other than man; however, prostate cancer is the most common non-skin cancer and the second leading cause of cancer deaths in man.

## ROLE OF ANDROGEN IN NORMAL PROSTATE

Growth of the prostate in man and in other species parallels the rise in serum testosterone which occurs at puberty (Figure 1). Castration prior to puberty prevents prostate growth as do 5α-reductase type II deficiency (Imperato-McGinley et al., 1979) and some mutations in the androgen receptor (AR) (McPhaul et al., 1993). Raijfer and Coffey (1978) demonstrated that androgen plays a critical role prior to adulthood in determining adult prostate size in rats and dogs. It is thought that androgen imprinting determines the number of stem cells which will determine prostate size (Isaacs and Coffey, 1989). A recent study suggests that some ligands other than androgen can activate the AR and androgen-responsive genes (Culig et al., 1994). The physiological and pathological importance of this observation must be clarified. Finally, Prins and colleagues (1993) reported that brief exposure of newborn male rats to estrogen permanently restricted prostatic growth and androgen sensitivity.

Stromal-epithelial interactions are very important for normal and abnormal prostate development. Cunha (1992) demonstrated convincingly that many of the effects of androgen during prostate development are mediated by the stroma. Furthermore, he and his colleagues observed stromal mediated effects in the adult. We

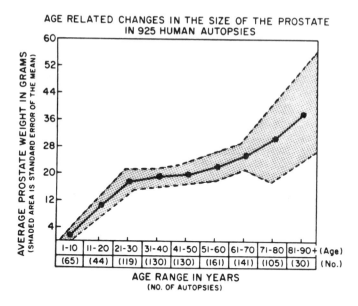

Figure 1.  Age related increase in  average weight of human male prostate.
Average  prostatic weights (mean ± standard  error  of mean) are presented
for 10- year intervals.  Prostates were obtained at autopsy from 925 samples
collected  from 5 separate studies  (Berry et al., 1984).

now know that growth factors secreted by stroma and epithelium express both
autocrine and paracrine effects (Steiner, 1993). Keratinocyte growth factor (KGF) is
a major stromal-derived growth factor which exerts paracrine effects on the
epithelium (Yan, 1992). Androgen stimulates growth of normal epithelial cells *in
vitro* only when they are co-cultured with stromal cells (Chang and Chung, 1989),
or when other growth factors are added to the media (Kusama, 1989).

Prostate size is determined in part by both androgen-mediated effects on
growth and androgen suppression of apoptotic genes (Schwartzman, 1993). The expression of many androgen-repressed genes is increased when the normal prostate is
deprived of androgen (Isaacs et al., 1992). As in animals, androgen deficiency in
young adult men results in involution of the prostate.

## ROLE OF ANDROGEN IN PATHOLOGICAL CONDITIONS

Androgen is thought to be essential, but not sufficient, for the development
of benign prostatic hyperplasia (BPH) and prostate cancer. Androgen imprinting
during development could account for differences in the prevalence of prostatic
diseases. It is of interest that circulating levels of testosterone are higher in the first
trimester of pregnancy in black women as compared with white women, whereas,
SHBG and estradiol levels are similar (Henderson et al., 1987). Mean testosterone
and free testosterone levels are higher in 20 year old black men as compared with
age-matched white men (Ross et al., 1986). Although Japanese men of this age have
similar levels of testosterone, they have lower levels of 5α-reduced metabolites (Ross

et al., 1992). Lower levels of 5α-androstanediol also have been observed in Hong Kong Chinese men (Lookingbill, 1991). Reduced 5α-reductase activity could account for differences in body hair and prostatic disease.

Testosterone is the major circulating androgen, and DHT, the 5α-reduced metabolite, is the major prostatic androgen. Studies correlating serum and prostatic concentrations of androgen or prostatic concentrations of androgen and BPH volume are limited (Osegbe and Ogunlewe, 1988; Montie and Pienta, 1994). Many cross-sectional studies have assessed sex hormones and sex hormone binding globulin levels during aging. Gray and colleagues (1991) examined a population-based group of 415 disease-free men and 1294 men who had one or more diseases which might affect circulating hormone levels. They found that SHBG increased by 1.2%/year, total testosterone decreased by 0.4%/year and estradiol and dihydrotestosterone levels were not changed significantly by aging. However, the DHT metabolites, androstanediol and androstanediol-glucuronide decreased 0.8%/year and 0.6%/year, respectively. In the prospective Physician's Health Study, a positive correlation between surgery for BPH and serum sex steroid levels was observed only for estradiol following adjustment for non-hormonal factors (Gann et al., 1995). BPH volume in 64 men undergoing prostatectomy for prostate cancer correlated positively with free testosterone, estradiol and estrone levels (Partin, 1991). These authors speculated that the age-related fall in androgen levels may reduce the number of men who develop clinical BPH.

Concentrations of DHT in normal prostate epithelium were higher than in normal stroma, and DHT levels in normal prostate epithelium and stroma were higher than in BPH epithelium and stroma (Kreig, 1993). Epithelial DHT decreased with age, but stromal DHT did not. Estradiol and estrone concentrations were higher in BPH stroma than epithelium and levels in BPH tissue were higher than those in normal tissue. These changes resulted in a higher estrogen/androgen ratio, particularly in the stroma of BPH nodules.

Attempts to correlate serum testosterone with prostate cancer have given inconsistent results. Increased mean serum testosterone and T/DHT ratios have been reported in prostate cancer patients (Ghanadian, 1979). However, Meikle and co-workers (1982) reported that familial prostate cancer patients had lower serum testosterone levels than controls. Similar testosterone levels in patients and controls have been reported in both Dutch and Japanese studies (de Jong et al., 1991). Nigerian black patients may have lower testosterone levels than age-matched Nigerian controls or American black patients, but this may be related to the severity of their disease (Ahluwalia, 1981).

## BENIGN PROSTATIC HYPERPLASIA

Benign prostatic hyperplasia has been described as having a pathological phase and a clinical phase (Isaacs and Coffey, 1989). The pathological phase probably begins before age 30 (Figure 2).

Most (>80%) men will develop microscopic BPH by age 80. The age-spe-

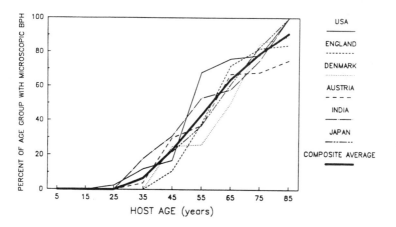

Figure 2. Age-specific prevalence of microscopic BPH in various geographic male populations. The composite average was obtained by
averaging six studies (Isaacs and Coffee, 1989).

cific prevalence of clinically diagnosed BPH correlates with age-specific autopsy
prevalence (Isaacs and Coffey, 1989; Arrighi et al., 1991). Approximately 50% of
men develop macroscopic BPH, but only half of them (approximately 25% of all
men who live to age 80) go on to develop clinical BPH which requires treatment.
The incidence in blacks and whites is thought to be similar (D'Aunoy et al., 1939).
However, the prevalence of clinical BPH in Japanese men appears to be lower
(Watanabe, 1986).

## PATHOGENESIS OF BPH

Progress has been made in our understanding of BPH, but uncertainty
remains as to the events in the development of BPH. The DHT thesis proposed that
BPH tissue contained higher concentrations of DHT than normal tissue. However,
prostatic concentrations of DHT do not appear to differ with those found in normal
prostate removed at surgery   (Walsh et al., 1983; Kreig et al., 1993).   Nuclear
concentrations of the AR may be increased (Barrack et al., 1983), but the mRNAs
for the AR and the estrogen receptor are reduced in BPH nodules as compared with
controls (Bonnet et al., 1993).   While there is evidence that estrogen can exert
stimulatory effects on the stroma (El Etreby, 1993), measurements of cytosolic and
nuclear concentrations of estradiol revealed similar concentrations in BPH glands
that were predominantly glandular and those that were predominantly stromal
(Mobbs et al., 1990).   This is important since BPH is primarily a disease of the
stroma (Rohr and Bartsch, 1980; Shapiro et al., 1992). In conclusion, the evidence
supports a role for androgen and possibly estrogen in the development and maintenance of BPH, but other factors must also be involved.

Activation of the stroma and disregulation of some growth factors has been reported by several groups (Steiner, 1993). These observations are consistent with the theory that BPH is due to a reawakening of the stroma (McNeal, 1978). BPH tissue has increased expression of bFGF and TGF-$\beta$2 (Mydlo et al., 1988; Mori et al., 1990). TGF-$\beta$1 staining is most intense in the stroma of BPH nodules (Thompson et al., 1992). Altered secretion of IGF II BPs and increased synthesis of the mRNA for IGF-II by cultured BPH stromal cells has been reported (Cohen et al., 1994).

Issacs and Coffey (1989) have proposed that BPH results from an expansion of the stem cell population. This could result from exposure to increased androgen during development of the stem cell population or it could result from changes in the stem cell population that occur after adulthood.

It also is possible that BPH results from reduced cell death and a prolonged cell life span rather than or in addition to increased mitotic activity. Using measurements of superoxide dismutase activity, the average life span of BPH epithelial cells has been estimated to exceed 2 years and that of BPH stromal cells to be more than 30 years (Tunn et al., 1989). Estradiol potentiates the effects of androstanediol or DHT in causing large hyperplastic prostates in the dog, but this combination reduces DNA synthesis, suggesting that it may enhance hyperplasia by reducing cell death (Barrack and Berry, 1987).

## WILL TESTOSTERONE TREATMENT INCREASE BPH IN NORMAL MEN?

There are several animal models which suggest that pharmacologic doses of testosterone can cause BPH, and once established, BPH can be maintained by physiologic levels of testosterone. It is well known that a form of BPH can be induced in dogs and non-human primates (Walsh and Wilson, 1976; DeKlerk et al., 1979; Karr et al., 1984). Prostatic hyperplasia in the mouse has been induced by implanting fetal urogenital sinus tissue into syngeneic mouse prostate (Sikes et al., 1990). A transgenic mouse prostate hyperplasia model has been developed using a MMTV-Int-2 construct (Tutrone et al., 1993). Nude mice also have been used as hosts for BPH xenografts (Claus et al., 1993). Interestingly, each of the mouse models of prostatic hyperplasia is sensitive to androgen ablation, but the transgenic model is not sensitive to 5$\alpha$-reductase inhibitors.

Reports of the effects of exogenous androgen on human prostate are limited. Androgen replacement of hypogonadal men does increase prostate volume as assessed by transrectal ultrasound (Sasagawa et al., 1990; Behre et al., 1994). I know of no long term evidence that androgen replacement increases the incidence of BPH over that observed in eugonadal men. Weekly administration of 200 mg of testosterone enanthate for 12 months was associated with an increase in prostate volume in 4 of 5 men (Wallace et al., 1993). However, the long-term effects of pharmacologic doses of androgen on the human prostate are unknown.

## ANDROGEN INHIBITION AND BPH

Several medical therapies have demonstrated modest effectiveness in the treatment of BPH (Oesterling, 1995). Finasteride, a 5α-reductase inhibitor that primarily inhibits the type II isoenzyme, provides effective treatment for some symptomatic patients. A 5 mg dose of finasteride reduced dihydrotestosterone levels in the prostate by 85% (Geller and Sionit, 1992). Treatment for one year increased maximum urine flow rates 1.6 ml/second and prostate volume was reduced 19% when compared with controls (Gormley et al., 1992; Stoner, 1994). GnRH agonists (Eri and Tveter, 1993) which reduce both DHT and testosterone and the anti-androgen, flutamide (Stone and Clejan, 1991), have had effects similar to finasteride on prostate volume and urine flow. Both of these approaches would be expected to affect other androgen-dependent tissues, and would not be acceptable for long-term therapy of "benign" disease.

## PROSTATE CANCER

It is estimated on the basis of autopsy data that 30% of white and black men in the United States over age 45 have latent prostate cancer (Breslow, 1977; Guileyardo et al., 1980). The prevalence of latent prostate cancer varies from 20% in Japanese to 37% in some Europeans and American blacks (Yatani et al., 1982). However, there are much larger racial differences in the incidence of clinical prostate cancer (Table 1). It is estimated that prostate cancer will cause 36% (244,000) of all new cancers in 1995 (Wingo et al., 1995). Prostate cancer is the second leading cause of cancer deaths (40,400 projected for 1995) in the United States. The 1985 SEER data indicated that the incidence of prostate cancer is 50% higher and the survival is 10% poorer in blacks (Mebane et al., 1990). We currently only have clues which may help to identify factors which cause latent prostate cancer to become clinically important.

Environmental factors must be important since in 1970 the incidence of prostate cancer in Nigerian blacks was 10.2 vs 99.4/100,000 for blacks in the United States (Ahluwalia et al., 1981). Japanese men living in Japan have a low incidence of prostate cancer, but this increases in Japanese immigrants to Hawaii (Yatani et al., 1982).

## MOLECULAR BASIS OF CARCINOMA OF THE PROSTATE

Current concepts of prostate cancer envision multiple genetic alterations as cells become premalignant, malignant, and metastatic (Sugimura, 1992). Sporadic prostate cancers frequently have cytogenetic changes in chromosomes 8p, 10q, 13q, 16q, 17p, and 18q. It is likely that tumor suppressor genes or oncogenes will be found on some of these chromosomes (Peehl, 1992; Bookstein, 1992). There is evidence that hereditary prostate cancer is caused by an autosomal dominant gene which has a frequency of 0.36% in the white population (Carter et al., 1992). Hereditary prostate cancer could account for up to 9% of prostate cancers. This gene also may be involved in sporadic prostate cancers.

Table 1

Worldwide Prostate Cancer 1988-1991
Age-Adjusted Death Rates per 100,000 Population

| Country | Prostate Cancer |
|---|---|
| Switzerland | 22.5 |
| Norway | 21.7 |
| Sweden | 20.4 |
| Iceland | 19.4 |
| Netherlands | 18.3 |
| Denmark | 18.1 |
| France | 17.3 |
| Australia | 17.2 |
| Canada | 16.9 |
| United States of America | 16.8 |
| England | 16.6 |
| Germany | 15.9 |
| Italy | 11.5 |
| Mexico | 10.6 |
| Israel | 8.6 |
| Greece | 8.1 |
| Singapore | 4.2 |
| Japan | 3.8 |
| Hong Kong | 2.6 |

Data compiled from Cancer Statistics 45:28, 1995

Pathologists utilize morphological changes in the nucleus to determine if a cell is malignant. These morphological changes are determined by changes in the nuclear matrix which represents the structural component of the nucleus. Specific nuclear matrix proteins have been identified which are unique to prostate cancer (Partin et al., 1993). Some of these proteins may provide more specific diagnostic markers.

## WILL TESTOSTERONE TREATMENT OF MEN WITHOUT KNOWN PROSTATE CARCINOMA INCREASE THE RISK OF INDUCTION OR PROGRESSION OF OCCULT CARCINOMA OF THE PROSTATE?

This is a crucial question! We do not have a definitive answer. As might be expected, some hypogonadal men have had clinical prostate cancers detected after androgen replacement was initiated (Jackson et al., 1989). The data from the case control studies which have been summarized correlating serum levels of androgens and estrogens with prostate cancer suggest that minor hormonal changes within the physiologic ranges are unlikely to increase the risk of developing prostate cancer. However, we must consider the possibility that normalization of serum testosterone in hypogonadal men, or super-physiological levels of androgen in normal men, could enable latent prostate cancer to become clinical cancers.

It may be possible to use an animal model of prostate cancer to gain information relevant to this question. Hormonally induced interstitial testicular tumors and dorsolateral lobe prostate adenocarcinoma have been observed in intact rats para-biosed to castrated rats (Brown, 1979). Prostate cancer can be induced in Noble rats by pharmacologic doses of testosterone, and this is potentiated by estrogen (Noble, 1977; Ofner, 1992). Dysplastic dorsolateral prostate lobes had increased mRNA levels of h-ras and k-ras oncogenes (Yu et al., 1993). High dose testosterone pro-pionate also potentiates development of prostate cancer in the dorso-lateral prostate of F334 intact rats pretreated for 20 weeks with 3, 2'-dimethyl-4-aminobiphenyl (Shirai et al., 1994). Transfection of ras and myc oncogenes into fetal mouse urogenital mesenchyme and epithelium has proven to be a useful model of prostate cancer (Thompson, 1989). The SV-40 large T antigen has been targeted to mouse prostate using a probasin promoter (Greenberg, personal communication). These transgenic animals have a high incidence of prostate cancer. The development of aggressive prostate cancer in mouse models is dependent upon androgen, but careful studies correlating serum and tissue levels of testosterone, DHT, estradiol and estrone have not been conducted.

Immunocompromised mice have been used to study the *in vivo* effects of androgen and stroma on tumorogenicity of LNCAP, PC-EW and PC-82 prostate cancer cell lines (Lim et al., 1993; Van Weerden et al., 1993). As anticipated, these studies demonstrate that tumorogenicity of androgen-dependent cell lines is in-hibited by androgen ablation. Of great interest is the observation that tumorogenicity of LNCAP cells is enhanced by co-inoculation with bone or prostate-derived fibroblasts (Gleave et al., 1991). It is likely that these fibroblasts have androgen receptors.

It is possible that androgens which cannot be reduced by $5\alpha$-reductase would have less effect on the prostate and still retain androgenicity in other androgen-dependent organs. Such androgens would be preferable for androgen replacement and contraception. An androgen like $7\alpha$-methyl-19-nortestosterone has been pro-posed for these reasons (Sundaram et al., 1994).

It also is possible that chemopreventive measures can be undertaken to reduce risk of prostate cancer and BPH in the presence of normal serum testosterone levels. A large multicenter trial is now underway to determine if a $5\alpha$-reductase inhibitor will delay or prevent the development of clinical BPH and prostate cancer in normal men (Brawley et al., 1994).

## ANDROGEN ABLATION IN THE MANAGEMENT OF PROSTATE CARCINOMA

The pioneering work of Huggins (1940) has provided rationale for the most effective treatment of advanced prostate carcinoma. Preliminary observations indi-cate that 10-15% of men with stage B disease can have their disease consolidated by androgen-ablative therapy prior to surgery (Schulman, 1994). Surgical castration or medical treatment with a GnRH agonist in combination with an anti-androgen is now the accepted treatment for metastatic disease (Crawford et al., 1989; Bertagna et al., 1994; Denis, 1994). These forms of androgen ablation cause apoptotic cell death of androgen-dependent cells. Unfortunately, initial responses to androgen ablation are not maintained and metastatic disease eventually becomes androgen-independent. In some cases mutations in the AR are associated with androgen-independence, but most prostate carcinomas remain AR positive (Newark et al., 1992). However, immunostaining of the AR may be more heterogeneous in advanced cancers, and this technique does not exclude mutations in the AR. Transfection of a normal AR into AR negative cell lines makes the cells more differentiated and growth rates are reduced in the presence of androgen (Yuan et al., 1993; Marcelli et al., 1995). Recent observations indicate that it is possible to induce apoptosis in both proliferating and resting androgen-insensitive cells with chemical agents (Kyprianou et al., 1994; Furuya and Isaacs, 1994). Such observations suggest therapy aimed at specific genes or mitotic events may improve therapy of advanced prostate carcinoma.

# DEVELOPMENT OF CRITERIA TO MONITOR RISK OF PROSTATE CARCINOMA IN TESTOSTERONE CLINICAL TRIALS

Treatment of aging androgen deficient men with androgen and using an androgen alone or in combination with another agent as a male contraceptive provide opportunities for treating large numbers of men with exogenous androgen. The possibilities of administering androgen at an age when BPH may first begin and at an age in which the prevalence of latent prostate cancer is increasing make it imperative that we develop and implement effective criteria for monitoring the prostate for BPH and prostate cancer.

Current techniques for assessing BPH include the history of symptoms of bladder outlet obstruction and of irritative symptoms during urination. The digital rectal examination can provide some information about prostate size, but enlargement of the transitional zone of the prostate may not be recognized on physical examination. Assessment of peak and average urine flow rates are helpful, but imprecise, and an increase in post-voiding residual urine volume is a late finding. Estimation of prostate volume, including the periurethral area with transrectal ultrasound of the prostate, is a more precise measurement. It causes some discomfort to patients and volume may not correlate well with symptoms.

Detection of small prostate cancers has been improved by the widespread use of the prostate specific antigen (PSA) assay. Its limitations, however, are important to recognize. Twenty-five percent of patients with prostate cancer have normal levels of PSA, and elevation may be seen with prostatitis and BPH. While digital rectal examination and transrectal ultrasound complement this test in detecting prostate cancer, differentiation of benign from malignant lesions requires prostate biopsy. Development of more specific and more sensitive serum markers of prostate cancer and identification of prostate cancer genes in familial prostate cancer should help to identify early stage prostate cancer.

It may be that administration of an androgen which is less stimulatory to the prostate or the combined use of androgen with a chemopreventive agent, such as a $5\alpha$-reductase inhibitor, a retinoic acid analogue, or a vitamin D analogue, will ultimately enable us to use androgen as a male contraceptive or to offer it for replacement therapy without undue concern for causing either clinical BPH or clinical prostate cancer.

# REFERENCES

Ahluwalia B, Jackson MA, Jones GW, Williams AO, Rao MS, Rajguru S (1981): Blood hormone profiles in prostate cancer patients in high-risk and low-risk populations. Cancer 48:2267-2273.

Arrighi HM, Metter EJ, Guess HA, Fozzard JL (1991): Natural history of benign prostatic hyperplasia and risk of prostatectomy. Urology Supplement 38:4-8.

Barrack ER, Berry SJ (1987): DNA synthesis in the canine prostate: Effects of androgen and estrogen treatment. Prostate 10:45-56.

Barrack ER, Bujnovszky P, Walsh PC (1983): Subcellar distribution of androgen receptors in human normal, benign hyperplastic, and malignant prostatic tissues: Characterization of nuclear salt-resistant receptors. Cancer Res 43:1107.

Behre HM, Bohmeyer J, Nieschlag E (1994): Prostate volume in testosterone-treated and untreated hypogonadal men in comparison to age-matched normal controls. Clin Endocrinol 40:341-349.

Berry SJ, Coffey DS, Walsh PC, Weing LL (1984): The development of human benign prostatic hyperplasia with age. J Urol 132:474.

Bertanga C, DeG'ery A, Hucher M, Francois JP, Zanirato J (1994): Efficacy of the combination of nilutamide plus orchidectomy in patients with metastatic prostate cancer. Br J Urol 73:396-402.

Bonnet P, Reiter E, Bruyninx M, Sente B, Dombrowicz D, de Leval J, Closset J, Hennen G (1993): Benign prostatic hyperplasia and normal prostate aging: differences in types I and II 5 alpha-reductase and steroid hormone receptor messenger ribonucleic acid (mRNA) levels, but not in insulin-like growth factor mRNA levels. J Clin Endocrinol Metab 77:1203-1208.

Bookstein R, Allred DC (1992): Recessive oncogenes. Cancer Suppl. 71:1179-1186.

Brawley OW, Ford LG, Thompson I, Perlman JA, Kramer BS (1994): 5-Alpha-reductase inhibition and prostate cancer prevention. Cancer Epidemiology, Biomarkers and Prevention 3:177-182.

Breslow N, Chan CW, Dohm G, Drury RAB, Franks LM, Geller B, Lee YS, Lundberg S, Sparke B, Sternby NH, Tulinius H (1977): Latent carcinoma of prostate at autopsy in seven areas. Int J Cancer 20:680-688.

Brown CE, Warren S, Chute RN, Ryan KJ, Todd RB (1979): Hormonally induced tumors of the reproductive system of parabiosed male rats. Cancer Res 39:3971-3976.

Carter BS, Beaty TH, Steinberg GD, Childs B, Walsh PC (1992): Mendelian inheritance of familial prostate cancer. Proc Natl Acad Sci USA 89:3367-3371.

Chang S-M, Chung LWK (1989): Interaction between prostatic fibroblast and epithelial cells in culture: Role of androgen. Endocrinology 125:2719-2727.

Claus S, Aumuller G, Tunn S, Senge T, Schultze H (1993): Influence of hormone application by subcutaneous injections or steroid-containing silastic implants on human benign hyperplastic prostate tissue transplanted into male nude mice. Prostate 22:199-215.

Cohen P, Peehl DM, Baker B, Liu F, Hintz RL, Rosenfeld RG (1994): Insulin-like growth factor axis abnormalities in prostatic stromal cells from patients with benign prostatic hyperplasia. J Clin Endocrinol Metab 79:1410-1415.

Crawford ED, Eisenberger MA, McLeod DG, Spaulding JT, Benson R, Dorr FA, Blumenstein BA, Davis MA, Goodman PJ (1989): A controlled randomized trial of leuprolide with and without flutamide in prostatic carcinoma (published erratum). N Engl J Med 321:419-424.

Culig Z, Hobisch A, Cronauer MV, Radmayr C, Trapman J, Hittmair A, Bartsch G, Klocker H (1994): Androgen receptor activation in prostatic tumor cell lines by insulin-like growth factor-4, keratinocyte growth factor, and epidermal growth factor. Cancer Res 54:5474-5478.

Cunha GR, Alarid ET, Turner T, Donjacour AA, Boutin EL, Foster BA (1992): Normal and abnormal development of the male urogenital tract. J Andrology 13:465-475.

D'Aunoy R, Schenken JR, Burns EL (1939): The relative incidence of hyperplasia of the prostate in the white and colored races in Louisiana. South Med J 32:47-56.

de Jong FH, Oishi K, Hayes RB, Boganowicz JF, Raatgever JW, van der Maas PJ, Yoshida O, Schroeder FH (1991): Peripheral hormone levels in controls and patients with prostatic cancer or benign prostatic hyperplasia; results from the Dutch-Japanese case-control study. Cancer Res 51:3445-3450.

Denis L (1994): Role of maximal androgen blockade in advanced prostate cancer. Prostate Suppl 5:17-22.

El Etreby MF (1993): Atamestane: an aromatase inhibitor for the treatment of benign prostatic hyperplasia. A short review. J Steroid Biochem Molec Biol 44(4-6):565-572.

Eri LM, Tveter KJ (1993): A prospective, placebo-controlled study of the luteinizing hormone-releasing hormone agonist leuprolide as treatment for patients with benign prostatic hyperplasia. J Urol 150:359-364.

Furuya Y, Isaacs JT (1994): Proliferation-dependent vs. independent programmed cell death of prostate cancer cells involves distinct gene regulation. Prostate 25:301-309.

Gann PH, Hennekens CH, Longcope C, Verhoek-Oftedahl W, Grodstein F, Stampfer MJ (1995): A prospective study of plasma hormone levels, nonhormonal factors, and development of benign prostatic hyperplasia. Prostate 26:40-49.

Geller L, Sionit L (1992): Castration-like effects on the human prostate of a 5 alpha-reductase inhibitor, finasteride. J Cellular Biochem Suppl 1 6H:109.

Ghanadian R, Puah CM, O'Donoghue EPN (1979): Serum testosterone and dihydrotestosterone in carcinoma of the prostate. Br J Cancer 39:696-699.

Gleave M, Hsieh JT, Gao CA, von Eschenbach AC, Chung LW (1991): Acceleration of human prostate cancer growth in vivo by factors produced by prostate and bone fibroblasts. Cancer Res 51:3753-3761.

Gormley GJ, Stoner E, Bruskewitz RC et al (1992): The effect of finasteride in men with benign prostatic hyperplasia. N Engl J Med 327: 1185-1191.

Gray A, Feldman HA, McKinlay JB, Longcope C (1991): Age, disease, and changing sex hormone levels in middle-aged men: results of the Massachusetts Male Aging Study. J Clin Endocrinol Metab 73:1016-1025.

Gulleyardo JM, Johnson WD, Welsh RA, Akazaki K, Correa P (1980): Prevalence of latent prostate carcinoma in two U.S. populations. JNCI 65:311-316.

Henderson BE, Bernstein L, Ross RK, Depue RH, Judd HL (1987): The early *in utero* estrogen and testosterone environment of blacks and whites: Potential effects on male offspring. Br J Cancer 57:216-218

Huggins C, Stevens RA (1940): The effect of castration on benign hypertrophy of the prostate in man. J Urol 43:705.

Isaacs JT, Coffey DS (1989): Etiology and disease process of benign prostatic hyperplasia. Prostate Suppl 2:33-50.

Isaacs JT, Lundmo PI, Berges R, Martikainen P, Kyprianou N, English HF (1992): Androgen regulation of programmed death of normal and malignant prostatic cells. J Androl 13:457-464.

Jackson JA, Waxman J, Spiekerman AM (1989): Prostatic complications of testosterone replacement therapy. Arch Intern Med 149:2365-2366.

Karr JP, Kim U, Resko JA, Schneider S, Chai LS, Murphy GP, Sandberg AA (1984): Induction of benign prostatic hypertrophy in baboons. Invest Urol 23:276.

Krieg M, Nass R, Tunn S (1993): Effect of aging on endogenous level of 5α-dihydrotestosterone, testosterone, estradiol and estrone in epithelium and stroma of normal and hyperplastic prostate. J Clin Endocrinol Metab 77:375-381.

Kusama Y, Enami J, Kano Y (1989): Growth and morphogenesis of mouse prostate epithelial cells in collagen gel matrix culture. Cell Biol Int Rep 13:569-575.

Kyprianou N, Bains AK, Jacobs SC (1994): Induction of apoptosis in androgen-independent human prostate cancer cells undergoing thymineless death. Prostate 25:66-75.

Lim DJ, Liu XL, Sutkowski DM, Braun EJ, Lee C, Kozlowski JM (1993): Growth of an androgen-sensitive human prostate cancer cell line, LNCaP, in nude mice. Prostate 22:109-118.

Lookingbill DP, Demers LM, Wang C, Leung A, Rittmaster RS, Santen RJ (1991): Clinical and biochemical parameters of androgen action in normal healthy Caucasian versus Chinese subjects. J Clin Endocrinol Metab 72:1242-1248.

McPhaul MJ, Marcelli M, Zoppi S, Griffin JE, Wilson JD (1993): The spectrum of mutations in the androgen receptor gene that causes androgen resistance. J Clin Endocrinol Metab 76:17-23.

Marcelli M, Haidacher SJ, Plymate SR, Birnbaum RS (1995): Altered growth and insulin-like growth factor-binding protein-3 production in PC3 prostate carcinoma cells stably transfected with a constituitively active androgen receptor complementary deoxyribonucleic acid. Endocrinology 136: 1040-1048.

McNeal JE (1978): Origin and evolution of benign prostatic enlargement. Invest Urol 15:340-345.

Mebane C, Gibbs T, Horm J (1990): Current status of prostate cancer in North American black males. J Natl Med Assn 82:782-788.

Meikle AW, Stanish WM (1982): Familial prostatic cancer risk and low testosterone. J Clin Endocrinol Metab 54:1104-1108.

Mobbs BG, Johnson IE, Liu Y (1990): Quantitation of cytosolic and nuclear estrogen and progesterone receptor in benign, untreated, and treated malignant human prostatic tissue by radioligand binding and enzyme-immunoassays. Prostate 16:235- 244.

Montie JE, Pienta KJ (1994): Review of the role of androgenic hormones in the epidemiology of benign prostatic hyperplasia and prostate cancer. Urology 43:892-899.

Mori H, Maki M, Oishi K, Jaye M, Igarashi K, Yoshida O, Hatanaka M (1990): Increased expression of genes for basic fibroblast growth factor and transforming growth factor type beta 2 in human benign prostatic hyperplasia. Prostate 16:71-80.

Mydlo JH, Michaeli J, Heston WDW, Fair WR (1988): Expression of basic fibroblast growth factor mRNA in benign prostatic hyperplasia and prostatic carcinoma. Prostate 13:241-247.

Newmark JR, Hardy DO, Tonb DC, Carter BS, Epstein JI, Isaacs WB, Brown TR, Barrack ER (1992): Androgen receptor gene mutations in human prostate cancer. Proc Natl Acad Sci USA 89:6319-6323.

Noble RL (1977): The development of prostatic adenocarcinoma in Nb rats following prolonged sex hormone administration. Cancer Res 37:1929-1933.

Oesterling JE (1995): Benign prostatic hyperplasia. N Engl J Med 332:99-109.

Ofner P, Bosland MC, Vena RL (1992): Differential effects of diethylstilbestrol and estradiol-17 beta in combination with testosterone on rat prostate lobes. Toxicol Appl Pharmacol 112:300-309.

Osegbe DN, Ogunlewe JO (1988): Androgen concentration in blacks with benign and malignant prostatic disease. J Urol 140:160-164.

Partin AW, Oesterline JE, Epstein JI, Horton R, Walsh PC (1991): Influence of age and endocrine factors on the volume of benign prostatic hyperplasia. J Urol 145:405-409.

Partin AW, Getzenberg RH, CarMichael MJ, Vindivich D, Yoo J, Epstein JI, Coffey DS (1993): Nuclear matrix protein patterns in human benign prostatic hyperplasia and prostate cancer. Cancer Res 53:744-746.

Partin AW, Coffey DS (1994): Benign and malignant prostatic neoplasms: Human studies. Recent Prog Horm Res 49:293-330.

Peehl DM (1992): Oncogenes in prostate cancer. Cancer 71:1159-1164.

Prins GS, Woodham C, Lepinske M, Birch L (1993): Effects of neonatal estrogen exposure on prostatic secretory genes and their correlation with androgen receptor expression in the separate prostate lobes of the adult rat. Endocrinology 132:2387-2398.

Raifer J, Coffey DS (1978): Sex steroid imprinting of the immature prostate: Long-term effect. Invest Urol 16:186-190.

Rohr HP, Bartsch G (1980): Human benign prostatic hyperplasia: A stromal disease? Urology 16:625-633.

Ross RK, Bernstein L, Judd H, Hanisch R, Pike M, Henderson B (1986): Serum testosterone levels in healthy young black and white men. JNCI 76:45-48.

Ross RK, Bernstein L, Lobo RA, Shimizu H, Stanczyk FZ, Pike MC, Henderson BE (1992): 5-alpha-reductase activity and risk of prostate cancer among Japanese and US white and black males. Lancet 339:887-889,

Sasagawa I, Nakada T, Kazama T, Satomi S, Terada T, Katayama T (1990): Volume change of the prostate and seminal vesicles in male hypogonadism after androgen replacement therapy. Int Urol Nephrol 22:279-284.

Schulman CC (1994): Neoadjuvant androgen blockade prior to prostatectomy: a retrospective study and critical review. Prostate Suppl 5:9-14.

Schwartzman RA, Cidlowski JA (1993): Apoptosis: The biochemistry and molecular biology of programmed cell death. Endocrine Rev 14:133-151.

Shapiro E, Becich MJ, Hartanto V, Lepor H (1992): The relative proportion of stromal and epithelial hyperplasia is related to the development of symptomatic benign prostate hyperplasia. J Urol 147:1293-1297.

Shirai T, Sano M, Imaida K, Takahashi S, Mori T, Ito N (1994): Duration dependent induction of invasive prostatic carcinomas with pharmacological dose of testosterone propionate in rats pretreated with androgen-independent carcinomas after castration. Cancer Lett 83:111-116.

Sikes RA, Thomsen S, Petrow V, Neubauer BL, Chung LW (1990): Inhibition of experimentally induced mouse prostatic hyperplasia by castration or steroid antagonist administration. Biol Reprod 43:353-362.

Steiner MS (1993): Role of peptide growth factors in the prostate: A review. Urology 42:99-110.

Stone NN, Clejan SJ (1991): Response of prostate volume, prostate-specific antigen, and testosterone to flutamide in men with benign prostatic hyperplasia. J Andrology 12:376-380.

Stoner, Elizabeth (1994): 5$\alpha$-reductase inhibitors for the treatment of benign prostatic hyperplasia. Rec Prog Horm Res 49:285-292.

Sugimura T (1992): Multistep carcinogenesis: A 1992 perspective. Science 258:603-606.

Sundaram K, Kumar N, Bardin CW (1994): 7 alpha-methyl-19-nortestosterone: an ideal androgen for replacement therapy. Recent Prog Horm Res 49:373-376.

Thompson TC, Southgate J, Kitchner G, Land H (1989):Multi-stage carcinogenesis induced by ras and myc oncogenes in a reconstituted organ. Cell 56:917-930.

Thompson TC, Truong LD, Timme TL et al (1992): Transforming growth factor $\beta$1 as a biomarker for prostate cancer. J Cell Biochem (Suppl) 16H:54-61.

Tunn S, Nass R, Ekkernkamp A, Schultze H, Krieg M (1989): Evaluation of average life span of epithelial and stromal cells of human prostate by superoxide dismutase activity. Prostate 15:263-271.

Tutrone RF Jr, Ball RA, Ornitz DM, Leder P, Richie JP (1993): Benign prostatic hyperplasia in a transgenic mouse: a new hormonally sensitive investigatory model. J Urol 149:633-639.

van Weerden WM, van Kreuningen A, Elissen NM, Vermeij M, De Jong FH, van Steenbrugge GJ, Schroeder FA (1993): Castration induced changes in morphology, androgen levels, and proliferative activity of human prostate cancer tissue grown in athymic nude mice. Prostate 23:149-164.

Walsh PC, Wilson JD (1976): The induction of prostatic hypertrophy in the dog with androstanediol. J Clin Invest 57:1093-1097.

Walsh PC, Hutchins GM, Ewing LL (1983): Tissue content of dihydrotestosterone in human prostatic hyperplasia is not supranormal. J Clin Invest:72:1772-1777.

Watanabe H (1986): Natural history of benign prostatic hypertrophy. Ultrasound Med Biol 12:567-571.

Wingo PA, Tong T, Bolden S (1995): Cancer Statistics, 1995. CA-Cancer J Clin 45:8-30.

Yatani R, Chigusa I, Akazaki K, Stemmermann GN, Welsh RA, Correa P (1982): Geographic pathology of latent prostatic carcinoma. Int J Cancer 29:611-616.

Yan G, Fukabori Y, Nikolaropoulos S, Wang F, McKeehan WL (1992): Heparin-binding keratinocyte growth factor is a candidate stromal-to-epithelial-cell andromedin. Mol Endocrinol 6:2123-2128.

Yu M, Leav BA, Leav I, Merk FB, Wolfe HJ, Ho SM (1993): Early alterations in ras protooncogene mRNA expression in testosterone and estradiol-17 beta induced prostatic dysplasia of noble rats. Lab Invest 68:33-44.

Yuan S, Trachtenberg J, Mills GB, Brown TJ, Xu F, Keating A (1993): Androgen-induced inhibition of cell proliferation in an androgen-insensitive prostate cancer cell line (PC-3) transfected with a human androgen receptor complementary DNA. Cancer Res 53:1304-1311

# 9

# ROLE OF ANDROGENS IN NORMAL AND MALIGNANT GROWTH OF THE PROSTATE

**John T. Isaacs**

**Professor of Oncology and Urology**
**The Johns Hopkins Oncology Center**
**The Johns Hopkins University School of Medicine**
**Baltimore, Maryland 21231**

Multiple malignant steps are necessary for a normal cell to give rise to a fully malignant cancer cell. The majority of prostatic cancers are derived from the secretorially active, androgen dependent, glandular epithelial cells in the prostate. With regard to prostatic carcinogenesis, it is known that androgens have at least a permissive role in this malignant process since: (1) prepubertal orchiectomy prevents the clinical development of prostatic cancer, and (2) clinically established prostatic cancers often respond to androgen ablation (Isaacs., 1994). In an intact adult male, the supply of androgens regulates a balance between cell death and proliferation of the prostatic glandular cells so that neither overgrowth nor involution of the gland normally occurs. Organ homeostasis is achieved by the balancing of two distinct processes, one responsible for initiating DNA synthesis and cell proliferation (i.e., agonistic effect of androgen), and the other responsible for inhibiting cell death (i.e., antagonistic effect), with both processes being under androgynic control (Isaacs et al., 1992). The importance of this chronic repression of prostatic glandular death by androgens is demonstrated by the dramatic increase in the death of these cells following androgen ablation induced by surgical castration. Such androgen ablation results in the activation of an energy dependent process of cellular suicide termed programmed or apoptotic cell death (Isaacs et al., 1992). This programmed cell death (PCD) process involves an epigenetic reprogramming of the cell resulting in a biochemical cascade in which the production of novel proteins leads to a chronic elevation in the intracellular free calcium ($Ca_i$) concentration (Isaacs et al., 1992; Furuya and Isaacs, 1993). Such an elevation in $Ca_i$ activates endonucleases within the cell nucleus to degrade the genomic DNA into functionless fragments. Such DNA fragmentation is then followed by cellular fragmentation into apoptotic bodies (Isaacs et al., 1992).

The observation that androgen is chronically required for prostatic carcinogenesis does not establish whether or not, besides maintaining the glandular

*Pharmacology, Biology, and Clinical Applications of Androgens*, edited by Shalender Bhasin et al.
ISBN 0-471-13320-5 © 1996 Wiley-Liss, Inc.

cells by stimulating cell proliferation and blocking cell death, androgens have additional carcinogenic abilities for prostatic glandular cells. Regardless of this uncertainty, it should be possible to reduce the risk of prostatic glandular cells undergoing both the initiation and promotional stages of carcinogenesis by lowering the androgenic influences of these cells, thus decreasing the number of prostatic glandular cells at risk and decreasing the proliferative drive on these cells. Usually such reduction in androgenic effects is achieved by reducing the blood levels of testosterone by either surgical or medical means. Unfortunately, such a systemic reduction in the circulating testosterone level has undesirable side effects including sterility, impotence, decreased libido, hot flashes, increased breast tenderness and loss of the anabolic effect of androgen upon muscle mass. Based upon these quality of life issues, systemic reduction of blood testosterone is unlikely to be very useful as an approach to chemoprevention of prostatic cancer.

Within the prostate, testosterone is rapidly converted irreversibly to $5\alpha$-dihydrotestosterone (DHT) by the membrane bound NADPH-dependent delta$^4$-3-ketosteroid $5\alpha$-oxidoreductase (i.e., $5\alpha$-reductase). A series of studies by a large variety of independent investigators has demonstrated that the major intracellular mediator of androgen action in the prostate is DHT rather than testosterone, and the $5\alpha$-reductase conversion of testosterone to DHT functions as a means of amplifying androgenic stimulation in the prostate (Isaacs, 1994). Recently a series of $5\alpha$-reductase inhibitors (e.g., finasteride, episteride) have been synthesized which can effectively inhibit the *in vivo* production of DHT and thereby lower its intraprostatic concentration without lowering serum testosterone. In experimental rodent models, treatment with such $5\alpha$-reductase inhibitors lowers prostatic tissue DHT which results in inhibition on prostatic cell proliferation and activation of prostatic cell death leading to involution of the normal prostate (Lamb et al., 1992). Such $5\alpha$-reduction inhibitor treatment does not result in a lowering of serum testosterone. Treatment with $5\alpha$-reductase inhibitors does not produce, however, as rapid or as extensive an involution of the normal rat prostate as surgical orchiectomy (Lamb et al., 1992). One explanation for this difference is that, unlike castration which reduces all androgens in the prostate (i.e., testosterone, DHT, and their metabolites) treatment with $5\alpha$-reductase inhibitors reduces DHT and its metabolites while increasing testosterone within the normal prostate. These results suggest that testosterone itself (without conversion) can have androgenic effects if the tissue levels are high enough.

Based upon these and other experimental studies of the *in vivo* response of the normal prostate, the potential of $5\alpha$-reductase inhibitors as chemopreventive agents for prostatic carcinogenesis was tested. To do this, 90 day old Lobund Wistar male rats were injected IV with 50 mg/kg of the direct acting carcinogen, N-methyl-nitroso-urea (MNU) and 1 week later implanted SQ with silastic tubing filled with testosterone propionate (TP) according to the protocol developed by Dr. Morris Pollard (Pollard et al., 1989). The TP implants raise and chronically maintain the serum testosterone by 5-6 fold and were replaced every two months. Using this protocol, 90% of these male rats developed adenocarcinomas of the male sex accessory tissue (i.e. 2/3 were of seminal vesicle origin and 1/3 of either the anterior or dorsal lobe of the prostate) within 1 year of MNU exposure. If such MNU/TP exposed rats were begun on daily treatment with a potent, product type of 5a-reductase inhibitor (i.e. at an oral dose of 25 mg/kg/day) starting three weeks after MNU exposure, only 50% of the animals develop such carcinomas of the male sex accessory glands within 1 year of MNU exposure. These results demonstrate that chronic treatment with an effective 5α-reductase inhibitor can have chemopreventive effects upon prostatic carcinogenesis.

Metastatic prostatic cancers, like the normal prostates from which they arise, are sensitive to androgenic stimulation of their growth. This is due to the presence of androgen dependent prostatic cancer cells within such metastatic patients. These cells are androgen dependent since androgen stimulates their daily rate of cell proliferation [i.e. Kp] while inhibiting their daily rate of death [i.e. Kd] (Kyprianou et al., 1990). In the presence of adequate androgen, continuous net growth of these dependent cells occurs since their rate of proliferation excesses their rate of death. In contrast, following androgen ablation, androgen dependent prostatic cancer cells stop proliferating and activate their programmed cell death [i.e. apoptosis] pathway (Kyprianou et al., 1990). This activation results in the elimination of these androgen dependent prostatic cancer cells from the patient since under these conditions their death rate value now excesses their rate of proliferation. Due to this elimination, eighty to ninety percent of all men with metastatic prostatic cancer treated with androgen ablation therapy have an initial positive response (Crawford et al., 1989). Eventually, all of these patients relapse to a state unresponsive to further anti-androgen therapy, no matter how completely given (Crawford et al., 1989). This is due to the heterogeneous presence of androgen independent prostatic cancer cells within such metastatic patients. These latter cells are androgen independent since their rate of proliferation excesses their rate of cell death even after complete androgen blockage is performed.

Since metastatic prostatic cancers are heterogeneously composed of both androgen dependent and independent cancer cells, such androgen ablation is not curative since it does not eliminate the androgen independent cancer cells. Thus, non-hormonal chemotherapeutic agents have been given to such hormonally failing patients unfortunately with very little success (Raghaven et al., 1988). This is paradoxical in the rapidly proliferating androgen-independent cancer cells *in vitro* can be induced to undergo apoptosis in response to a variety of antiproliferative chemotherapeutic agents which disrupt progression through the cell cycle demonstrating that these cells are not fundamentally resistant to activation of programmed death. In fact, proliferating cells are prone to undergo PCD in response to perturbations in the proliferative cell cycle. The process of PCD itself in such perturbed cells has been proposed to reflect a defective execution of the proliferative cell cycle. Unfortunately, however, the rate of proliferation of human prostatic carcinoma cells *in vivo* is quite low (1-2%)/days, limiting the therapeutic usefulness of treatment strategies whose activation of the PCD pathway(s) requires perturbation of the cell cycle (Berges et al., 1995). The critical issue for advanced prostate cancer treatment therefore is whether it is possible to induce PCD in proliferatively quiescent ($G_0$) cancer cells or whether these cells need to be recruited into a perturbed cell cycle.

To determine whether androgen ablation induced PCD of prostatic glandular cells involves recruitment of nonproliferating cells into a perturbed proliferative cell cycle rat ventral prostates were assessed temporally following castration for several stereotypical molecular stigmata of entry into the proliferative cell cycle (Furuya et al., 1995). Northern blot analysis was used to assess levels of transcripts from genes characteristically activated: (1) during the transition from quiescence ($G_0$) into $G_1$ of the proliferative cell cycle (cyclin $D_1$, and cyclin C); (2) during the transition from $G_1$ to S (cyclin E, cdk2, thymidine kinase, and H4 histone); and (3) during progression through S (cyclin A). While levels of each of these transcripts increased as expected in prostatic glandular cells stimulated to proliferate by administration of exogenous androgen to previously castrated rats, levels of the same transcripts decreased in prostatic glandular cells induced to undergo PCD following androgen withdrawal (Furuya et al., 1995). Likewise, androgen ablation induced PCD of prostatic glandular cells was not accompanied by retinoblastoma (Rb) protein phosphorylation characteristic of progression from $G_1$ to S. This is consistent with a decrease in the number of cells entering S cells using $^3$H-thymidine radioautography. Nuclear run on assays demonstrated that there is no increase in the prostatic rate of transcription of the c-*myc* and c-*fos* genes following castration. Northern and Western blot analysis also demonstrated that there is no increase in the prostatic p53 mRNA or protein content per cell following androgen ablation. Likewise, following castration there is no enhanced prostatic expression of the WAF1/CIP1 gene, a gene whose expression is known to be induced by either increased p53 protein levels or entrance into $G_1$ (Furuya et al., 1995). These results demonstrate that prostatic glandular cells undergo PCD in $G_0$ without recruitment into $G_1$ phase of a defective cell cycle and that an increase in p53 protein or its function are not involved in this death process (Berges et al., 1993; Furuya et al., 1995).

These combined results demonstrate that androgen ablation induced programmed death of prostatic glandular cells does not involve recruitment into a defective cell cycle. Instead, such cell death involves recruitment of proliferatively quiescent $G_0$ prostatic glandular cells into an alternative pathway of programmed (apoptotic) cell death. This programmed cell death pathway involves three phases. During the first phase, denoted as $D_1$ in the figure below, epigenetic reprogression occurs in which there is decreased mRNA expression of secretory protein coupled with induction of new gene expression [e.g. TRPM-2, $TGFb_1$, calmodulin, $\alpha$-pothymosin, etc.] and increased protein synthesis of these newly expressed genes (Isaacs et al., 1994). Such epigenetic reprogramming of the cell results in an influx of extracellular calcium ($Ca^{2+}$), thus raising the intracellular free $Ca^{2+}$-$Mg^{2+}$ dependent endonucleases present within the nucleus of these cells. This is coupled with a decrease in the nuclear histone and polyamine content which enhances the accessibility of the linker region between nucleosomes to the activated nucleases (Isaacs et al., 1994). This activation occurs during progression into the second phase of PCD, denoted as F in figure below. During the F phase, DNA fragmentation begins in the linker region, initially producing 50-300 Kb size pieces. While these large size DNA fragments themselves are lethal of the cell, they are nonetheless further degraded into nucleosomal size pieces. Following DNA fragmentation, the cell itself becomes fragmented into apoptotic bodies which are then phagocytosed by macrophages and/or neighboring epithelial cells. This third phase of PCD is denoted as $D_2$ in the figure below. Thus prostatic glandular cells have three possible options. These cells can be: (1) metabolically active (i.e.

secretory) but not undergoing either proliferation or death, (2) undergoing cell proliferation ($G_0 \rightarrow$ mitosis), or (3) undergoing cell death (i.e. $G_0 \rightarrow$ cell death). That each of these three pathways is distinct has been demonstrated based upon the differential gene expression characteristic of each of the three options (Isaacs et al., 1994).

Androgen-independent prostatic cancer cells do not activate the program of cell death following androgen ablation due to a defect in the initiation step. Even with this defect, however, these cells still retain the ability to undergo programmed cell death if initiated by non-androgen ablation methods. This has been demonstrated using a series of androgen-independent prostatic cancers established as continuously growing *in vitro* cell lines. For example, when androgen-independent, highly metastatic, anaplastic prostatic cancer cells have been treated *in vitro* with a variety of non-androgen ablative agents that inhibit thymidylate synthetase and thus induce "thymine-less death" of the cells. This "thymine-less death" requires these cells to be proliferating and the cells die during progression through the cell cycle due to inhibition of DNA synthesis while cellular production of both RNA and protein continues (Furuya and Isaacs, 1994).

Additional studies have demonstrated that programmed death of the androgen independent prostatic cancer cells can also be induced in a manner which, unlike thymine-less death, does not require entrance and progression through the cell cycle (Martikainen et al., 1991; Furuya and Isaacs, 1994; Furuya et al., 1994). Such cell proliferation independent programmed death can be induced in androgen independent prostatic cancer cells if $Ca_i$ is chronically elevated 2-3 fold for more than 12 hr by exposure to either the $Ca^{2+}$ ionophore, ionomycin (Martikainen et al., 1991), or the sesquiterpene lactone, thapsigargin (Furuya et al., 1994). Thapsigargin

## Cell Cycle

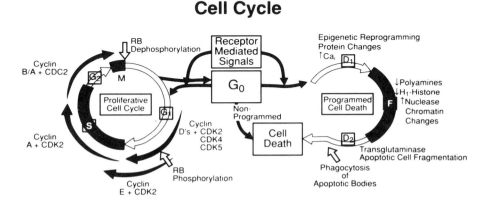

Figure 1

(TG), is a cell permeable, potent inhibitor ($IC_{50}$ = 30nM) of endoplasmic reticulum (ER) $Ca^{2+}$ pumps within androgen-independent PC cells of both rodent (AT-3) and human (TSU, PC-3, DU-145) origin (Furuya et al., 1994). TG treatment depletes the ER pool of $Ca^{2+}$ resulting within minutes in a 3-4 fold elevation in intracellular free $Ca^{2+}$ ($Ca_i$) which generates a diffusible messenger increasing permeability of the plasma membrane allowing influx of extracellular $Ca^{2+}$ sustaining elevation in $Ca_i$ for hrs. This leads to morphological changes and new protein synthesis within 6-12 hr. Within 24 hr, cells arrest in $G_0$ and irreversibly lose proliferative ability. During the next 24-48 hr, the $G_0$ cells fragment their DNA and undergo fragmentation into apoptotic bodies (Furuya et al., 1994).

Since these prostatic cancer cell lines have an exceptionally high rate of proliferation *in vitro*, this raised the issue of whether activation of PCD by TG requires cells to be inhibited during progression through the cell cycle or whether cells neither in nor attempting to enter the cycle (i.e. proliferative quiescent $G_0$ cells) can be induced to undergo PCD by TG treatment. To resolve this question, human prostatic cancer tissue obtained from prostatectomy specimens was collagenase dissociated to produce organoids which were then cultured in serum-free defined media. In these culture cells in organoids initially attach and undergo a limited number of cell divisions. During a 1-2 week culture period, cells become confluent, stop proliferating as determined by $^{14}$C-thymidine incorporated and flow cytometric analysis, and entered a proliferatively quiescent $G_0$ state determined by Ki67 immunostaining in which they remain viable for more than a month. Treatment with 500nM TG results in morphological changes within 24 hours, and cytotoxic effects within 2-4 days. In contrast, treatment of such $G_0$ cultures with 10 mM of the proliferation dependent cytotoxic agent, 5-fluorodeoxyuridine had no effect. These results demonstrate that TG can induce the PCD of $G_0$ human prostatic cancer cells without requiring them to attempt to enter the cell cycle. In conclusion, these studies have identified both a new target (i.e. ER $Ca^{2+}$ pumps) and a new agent (i.e. TG) which offer a novel approach to the elimination of androgen independent cancer cells in advanced PC without requiring these cells from entering or progression through the proliferation cell cycle.

## REFERENCES

Berges RR, Furuya Y, Jacks T, English H, Isaacs, JT (1993): Cell proliferation, DNA repair, and p53 function are not required for programmed death of prostatic glandular cells induced by androgen ablation. Proc Natl Acad Sci (USA) 90:8910-8914.

Berges RR, Vukanovic J, Epstein JI, CarMichel M, Cisek L, Johnson DE, Veltri RW, Walsh PC, Isaacs JT (1995): Implication of the cell kinetic changes during the progression of human prostatic cancer. Clinical Cancer Res 1:473-480.

Crawford ED, Eisenberger MA, McLeod DC, Spaulding J, Benson R, Dorr FA, Blumenstein BA, Davis MA, Goodman PJ (1989): A controlled randomized trial of leuprolide with and without flutamide in prostatic cancer. New Engl J Med 321:419-424.

Furuya Y, Isaacs JT (1993): Differential gene regulation during programmed death (apoptosis) versus proliferation of prostatic glandular cells induced by androgen manipulation. Endocrinol 133:2660-2666.

Furuya Y, Isaacs JT (1994): Proliferation dependent versus independent programmed cell death of prostatic cancer cells involving distinct gene regulation. Prostate 25:301-309.

Furuya Y, Lundmo P, Short AD, Gill DL, Isaacs JT (1994): The role of calcium, pH, and cell proliferation in the programmed (apoptotic) death of androgen-independent prostatic cancer cells Induced by thapsigargin. Cancer Res 54:6167-6175.

Furuya Y, Walsh JC, Lin X, Nelson WG, Isaacs JT (1995): Androgen ablation induced programmed death of prostatic glandular cells does not involve recruitment into a defective cell cycle or p53 induction. Endocrinol 136:1898-1906.

Isaacs JT, Lundmo PI, Berges R, Martikainen P, Kyprianou N, English HF (1992): Androgen regulation of programmed death of normal and malignant prostatic cells. J Andrology 13:457-464.

Isaacs JT (1994): Role of androgens in prostatic cancer. Vitamins and Hormones 49:433-502.

Isaacs JT, Furuya Y, Berges R (1994): The role of androgen in the regulation of programmed cell death/apoptosis in normal and malignant prostatic tissue. Seminar in Cancer Biol 5:391-400.

Kyprianou N, English H, Isaacs JT (1990): Programmed cell death during regression of the PC-82 human prostate cancer following androgen ablation. Cancer Res 50:3748-3752.

Lamb JC, English H, Levandoski PL, Rhodes GR, Johnson RK, Isaacs JT (1992): Prostatic involution in rats induced by a novel 5α-reductase inhibitor, SK&F 105657: role for testosterone in the androgenic response. Endocrin 130:685-694.

Martikainen P, Kyprianou N, Tucker RW, Isaacs JT (1991): Programmed death of non-proliferating androgen independent prostatic cancer cells. Cancer Res 51:4693-4700.

Pollard M, Luckert PH, Synder DL (1989): The promotional effect of testosterone on induction of prostate cancer in MNU-sensitized L-W rats. Cancer Lett 45:209-212.

Raghaven D (1988): Non-hormone chemotherapy for prostate cancer: principles of treatment and application to the testing of new drugs. Seminars in Oncology 15:371-389.

# 10

# ANDROGEN INHIBITION AND BPH

**Jack Geller**

**Department of Medical Education**
**Mercy Hospital and Medical Center**
**Adjunct Professor of Medicine**
**University of California**
**San Diego, CA 92103-2180**

## ANDROGEN INHIBITION AND BPH

The human prostate is an androgen dependent organ. Therefore, anything that blocks androgen mediated biological action will have major effects on both the normal development of the prostate, and on the subsequent changes in prostate size that commonly occur with aging.

Androgen mediated action is demonstrated in Figure 1. It depends upon the secretion of androgens by both the testes and the adrenal cortex. The major adrenal androgens are DHEA, DHEA sulfate and androstenedione. Both adrenal and testicular androgens diffuse into prostate cells where they are acted upon by enzymes. 5α-reductase converts testosterone to dihydrotestosterone within the prostate. DHT is the predominant and the most biologically potent androgen in the prostate with levels approximately 20 times higher than T.

Adrenal androgens are converted into DHT in the prostate by multiple enzymatic steps. This conversion requires an obligatory 5α-reductase step. Approximately 75% of the DHT in the prostate is derived from the testes and 25% from the adrenal cortex (Geller, 1990) Enzymes that further metabolize DHT by reduction to androstenediols and triols or by oxidation to androstenedione are also present in prostate tissue (Figure 2).

After conversion to DHT, there is binding of the DHT to the androgen receptor; the steroid-receptor complex is then translocated to the nucleus where the complex binds to an acceptor site, which then regulates genomic function, including protein synthesis and replication.

Historically inhibition of androgen has been utilized for many centuries in societies in which eunuchs played a role. This includes the Skoptzys in the Caucasus region of Russia where ritual castration was practiced after age 35. There are reports from a German pathologist that BPH in the Skoptzys was rare, if not unknown, because of this ritual castration. In addition, it is well known that the Chinese dynasties practiced castration and eunuchs played a major role in those societies. Professor Wu Jie-Ping reported (Wu, 1987) that among the last 26 surviving eunuchs from the Qing Chinese Dynasty which ended in 1911, none had

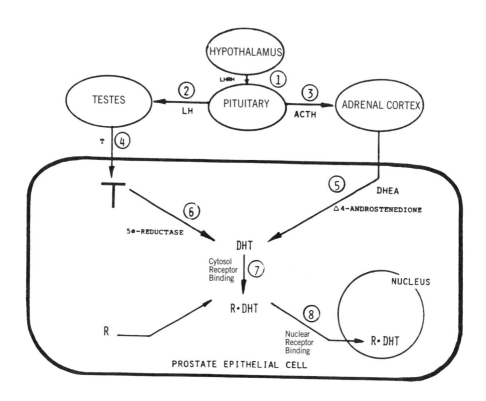

Figure 1. Multiple factors contributing to androgen mediated action. Pathway for synthesis is shown; primary loci at which various androgen withdrawal therapies block androgen action are indicated by numbers as follows: surgical castration, 4; medical castration with progestational antiandrogens, 2, 3, 4, 6, 7; androgen blockade with pure antiandrogens, 7; medical castration with gonadotropin-releasing hormone (GnRH) agonist, 1; androgen blockade with 5α-reductase inhibitors, 5 and 6; no therapy, 8. (LHRH = Luteinizing hormone-releasing hormone; LH = luteinizing hormone; ACTH = adrenocorticotropic hormone; T = testosterone; DHEA = dehydroepiandrosterone; R = androgen receptor; R . DHT = androgen receptor-steroid complex)

clinical obstructive symptoms of BPH and the prostate was either nonpalpable (3/4 of the patients) or very small (the remainder of the patients).

Probably the most careful study in the literature regarding the effects of castration or hypopituitarism on the histologic process of BPH was recorded by Dr. Robert Moore (Moore, 1944) who did post-mortem studies of the prostates of 28 patients who were castrated or hypopituitary prior to age 40 and who lived into the BPH age group. Moore could not find a single example of histologic BPH in a group of patients in whom more than 50% of the sections would have been expected to show this pathology.

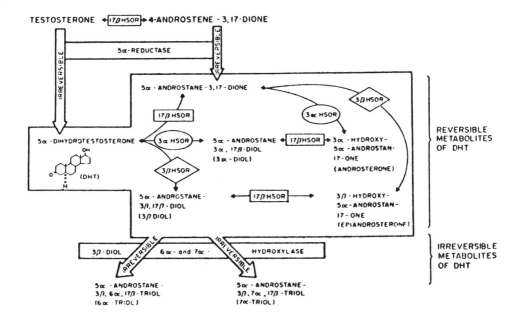

Figure 2. Overview of the pathways for androgen metabolism in the human prostate.

Since the development over the last two decades of a variety of drugs, or surgical techniques which block androgen mediated action at various sites, we have been able to study the effects of androgen inhibition on prostate size using quantitative end points, such as ultrasound or MRI. The effects of five such techniques on prostate size in patients with BPH is shown in Table 1. These techniques include surgical castration, GNRH agonists, steroidal and non-steroidal anti-androgens and a 5α-reductase inhibitor. Note that none of these techniques represents a total androgen blockade since either adrenal androgens were not inhibited, as in the case of castration and GNRH agonists, or there was an incomplete blockade of androgens with the other techniques. Although four of five androgen inhibitors block both DHT and T activity or production, the common denominator for the reduction in prostate size is inhibition of DHT, since finasteride, although the best inhibitor of DHT, increases prostatic T five-fold. Nevertheless, despite the imperfect androgen blockade induced by these five techniques, the prostate shrinks significantly three to six months following institution of each of these treatments.

None of the drugs, except for finasteride, is suitable for clinical use however, because of side effects which include either impotence, gynecomastia or gastrointestinal disturbances. Finasteride has minimal side effects with a 5-10% incidence of sexual side effects at most (Gormley et al., 1992). Only a small number of

Table 1

## EFFECT OF ANDROGEN WITHDRAWAL ON PROSTATE SIZE

| Androgen Blockers | Mean % ⇓ in Prostate Volume (Type of Measurement) | Average Time for Maximal Decrease in Size | Large Double-Bind Studies of Clinical Effects |
|---|---|---|---|
| 1. Surgical Castration | 30% (Trus) | 3-6 months | No |
| 2. Progestational Anti-Androgens (cyproterone acetate) | 30% (Trus) | 3-6 months | No |
| 3. Flutamide | 40% (Trus) | 3-6 months | No |
| 4. GNRH agonists | 25% (Trus) | 3-6 months | No |
| 5. 5α-reductase Inhibitors (Finasteride) | 20% (MRI) | 3-6 months | Yes |

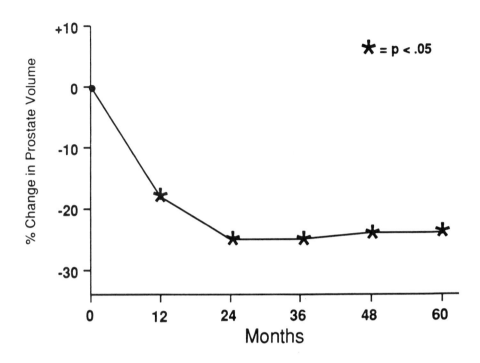

Figure 3. The percentage change in prostate volume from baseline shown on the vertical axis in relationship to time shown on the horizontal axis. P values at each year interval are indicated and an asterisk is shown for statistically significant changes ($p < 0.05$).

patients, often without controls, have been studied following treatment with surgical castration, GNRH agonists, steroidal and non-steroidal antiandrogens. In the case of finasteride, however, there have been a large number of patients studied, including placebo-controlled randomized trials (Gormley et al., 1992; Stoner, 1994). Data on five year follow-up of continuous therapy is available (Geller, 1994). These studies conclusively show that finasteride decreases prostate size, improves maximum urinary flow rates and decreases clinical symptoms of prostatism (Gormley et al., 1992; Stoner, 1994; Geller, 1994). (See Figures 3, 4, and 5).

Major support for the critical role of volume in relationship to changes in pressure-flow relationships in patients with BPH is provided by the work of Tammela et al., who have shown an inverse relationship between change in prostate size and urodynamic improvement in patients treated with finasteride in randomized, placebo-controlled, double-blind studies (Tammela et al., 1993). In human studies in which androgen mediated action is blocked, as well as in animal studies, the

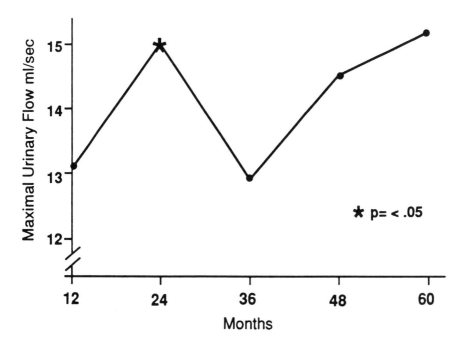

Figure 4. Changes in maximum urinary flow rate in ml/sec, shown on the vertical axis in relationship to months following therapy shown on the abscissa. Note that the baseline value begins at 12 months since no reliable pre-therapy baseline was obtained. Statistically significant changes are indicated with the p value of less than 0.05 and asterisk.

decrease in prostate size following such inhibition appears to be related to the process of apostasis. Kyprianou and Isaacs, (Isaacs et al., 1992) as well as others, have clearly shown that following castration and a decrease in plasma androgens, the testosterone repressed prostate message gene (TRPM) is activated, resulting in apostasis as an active biological process induced by this gene. Studies by Rittmaster (1994) have shown that following six to eight weeks of finasteride, transglutaminase as a marker for apostasis, was found in surgically resected prostate tissue. Rittmaster's study appears to be the first demonstration of this phenomenon in human prostate tissue following finasteride.

The fact that five year follow-up in patients treated with finasteride shows a sustained inhibition of prostatic growth suggests that a level of tissue androgen action below a certain biological threshold inhibits the ability of the prostate to

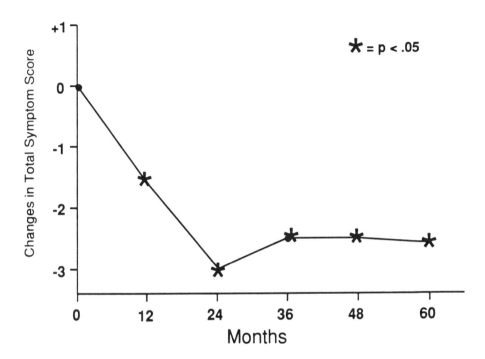

Figure 5. The average change in clinical symptom score in units (as described in Methods and Materials) on the vertical axis in relationship to time in months shown on the abscissa. Note the significant decrease in symptom score at all time points over 60 months.

grow. We don't yet have scientific information regarding the relative effects of androgen withdrawal on epithelial vs. stromal cell proliferation; this remains for the future. It does appear that in patient's with BPH, a sustained inhibition of prostate growth with androgen withdrawal is possible for at least five years.

## REFERENCES

Geller J (1990): Effect of finasteride, a 5α-reductase inhibitor on prostate tissue androgens and prostate specific antigen. Clin Endocrinol Metab 71:1552-1555.
Geller J (1994): Five-year follow-up of patients with BPH treated with finasteride. Accepted for publication Eur Urol.

Gormley JG, Stoner E, Bruskewitz RC, Imperato-McGinley J, Walsh PC, McConnell JD, Andriole GL, Geller J, Bracken BR, Tenover JS, Vaughan ED, Pappas F, Taylor A, Binkowitz B, Ng J and the Finasteride Study Group (1992): The effect of finasteride in men with benign prostatic hyperplasia. N Eng J Med 327:1185-91.

Isaacs JT, Lundmo PI, Berges R, Martikainen P, Kyprianou N, English HF (1992): Androgen regulation of programmed death of normal and malignant prostatic cells. J Androl 13:457-464.

Moore R (1944): Benign hypertrophy and carcinoma of the prostate. Surgery 16:152-167.

Rittmaster R (6/15/94): Temporal changes showing atrophy and cell death in the prostates of men treated with finasteride. The Endocrine Society Program and Abstracts, 7th Annual Meeting, Anaheim, CA, abstract #1320.

Stoner E (1994): Three-year safety and efficacy data on the use of finasteride in the treatment of benign prostatic hyperplasia. Accepted for publication in J Urol.

Tammela TLJ, Kontturi MJ (1993): Urodynamic effects of finasteride in the treatment of bladder outlet obstruction due to benign prostatic hyperplasia. J Urol 149:342-344.

Wu Jie-ping, Fang-Liu G (1987): The prostate 41-65 years post castration -an analysis of 26 eunuchs. Chin Med J 100(4):271-72.

# 11

# ANDROGEN SUPPLEMENTATION CAUSES BPH

Jon L. Pryor

Departments of Urologic Surgery and
Cell Biology/Neuroanatomy
University of Minnesota
Minneapolis, Minnesota   55455

## INTRODUCTION

Benign Prostatic Hyperplasia (BPH) is an enlargement of the prostate gland that occurs from hyperplasia of the glandular and stromal elements.  This can result in symptoms of frequency, nocturia, hesitancy, urinary tract infections, and can lead to the inability to void and possible renal failure.  BPH plagues 50% of men over the age of 50 and is thought to be responsible for one billion dollars a year of medical costs in the U.S.  Needless to say, understanding the etiology of BPH, developing new treatments for this disease, and determining preventive therapy for BPH is essential, both for cost effective medicine, and for the overall improvement of male health care.  In this section we will review the evidence for androgen supplementation in men as a cause for BPH.

## ANDROGEN DEPENDENCE OF BPH

According to Luke and Coffey, the androgen dihydrotestosterone (DHT) is of "paramount importance for growth within the prostate" (Luke and Coffey, 1994).  DHT is formed from the reduction of testosterone by 5-alpha-reductase.  Though DHT is of low plasma concentration, it is the primary androgen in the prostate and is found five-fold higher than testosterone.  In addition, DHT is known to be 1.5 to 2.5 times as potent as testosterone in bioassay systems.

It has been shown that without androgens, BPH does not develop (Huggins and Stevens, 1940).  Pre-pubertal castration has been shown to prevent the development of BPH.  In addition, genetic diseases that block androgen action have also been shown to prevent prostatic growth.

Since DHT is essential for prostatic growth and function, and without DHT, the patient does not develop BPH, elevated levels of DHT has been considered a cause of BPH.  However, the DHT levels in the peripheral prostate has been shown

*Pharmacology, Biology, and Clinical Applications of Androgens,* edited by Shalender Bhasin et al.
ISBN 0-471-13320-5 © 1996 Wiley-Liss, Inc.

to be similar in normal, compared to hyperplastic tissues, and DHT levels did not correlate with age (Walsh et.al., 1983). This suggests that other factors besides DHT, are involved in the etiology of BPH.

## ESTROGEN EFFECTS ON THE PROSTATE

Estrogens are thought to be involved in the etiology of BPH. For example, in the presence of estrogens, androstenediol causes profound BPH in young castrated dogs (Walsh and Wilson, 1971). Estrogen has also been shown to increase andro-gen receptors in the dog prostate (Moore et al., 1979). However, estradiol alone has been shown not to cause BPH (Levine et al., 1991). Estrogens can be synthesized from testosterone and androstenedione. This occurs by aromatase which has been shown to be present primarily in the prostatic stroma (Matzkin and Soloway, 1992). Interestingly, aromatase activity has been shown to increase with age (Hemsell et al., 1974).

## EVIDENCE THAT ANDROGEN SUPPLEMENTATION STIMULATES BPH

Though DHT administration to dogs causes BPH (Gloyna, 1970), there are species differences between dog and human prostate (Isaacs and Coffey, 1989) that prevents extrapolating these results to the human. There are virtually no prospec-tive, controlled, long-term studies on testosterone adminstration to humans with evaluation for the development of BPH. In a controlled, short-term study in hu-mans, testosterone was given to 13 men who had low testosterone (Tenover, 1992). These men were treated with both testosterone and a placebo (cross-over study) for a 3 month course. There was a sustained increase in the marker prostatic specific antigen (PSA) noted in the group treated with testosterone. Since PSA density (PSA serum/prostate volume) is similar between normal and hyperplastic prostate tissue (Wolff et al., 1994), the elevated PSA level correlates to an increase in prostate vol-ume or size.

## EVIDENCE THAT SUPPRESSION OF TESTOSTERONE DECREASES BPH

A.      Treatment with 5 alpha-reductase inhibitors such as finasteride (Proscar$^{TM}$) has been shown to decrease prostatic DHT by 90% (McConnel et al., 1989). Clinical trials suggest that treatment with this medication results in a decrease in prostatic size by approximately 30% (Proscar study group, 1990).

B.      Treatment with a LHRH agonist to suppress LH secretion from the pituitary and subsequent testosterone production by Leydig cells results in subse-quent decrease in DHT in the prostate. The LHRH agonist Nafarelin has been shown to decrease prostate size by 24% and result in an improvement in symptoms in 3 of 9 patients (Peters and Walsh, 1987).

C.      The antiandrogen flutamide has been shown to decrease prostatic volume by 23% after 3 months of therapy (Stone et al., 1989).

## CONCLUSIONS

The prostate needs DHT for function and growth. The primary source of DHT is from the reduction of serum testosterone. Therefore, serum testosterone is necessary for the development of BPH. Since 30% of patients show decrease in prostatic size from androgen ablation (anti-androgens, LHRH agonists, or 5 alpha-reductase inhibitors), this provides indirect evidence that testosterone has at least a permissive effect on the development of BPH. Finally, in one of the few studies where testosterone supplementation is given over a short period of time, there was a statistically significant and sustained increase in the prostatic marker PSA (Tenover, 1992) which should correlate to an increase in prostate size. Clearly, longer term studies with testosterone supplementation and determining its effect on prostatic function and size is necessary to resolve this issue.

## REFERENCES

Gloyna RE, Siiteri PK, Wilson JD (1970): Dihydrotestosterone in prostatic hypertrophy. II. The formation and content of dihydrotestosterone in the hyper-trophiccanine prostate and the effect of dihydrotestosterone on prostatic growth in the dog. J Clin Invest 49:1746-1793.

Hemsell DL, Grodin JM, Brenner PF, Siiteri PK, MacDonald PC (1974): Plasma precursors of estrogen. II. Correlation of the extent of conversion of plasma an drostenedione to estrone with age. J Clin Endocrinol Metab 38:476-479.

Huggins C, Stevens R (1940): The effect of castration on BPH in man. J Urol 43:705.

Isaacs JT, Coffey DS (1989): Etiology and disease process of benign prostatic hy-perplasia. Prostate 2:33-50.

Levine AC, Kirschenbaum A, Droller M, Gabrilove JL (1991): Effect of the addi-tion of estrogen to medical castration on prostatic size, symptoms, histology and serum prostate specific antigen in 4 men with benign prostatic hypertrophy. J Urol 146:790-793.

Luke MC, Coffey DS (1994): The male sex accessory tissues structure, androgen ac-tion, and physiology. In: Knobil E, Neill JD, eds. The physiology of repro-duction. New York, Raven Press, Ltd.

Matzkin H, Soloway MS (1992): Immunohistochemical evidence of the existence and localization of aromatase in human prostatic tissues. Prostate 21: 309-314.

McConnell JD, Wilson JD, George FW, Geller J, Walsh PC, Ewing LL, Issacs J, Stoner E (1989): An inhibitor of 5 alpha-reductase, MK-906, suppresses prostatic dihydrotestosterone in men with benign prostatic hyperplasia. J Urol 141: 299A.

Moore RJ, Gozak JM, Wilson JD (1979): Regulation of cytoplasmic dihydrotestosterone binding in dog prostate by 17βestradiol. J Clin Invest 63:351-357.

Peters CA, Walsh PC (1987): The effect of nafarelin acetate, a luteinizing-hormone-releasing hormone agonist, on benign prostatic hyperplasia. N Engl J Med 317:599-604.

The PROSCAR Study Group (Jan. 17, 1990): Treatment of benign prostatic hyperplasia (BPH) with PROSCAR, a 5 alpha-reductase (5α) inhibitor. Abstract of Workshop Conference on Androgen Therapy: Biologic and Clinical Consequences. Marco Island, FL.

Stone N, Ray PS, Smith JA et. al. (1989): A double blinded randomized controlled study of the effect of flutamide on benign prostatic hyperplasia: Clinical efficacy. J Urol 141:240A.

Tenover J S (1992): Effects of testosterone supplementation in the aging male. J. Clin Endocrinol. Metab 75:1092-1098.

Walsh PC, Hutchins GM, Ewing LL (1983): Tissue content of dihydrotestosterone in human prostatic hyperplasia is not supranormal. J Clin Invest 72:1772-1777.

Walsh PC, Wilson JD (1971): The induction of prostatic hypertrophy in the dog with androstenediol. J Clin Invest 57:1093-1097.

Wolff JM, Scholz A, Boeckmann W, Jakse G (1994): Differentiation of benign prostatic hyperplasia and prostate cancer employing prostatic specific antigen density. Eur Urol 25:295-298.

# DISCUSSION: ANDROGEN AND THE PROSTATE
## Chairpersons: Glenn Cunningham, Hermann Behre

**Stephen J. Winters:** Dr. Coffey, I was interested in your finding that in the castrated beagle, the combination of DHT and estradiol caused BPH, but the combination of T and estradiol did not. One of the differences between T and DHT is their relative binding to SHBG. Whereas most of the DHT in the circulation is SHBG bound, only about half of the T is SHBG-bound. Membrane receptors for SHBG have been described. One can invoke the hypothesis that the difference between the T and DHT result is the amount of SHBG bound androgen. Secondly, can you explain how androstenediol plus estradiol stimulates prostate growth.

**Donald Coffey:** The first part of your question deals with the relative amounts or loosely bound and free T and DHT; we absolutely have to do this on these dogs. We have done it on some of the earlier dog studies and we don't think this is the entire answer. Anybody who says that BHP is increasing growth, has not measured DNA synthesis in BPH. A BPH has less DNA synthesis in it than a normal prostate does. John Isaac can hardly find the myotonic spindle in some BPH tissue. It looks like estrogen decreases the death rate. The androgens cause an increase in the amount of DNA in that prostate. When you add estrogens to that it decreases the death rate.

**Richard Horton:** Dr. Geller, it is disappointing to see finasteride action, (prostate size) reach a plateau between 6 and 12 months of therapy. The control group was only followed for one year. Is there any data in the literature on a control group in terms of prostate changes during four or five years? The second question is, whether you have seen any change in nocturia between the control and the Finasteride treated group?

**Jack Geller:** The answer to your first question is that I really don't think there is any information available. There isn't a good control group available yet. There is a four year double-blind study ongoing in which the control group is being kept in for four years. Perhaps we will know the results in another year and a half. I think the seven year chemotherapy prevention trial may provide some of that information as well, but that study is just beginning. In response to your second question, nocturia is in the symptom score as one of the seven symptoms. I don't think it has been dissected out from the other symptoms in a large group of patients. It is simply expressed as part of the symptom score and the symptom score does improve. I think irritable symptoms, of which nocturia is a representation, are harder to improve than are the obstructive symptoms. My guess is, there is a less effect on irritative than obstructive symptoms, but I don't know of any data that particularly addresses nocturia.

**Wayne Meikle:** My comment has to do with whether androgen therapy will cause BPH. We have had the opportunity of studying about 30 men during a period of androgen withdrawal from their former treatment and then measuring prostate size by ultrasound. After about eight weeks there is about a 20% reduction in prostate size, which is then restored to the original size after another eight weeks on androgen therapy. Over a year's period of observation the glands really did not increase, consistent with your observations. At least during a period of one year, androgen therapy doesn't cause BPH or continued prostate growth. My question to this distinguished panel is, why don't you get continued growth with therapy with androgens? Why does it stop at a certain level?

**John Isaacs:** Drs. Craig Perter and Patrick C. Walsh, gave men that had BPH and were not good surgical candidates for a surgical management of BPH LHRH analogues and watched the regression of the prostate. They also biopsied these men to document that this regression was actually due to a decrease in cell content. The importance of the observation is that when they stopped giving the LHRH analogue, there was a phase of rapid prostatic regrowth. The 25% decrease in prostatic volume during LHRH analogue treatment was restored within three months after stopping the drug. In fact, most of it was restored within six weeks. Once it had reached the restored size, the prostate stopped growing. This suggests that whatever the control mechanism for size prostate, it is already in place in the BPH tissue and is not removed by regressing the gland. Thus, temporary decrease in blood androgen levels did not get rid of the root cause of the BPH overgrowth. One of the things that is interesting is the remarkably low rate of cell proliferation and death in the normal prostate. When you see a patient who has been on LHRH analogue or other medical ablation and their prostate regresses by 30-40% and then you stop giving the treatment, you see a regrowth in a period of six or eight weeks, Thus, the gland has the potential to grow rapidly if you decrease  the number of androgen dependent cells, which you have eliminated, leaving just the stem cells and transient cells. These remaining cells have the potential for very rapidly expanding, but once they expand back to the original cell number set growth ceases. Thus the total cell number is dependent upon the number of stem cell units and if you don't have more of those units, you are not going to overgrow.

**V.A. Grinvald:** I have two questions to Dr. Geller. Number one, what is your experience about the influence of long-term treatment with finasteride on potency in BPH patients? Second question is, how Finastride masks the growth of cancer in patients with BPH?

**Jack Geller:** The potency problem is difficult in the BPH age group because there is a spontaneous decrease in sexual function with aging. In our experience the majority of complaints of sexual dysfunction on Finasteride turned out not to be drug related. The quoted statistics of sexual dysfunction on Finasteride indicates that approximately 5% of patients develop impotence and erectile dysfunction. It is a small number. I think you have to be careful before you attribute sexual dysfunction to the drug; you must give patients a drug holiday and possibly re-challenge if you really want to know. Finasteride lowers the level of PSA by an average of 50% after 6-12 months. I think if you use the PSA levels in a Finasteride-treated patient at the end of the year, as your new baseline, it doesn't mask prostate cancer at all, because you simply follow that new baseline. If that baseline stays stable, what ever it may be, you should follow PSA levels thereafter on a yearly basis; if it rises approximately .75 nanograms/ml. during the year, then refer the patient for a workup for cancer. One should never treat a patient medically for BPH without first ruling out prostate cancer; that is essential. If you do that and if you follow your PSA yearly, there should not be any difficulty.

**Glenn Cunningham:** I wanted to comment on the effects of finasteride on erectile function. We have done a double blind, placebo-controlled study with finasteride in 20 men. We were unable to see any consistent effect of finasteride on a number of different NPT parameters including penile rigidity. There was no reported change in libido.

**Eberhardt Nieschlag:** I would like to come back to the introduction. Dr. Cunningham, you mentioned that the final prostate size may be determined by imprinting through androgens. My question would be, when does that imprinting take place? In order to make the answer somewhat easier for you, I would like to mention a study which we just concluded. We wanted to investigate whether puberty may be that time of "imprinting". As you know, in clinical medicine we are limited with the experiments we can do, but doctors do "experiments" with over-tall boys and treat them in early puberty with high doses of testosterone for up to two years. One might expect that if the time of puberty is the time of imprinting that, then the prostates of the treated over-tall boys may be larger in later life. About ten to 12 years after the treatment, we re-investigated about 50 of these boys and compared them with age-matched controls. Their prostates were equal in size. So puberty does not seem to be the time of that imprinting. Can you then tell us when that imprinting takes place?

**Glenn Cunningham:** I think this is an important question. The data that I was referring to was that of Coffey and Isaacs. There is one other paper that I did not mention and that is by Gail Prins; she has shown in the rat that exposure to estrogen will reduce the potential size of the prostate in adult rats. The situation in the boys is important. Although I am not sure that you answered the question in terms of BPH. It may be that you have not followed those individuals long enough. I think it would be interesting to know what would happen, lets say, to individuals who have had delayed puberty and late treatment, or individuals who have GnRH deficiency and late treatment. Do they have the same incidence of BPH and prostate cancer? I think that would be very interesting to know.

**John Isaacs:** We have such a biological experiment ongoing, it is called professional football. There are professional football players who, starting as high school students, have taken high doses of testosterone to build up their bodies for years. You would think that if androgen alone was as potent as many people believe it to be to induce these conditions, then we would be seeing precocious development of both prostate cancer and also BPH in a relatively substantial number of these potential football players who have taken incredible doses of testosterone for many years. So far, this has not been observed.

**David Handelsman:** I wondered if Dr. Coffey would comment on the question whether BPH occurs in the non-human primate. As you pointed out there are no other species apart from the dog that get BPH spontaneously, but what I wondered is, how carefully has BPH been searched for the non-human primate?

**Donald Coffey:** There are a lot of zoo studies that have been done in which aged animals are autopsied in the zoos. The bottom line is that there is some atypia, but there is no frank BPH in other species.

**Bernard Robaire:** The administration of a combined formulation of testosterone and estradiol as proposed by Ewing et al. for male contraception is becoming more attractive. The use of estradiol in women as a cardioprotective therapy is now being strongly recommended by many groups for the management of menopause. In Dr. Coffey's studies on dogs, are you investigating the changes in serum lipids as a function of therapy and changes taking place in the vessels?

**Donald Coffey:**  We are not and that is why I am appealing to people who might want to be involved in our studies to contact us.

**Bernard Robaire:**  My second question is for John Isaacs. What you showed is very nice with the increasing low doses of testosterone and the plateau that is reached with 2.5 cm. testosterone implants, but if testosterone is increased to very high doses, with doses of testosterone going up to 10, 15, 20 cm. implants, you will get a further increase in weight. Not a very big increase, but up to about 50 - 60% beyond what you find with the 2.5 cm implant. Is that additional increase in tissue weight hyperplasia or hypertrophy? Have you looked at that specific cell type?

**John Isaacs:**  Yes, and we think it is hypertrophy. If you take young rats and give them exogenous androgen, you can make not only their prostate wet weight, but also DNA content increases more than that observed in age-matched untreated animals. If you follow the natural aging process, it takes about eight to nine months for the rat prostate to grow up to its maximum cell number. If one compares the maximal cell number in the treated aging rats as the final end point, we could never, regardless of what dose of androgen or estrogen combinations was used, drive the DNA content higher.

**Bruno de Lignieres:**  I am an endocrinologist working in Necker Hospital in Paris. I would like to make a specific comment on the influence of dihydrotestosterone and estradiol, because in France we have a specific opportunity to treat patients with DHT. I have followed 94 men, 63 years old as a mean, well in the BPH age. During treatment with the transdermal DHT, they had  very high levels of circulating DHT, something like 5 ng/ml as a mean. Their testosterone serum level decreased to less than 1 ng/ml and estradiol decreased to 50% baseline. In this situation we have observed no increase in prostate size. Actually, we have measured a small but significant reduction of 12% in mean prostate volume and 7% in PSA. In this situation with very high levels of DHT and very low levels of estradiol, there is no visible stimulation of prostate in French men.

**Hermann Behre:**  Could you please add how long the mean duration of treatment was?

**Bruno de Lignieres:**  The mean duration of treatment was 2.5 years, but we have some of these patients treated for 2.5 to 10 years. A small part of this group has been on DHT for more than ten years.

**Hermann M. Behre:**  Did you measure PSA?

**Bruno de Lignieres:**  Yes. We get a mean decrease of 6.9%, which is small but is significant. Unfortunately, we don't have any control group in this situation. The reason why I don't believe it is a placebo effect is because the decrease in PSA and prostate size is directly related to DHT level. The patients having no increase or minimal increase in serum DHT don't have any decrease in PSA.

**Jon Pryor:**  I think these studies are very important, but it reminds me of some methodologic problems in the previous literature and some concerns for future studies: The importance of assessing signs and symptoms. Using the AUA (American Urological Association) Symptom Score, which has been discussed before, a subjective index that allows us to quantitate patient complaints, such as nocturia, frequency and hesitancy. This AUA Symptoms Score, assessing prostate size by transrectal ultrasound, obtaining PSA levels, and having control groups, should be important components of studies investigating the effect of testosterone on the prostate. Let us keep this in mind as we review the literature and design future studies.

**Hermann Behre:** In the study I showed you before, when we looked at the long-term testosterone treated hypogonadal patients, we had a subgroup of patients treated with transdermal scrotal testosterone. In this subgroup the serum DHT was higher than the normal range with mean levels of 3.1 nmol per liter. In these patients there was no difference in prostate volume compared to those patients treated with other testosterone preparations resulting in mean DHT levels of 1 nmol/l. The same is true for PSA. It was similar in the transdermal testosterone treated patients compared to patient treated with other testosterone preparations.

**Ronald Swerdloff:** One point that was brought out in the presentation regarding the rapid involution in prostate size in pharmacologically induced androgen deficiency and the rapid return in prostate size with androgen treatment is of great practical importance to investigators, regulatory agencies and pharmaceutical companies involved in androgen trials. Often when we do clinical studies on assessing the effects of androgen treatment, we take a group of men that are hypogonadal, wash them out from their previous androgen treatment, obtain a baseline at that time, treat the subjects with androgens and follow them for a period of time. If the washout time of eight weeks is sufficient to produce an involution of the prostate up to 20%, that means you are going to begin in a control situation of prostate involution and the androgen treatment, which really represents a return to the baseline. I think that it is an important point for our regulatory people to consider in evaluating potential adverse effects of testosterone on the prostate.

**Jean Wilson:** I wanted to make a couple of comments. One, the reason androstenediol works is that it is an efficient precursor of DHT. For that reason, I still don't understand why testosterone plus estradiol does not work, because testosterone is also a precursor of DHT. I also believe that the question about what limits prostate growth is being phrased totally the wrong way. It may be that the number of stem cells determines that a prostate will be 70 grams rather than 170 grams, but the fact remains that the prostate of the human, and the dog, and a very few other species, are almost unique in the biological kingdom in the sense that they do not have a limited growth response to androgen. In other androgen dependent tissues, like the penis for example, an explosive growth occurs at the time of puberty, and then growth ceases. No matter how much additional androgen you get, you don't get any additional growth. A similar phenomenon occurs in the prostate of most species. The unique feature of the dog and human prostates, is that growth does not cease. It slows down, but it does not cease. What is the difference between the human and dog prostates and those of other species?

**Donald Coffey:** Your points are well taken and emphasize how much we have yet to learn about steroid rejuvenation of the prostate.

**F. H. Schröder:** Dr. Behre, you presented data comparing prostates in terms of size and PSA values that were derived from a controlled group and another set that was derived from a group of patients who had androgen substitutions. I agreed with everything you showed and I agree that the sizes of the prostates you showed are similar, but you said they were comparable to normal and I don't agree with that. In your slide there were large numbers of patients in both the control groups and your substitution group that had prostatic size above 30 grams. I don't believe these prostates can be called normal. What your slide shows is that in some of these men you have been inducing or maintaining BPH. You cannot consider a 40 gram gland as a normal prostate.

**Hermann Behre:** The intention of our study was to compare prostate volume in long-term testosterone treated men to men selected randomly from the general population. We were interested if prostate volume in testosterone treated hypogo- nadal men is similar or even larger in that of control men. As a result, the prostate volume, PSA, and uroflow parameters were similar in both groups.

# 12

# IMPACT OF ETHNIC, NUTRITIONAL, AND ENVIRONMENTAL FACTORS ON PROSTATE CANCER

**Fritz H. Schröder**

**Professor and Chairman, Department of Urology**
**Erasmus University and Academic Hospital**
**P.O. Box 1738, 3000 DR**
**Rotterdam, The Netherlands**

## INTRODUCTION

Large geographical variations in incidence and mortality of prostate cancer are probably the most important epidemiological lead, indicating that environmental factors play a role in the pathogenesis of prostate cancer. The most pronounced differences as evident from Figure 1 are seen between ethnic Japanese and Chinese living in their own countries on one side, and men living in the "Western world" on the other side. The difference in incidence between these groups amounts to a factor of 10-15. Astonishingly, the incidence of prostate cancer in African-Americans again is roughly by a factor of two higher than in white Americans living under the same circumstances.

## RACIAL VARIATION OF PROSTATE CANCER INCIDENCE AND MORTALITY

Why then should these differences be explained by environmental factors, such as diet, sexual habits, drinking habits, use of vitamins, etc., and not by the obvious racial differences which exist between these geographic areas? The strongest, and also the most recognized evidence, lies in the fact that migrants seem to develop the pattern of incidence and mortality of prostate cancer of the area they move to, and do not retain the patterns of their home country, which might then be considered to be determined by the Japanese, Chinese, or African race.

*Pharmacology, Biology, and Clinical Applications of Androgens,* edited by Shalender Bhasin et al.
ISBN 0-471-13320-5 © 1996 Wiley-Liss, Inc.

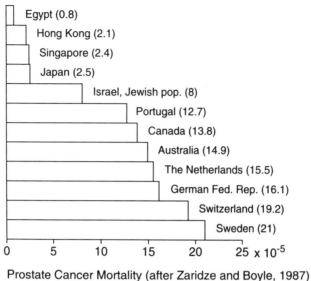

Prostate Cancer Mortality (after Zaridze and Boyle, 1987)

Figure 1. Incidence of Prostate Cancer World Wide - Geographical Variation (Adapted from Zaridze and Boyle, 1987).

## What Is the Evidence?

Akazaki and Stemmermann (1973) carried out a comparative study of latent prostate cancer in native Japanese, and Japanese who migrated to Hawaii. They found that while the prevalence of focal disease (non-invasive carcinoma) remained unchanged, the prevalence of larger cancers was higher in Hawaiian Japanese. In first generation migrants, the prevalence went to about one half of the native Hawaiians; the prevalence of such lesions increased further in second generation Hawaiian Japanese. Breslow (1977) and his associates of a WHO working group carried out an autopsy study of latent carcinoma of the prostate in 7 areas of the world, which resulted in very similar findings: the group confirmed that there is a very high prevalence of **focal** lesions, which is rather uniform in areas of the world which have a low or a high incidence of clinical prostate cancer. The prevalence of **latent** extensive tumors, however, was positively correlated with a high incidence of clinical prostate cancer in the corresponding regions. Probably the most classical reference on the issue of latent carcinoma of the prostate is the paper by Franks (1954), who established a strong age-dependence of the presence of latent prostate carcinoma in a large autopsy series. At age 60, in his autopsy series, the prevalence averages 32.2%. Interesting enough, in the study by Breslow et al., an age-dependence of the incidence of small latent tumors could not be established. Unfortunately, only little information on African blacks living in Africa is available. A more recent study comparing the incidence rates of cancers of the colon, rectum, female breast and of the prostate among native Chinese living in Shanghai, Chinese Americans and the American population was reported by Yu et al. (1991). The study showed that the rate of prostate cancer was 26 times higher in Americans than in Chinese. The rates for Chinese Americans were intermediate.

In spite of several studies addressing this problem directly, the reasons for these strong differences are still unclear. The independently high prevalence of focal latent carcinoma in autopsy series, even in those countries with a low clinical incidence of prostate cancer on one side, and in those countries with a high clinical incidence on the other side, have led to the hypothetical differentiation between a phase of initiation and promotion of prostate cancer. In this working hypothesis, the factors leading to initiation of focal prostate cancer would be independent of race and geography. Promotion, however, which would lead to the more advanced latent carcinomas paralleling a high clinical incidence, would be dependent on factors related to geography and environment in the widest sense. Unfortunately, up to now, it has not been possible to identify these factors with accuracy. Recent data derived from the "Dutch Japanese case-control study of prostate cancer" reported by Yamabe et al. (1986), compared the autopsy prevalence of prostate cancer incidentally found at the time of surgery for BPH in Dutch and Japanese men. In this study a very similar incidence of focal and more extensive lesions were found in the Japanese and Dutch sample amounting to 12-14%. This may reflect the increasing incidence of clinical PC in Japan and an indication of 'Westernization' of Japanese life style.

## INITIATION AND PROGRESSION OF PROSTATE CANCER

The morphological, functional, and genetic changes observed in the process of progression of prostate cancer from precursor lesions to the fully manifest metastatic disease, is compatible with a multistep event, which is probably governed by a series of different unidentified mutations. In this contribution, only the clinical and epidemiological aspects of this process are dealt with. Table 1 gives an indication of the phenotypic events and their possible time sequence.

## Initiation

Only recently, appropriate studies have been done which clearly establish a pattern of inheritance of prostate cancer. In two large case-control studies reported by Steinberg et al. (1990), and Spitz et al. (1991), specific empiric risk estimates associated with different family histories were established. Both studies showed similar increase of the relative risk of developing clinical prostate cancer for first degree relatives (2.0-2.4), and second degree relatives (1.7-2.1). Steinberg et al., in addition, found that the odds ratio went up to 8.8 if a first and second degree relative had prostate cancer, and that relative risk increased if relatives had prostate cancer with early onset. Carter et al. (1992) also reported the results of a segregation analysis carried out on the 691 families initially used in the case-control study of Steinberg et al. (1990). A segregation analysis is a statistical methodology which can

Table 1. Biological Progression of Prostate Cancer

| Initiation | Normal Epithelial Cell | | Factors | Duration |
|---|---|---|---|---|
| | Transition zone (20%) | Peripheral zone (80%) | Inheritance unknown | unknown |
| | ↓ | ↓ | | |
| ↓ | Atypical adeno-matous hyper-plasia (AAH) | Focal carcinoma Prostatic intraepithelial neoplasia (PIN) | | ± 13 years |
| | ↓ | ↓ | | |
| Promotion ↓ | ↓ | ↓ | | |
| | Transition zone cancer | Palpable or visible carcinoma | Inheritance Androgens Diet Vitamin A | Time to M1 averages ± 10 years |
| | ↓ | ↓ | | |
| | ? | Nodal metastases ↓ M1 disease | Unknown | |
| | | ↓ | | Average 18 months |
| | | Endocrine independence | | 8-12 mo. till death |
| | | ↓ | | |
| | | Small cell carcinoma | "Paracrine promotion" | Unknown |

be used to identify a Mendelian mutation at a single locus and to determine the specific mode of inheritance. The results revealed autosomal dominant inheritance which leads to the early onset of prostate cancer. It is estimated that 43% of those tumors that surface clinically below the age of 55 years, and 9% of all prostate cancers may be inherited. The genetic alteration, which is associated with hereditary prostate cancer, has not yet been identified. The epidemiologic and clinical features of hereditary prostate cancer have recently been reviewed by Carter et al. (1993). The authors conclude that the clinical and pathological features of hereditary sporadic prostate cancer are similar. Screening for clinical prostate cancer in high-risk families at early age of onset is advised as part of their conclusions. It is completely unknown at this time whether inheritance only impacts on clinical prostate cancer and how frequently it may play a role in the initiation of this disease. This problem can only be unravelled after the underlying genetic changes have been identified.

## Race, Age, and Endocrine Status

There is no literature evidence that racial and ethnic backgrounds have an impact on the prevalence of the focal lesions which are considered the result of the unknown initiation process. Most autopsy studies describe a strong age-dependence of latent prostate cancer. The incidence and mortality of clinical prostate cancer is also age-dependent as recently elaborated for all European countries by Møller Jensen, et al. (1990). The incidence of prostate cancer roughly doubles with each 5 year age advancement. In a recent autopsy study of 152 prostate glands of young African American and white American men in the Detroit area, Sakr et al. (1993) found an alarmingly high prevalence of prostatic intraepithelial neoplasia (PIN). Grade 3 PIN was usually associated with histological cancer. Some of these lesions, and also some of the latent focal carcinomas, were found during the third and fourth decade of life. The prevalence of the PIN lesions also increased with age. There was no difference in the incidence of precursor lesions between the black and white population of this study.

The endocrine status of men at risk, and its role as a possible determinant of prostate cancer incidence, is difficult to investigate. Evidence has remained anecdotal. Documentation concerning the medical finding in Chinese eunuchs and inmates of American prisons who were castrated because of sexual criminality, do not produce conclusive information concerning the question whether the absence of the androgenic stimulus will have an impact on prostate cancer incidence. Case descriptions are related by Lippsett (1979) and by Boccon Gibod et al. (1991), who described the scarceness and the occasional occurrence of prostate cancer in men after decades of testicular androgen deprivation. In the latter case, castration was carried out at age 35, prostate cancer was seen 40 years later.

In summary, it is unknown at this time what initiates prostate cancer. The equal prevalence of focal disease in different geographic areas and races precludes such predispositions. Much less information is available on prostatic intraepithelial neoplasia (PIN). The role of endocrine factors is unclear. The role of the endocrine status in the promotion phase will be discussed later.

## Promotion

In our present understanding of the pathogenesis of prostate cancer, some of the precursor lesions, for unknown reasons, develop into clinically relevant prostate cancer and are eventually diagnosed as locally confined or advanced disease. The hypothetical factors which cause this process are called promoting factors, the process itself is called promotion.

In most European countries the life time risk of a man to develop prostate cancer is in the range of 4%, his chance of dying of it amounts to about 2%. The discrepancy between incidence and mortality is due to the frequent occurrence of intercurrent deaths in the age groups involved, and with a tumor which often has a relatively long clinical course. Median times to prostate cancer death for men who are diagnosed with non-metastatic prostate cancer, and with metastatic prostate cancer, are in the range of 10-15 years respectively, 3-4 years. Prostate cancer incidence has been increasing for a number of decades, a much more moderate increase of prostate cancer mortality is also seen, at least in most European countries. Further increase of prostate cancer incidence is predicted (Boyle, 1992). Some of these data are summarized in Table 2. This true increase of prostate cancer incidence needs to be differentiated from the very rapid increase in incidence which is seen in countries where population-based screening is recommended and carried out. In the United States, this has led to a sharp increase of the numbers of locally confined cases and of prostate cancer incidence since 1989, as recently reviewed for the area of Rochester, Minnesota by Corder et al. (1994). This increase is mainly due to the use of prostate specific antigen (PSA), in combination with rectal examination and transrectal ultrasonography (TRUS) in large parts of the male population. Similar findings were obtained on the basis of the surveillance, epidemiology and end results program (SEER), of the United States National Cancer Institute, and described by Lu-Yao and Greenberg (1994). As a result of these activities, the discrepancy between prostate cancer incidence and mortality in the United States has now risen to 5/1. Muir et al. (1991) described a slow increase in prostate cancer, especially in Asia, but also in most western countries. The increase of prostate cancer incidence and mortality in Japan is in line with the observation of Yamabe et al. (1986) who showed in a comparative pathological study that the

Table 2. Cancer of the Prostate in EC, Numbers of New Cases in Males Aged 65+ (after P. Boyle, 1992)

| Country | 1990 | 2000 | 2010 | 2020 |
|---|---|---|---|---|
| Belgium | 2,796 | 3,156 | 3,248 | 3,939 |
| Denmark | 1,120 | 1,120 | 1,307 | 1,596 |
| France | 16,444 | 19,507 | 20,497 | 26,157 |
| FR Germany | 17,658 | 21,727 | 27,416 | 28,927 |
| Italy | 11,321 | 13,510 | 14,836 | 16,313 |
| Netherlands | 3,559 | 4,087 | 4,861 | 6,512 |
| Spain | 8,056 | 9,938 | 10,454 | 11,933 |
| United Kingdom | 14,125 | 14,421 | 15,352 | 18,099 |
| Total EC | 79,453 | 92,240 | 102,341 | 118,175 |
| Canada | 6,494 | 7,784 | 9,391 | 12,927 |

incidence of locally extensive, latent, carcinoma is similar in the regions of Rotterdam and Kyoto.

While epidemiological figures and morphological findings are compatible with the hypothesis of initiation and promotion, it has been difficult up to now to clearly delineate promoting factors. Dramatic geographical differences in the use of foodstuffs and population trends toward more vegetarian nourishment exist around the world and seem to parallel the geographical differences in the incidence and mortality of prostate cancer. Reviews are available by Wynder et al. (1971) and Flanders (1984). Adlercreutz (1990) presents a complete overview concerning the available facts relating Western style diet to prostate cancer and to hormonal changes, which may play an important role in the promotion of disease progression.

## DIET, HORMONAL STATUS, AND PROSTATE CANCER

An indirect but effective approach to further investigate the relationship of diet and cancer incidence is the study of international variations of the utilization of food stuffs in comparison with cancer mortality. Such a study was carried out by Rose et al. (1986) for carcinoma of the breast, ovary, prostate and colon. The per capita consumption of certain food stuffs is compared with prostate cancer mortality in incidence countries throughout the world. The results are given in Figure 2. Obviously, evidence produced in this way can only be indirect and does not preclude the necessity of directly establishing the effect of dietary habits through case control or cohort studies. Since caloric intake per day and per capita is a standard parameter, there is always a trade-off between food stuffs. For example, in countries with a more vegetarian diet, caloric intake, which is not based on the consumption of milk, milk products and animal fat, has to be covered by alternative sources. These are often vegetarian and rich in biological fibers, lignans, and plant estrogens, which in itself could have a protective effect as postulated by Adlercreutz et al. (1988).

### Possible Mechanisms of Prostate Cancer Promotion

Hämäläinen et al. (1984) studied the effect of a switch from a regular diet to a vegetarian diet on plasma hormones in 30 young Finnish males. These 30 males were placed on a semi-vegetarian diet in which only 25% of the energy was supplied by animal fats. The investigators noted a significant, reversible decrease in free and overall plasma testosterone, which for the latter amounted to a change from $22.7 \pm 1.1$ to $19.3 \pm 1.2$ nmol/l, but no significant effect on serum estradiol, serum 5-alpha-dihydrotestosterone (DHT), LH or adrenal hormones. In absence of a pituitary response, the authors postulate that probably testicular hormone production is influenced by a drastic decrease in serum cholesterol and lipoprotein levels observed in the same experiment. As will be discussed later, presently available evidence establishes at least a permissive role of androgens in the promotion of prostate cancer. The dietary effect of a low fat, vegetarian diet could be mediated through a decrease of androgen levels. Interestingly, in the Dutch-Japanese case-control study of prostate cancer, de Jong et al. (1991) found a similar significant difference in plasma testosterone between large Dutch and Japanese samples of age matched males. Unfortunately, these differences were not seen between men with prostate cancer and the respective controls.

Another possible mechanism influencing prostate cancer promotion could be the presence or absence of plant estrogens. These substances (examples are equol, dadzein and enterolactone) are present in fiber-rich vegetarian and semi-vegetarian food and could explain a possible protective effect of such diets. These weekly estrogenic substances grouped as lignans and isoflavonoids bind to the estrogen receptor and could thereby modify the biological action of estradiol at the level of the genome. These substances could also have a similar effect at the level of the androgen receptor and could decrease androgen production by interference with the pituitary testicular feedback mechanism. Estrogens, on the other hand, could also have a promoting role. Their carcinogenic effect at the level of microtubular proteins has been shown by Epe et al. (1989).

Schwartz and Hulka (1990) developed the hypothesis that ultraviolet light, promoting higher levels of vitamin D, may be protective for clinical prostate cancer. Hanchette and Schwartz (1992) presented further evidence on this issue. They found that mortality rates from prostate cancer in the Unites States are inversely correlated with ultraviolet radiation. Experimental studies exploring the effect of vitamin D on prostate cancer growth are in progress.

A protective effect of vitamin A on organ cultures of prostate transformed by carcinogens was first explored by Lasnitzki et al. (1955). The epidemiological literature on vitamin consumption, vitamin A and beta-carotene blood levels, and their possible protective effect is suggestive but remains contradictory, and therefore inconclusive.

Promotion by changes in the endocrine status of men has not been shown, but cannot entirely be excluded at this time. Since the prostate itself has the capability of metabolising and binding androgens at higher levels than plasma concentrations, differences in tissue levels were thought early on to be the most relevant parameter. This, however, has also not been shown. Literature evidence has recently been reviewed by Schröder et al. (1990). Available data are compatible with the view that androgens are permissive at least, although evidence that absence of androgens does not permit prostate cancer to develop is not strong either. Suppression of intraprostatic DHT by the use of a $5\alpha$-reductase inhibitor is presently used in a large endocrine prevention study. Data resulting from this protocol should help to further elucidate the role of androgens in the promotion of prostate cancer. The issue of androgenic stimulation of prostatic carcinogenesis will be more extensively dealt with elsewhere in this volume.

## Recent Epidemiological Studies

The recent epidemiological literature is very large; a complete review is not within the scope of this contribution. Developments within the last 5 years will be summarized. For the non-epidemiologist observer of this literature, it is confusing that data are often not only equivocal, but contradictory.

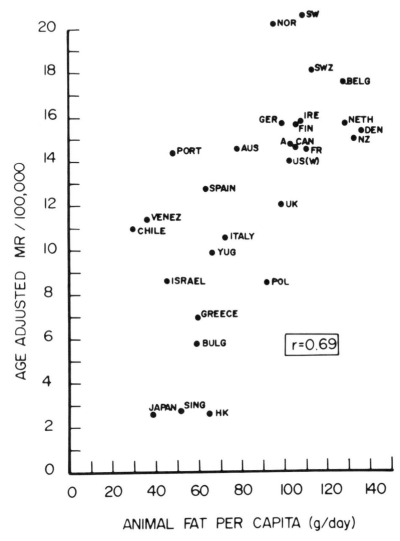

Correlation between age-adjusted prostate cancer mortality rates for 29 countries and available animal fat *per capita.*

Rose et al. 1986 (with permission)

Figure 2. Animal Fat Consumption and Prostate Cancer Mortality - Geographical Variation.

## Animal Fat and Meat

Animal fats may be promoting factors, polyunsaturated fatty acids coming from plant and fish may be protective. La Vecchia et al. (1991) described a relative risk of 5 (95% CI 1.5 - 16.6) for men who regularly utilize more than 2 glasses of milk per day. Le Marchand et al. (1994) in a cohort study of 20316 Hawaiian men found slightly elevated relative risks of developing clinical prostate cancer with a high intake of beef, milk, and animal products in general. The effect was more pronounced in older men. In a prospective case-control study of dietary fat and the risk of prostate cancer, Giovannucci et al. (1993) found a markedly increased relative risk (2.54, 95% CI 1.21 - 5.77, p = 0.02) for overconsumption of red meat. The slightly elevated relative risk for high, versus low consumption of animal fat, was not statistically significant. The results of this large case-control study support the hypothesis that animal fat, especially fat from red meat, leads to an elevated risk of prostate cancer. Hankin et al. (1992) in the Hawaiian cohort study found that a reduction of fat consumption from the highest to the lowest cohort would lead to a 10-20% decrease in the risk of prostate cancer. Giovannucci et al. (1993) and Hankin et al. (1992), recommend a reduction of dietary saturated fat as a preventive measure for prostate cancer. Hankin also recommended the same reduction for carcinoma of the breast and lung cancer. Other studies, which show a positive correlation between dietary animal fat intake and a higher relative risk of prostate cancer, are those by Talamini et al. (1992), West et al. (1991), and Bravo et al. (1991). The analysis of dietary habits in the Dutch-Japanese case-control study were reported for the Japanese part by Oishi et al. (1988). In this study, no risk correlation was found between cases and controls for the intake of carbohydrates, protein, fat, total calories, fibers, vitamin B and vitamin C.

## Vitamins

Le Marchand et al. (1991), who had previously described a positive association between beta-carotene intake and prostate cancer risk, could not confirm this finding in another study where vegetable-related vitamin consumption, after the exclusion of papaya, was not associated with an elevated cancer risk. They concluded that the positive association with beta-carotene intake among older men, which was previously reported, was essentially due to the greater papaya consumption of cases in comparison to controls. Reichman et al. (1990) found in the National Health and Nutrition Examination Survey among 2,440 study subjects, 84 men who developed prostate cancer. The mean level of serum vitamin A was significantly lower in prostate cancer cases than in controls. There was an elevated risk of prostate cancer associated with the lowest quartile of serum vitamin A. Hayes et al. (1988) found a similar correlation between plasma retinol and prostate cancer in the Dutch-Japanese case-control study. Also, Hsing et al. (1990) described an inverse relation between serum retinol levels and the risk of prostate cancer.

Willett and Hunter (1994) presented an extensive review of vitamin A and cancers of the breast, large bowel, and prostate. The emerging picture is that vitamin

A intake has no impact, but that low retinol serum levels are associated with a higher prostate cancer risk.

## Vasectomy, Smoking, and Other Factors

Extensive literature has developed around the question of whether vasectomy promotes prostate cancer, after the provocating and controversial publications of Giovannucci (1993-I and -II), which give the results of a prospective and a retrospective study. The risk to develop prostate cancer later was in the range of 2 fold if a vasectomy had been performed. The risk increased with the time that elapsed after vasectomy. Relative risks varied between 1.66 and in the extreme group 2.89. An elevated risk of dying of prostate cancer was not shown in either one of the studies. If this connection is confirmed, a doubling of the relative risk may be associated with early vasectomy. One has to keep in mind that a doubling of the relative risk also occurs with every age increase of 5 years in men above the age of 50. The data by Giovannucci are supported by studies of Hayes et al. (1993), Mettlin et al. (1990), and Rosenberg et al. (1990). A large retrospective cohort study by Nienhuis et al. (1992) was not confirmatory. A conclusive mechanism that could explain a higher incidence of prostate cancer after vasectomy is not available.

Smoking and alcohol consumption have been extensively studied. Virtually all studies come to the conclusion that prostate cancer risk is not influenced by cigarette smoking and alcohol consumption. Very recent reports, which also include reviews of the issue are those by Hayes et al. (1994), Van der Gulden et al. (1994), and Hiatt et al. (1994).

Studies on socioeconomic status, physical activity, physical characteristics and occupation have been carried out but did not produce convincing evidence of an association with prostate cancer. Also, studies on sexual activity and sexual frustration have produced contradictory results and no clear evidence of protective effects or risk increase. This was also true within the Japanese part of the Dutch-Japanese case-control study as reported by Oishi et al. (1990).

## CONCLUSIONS

Strong evidence from autopsy data and epidemiological investigations suggests that in the pathogenesis of prostate cancer, initiation and promotion should be differentiated. The factors responsible for both processes are incompletely understood. Morphologically, the initiation step is correlated with a very high, geographically non-variable autopsy prevalence of precursor lesions, such as focal carcinoma, and prostatic intraepithelial neoplasia (PIN). A high prevalence in autopsy studies of more extensive, latent cancer, correlates with a high incidence of clinical prostate cancers in those geographic areas which can be described as "the Western world". Migrants from areas of low prostate cancer incidence to prevalence of high incidence will adopt the pattern of prostate cancer incidence of their new living areas. Racial factors are not likely to play a major role in the initiation and progression of prostate cancer.

9% of human prostate cancer may be hereditary. This proportion may be as high as 25% if prostate cancer develops below the age of 55. The incidence of preclinical and clinical variations of prostate cancer is strongly age-dependent. The autopsy prevalence averages ±30%, lifetime prevalence of the clinical disease amounts to ±4%; in European countries, half of these men die of prostate cancer. Most precursor lesions will never become clinically relevant.

The strong, geographical variations in clinical prostate cancer incidence can only be explained by environmental factors, which may be related to the endocrine status of the respective male population . It has been observed that a predominantly vegetarian diet is associated with lower plasma testosterone levels than a "Western diet". The differences could, on one side, be explained by a promoting effect of food stuffs containing animal fat. On the other hand, in vegetarian diets, the fat-related calorie intake is replaced by fiber-rich products, which may be protective. This protective effect may be related to the presence of estrogenic plant hormones.

Other "environmental factors" such as vasectomy, smoking, socioeconomic status, and sex, are discussed.

## REFERENCES

Adlercreutz H, Höckerstedt K, Bannwart C, Bloigu S, Hämäläinen E, Fotsis T, Ollus A (1987): Effect of dietary components, including ligands and phytoestrogens, on enterohepatic circulation and liver metabolism of estrogens and on sex hormone binding globulin (SHBG). J Steroid Biochem 27 (4-6): 1135-1144.

Adlercreutz H (1988): Ligands and phytoestrogens. Possible preventive role in cancer. Front Gastrointest Res 14: 165-176.

Adlercreutz H (1990): Western diet and Western diseases: some hormonal and biochemical mechanisms and associations. Scand J Clin Lab Invest (Suppl 201): 3-23.

Akazaki K, Stemmermann GN (1973): Comparative study of latent carcinoma of the prostate among Japanese in Japan and Hawaii. J Nat Cancer Inst 50: 1137-1144.

Boccon-Gibod L, Dauge MC, Billebaud T, Sibert A, Baron JC, Nahoul K (1991): Prostate cancer in a 75-year-old man after four decades of testicular androgen deprivation. Eur Urol 20: 81-84.

Boyle P (1992): Epidemiology of prostate disease - cancer, BPH. Oral Communication "Prostate Cancer 2000", Milan, 15.10.1992.

Bravo MP, Castellanos E, del Rey Calero J (1991): Dietary factors and prostatic cancer. Urol Int 46: 163-166.

Breslow N, Chan CW, Dhom G, Drury RAB, Fraks LM, Gellei B, Lee YS, Lundberg S, Sparke B, Sternby NH, Tulinius H (1977): Latent carcinoma of prostate at autopsy in seven areas. Int J Cancer 20: 680-688.

Carter HB, Morrell CH, Pearson JD, Brant LJ, Plato CC, Metter EJ, Chan DW, Fozard JL, Walsh PC (1992): Estimation of prostatic growth using serial prostate-specific antigen measurements in men with and without prostate disease. Cancer Res 52: 3323-3328.

Carter BS, Bova S, Beaty TH, Steinberg GD, Childs B, Isaacs WB, Walsh PC (1993): Hereditary prostate cancer: epidemiologic and clinical features. J Urol 150: 797-820.

Corder EH, Chute CG, Guess HA, Beard CM, O'Fallon WM, Lieber MM (1994): Prostate cancer in Rochester, Minnesota (USA), from 1935 to 1989: increase in incidence related to more complete ascertainment. Cancer Causes Control 5: 207-214.

de Jong FH, Oishi K, Hayes RB, Bogdanowicz JF, Raatgever JW, van der Maas PJ, Yoshida O, Schröder FH (1991): Peripheral hormone levels in controls and patients with prostatic cancer or benign prostatic hyperplasia: results from the Dutch-Japanese case-control study. Cancer Res 51: 3445-3450.

Epe B, Harttig UH, Schiffmann, Metzler M (1989): Microtubular proteins as cellular targets for carcinogenic estrogens and other carcinogens. In: "Mechanisms of Chromosome Distribution and Aneuploidy". New York: Alan R. Liss Inc, pp 345-351.

Flanders WD (1984). Review: prostate cancer epidemiology. Prostate 5: 621-629.

Franks LM (1954): Latent carcinoma of the prostate. J Path Bact 68: 603-616.

Giovannucci E, Ascherio A, Rimm EB, Colditz GA, Stampfer MJ, Willett WC (1993-I): A prospective cohort study of vasectomy and prostate cancer in US men. JAMA 269: 873-877,.

Giovannucci E, Tosteson TD, Speizer FE, Ascherio A, Vessey MP, Colditz GA: (1993-II): A retrospective cohort study of vasectomy and prostate cancer in US men. JAMA 269: 878-882.

Giovannucci E, Rimm EB, Colditz GA, Stampfer MJ, Ascherio A, Chute CC, Willett WC (1993): A prospective study of dietary fat and risk of prostate cancer. J Natl Cancer Inst 85: 1571-1579.

Hämäläinen E, Adlercreutz H, Puska P, Pietinen P (1984): Diet and serum sex hormones in healthy men. J Steroid Biochem 20: 459-464.

Hanchette CL, Schwartz GG (1992): Geographic patterns of prostate cancer mortality. Evidence for a protective effect of ultraviolet radiation. Cancer 70: 2861-2869.

Hankin JH, Zhao LP, Wilkens LR, Kolonel LN (1992): Attributable risk of breast, prostate, and lung cancer in Hawaii due to standard fat. Cancer Causes Control 3: 17-23.

Hayes RB, Bogdanowicz JFAT, Schröder FH, A de Bruijn, Raatgever JW, Maas PJ van der, Oishi K, Yoshida O (1988): Serum retinol and prostate cancer. Cancer 62: 2021-2026.

Hayes RB, Pottern LM, Greenberg R, Schoenberg JB, Swanson GM, Liff J, Schwartz AG, Brown LM, Hoover RN (1993): Vasectomy and prostate cancer in US blacks and whites. Am J Epidemiol 137: 263-269.

Hayes RB, Pottern LM, Swanson GM, Liff JM, Schoenberg JB, Greenberg RS, Schwartz AG, Brown LM, Silverman DT, Hoover RN (1994): Tobacco use and prostate cancer in blacks and whites in the United States. Cancer Causes Control 5: 221-226.

Hiatt RA, Armstrong MA, Klatsky AL, Sidney S (1994): Alcohol consumption, smoking and other risk factors and prostate cancer in a large health plan cohort in California (United States). Cancer Causes Control 5: 66-72.

Hsing AW, Comstock GW, Abbey H, Polk BF (1990): Serologic precursors of cancer. Retinol, carotenoids, and tocopherol and risk of prostate cancer. J Natl Cancer Inst 82: 941-946.

Jensen OM, Estève J, Møller H, Renard H (1990): Cancer in the European Community and its members states. Eur J Cancer 26: 1167-1256.

La Vecchio C, Negri E, d'Avanzo B, Franceschi S, Boyle P (1991): Dairy products and the risk of prostatic cancer. Oncology 48: 406-410.

Lasnitzki I (1955): The influence of a hypervitaminosis on the effect of 20-Methylcholanthrene on mouse prostate glands grown in vitro. Brit J Cancer 9: 434-441.

le Marchand L, Hankin JH, Kolonel LN, Wilkens LR (1991): Vegetable and fruit consumption in relation to prostate cancer risk in Hawaii: a reevaluation of the effect of dietary beta-carotene. Am J Epidemiol 133: 215-219.

le Marchand L, Kolonel LN, Wilkens LR, Myers BC, Hirohata T (1994): Animal fat consumption and prostate cancer: a prospective study in Hawaii. Epidemiol 5: 276-282.

Lipsett B (1979): Interaction of drugs, hormones and nutrition in the causes of cancer. Cancer 43: 1967-1981.

Lu-Yao GL, Greenberg ER (1994): Changes in prostate cancer incidence and treatment in USA. Lancet 343:251-254.

Mettlin C, Natarajan N, Huben R (1990): Vasectomy and prostate cancer risk. Amer J Epidemiol 132 (6): 1056-1061.

Muir CS, Nectoux J, Staszewski J (1991): The epidemiology of prostatic cancer. Geographic distribution and time-trends. Acta Oncol 30 (2): 133-140.

Nienhuis H, Goldacre M, Seagroatt V, Gill L, Vessey M (1992): Incidence of disease after vasectomy: a record linkage retrospective cohort study. BMJ 304: 743-746.

Oishi K, Okada K, Yoshida O, Yamabe H, Ohno Y, Hayes RB, Schröder FH (1988): A case-control study of prostatic cancer with reference to dietary habits. Prostate 12: 179-190.

Oishi K, Okada K, Yoshida O, Yamabe H, Ohno Y, Hayes RB, Schröder FH, Boyle P (1990): A case-control study of prostatic cancer in Kyoto, Japan: sexual risk factors. Prostate 17: 269-279.

Reichman ME, Hayes RB, Ziegler RG, Schatzkin A, Taylor PR, Kahle LL, Fraumeni JF Jr (1990): Serum vitamin A and subsequent development of prostate cancer in the first National Health and Nutrition Examination Survey Epidemiologic Follow-up Study. Cancer Res 50 (8): 2311-2315.

Rose DP, Boyar AP, Wynder EL (1986): International comparisons of mortality rates for cancer of the breast, ovary, prostate, and colon, and per capita food consumption. Cancer 58: 2363-2371.

Rosenberg L, Palmer JR, Zauber AG, Warshauer ME, Stolley PD, Shapiro S (1990): Vasectomy and the risk of prostate cancer. Am J Epidemiol 132: 1051-1055.

Sakr WA, Haas GP, Cassin BF, Pontes JE, Crissman JD (1993): The frequency of carcinoma and intraepithelial neoplasia of the prostate in young male patients. J Urol 150: 379-385.

Schröder FH: Androgens and carcinoma of the prostate. In Nieschlag E, Behre HM (eds): "Testosterone. Action Deficiency Substitution". Berlin/Heidelberg: Spinger-Verlag, pp 245-260.

Schwartz GG, Hulka BS (1990): Is vitamin D deficiency a risk factor for prostate cancer? Anticancer Res 10: 1307-1311.

Spitz MR, Currier RD, Fueger JJ, Babaian RJ, Newell Gr (1991): Familial patterns of prostate cancer: a case-control analysis. J Urol 146: 1305-1307.

Steinberg GD, Epstein JI, Piantadosi S, Walsh PC (1990): Management of stage D1 adenocarcinoma of the prostate: the Johns Hopkins experience 1974 to 1987. J Urol 144: 1425-1432.

Talamini R, Franceschi S, La Vecchia C, Serraino D, Barra S, Negri E (1992): Diet and prostatic cancer: a case-control study in Northern Italy. Nutr Cancer 18: 277-286.

van der Gulden JW, Verbeek AL, Kolk JJ (1994): Smoking and drinking habits in relation to prostate cancer. Brit J Urol 73 (4): 382-389.

West DW, Slattery ML, Robinson LM, French TK, Mahoney AW (1991): Adult dietary intake and prostate cancer risk in Utah: a case-control study with special emphasis on aggressive tumors. Cancer Causes Control 2 (2): 85-94.

Willett WC, Hunter DJ (1994): Vitamin A and cancers of the breast, large bowel and prostate: epidemiologic evidence. Nutr Rev 52: 53-59.

Wynder EL, Mabuchi K, Whitmore W (1971): Epidemiology of cancer of the prostate. Cancer 28: 344-360.

Yamabe H, ten Kate FJW, Gallee MPW, Schröder FH, Oishi K, Okada K, Yoshida O (1986): Stage A prostatic cancer: a comparative study in Japan and The Netherlands. World J Urol 4: 136-140.

Yu H, Harris RE, Gao YT, Gao R, Wynder EL (1991): Comparative epidemiology of cancers of the colon, rectum, prostate and breast in Shanghai, China versus the United States. Int J Epidemiol 20: 76-81.

# 13

# DOES TESTOSTERONE TREATMENT INCREASE THE RISK OR INDUCTION OF PROGRESSION OF OCCULT CANCER OF THE PROSTATE?
Point - Counterpoint Position

**Fritz H. Schröder**

**Professor and Chairman, Department of Urology**
**Erasmus University and Academic Hospital**
**PO Box 1738, 3000 DR**
**Rotterdam, The Netherlands**

## INTRODUCTION

Prostate cancer occurs in several pre-clinical entities which can be morphologically identified. Their description, their prevalence in autopsy and clinical findings, as well as their possible relationship to clinical prostate cancer, have been discussed by the same author elsewhere in this issue. On the basis of epidemiological data, which show that focal lesions are equally frequent throughout the world, while more extensive prostate cancer varies geographically, it is very sensible to differentiate in the pathogenesis of this disease between a phase of initiation and a subsequent phase of promotion, which is governed by unknown environmental factors. From recent epidemiological data, which are summarised in the same contribution, it becomes more and more likely that either dietary animal fat consumption is a promoting factor, or that the trade-off in terms of calorie intake that is made in fiber-rich and plant estrogen-rich predominantly vegetarian diets, is protective.

## INITIATION OF PROSTATE CANCER

There is no evidence that the endocrine status of men impacts on the prevalence of precursor lesions, such as focal carcinoma, atypical adenomatous hyperplasia (AAH), or prostatic intraepithelial neoplasia (PIN). The fact that geographical variations of these lesions have not been reported in the relevant and available autopsy studies also allows to conclude that environmental factors, such as diet, which may be related to endocrine status, do not influence the process of

*Pharmacology, Biology, and Clinical Applications of Androgens,* edited by Shalender Bhasin et al.
ISBN 0-471-13320-5 © 1996 Wiley-Liss, Inc.

initiation. Unfortunately, the only two large studies available in the literature on longitudinal observations of castrated men are not conclusive, with respect to the possible occurrence of prostate cancer. These studies relate to Chinese eunuchs as reported by Von Wagenseil (1933), and to the population described by Hamilton and Mestler (1969), who reported on the fate of 1799 male inmates of the United States penal institutions who were castrated after crimes related to sexual aggressiveness. Conclusive data which would show an impact of the androgenic status on the prevalence of precursor lesions are not available. If one assumes that the promotional effect of diet may be related to endocrine factors, certainly the lack of a regional geographic variation in the distribution of such lesions would preclude a role of the factors involved in the pathogenesis of the precursor lesions.

## Promotion of Human Prostate Cancer

At the level of the genome, promotion is likely to be a multi-step event. This is also reflected in the different phenotypic appearances of prostate cancer (focal, invasively growing endocrine-dependent, metastasizing and endocrine-dependent, metastatic, and endocrine-independent). The differences in geographic distribution of the locally more advanced latent cancers or the clinically relevant prostatic carcinomas, testifies to the presence of external factors impacting on promotional steps. Promotion is possible at several levels of the path of progression of this disease. Neither the genetic steps, nor the exact mechanisms of promotion are firmly established. The crucial questions whether androgens can stimulate precursor lesions to grow and to develop into the phenotype of clinical prostate cancer has to remain unanswered at this time. Also, the question whether exogenous androgen supplementation would have a different effect from circulating natural androgens, cannot be answered.

## Androgens Stimulate Established Prostate Cancer

Endocrine-dependent human prostate cancer (the PC-82 and EW-models) are stimulated by exogenous androgens in their growth in a dose-dependent fashion (Van Weerden, 1991). Fowler and Whitmore (1981) have shown that metastatic prostatic cancer exacerbates after stimulation with exogenous testosterone. There is evidence that even hormone-independent, metastatic prostate cancer can be stimulated by exogenous testosterone. Similar observations were made by Manni et al. (1987) who applied androgen depletion and repletion regimens to synchronise prostate cancer cell populations for more effective chemotherapy.

Athletes and body-builders using steroid hormones have been reported to develop aggressive prostate cancer at a young age by Roberts and Esseningh (1986), and Wemyss-Holden et al. (1994). Exogenous androgen supplementation in castrated or pan-hypopituitaric men can induce and maintain benign prostatic hyperplasia (BPH). Statistical information on these issues is unavailable; evidence remains anecdotal but is firm in the reported cases.

Few mechanisms are known which could explain a stimulation of prostatic carcinogenesis by androgens. These include androgen hypersensitivity as observed in clonal populations of the androgen-dependent Shionogi mouse mammary carcinoma line by Labrie et al. (1988). Androgen hypersensitivity could be caused by androgen receptor magnification or by mutations of the androgen receptor. Important in this context may be the observation of Geller et al. (1984) and Bélanger et al. (1989), that prostatic tissue is capable after castration to accumulate 5α-dihydrotestosterone to higher levels than would be expected according to serum concentrations of testosterone.

## Diet-Related Endocrine Changes

Probably the strongest available evidence giving an explanation for geographic variations in prostate and breast cancer incidence relates to a diet. Adlercreutz et al. (1991) have not only pointed out but have also extensively studied possible mechanisms which may explain why regions where a "Western diet" is common, show a higher incidence of clinical prostate cancer. This author reviews the possible mechanisms which may relate to a decrease of hepatic elimination of circulating steroids in humans who use a diet rich in animal fats, but also to a protective effect of fiber-rich diets which may be mediated by phytoestrogens, such as lignans and isoflavonoids. Some of these poorly explored and understood plant estrogens may in fact act as anti-estrogens. They may inhibit steroid action at the level of androgen and type 2 estrogen receptors and thereby modulate the effect of circulating estrogens. The same group observed that the temporary use of a vegetarian diet in Finnish men leads to a significant decrease of plasma testosterone and an increase of steroid hormone binding globulin (SHBG) levels (Hämäläinen et al., 1984). De Jong et al. (1991) found significantly lower plasma testosterone levels in Japanese men as compared to Dutch men in the Dutch-Japanese case-control study of prostate cancer. These differences were, however, not found between cases and controls. Several authors have studied plasma hormones in prostate cancer patients in comparison to normal controls, or patients with benign prostatic hyperplasia. Ranniko and Adlercreutz (1983) found significantly lower plasma testosterone and estradiol levels in men with prostate cancer. Their sample, however, was not age-controlled. Two more recent studies and a review are available on the same issue. Hsing and Comstock (1993), and Andersson et al. (1993) did not find significant differences between prostate cancer cases and appropriate controls, as far as SHBG is concerned. The review paper by Montie and Pienta (1994) is confirmatory. Still, considering the mechanism of action of phytoestrogens, the strong possibility of a causative relationship cannot be excluded at this time. If these findings are confirmed, they provide evidence that small changes in the androgenic status of men can lead to large differences in PC incidence.

An interesting observation has been reported by Wallace et al. (1993) with relation to androgen stimulation of prostate-specific antigen (PSA). PSA is an androgen-dependent protein which is found in normal and abnormal prostatic epithelial tissue. During a study of a prototype regimen of 200 mg testosterone enanthate i.m. weekly, as a potential male contraception regimen, significant changes in plasma hormones were observed. Despite a sustained rise in serum levels of testosterone and dihydrotestosterone during treatment, there was no significant change in concentrations of PSA.

## CONCLUSIONS

Considering the available evidence, it is quite unlikely that the initiation phase of the pathogenesis of prostate cancer is influenced by androgens. Considerable evidence, however, exists that androgens may have an impact on the steps which characterize promotion and progression of the disease through its biological development. There is equivocal evidence that pre-existing prostate cancer is stimulated by androgens to grow. This must also be assumed for cancers that still remain clinically latent but have reached a stage that exceeds the size and characteristics of the precursor lesions. The prevalence of high volume (> 0.5 ml) disease is not exactly known at this time but emerges as a finding from wide-spread screening efforts in the United States. Steroids used by body-builders and athletes, which has led to aggressive prostate cancer in a number of very young men, seems to indicate that precursor lesions can be promoted to clinical disease by the use of androgenic steroids. There is evidence that a diet rich in animal fats leads to higher plasma testosterone levels in males than a semi-vegetarian or vegetarian diet. Increasing epidemiological evidence points in the direction that the trade-off in caloric intake between animal fats and vegetarian food stuffs offers the best possible explanation for the geographic variations in clinical prostate cancer incidence.

The possibility that androgen supplementation promotes prostate cancer cannot be excluded at this time.

## REFERENCES

Adlercreutz H (1991): Diet and sex hormone metabolism. Chapter 6. In: Rowland IR (Ed) "Nutrition, Toxicity, and Cancer". Boca Raton, USA: CRC Press Inc., pp 137-195.

Andersson SO, Adami HO, Bergström R, Wide L (1993): Serum pituitary and sex steroid hormone levels in the etiology of prostatic cancer - population-based case-control study. Brit J Cancer 68: 97-102.

Bélanger B, Bélanger A, Labrie F, Dupont A, Cusan L, Monfette G (1989): Comparison of residual C-19 steroids in plasma and prostatic tissue of human, rat and guinea pig after castration: unique importance of extratesticular androgens in men. J Steroid Biochem 32: 695-698.

de Jong FH, Oishi K, Hayes RB, Bogdanovicz J, Raatgever J, vad der Maas PJ, Yoshima O, Schröder FH (1991): Peripheral hormone levels in controls and patients with prostatic cancer or benign prostatic hyperplasia: results from the Dutch-Japanese case-control study. Cancer Res 51: 3445-3450.

Fowler JE, Whitmore WF (1981): The response of metastatic adenocarcinoma of the prostate to exogenous testosterone. J Urol 126: 372-375.

Geller J, Albert JD, Nachtsheim DA, Loza D (1984): Comparison of prostatic cancer tissue Dihydrotestosterone levels at the time of relapse following orchiectomy or estrogen therapy. J Urol 132: 693-696.

Hämäläinen E, Adlercreutz H, Puska P, Pietinen P (1984): Diet and serum sex hormones in healthy men. J Steroid Biochem 20: 459-464.

Hamilton JB, Mestler GE (1969): Mortality and survival: comparison of eunuchs with intact men and women in a mentally retarded population. J Gerontol 24: 395-411.

Hsing AW, Comstock GW (1993): Serological precursors of cancer: serum hormones and risk of subsequent prostate cancer. Cancer Epidemiol Biomarkers Prev 2: 27-32.

Labrie F, Veilleux R, Fournier A (1988): Low androgen levels induce the development of androgen-hypersensitive cell clones in Shionogi mouse mammary carcinoma cells in culture. J Natl Cancer Inst 80: 1138-1147.

Manni A, Santen RJ, Boucher AE, Lipton A, Harvey H, Simmonds M, Gordon R, Rohner T, Drago J, Wettlaufer J, Glode LM (1987): Androgen depletion and repletion as a means of potentiating the effects of cytotoxic chemotherapy in advanced prostate cancer. J Steroid Biochem 27: 551-556.

Montie JE, Pienta KJ (1994): Review of the role of androgenic hormones in the epidemiology of benign prostatic hyperplasia and prostate cancer. Urology 43: 892-999.

Ranniko S, Adlercreutz H (1983): Plasma estradiol, free testosterone, sex hormone binding globulin binding capacity, and prolactin in benign prostatic hyperplasia and prostatic cancer. Prostate 4: 223-229.

Roberts JT, Esseningh (1986): Adenocarcinoma of prostate in 40-year-old body-builder. Lancet 8509 (Vol II): 742

van Weerden WM, van Steenbrugge GJ, van Kreuningen A, Moerings EP, de Jong FH, Schröder FH (1991): Assessment of the critical level of androgen for growth response of transplantable human prostatic carcinoma (PC-82) in nude mice. J Urol 145: 631-634.

Wagenseil F von (1933): Chinesische Eunuchen (Zugleich ein Beitrag zur Kenntnis der Kastrationsfolgen und der rassialen und körperbaulichen Bedeutung der anthropologischen Merkmale). Zeitschr Morphol Anthrol 32: 415-468.

Wallace EM, Pye SD, Wild SR, Wu FCW (1993): Prostate-specific antigen and prostate gland size in men receiving exogenous testosterone for male contraception. Int J Androl 16: 35-40.

Wemyss-Holden SA, Hamdy FC, Hastie KJ (1994): Steroid abuse in athletes, prostatic enlargement and bladder outflow obstruction - is there a relationship? Brit J Urol 74: 476-478.

# 14

# DEVELOPMENT OF CRITERIA TO MONITOR THE OCCURRENCE OF PROSTATE CANCER IN TESTOSTERONE CLINICAL TRIALS

Peter J. Snyder

Department of Medicine
University of Pennsylvania School of Medicine
Philadelphia, PA 19104

## INTRODUCTION

As men age, their serum testosterone concentrations decrease, leading to the suggestion that this decrease may be a cause of the decreases in libido, energy, muscle mass, bone mineral density, etc., that also occur with increasing age. To test this possibility, studies are now underway to increase the serum testosterone concentrations of elderly men to those of young men and determine if the increase can reverse some of these phenomena of aging. Increasing the serum testosterone concentrations of elderly men, however, could increase their risk of prostate cancer, because many men apparently harbor clinically silent prostate cancers, and because prostate cancer is, to some extent, a testosterone-dependent disease. Consequently, investigators who increase the serum testosterone concentrations of elderly men need to screen the men for the presence of prostate cancer before entry into the study and monitor them for newly detectable prostate cancer during the course of the study.

## HIGH PREVALENCE OF CLINICALLY SILENT PROSTATE CANCER

Although prostate cancer is the second leading cause of cancer deaths among men in the United States, what may be of greater significance for the purposes of an investigator contemplating a study of the effect of testosterone treatment of elderly men is the prevalence of clinically silent prostate cancer. Several autopsy series show that men who died in their 70s and 80s of unrelated causes, harbored clinically silent prostate cancer (Franks, 1977). (These autopsy studies were all conducted before the advent of PSA measurement, so some of these cancers might

*Pharmacology, Biology, and Clinical Applications of Androgens,* edited by Shalender Bhasin et al.
ISBN 0-471-13320-5 © 1996 Wiley-Liss, Inc.

have been detected within the person's lifetime had PSA been available then.) The potential relevance for studies of the effect of testosterone in elderly men is the possibility that testosterone treatment might stimulate the growth of these prostate cancers.

## PROSTATE CANCER IS TESTOSTERONE-DEPENDENT

Huggins demonstrated more than fifty years ago the testosterone dependence of prostate cancer when he found that castration of men with metastatic prostate cancer decreased the size and activity of the metastases, as demonstrated by a fall in their serum prostatic acid phosphatase concentrations (Huggins and Hodges, 1941). Subsequently, castration became a standard treatment for metastatic prostate cancer. Currently, castration is being replaced as treatment for metastatic prostate cancer by other modalities based on its testosterone dependence. One treatment is to decrease testosterone secretion by decreasing LH secretion by administration of superactive agonist of GnRH. Another is to block the action of testosterone by administration of a testosterone receptor antagonist. Both may be used together (Iverson et al., 1990). What is of special concern with regard to increasing the testosterone concentrations of elderly men is that the incidence of clinically apparent prostate cancer increases with increasing age, even though their serum testosterone concentrations decrease.

## ELDERLY MEN ARE HYPOGONADAL

For many years it was controversial as to whether or not men's serum testosterone concentrations decreased with increasing age. A study of Bremner and collaborators appeared to resolve the controversy by demonstrating that the serum testosterone concentrations of young men exhibit a diurnal variation, with a peak at about 8 A.M. and a nadir at about 8 P.M., but elderly men do not exhibit such a variation (Bremner et al., 1983). Consequently, studies of the effect of age on serum testosterone in which testosterone is sampled early in the morning are more likely to show a difference between young and old men that studies in which sampling is in the afternoon. Several studies in which testosterone was sampled in the morning do show such a difference (Purifoy et al., 1981; Deslypere and Vermeulen, 1984; Tenover et al., 1987).

## THE DILEMMA

We now reach the dilemma: If elderly men are hypogonadal and often also harbor clinically silent prostate cancers, and if the growth of prostate cancer is dependent on testosterone, will increasing their serum testosterone concentrations to those of young men stimulate the growth of their prostate cancers? The answer to this question is not yet known.

# HOW TO SCREEN MEN FOR PROSTATE CANCER BEFORE THEY ENTER A STUDY IN WHICH THEIR SERUM TESTOSTERONE CONCENTRATIONS WILL BE INCREASED

There is little question that elderly men who are to enter a study in which their serum testosterone concentrations are to be raised should be screened to exclude those who have prostate cancer. There is also little question that this screening should include a history of prostate cancer and a digital rectal examination, and those whose examination shows a prostate nodule should be referred for urologic consultation and a prostate biopsy. There is probably also little question that the screening should include a measurement of prostate specific antigen (PSA), because the rate of detection of prostate cancer using both the digital rectal examination and PSA is significantly greater than either alone (Figure 1) (Catalona et al., 1994b). Adding a transrectal ultrasound, however, increases the rate of detection by only a small additional amount. What exclusion value of PSA should be used is less certain. For several years a PSA of <4 ng/mL has been considered normal for men of all ages, and values of >4 ng/mL have been shown to have greater risk of prostate

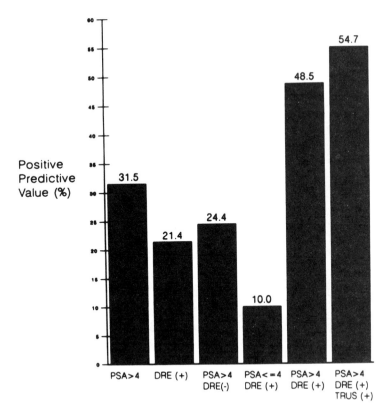

Figure 1. Positive predictive value of digital rectal examination (DRE), prostate specific antigen (PSA), and transrectal ultrasound (TRUS) (Catalona et al., 1994).

cancer. One approach, therefore, would be to exclude all men whose PSA is >4.0 ng/mL.

More recently, two other ways for using the PSA have been suggested. Both ways take into account that benign prostatic hypertrophy, as well as prostate cancer, increases the PSA. The first way takes into account the fact that virtually all men develop some degree of BPH as they age, and the BPH leads to a gradually increasing PSA concentrations with increasing age (Figure 2) (Oesterling et al., 1993), an increase that is apparently not related to prostate cancer. The suggestion has therefore been made that prostate cancer should be suspected not on the basis of the same PSA value for all ages but an age-adjusted range of values (Table 1) (Oesterling et al., 1993). Another study, however, showed that when prostate biopsies to detect prostate cancer are performed on the basis of the PSA concentration, the number of prostate biopsies performed for each cancer detected with a PSA of >4.0 ng/mL is similar for all age groups, suggesting that this value is best for men of all ages (Catalona et al., 1994b).

The second way of using the PSA takes into account the fact that prostate cancer causes a higher serum PSA concentration per volume of prostate cancer tissue than BPH does per volume of BPH tissue. The suggestion has therefore been made that prostate cancer should be suspected on the basis of the PSA, divided by the prostate volume as determined by transrectal ultrasound, called the "PSA density," rather than on the basis of the PSA alone (Benson et al., 1992). Similarly,

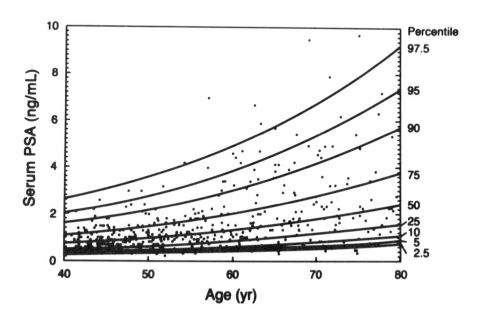

Figure 2. Increasing serum prostate specific antigen (PSA) concentrations with increasing age (Oesterling et al., 1993).

Table 1.   Age-Specific Ranges of Normal for Prostate Specific Antigen (PSA) (Oesterling et al., 1993).

### Age-Specific Reference Ranges*
### for Serum Prostate-specific Kantigen†

| Age (yr) | Serum PSA (ng/mL) | PSA density |
|----------|-------------------|-------------|
| 40-49 | 0.0-2.5 | 0.0-0.08 |
| 50-59 | 0.0-3.5 | 0.0-0.10 |
| 60-69 | 0.0-4.5 | 0.0-0.11 |
| 70-79 | 0.0-6.5 | 0.0-0.13 |

*Upper limit defined as the 95th percentile.
†PSA = prostate-specific antigen.

study candidates could be excluded on a  similar basis.  At lease one other study, however, appears  to show that the PSA density is a less sensitive means of detecting prostate cancer  than is the PSA alone (Smith and Catalona, 1994).  Although there may be merit to both of these alternatives to an age-invariate PSA alone as screening tests for elderly men entering a trial of testosterone, use of a PSA of <4.0 ng/mL alone is probably a more conservative approach.  Until and unless it is shown that testosterone treatment of elderly men does not increase the incidence of prostate cancer, use of a PSA $\leq$4 ng/mL alone is probably the best way to use PSA for screening.

## HOW TO MONITOR MEN FOR PROSTATE CANCER AFTER THEY ENTER A STUDY IN WHICH THEIR SERUM TESTOS-TERONE CONCENTRATIONS WILL BE INCREASED

After elderly men who do not have evidence of prostate cancer enter a testosterone trial, they need to be monitored for the possible development of prostate cancer, especially if the trial lasts for several years.  If a man develops a prostate nodule that was previously undetected or if his PSA increases above the "trigger" value, he should be referred for urologic evaluation and prostate biopsy.  The question again becomes, what should the trigger value for the PSA be?  Use of the same PSA value used for screening is not practical, since in normal men PSA tends to increase gradually with time (Oesterling et al., 1993), and the PSA fluctuates considerably from time to time.  Consequently, when the value for admission to the study is $\leq$4.0 ng/mL, and a subject has a pre-study value of  3.9 ng/mL, the PSA could well  become  >4 ng/mL within  the next three years, even if he does not develop prostate cancer.  Probably a better means of using the PSA to monitor subjects for  the possible development of  prostate cancer  is to us a rate of change criterion.

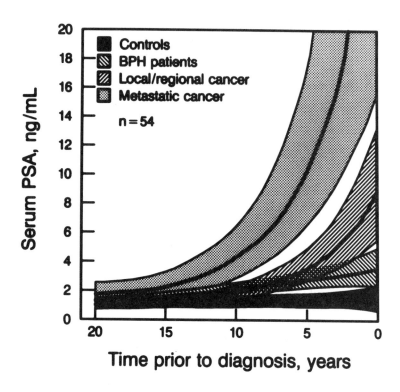

Figure 3. Serum prostate specific antigen (PSA) concentration in the years prior to the diagnosis of prostate cancer and other prostate diseases (Carter et al., 1992).

One study of PSA values over the course of several years showed that men who were found to have prostate cancer also had increases in PSA of >0.75 ng/mL/year over a two year period, but men who were not found to have prostate cancer had increases of <0.75 ng/mL/year during this time (Figure 3) (Carter et al., 1992). Another study confirmed the value of the sensitivity and specificity of the value of 0.75 ng/mL/year, but only for men whose initial value was ≤4.0 ng/mL and who were <70 years of age (Smith and Catalona, 1994). For men whose initial PSA was >4.0 ng/mL, an annualized rate of change of 0.4 ng/mL/year was found to be maximize sensitivity and specificity. For men who were >70 years of age, the rate of change of >0.75 ng/mL/year was less sensitive than in men <70, but no alternative value was found to more sensitive. For now, an annualized value of >0.75 ng/mL/year for a two year period for all ages appears to be the best criterion available.

## SUMMARY

Investigators conducting trials of testosterone treatment of elderly men to determine if it has beneficial effects should screen the men for prostate cancer before entering them in the study and monitor those who enter the study for the possible development of prostate cancer, because prostate cancer is, to some extent, testosterone dependent. Screening should include a digital rectal examination and a PSA. Finding a prostate nodule should lead to urologic consultation. Subjects who have an elevated PSA should be excluded. Using a PSA value of 4.0 ng/mL as the upper limit of normal would be conservative; alternatively, an age-adjusted range of normal or a PSA density could be used. Subjects who qualify for and enter the study should also be monitored by digital rectal examination and PSA. An annualized rate of change of >0.75 ng/mL/year for two years should lead to urologic evaluation and prostate biopsy.

## REFERENCES

Benson MC, Whang IS, Olsson CA, et al. (1992): The use of prostate specific antigen density to enhance the predictive value of intermediate level of serum prostate specific antigen. J Urol 147:817-821.

Bremner WJ, Vitiello MV, Prinz, PN (1983): Loss of circadian rhythmicity in blood testosterone levels with aging in normal men. J Clin Endocrinol Metab 56:1278-1281.

Carter HB, Pearson JD, Metter EJ, et al. (1992): Longitudinal evaluation of prostate-specific antigen levels in men with and without prostate disease. JAMA 167: 2215-2220.

Catalona WJ, Richie JP, deKernion JB, et al. (1994): Comparison of prostate specific antigen concentration versus prostate specific antigen density in the early detection of prostate cancer: receiver operating characteristic curves. J Urol 152:2031-2036.

Catalona WJ, Richie JP, Ahmann FR, et al. (1994): Comparison of digital rectal examination and serum prostate specific antigen in the early detection of prostate cancer: results of a multicenter clinical trial of 6,630 men. J Urol 151: 1283-1290.

Catalona WJ, Hudson MA, Scardino PT, et al. (1994): Selection of optimal prostate specific antigen cutoffs for early detection of prostate cancer: receiver operating characteristics curves. J Urol 152:3037-2041.

Deslypere JP, Vermeulen A (1984): Leydig cell function in normal men: effect of age, life-style, residence, diet and activity. J Clin Endocrinal Metab 59:955-962.

Franks LM (1977): Etiology and epidemiology of human prostatic disorders. Urologic Pathology: The Prostate. Tannenbaum M, Ed. Lea and Feiger, Philadelphia, p 23.

Huggins C, Hodges CV (1941): Studies on Prostatic Cancer I. The effect of castration, of estrogen and of androgen injection on serum phosphatases in metastatic carcinoma of the prostate. Cancer Res 1: 293-297.

Iversen P, Christensen MG, Feriis E, et al. (1990): A phase III trial of zoladex and flutamide versus orchiectomy in the treatment of patients with advanced carcinoma of the prostate. Cancer 66: 1058-1066.

Purifoy FE, Koopmans LH, Mayes DM (1981): Age differences in serum androgen levels in normal adult males. Hum Bio 53:199-511.

Smith DS, Catalona WJ (1994): Rate of change in serum prostate specific antigen levels as a method for prostate cancer detection. J Urol 152: 1163-1167.

Tenover JS, Matsumoto AM, Plymate SR, Bremner WJ (1987): The effects of aging in normal men on bioavailable testosterone and luteinizing hormone secretion: response to clomiphene citrate. J Clin Endocrinol Metab 65: 1118-1126.

# DISCUSSION: ANDROGEN AND PROSTATE CANCER
## Chairpersons: Glenn Cunningham, Hermann Behre

**Ronald Swerdloff:** This is an opportunity to ask this outstanding panel to refocus on several areas of concern that have remained since the last meeting in Marco Island. It is noteworthy that since our meeting four and a half years ago, we have begun long-term studies on androgen treatment of elderly men that previously would not have been identified as requiring androgen replacement. Secondly, we have demonstrated that androgen treatment, either alone or in combination with other agents, has the potential to block spermatogenesis sufficiently to be considered as part of an experimental contraceptive regimen which implies treatment of otherwise healthy people for long periods of time. We have also increased our treatment of adolescent boys and young men with testosterone for delayed sexual maturation. One question that we are asking is, what are the implications of androgen treatment on future development of BPH and/or prostate cancer? Do we have sufficient evidence on safety to allow us to proceed with longer term studies? If we go forward, how do we monitor these situations?

**Donald Coffey:** First of all, you asked for opinions and this is what we are going to give, because we do not have the answer to this. I think that androgen based male contraceptives are probably safer than oral contraceptives for the female. The second thing is, the female oral contraceptives protect against benign breast disorders. I have always been interested in that and I think that androgen contraceptives may provide BPH protection in adults. However, if you give androgens to people that have prostate tumors, that is not a good thing. Dr. Whitmore gave androgens to patients who had cancer and these patients had excruciating pains. I want to point out that occurred within hours and that was before there could be any tumor growth. Patients with bone pain due to metastatic prostate cancer have improvement in their pain within hours after castration. We believe that the pain is due to proteolytic proteins secreted by the prostate.

**Fritz Schröder:** I do not have an explanation for the very quick pain relief and I would like to comment on the monitoring of these patients. I think the monitoring would actually have to be done before hand and we should differentiate between very young men and the older men. In the very young men, the prevalence of precursor lesions may be smaller. The proposal of monitoring these people has to be very carefully considered. First of all, even in radical prostatectomy series, about 30% of men do not have an elevated PSA. Also in the screening studies that use all three available screening tests, about 30% of men are identified that do have a PSA that is below 4 (considered normal). So the PSA alone would not be sufficient to monitor these men and it would have to be at least accompanied by digital rectal examinations. If you consider the possibility of androgen treatment stimulating subclinical prostate cancer, you may have to consider the possibility that you may identify the tumor earlier and treat it earlier. I was very surprised, together with all of the epidemiologists, about the high detection rates of lesions that are clinically significant. We thought in the beginning that with the screening, we would detect many lesions that are focal, but this is actually limited to less than 10%. Most of the lesions that are detected with the screening procedures are lesions that are larger than 0.5 cm$^2$

in volume and have a Gleason grade that is higher than that of the focal lesions. It is realistic to assume that in men in the age group between 55 and 75, who are treated with a supraphysiological concentration of androgens, one would stimulate prostate cancer somewhere between 2.5% and 3.5% of that population.

**John Isaacs:**  The most critical issues are going to be discussed tomorrow with regard to heart disease and other quality of life issues. If we are unwilling to lower serum testosterone in men who are 75 years of age and who happen to have a supraphysiological level of testosterone, then raising the serum testosterone levels moderately in men with subphysiological levels of testosterone does not seem to be so unreasonable. For example, if a man had serum testosterone which was above the norm, but he is otherwise healthy, would you want to give this man antiandrogens or castrate him to lower the androgen levels because of fears of prostate disease? Presently, such a man could be left untreated.

**Donald Coffey:**  If you had a hypothetical couple, each in their 20's, come in your office seeking contraceptive advice. They were trying to decide if she should go on an oral contraceptive or her husband use a testosterone-based male contraceptive. Which one would you be putting at risk; the man, by giving him a testosterone implant, or the woman by giving her a progesterone implant or oral birth control pills?

**Jean Fourcroy:**  We are having the same dialogue that we had 40 years ago in our considerations of risk related to estrogen treatment for women. We need to think just as seriously today about risk: benefit issues for androgens in men.

**Donald Coffey:**  But who do you think you would be putting at most risk?

**Jean Fourcroy:**  I am more worried about the risk of androgens in the male.

**Donald Coffey** - I think you are putting a 20-year-old woman at much more risk by giving her an oral contraceptive than you are the 20-year-old male. If the woman becomes 40 and you give her the oral contraceptive, you are really putting her at risk. If you give a 40 year-old male an implant, you are probably putting him at an increased risk, but is it any higher than it is for the female? I think the oral contraceptive risk is tolerable and a male-directed contraceptive with equal risk would also be acceptable if not ideal. We are talking about young people who are going to need greater options on birth control methods. And if you ask me what I am worried about with the use of androgens, it is not the later development of BPH and prostate cancer but the short-term problems of increased aggression.

**Jean Fourcroy:**  That is exactly where my concern is.

**Bernard Robaire:**  Dr. Coffey, do you think that because of the cardioprotective effects and prevention of osteoporosis that estrogens show in women, that the formulation of testosterone and estradiol proposed by Larry Ewing et al. should be revived in the context of contraceptive testing?

**Donald Coffey:**  We need a lot more work, but I do not think that there is anything there that bothers me so far that I have heard. What you have to come to hear is that you are going to pay some price for control of population, and we are willing to pay that price with oral contraceptives. A professor at Hopkins once said to the Safety Committee that every time a person reaches for an oral contraceptive, they might as well be reaching for a cyanide. That is how dangerous oral contraceptives were felt to be. You remember all of that. After our experience increased, we said that oral birth control treatment was not as good as peanut butter, but when you pick the right patient and right conditions, oral contraceptives can be used quite effectively and safely. I think we have to come to the same place with the male system. New, safe, and effective hormonal male contraceptives need to be developed. I do not believe that consensus about the induction of BPH and prostate cancer are compelling enough to prevent further development of androgen-based male methods. I think the biggest problem we are looking at is in severe overpopulation and aggression.

**John Isaacs:** One last statement about estrogens. Many urologists remember that time when they gave oral diethylstilbestrol for the treatment of prostatic cancer and saw an increase in cardiovascular side-effects. So, they think that estrogens are inherently bad. The point is that it has been demonstrated that if estrogens are given other than by oral delivery (for example, they are given by dermal patches or by subcutaneous depots), instead of increasing cardiovascular risks, they actually decrease them. I point you to the studies done in Sweden with Estraderm which is a 17B-estradiol polyphosphonate which can be given subcutaneously as a depot and lowers serum cholesterol and reduces cardiovascular risk, if anything. Estrogens from a cardiovascular standpoint can be either good or bad, depending how they are given. We have to reexamine how estrogens were formulated, how they were actually delivered, and what is known about the pharmacokinetics of that formulation. When you talk about combining estrogens with testosterone, I would prefer transdermal or parenteral over oral estrogens because of the first pass effect on the liver.

**Jean Wilson:** I would like to comment on a point Dr. Coffey has made. It is true that androgen abuse is not as bad as cocaine abuse, but it is premature to conclude that androgen abuse is harmless. There is not a single significant long-term follow-up of androgen abusers to ascertain the long-term implication for health. We simply do not know what the long-term complications are. But even if it were demonstrated there were no long-term complications to androgen abuse by athletes, it may not be relevant to the issue because the vast amount of androgen abuse by athletes is intermittent, and the real concern is the potential for harm by long-term continued use over many months to years. The vast majority of androgen abusers take the drugs intermittently and then go through periods of withdrawal; the percentage of body builders and power lifters who use it continuously is minuscule. And consequently, even if it were demonstrated that androgen as ordinarily abused is not harmful, that is not necessarily relevant to the issue of long-term androgen use in doses sufficient to suppress hypothalamic-pituitary functions. And consequently, I agree with Dr. Schröder that the issue is really a serious one and that the point that Dr. Snyder has made about the necessity of being certain that we are not having a bad effect on health. The fact that estrogens were not studied carefully at the start of either use is irrelevant because we have higher standards about drug testing now than we did then.

**Donald Coffey:** Oral contraceptives are not used forever either.

**Jean Wilson:** I did not say forever, I said long-term.

**Cargos Callegari:** In countries with high incidence of prostate cancer, would you recommend yearly PSA screening for all men over 40?

**Peter Snyder**: That is a very controversial area. The reason for the controversy is that although it is quite clear that PSA is a very effective way of detecting prostate cancer early, it is not clear whether detecting it early will influence the course of the disease.

# PART III: ANDROGEN EFFECTS ON THE BRAIN: COGNITIVE, SEXUAL, AND AGGRESSIVE BEHAVIOR

# 15

# ANDROGEN: EFFECTS ON THE BRAIN: COGNITIVE, SEXUAL, AND AGGRESSIVE BEHAVIOR, AN OVERVIEW

**Roger A. Gorski**

**Department of Anatomy & Cell Biology**
**Laboratory of Neuroendocrinology of the**
**Brain Research Institute**
**UCLA School of Medicine**
**Los Angeles, California 90095**

Although clinicians usually weigh the benefits of a given treatment or procedure against its potential risks, this is virtually impossible when potential risks are currently unknown. In such cases, an awareness of potential risks and a follow-up of treated individuals over time, should be standard procedure, but frequently is not because of the cost in time and effort. In the area of androgen therapy, attempts are being made to improve delivery systems and to increase the effectiveness of the hormone molecule as this therapy grows more popular for adolescents, aging men and even postmenopausal women. In addition, both male and female athletes and body builders commonly expose themselves to androgens to enhance their performance and appearance. Are there risks associated with androgen administration?

One might consider potential risks in terms of prostate cancer, bone and vascular physiology as is discussed in other sections of these proceedings. However, the focus of the present discussion is on a vastly different potential target for androgen action - *the brain*. In contrast to androgen action on other tissues where molecular, biochemical and physiological processes are paramount, three facts make studies of androgen action on the brain much more complex. First, is the marked anatomical, chemical, and functional heterogeneity and complexity of the brain itself. Second, gonadal hormones have two types of action on the brain: permanent, or *organizational,* and transient, or *activational.* (Note also, that activational effects could well be inhibitory in nature.) Although the organizational actions of gonadal hormones are probably limited to specific developmental stages, they clearly help determine the nature of the response to hormones in adulthood. Third, and perhaps the most important, is the fact that human behavior is modified by many non-hormonal influences, some of which are suggested in Figure 1. A person's behavior might be determined more by the sexual stereotype typical of his/her society or by

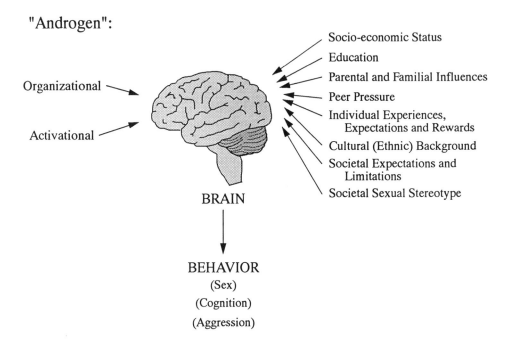

"Androgen":

Organizational

Activational

BRAIN

Socio-economic Status

Education

Parental and Familial Influences

Peer Pressure

Individual Experiences,
   Expectations and Rewards

Cultural (Ethnic) Background

Societal Expectations and
   Limitations

Societal Sexual Stereotype

BEHAVIOR
(Sex)
(Cognition)
(Aggression)

Figure 1. Some factors that may influence human behavior. Androgen is listed in quotation marks because of its potential to act as estradiol or dihydrotestosterone.

societal, parental and/or peer pressures, than by his/her hormones. When dealing with human beings, one cannot simply administer a hormone and observe its effects unaltered by parameters that are not easily controlled for, nor sometimes even recognized, by the clinician or investigator. Human behavior is the sum of many variables, androgens or hormones in general, are but one!

In the discussions to follow, basically four questions will be considered. Do androgens modify brain structure during development and in adulthood? Do androgens influence cognitive abilities? Do androgens contribute to aggressive or anti-social behavior? What components of the sexual behavior of the human male are sensitive to androgens? However, the fundamental question which underlies each of these discussions is quite explicit even though, at our present level of understanding, its answer remains elusive: Should one anticipate undesirable side effects of androgen therapy in any or all of these areas?

# 16

# ANDROGENS AND SEXUAL DIFFERENTIATION OF THE BRAIN

Roger A. Gorski

Department of Anatomy & Cell Biology
Laboratory of Neuroendocrinology of the
Brain Research Institute
UCLA School of Medicine
Los Angeles, California  90095

Although the question under consideration is whether androgen therapy could have undesirable effects on the brain in adolescent, adult, and aging individuals, it is useful to begin with a consideration of the fundamental concept of hormone-induced sexual differentiation of the brain.  Androgen therapy or androgen abuse would have the potential to affect prenatal development only if administered to or abused by a woman relatively early in pregnancy.   Nevertheless, a consideration of the process of the sexual differentiation of the brain highlights and documents the vast potential for hormone-induced alterations in brain function and structure and thus, serves as a model system to consider possible ramifications of clinical androgen therapy.   From the ovarian independent persistent vaginal cornification in mice exposed postnatally to estrogen (Bern et al., 1973), one might have predicted the occurrence of clear cell carcinoma of the vagina in women exposed prenatally to diethylstilbestrol (DES).  Whether the actions of androgen during the developmentally early sexual differentiation of the brain have a similar predictive value for androgen therapy remains to be determined.

## SEXUAL DIFFERENTIATION

In terms of the reproductive system, i.e., the internal sex organs (other than the gonads) and the genitalia, nature's blueprint for the mammal is female.   At fertilization, genomic events determine whether the zygote is male (XY) or female (XX) and the presence of a testis determining factor on the Y chromosome leads to the development of testes; and the role of the testes is critical for masculine sexual differentiation.   The testes produce Mullerian Duct Inhibiting Hormone which suppresses the development of this duct's derivatives (oviduct, uterus, and the deepest part of the vagina), and testosterone, which stimulates Wolffian Duct derivatives (epididymis, ductus deferens [vas], and seminal vesicles).  Enzymatic reduction of testosterone yields dihydrotestosterone (DHT), the hormone which

*Pharmacology, Biology, and Clinical Applications of Androgens*, edited by Shalender Bhasin et al.
ISBN 0-471-13320-5 © 1996 Wiley-Liss, Inc.

masculinizes the human male's external genitalia. Since nature's blueprint for the reproductive system is female, no major hormonal action appears to be necessary for the development of the female system, although this conclusion may not actually apply to the brain (see below).

A very similar process applies to the brain, at least in animals such as the rat, mouse, hamster and gerbil. Since it is not possible to provide an exhaustive list of citations to the literature in this brief review, the reader is referred to recent reviews for more complete documentation of the statements presented here (Döhler, 1991; Gorski, 1991, 1995; vom Saal et al., 1992). It is essentially proven that in these animals, functional characteristics of the brain that are typical of the male are imposed on the brain by testicular hormones acting during a critical developmental period which, in the rat, is perinatal. A host of functional parameters which are sexually dimorphic in adults, undergo this process of testicular hormone-dependent sexual differentiation. In rats, these include the potential to display masculine or feminine copulatory behaviors, the activity of a cyclic neural system which responds to estrogen by triggering a surge in gonadotropin-releasing hormone which in turn induces a surge of luteinizing hormone and ovulation. However, sexual differentiation also applies to the regulation of food intake and body weight, play behavior and learning performance and perhaps strategies (Williams and Meck, 1991).

Males and females of most species differ in a number of functional domains, but it is important to differentiate between functional sex differences imposed on the brain by the transient, or activational, effects of ovarian or testicular hormones, and those that are permanent, and the consequence of the organizational effects of gonadal steroids. Although this concept of activational versus organizational effects of these hormones on the brain was initially defined in behavioral terms, over time morphological effects of gonadal steroids were included in the organizational concept. Although there are distinct morphological components of brain sexual differentiation, as will be discussed below, it is no longer tenable to restrict the ability of gonadal hormones to modify neural morphology to the period or process of sexual differentiation.

Currently, there are over 12 reports of different structural sex differences in the central nervous system in terms of nuclear or regional volume and another 10 in terms of synaptic organization, just in the rat (Gorski, 1995). Moreover, it is likely that these numbers will increase with further research. One structural sex difference, the sexually dimorphic nucleus of the preoptic area (SDN-POA), has been studied rather extensively and has served as a model system to access possible mechanisms of hormone action on the structure of the developing brain. Moreover, as will be discussed below, the concept of the SDN-POA has, perhaps prematurely, been applied to the human brain. The SDN-POA and most of the reported volumetric sex differences in the rat brain, are larger in the male. Exceptions are the locus coeruleus (Guillamón et al., 1988), the parastrial nucleus (del Abril et al., 1990) and the anteroventral periventricular nucleus (AVPV; Bleier et al., 1982; Bloch and Gorski, 1988), which are larger in females.

The SDN-POA is clearly hormone-dependent although it must be emphasized that under physiological conditions, factors other than hormones, perhaps genomic factors, may play a role in SDN-POA development. However at least under the specific conditions of prolonged exposure perinatally to exogenous testosterone, hormones alone are sufficient to masculinize this nucleus fully (Döhler et al., 1982a). Note, however, that DES is as effective as testosterone (Döhler et al., 1982b). Although this masculinizing effect of estrogen initially came as somewhat of a surprise, it is now well documented that the masculinizing hormone of the rat brain is indeed estradiol, formed by the intraneuronal aromatization of testosterone secreted by the testes.

When RIAs were developed for steroid hormones, it was found that estrogen titers in the plasma of neonatal rats, both male and female, are high (Weisz and Gunsalus, 1973). Since estrogen appears to be the masculinizing hormone, this observation seemed to challenge the concept of the estrogen-dependent sexual differentiation of the rat brain. However, in rats, a liver protein, alpha fetoprotein (AFP) binds estradiol and has been proposed to protect the brain of both the female and male from the neural action of these high plasma titers of estrogen. However, the results of several experiments suggest that estrogen may, in fact, be required for the *normal development* and/or maturation of the female brain. In fact, it has been proposed that the actual role of AFP is, in animals in which the process of the sexual differentiation of the brain extends beyond parturition, to deliver estrogen to the brain so that female development can occur normally. Since AFP does not bind testosterone, in males this testicular hormone can enter neurons and be converted to additional estrogen which masculinizes the brain. It still has not been determined which of these processes really occurs; protection of the inherently feminine brain by AFP which binds and functionally sequesters estrogen, or the delivery by AFP of estrogen at a level that is required for the normal development of the female brain from a neuter or undifferentiated state. Whatever the role of estrogen in the female brain, both hypotheses propose that the *masculinization* of the brain in males is due to the action of estradiol derived from the aromatization of testosterone secreted by the testes.

Although the focus of this discussion is on androgen, the fact that at least in some processes, we are actually dealing with estrogen, is in the present context, not particularly significant. The enzyme aromatase will act on its substrate, testosterone, whether it is endogenous or administered during therapy! What does matter is whether or not the aromatization hypothesis applies to the sexual differentiation of the human brain, a question which in this author's opinion still remains unanswered.

The potential mechanism(s) of the action of testosterone-derived estrogen remains an area of active investigation. It is currently believed that steroid exposure prevents or limits neuronal death during development. However, this is most certainly not the only mechanism. The AVPV, for example, is larger in volume in females and rendered smaller by androgen exposure of the female (Ito et al., 1986). This observation is hardly compatible with the view that androgen exposure always prevents neuronal death. However, it also appears that the sex difference in AVPV volume does not develop until much later in development, i.e., peripubertally (Davis et al., 1993). It clearly appears that the mechanisms of the sexual differentiation of the SDN-POA and AVPV are different.

## SEX DIFFERENCES IN THE HUMAN BRAIN

Structural sex differences in the human brain do appear to exist. In terms of the hypothalamus, several structural sex differences have been reported. In fact, Hofman and Swaab (1989) have reported the existence of an SDN-POA in the human hypothalamus; it is larger in volume in males and contains more neurons than in females. However, in an independent study, Allen et al., (1989) evaluated four small nuclei which they labeled interstitial nucleus of the anterior hypothalamus (INAH), one-through-four. They found INAH-2 and INAH-3 to be larger in volume in males. These authors also believe that INAH-1, which they did not find to be sexually dimorphic, is the same nucleus called the SDN-POA by Hofman and Swaab (1989). This apparent discrepancy may relate to differences in analytical methods used in the two studies, or to the subjects whose brain tissue was analyzed. Study of detailed human brain anatomy may be complicated by possible degenerative changes that occur between the time of death and the fixation of brain tissue, which also must occur by diffusion rather than perfusion. Subsequently, LeVay (1991), using the methodology of Allen et al., (1989), confirmed that INAH-3 is larger in men than in women. He also confirmed that INAH-1 and INAH-4 are not sexually dimorphic. However, he did not find a significant sex difference in the volume of INAH-2. Given the potential problems with fixation of human brain tissue, subtle neuropathology and perhaps some variation in the human brain, depending on social or environmental factors, the reported sex differences in human brain structure must be confirmed by at least several independent laboratories and on independent groups of subjects from diverse social backgrounds.

As in the rat, a darkly-staining component of the bed nucleus of the stria terminalis has been reported to be larger in volume in the brains of men (Allen and Gorski, 1990). One indication of the variability in the human brain is the rather large number of studies which failed to confirm an initial report that the corpus callosum (CC) was larger in the human female brain (de Lacoste-Utamsing and Holloway, 1982). (See Hines (1990) and Allen et al., (1991) for a more complete discussion of possible sex differences in the CC.) In these various studies, the methods of analysis of regional variations in the CC were not always the same, nor were subjects of the two sexes necessarily age-matched. There are changes in the brain, and in the CC with aging, and although chronological age may not be the best index of the aging process, age-matching is the best tool currently available to control for age-related changes. Allen et al., (1991) analyzed the CC from magnetic resonance images of living individuals and used both published procedures to subdivide the CC into various regions and found no statistically significant sex differences. However, the posterior fifth of the CC, called the splenium, was more bulbous in shape in women than in men. This difference in shape could be due to the number of axons, their size and/or their degree of myelinization.

Another fiber pathway like the CC, but much smaller, is the anterior commissure (AC). Allen and Gorski (1991) reported the midsagittal area of the AC to be significantly larger in women. Finally, the massa intermedia, which connects the right and left hypothalamus across the third ventricle, is more often present in women, and when present in both sexes, is larger in area in women (Allen and Gorski, 1991).

The reported structural sex differences in the human brain are much smaller than many of those in the rat brain, especially the SDN-POA. They are also much more controversial and clearly in need of replication. Furthermore, there is no evidence that these structural sex differences are, or are not, influenced by hormones. Human beings live under dramatically different social and cultural conditions and these conditions might possibly affect brain structure.

## STRUCTURAL DIFFERENCES IN THE BRAIN OF THE MALE HOMOSEXUAL

Although an understanding of sex differences in the structure of the rat brain and how they arise is of value in and of itself, it is hoped that such understanding will also help scientists unravel the mysteries of the human brain. In this regard, if gonadal hormones masculinize the human brain, then the rat might be considered a useful model for understanding transsexualism, where an individual feels trapped in the body of the wrong sex. But what about the homosexual? It is clear that most homosexual men consider themselves male, and lesbians consider themselves female. How then could hormone-induced sexual differentiation of the brain contribute to the development of homosexuality?

In this regard, the results of studies of experimental animals strongly suggest that the process of sexual differentiation of the brain is divided into independent components: masculinization, de-feminization, de-masculinization and feminization. Thus, it is possible that some temporary alteration in hormone production by a fetus, or some perturbation of the pregnant woman (e.g., stress, drugs) might alter only one component of sexual differentiation, or perhaps only one facet of that component. Whether such an alteration could contribute to the development of homosexuality is currently purely speculative. Nevertheless, structural differences have been observed between the brains of homosexual and presumably heterosexual men. In fact, there have been four such reports.

The suprachiasmatic nuclei (SCN), which appear to regulate circadian rhythmicity, are larger and contain more neurons in homosexual men than in heterosexual men or women (Swaab and Hofman, 1990). However, this nucleus does not appear to differ in size between men and women (Hofman et al., 1988). Moreover, the SCN in the human brain is not prominent in Nissl preparations and the nucleus was identified, at least in part, by immunohistochemical staining for vasopressin. Currently, it is known that neuropeptide expression by neurons can be state dependent. Thus, it is possible that homosexual men may differ in terms of vasopressin expression rather than neuroanatomically. The second observation was that of LeVay (1991), who reported INAH-3 to be smaller in homosexual men than in apparently heterosexual men. Although the general region of the hypothalamus in which INAH-3 is located, has been implicated in the control of reproductive behavior in several species, there is no evidence to suggest that INAH-3 *per se* plays such a role, and no evidence that the volume of INAH-3 may be causally related to homosexuality. Since brain structure can be modified by experience and the environment, it may be that the volume of INAH-3 reflects a person's life style rather than causing it.

The mid-sagittal area of the AC is larger in women than in men (Allen and Gorski, 1991), and possibly even larger in homosexual men (Allen and Gorski, 1992). In this study there was a sufficient number of homosexual men who did not have AIDS (six), and an equal number of heterosexual men who did have this disease to analyze the data statistically; there was no indication that this disease affected the mid-sagittal area of the AC. The most recent report in this area adds yet another potential level of complexity - handedness. It was reported that the isthmus of the CC in right-handed homosexual men was significantly, although only borderline so, larger than that of right-handed heterosexual men (Scamvougeras et al., 1994). Since there may be some relationship between handedness and homosexuality (McCormick et al., 1990), the three previous studies, in which handedness was not taken into account may be misleading. However the relationship between left-handedness (defined as non-consistent right-handedness) and homosexuality is not particularly robust.

## ARE MORPHOLOGICAL EFFECTS OF GONADAL STEROIDS ON THE BRAIN RESTRICTED TO THE DEVELOPMENTAL PERIOD OF SEXUAL DIFFERENTIATION?

It is clear from the literature briefly reviewed above that in a number of mammalian species, exposure to testicular hormones during development leads to a masculine brain both in terms of its functional capacity and its structure. This process has led to the concept of the organizational and activational effects of gonadal hormones on the brain. If a woman abuses androgens or for whatever reason is given androgen therapy early in pregnancy, one might predict alterations in the sexual differentiation of her child's brain; but this must be viewed as relatively uncommon. However, the role of gonadal hormones in the sexual differentiation of the brain demonstrates the malleability of brain structure in the presence or absence of gonadal hormones. As indicated above, the permanent or organizational actions of testicular hormones have come to mean, at least in part, structural changes. During development, various tissues, including regions of the brain, undergo the process of "programmed cell death." Thus, during development, hormones may help determine which neurons survive this process and which die, but what about synaptology and connectivity of neurons which survive this process of cell death? Could it be that throughout life, there is the potential for hormone-dependent re-sculpturing of the detailed anatomy of the CNS? Would one expect androgen therapy in the adult to modify CNS structure?

The answer appears to be, Yes. Modification of neuronal structure is not limited to the period of sexual differentiation and need not be permanent, i.e., organizational. The CNS has a relatively high degree of plasticity in response to hormones, and androgen therapy can be expected to influence neuronal structure even in the adult.

Just as the process of the sexual differentiation of the brain offers a model of the potential morphological effects of gonadal hormones on the CNS, the songbird brain may serve as a model of similar hormonal effects during adult life. Within the song system of the zebra finch brain, there are a number of structural sex differences, some of which are quite marked (Nottebohm and Arnold, 1976). In this species only the males sing. Importantly, for our current consideration, during the non-breeding season the testes become quiescent and there is a decrease in the size of these brain regions. As the next breeding season approaches and the testes become active, brain nuclear volume increases, dendrites lengthen, and new synapses are formed (Nottebohm, 1981; DeVoogd, 1991)!

In rats, regeneration of the transected hypoglossal nerve is facilitated by androgen exposure (Yu and Yu, 1983). Even structures such as the SDN-POA (Bloch and Gorski, 1988) and its apparent homologue in the gerbil (Commins and Yahr, 1984), and the AVPV (Bloch and Gorski, 1988) can change in volume following hormonal manipulations. Such a change in volume may simply relate to a reduction in soma size due to inactivity, but it appears likely that such changes also reflect changes in synaptology (Arnold, 1992; Matsumoto, 1992). The ultimate in the malleability or plasticity of neuronal structure may be the observation that, at least within the hippocampus (Woolley and McEwen, 1992), there is significant remodeling of synapses over the course of the short estrous cycle in rats!

Thus, it appears quite likely that androgen therapy will alter CNS morphology even in adults. In aging men, one might expect androgen therapy to slow or even reverse CNS changes, due to the gradual fall in testosterone. Presumably, this might be beneficial. But what about the postmenopausal woman given androgen? In this author's opinion there is even a potential, more susceptible period of time: the peripubertal period.

In the field of the sexual differentiation of the brain, most emphasis has been placed on early development: the prenatal period in human beings, and in rats, the perinatal period. In one sense, scientists are forced to emphasize these periods to most clearly distinguish developmental or organization affects from those that are considered activational. However, given the more recent evidence of morphological effects of gonadal hormones during adulthood, one is forced to consider the time of puberty, when marked physical changes occur in the body and marked emotional changes related to sexual interest and arousal occur in the mind, as a time when gonadal hormones could have marked structural effects, probably not the survival or death of neurons, but certainly their connectivity. With the present focus on the effects of hormones early in development, there has been too little study of the possible effects of hormones at the time of puberty. Puberty may well be the time when the process of the sexual differentiation of the brain is completed or finalized.

Androgen therapy given to the adolescent must be carefully monitored, although, unfortunately, it may take years for any effects on personality, cognition, or sexual activity to appear. The psychological effects of markedly delayed puberty may well be traumatic and damaging, but it is quite possible that androgen therapy at this time will do more than mature the genitalia.

## SUMMARY

During the process of the sexual differentiation of the brain, testicular hormones exert profound effects on the CNS, including its very structure. The potential consequences to the child of a pregnant woman exposed to androgens are obvious, but such treatment is likely to be infrequent. The results of studies of the effects of gonadal hormones on the adult brain strongly suggest that the brain maintains a degree of hormonal plasticity throughout life. Androgen therapy in aging men might be assumed to stop or even reverse changes due to the gradual decrease in endogenous androgen levels. Androgen therapy in postmenopausal women is less predictable as to its effects on brain structure and function. Perhaps the most vulnerable time, other than the prenatal period, would be peripubertally. Obviously, clinicians cannot ignore prolonged puberty because of the psychological problems this can cause the individual and family. Nevertheless, further research is clearly needed to determine whether androgen therapy during this period will or will not produce alterations in brain structure, alterations that may well affect cognition, aggression, or sexual behavior, if not other factors such as personality.

## REFERENCES

Allen LS, Gorski RA (1990): A sex difference in the bed nucleus of the stria terminalis of the human brain. J Comp Neurol 302:697-706.

Allen LS, Gorski RA (1991): Sexual dimorphism of the anterior commissure and massa intermedia of the human brain. J Comp Neurol 312:97-104.

Allen LS, Gorski RA (1992): Sexual orientation and the size of the anterior commissure in the human brain. Proc Nat Acad Sciences USA 89:7199-7202.

Allen LS, Hines M, Shryne JE, Gorski RA (1989): Two sexually dimorphic cell groups in the human brain. J Neurosci 9:497-506.

Allen LS, Richey MF, Chai YM, Gorski RA (1991): Sex differences in the corpus callosum of the living human being. J Neurosci 11:933-942.

Arnold AP (1992): Hormonally-induced alterations in synaptic organization in the adult nervous system. Exp Gerontology 27:99-110.

Bern HA, Gorski RA, Kawashima S (1973): Long-term effects of perinatal hormone administration. Science 181:189-190.

Bleier R, Byne W, Siggelow I (1982): Cytoarchitectonic sexual dimorphisms of the medial preoptic and anterior hypothalamic areas in guinea pig, rat, hamster and mouse. J Comp Neurol 212:118-130.

Bloch GJ, Gorski RA (1988): Estrogen/progesterone treatment in adulthood affects the size of several components of the medial preoptic area in the male rat. J Comp Neurol 275:613-622.

Commins D, Yahr P (1984): Adult testosterone levels influence the morphology of a sexually dimorphic area in the Mongolian gerbil brain. J Comp Neurol 224:132-140.

Davis EC, Elihu N, Shryne JE, Gorski RA (1993): Evidence for post-pubertal onset of the volumetric sexual dimorphism and post-pubertal growth of the anteroventral periventricular nucleus of the rat hypothalamus. Soc Neurosci Abstr 19:1312.

del Abril A, Segovia S, Guillamón A (1990): Sexual dimorphism in the parastrial nucleus of the rat preoptic area. Dev Brain Res 52:11-15.

de Lacoste-Utamsing C, Holloway RL (1982): Sexual dimorphism in human corpus callosum. Science 216:1432.

DeVoogd TJ (1991): Endocrine modulation of the development and adult function of the avian song system. Psychoneuroendocrinology 16:41-66.

Döhler KD (1991): Pre- and postnatal influence of hormones and neurotransmitters on sexual differentiation of the mammalian hypothalamus. Internat Rev Cytology 131:1-57.

Döhler KD, Coquelin A, Davis F, Hines M, Shryne JE, Gorski RA (1982a): Differentiation of the sexually dimorphic nucleus in the preoptic area of the rat brain is determined by the perinatal hormone environment. Neurosci Lett 33:295-98.

Döhler KD, Hines M, Coquelin A, Davis F, Shryne JE, Gorski RA (1982b): Pre- and postnatal influence of diesthystilbestrol on differentiation of the sexually dimorphic nucleus in the preoptic area of the female rat brain. Neuroendocrinol Lett 4:361-365.

Gorski RA (1991): Sexual differentiation of the endocrine brain and its control. In Motta M (ed): "Brain Endocrinology." New York: Raven Press, pp. 71-104.

Gorski RA (1995): Gonadal hormones and the organization of brain structure and function. In Magnusson D (ed): "Nobel Symposium: Life-span Development of Individuals: A Synthesis of Biological and Psychological Perspectives." New York, Cambridge University Press (in press).

Guillamón A, De Blas MR, Segovia S (1988): Effects of sex steroids on the development of the locus coerulus in the rat. Develop Brain Res 40:306-310.

Hines M (1990): Gonadal hormones and human cognitive development. In Balthazart J (ed): "Hormones, Brain and Behavior in Vertebrates. 1. Sexual Differentiation, Neuroanatomical Aspects, Neurotransmitters and Neuropeptides. Basel: Karger, pp.51-63.

Hofman MA, Swaab DF (1989): The sexually dimorphic nucleus of the preoptic area in the human brain: a comparative morphometric study. J Anat 164:55-72.

Hofman MA, Fliers E, Goudsmit E, Swaab DF (1988): Morphometric analysis of the suprachiasmic and paraventricular nuclei in the human brain. J Anat 160:127-143.

Ito S, Murakami S, Yamanouchi K, Arai Y (1986): Perinatal androgen exposure decreases the size of the sexually dimorphic medial preoptic nucleus in the rat. Proc Japan Academy 62:408-411.

LeVay S (1991): A difference in hypothalamic structure between heterosexual and homosexual men. Science 253:1034-1037.

Matsumoto A (1992): Hormonally induced synaptic plasticity in the adult neuroendocrine brain. Zool Science 9:679-695.

McCormick CM, Witelson SF, Kinstone E (1990): Left-handedness in homosexual men and women: neuroendocrine implications. Psychoneuroendocrinol 15:69-76.

Nottebohm, F (1981): A brain for all seasons: cyclical anatomical changes in song control nuclei of the canary brain. Science 214:1368-1370.

Nottebohm F, Arnold AP (1976): Sexual dimorphism in vocal control areas of the songbird brain. Science 194:211-213.

Scamvougeras A, Witelson SR, Bronskill M, Stanchev P, Black S, Cheung G, Steiner M, Buck B (1994): Sexual orientation and anatomy of the corpus callosum. Soc Neurosci Abstr 20:1425.

Swaab DF, Hofman MA (1990): An enlarged suprachiasmatic nucleus in homosexual men. Brain Res 537:141-148.

vom Saal FS, Montano MM, Wang MH (1992): Sexual differentiation in mammals. In: Colborn T, Clement C (eds): "Chemically-induced alterations in sexual and functional development: the wildlife/human connection." Princeton, Princeton Scientific Pub, pp 17-83.

Weisz J, Gunsalus P (1973): Estrogen levels in immature female rats: true or spurious-ovarian or adrenal? Endocrinology 93:1057-1065.

Williams CL, Meck WH (1991): The organizational effects of gonadal steroids on sexually dimorphic spatial ability. Psychoneuroendocrinol. 16:155-176.

Woolley CS, McEwen BS (1992): Estradiol mediates fluctuation in hippocampal synapse density during the estrous cycle in the adult rat. J Neurosci 12:2549-2554.

Yu WA, Yu MC (1983): Acceleration of the regeneration of the crushed hypoglossal nerve by testosterone. Exp Neurol 80:349-360.

# 17

# ANDROGENS AND COGNITIVE FUNCTION

**Gerianne M. Alexander**

**Department of Psychology**
**University of New Orleans**
**New Orleans, Louisiana**

## INTRODUCTION

Research in animals has established that androgens influence the development of sex-typed behavior, including reproductive function and nonreproductive behaviors, such as complex maze learning and juvenile play (Beatty, 1984; Hines and Green, 1991). In humans, the possibility that androgens may also mediate sex-typed functions is consistent with findings that, in hypogonadal men, behaviors such as sexual desire and sexual fantasy depend on critical amounts of the hormone in adulthood ( O'Carroll et al., 1985). Other evidence suggests that androgens influence a masculine cognitive style characterized by high visuospatial ability and low verbal ability in men relative to that in women (Christiansen and Knussman, 1987). However, one area of current debate is the nature of the association between normal levels of androgens in adulthood and spatial function, which is variously proposed to be linear (Christiansen and Knussman, 1987) and curvilinear (Gouchie and Kimura, 1991). A third possibility is that there is a threshold effect of androgens on male behavior, similar to that proposed to explain most androgen-sexual behavior relations in men (Bancroft, 1988). According to the threshold property proposal, increments in levels of androgens above the bottom of the normal physiological range have no further enhancing effects on cognitive behavior.

## EVIDENCE OF TESTOSTERONE-COGNITIVE BEHAVIOR RELATIONS

### Animal Research

Research in rats has documented sex differences in behavioral processes underlying spatial memory (Williams and Meck, 1993). The use of a masculine strategy (i.e., use of geometric cues) is dependent on exposure to androgens during neonatal development (Williams et al., 1990). Testosterone (T) aromatized to estradiol appears to organize spatial function in the developing male by influencing

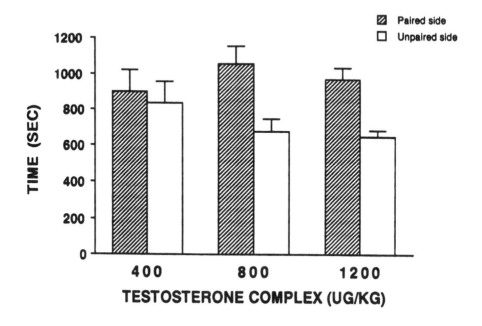

Figure 1. Testosterone Complex (UG/KG)

the development of brain structures subserving spatial function (e.g., hippocampus) (Williams and Meck, 1993; Roof and Havens, 1992). Experimental manipulation of androgen levels in adulthood does not affect the processing of spatial information, suggesting that, unlike sexual behavior, spatial function does not require exposure to critical amounts of hormone in adulthood (Williams and Meck, 1993)

Recently, we found evidence suggesting changes in androgen levels in adulthood may influence cognitive behavior in some instances. An effect of T on learning in male rats was observed in a study of the affective properties of the hormone (Alexander et al., 1994a). In that study, we employed the conditioned-place-preference paradigm, a procedure commonly used to evaluate the affective properties of other substances, such as psychostimulants (Reicher and Holman, 1977). The place-preference apparatus was a large box consisting of two conditioning compartments (one black and one white) and a smaller, central connecting compartment. Animals were randomly assigned to a pairing compartment (black or white) and an injection order (hormone on even days, or saline on even days). We induced acute elevations of plasma T in intact male rats by systemic administration of a recently developed testosterone-hydroxypropyl-B-cyclodextrin inclusion complex. This me-thod of hormone delivery results in a rapid increase in plasma T, with maximal serum concentrations in rats, peaking within one hour and decreasing to preinjection levels after about three hours (Taylor et al., 1989). Injections of saline or T-complex were administered before exposure to the pairing compartment. For example, if an animal received hormone injection prior to exposure to the black compartment, then it received saline injections before exposure to the white compartment on the subsequent day. In all, there were six hormone pairings and six saline pairings. On the test day, no hormones were injected and animals were allowed to move freely in the three compartments for 30 minutes.

In the conditioned-place-preference task, a drug's rewarding properties are inferred when animals spend more time during a drug-free test session in a location that was previously paired with drug treatment than in a location paired with administration of a vehicle solution. We found that male rats prefer the location where they previously received injections of the T-complex over the location where they previously received injections of saline (Figure 1). The finding that animals approach previously neutral stimuli (i.e., a distinct location) previously paired with T administration shows that the hormone has rewarding affective properties. This is consistent with human research showing positive correlations between rises in plasma T and self-reports of elation in male athletes (Booth et al., 1989) and with the proposal that anabolic steroids may have addictive properties and abuse potential in humans (Kashkin and Kleber, 1989).

The learning requirements of the place preference task must also be emphasized (Carr et al., 1989), as no hormone is injected on the test day, animals must associate specific cues in the apparatus with the rewarding affective properties of T to display a place preference. Given evidence of surges in T that normally occur following sexual activity in male rats (Harding, 1981), we suggest T may also facilitate the acquisition or expression of learned associations between previously neutral stimuli, such as environmental cues, and sexual activity.

Further support for a role of acute changes in gonadal hormones in animal learning comes from a recent study of estradiol and spatial memory. Briefly, we found that post-training intrahippocampal injection of an estradiol-complex enhanced spatial memory in intact male rats (Alexander et al., 1994b). These enhancing effects of estradiol on spatial learning are consistent with the proposal that T-derived estradiol determines sex differences in spatial function (Williams and Meck, 1993).

In sum, animal research supports an organizational effect of androgens on spatial function. These studies suggest that manipulations of absolute levels of hormones in adulthood (i.e., castration and hormone replacement) do not affect spatial processing in male rats. However, recent evidence suggests that manipulation of hormone levels in adulthood has affective properties (Alexander et al., 1994a) and facilitates memory storage processes (Alexander et al., 1994b).

## Human Research

In general, men perform visuospatial tasks more accurately than do women, whereas women excel at verbal tasks (Linn and Petersen, 1985; Maccoby and Jacklin, 1974). Nonhormonal factors, such as sex differences in play experiences, may facilitate the acquisition or development of spatial function and may contribute to sex differences on visuospatial tasks ( Serbin and Connor, 1979). However, in females exposed prenatally to levels of androgens usually associated with male development because of congenital adrenal hyperplasia, enhanced visuospatial ability has been reported (Resnick et al., 1986). Moreover, in males presumably exposed to low levels of androgens during perinatal period because of idiopathic hypogonadotrophic hypogonadism, reduced visuospatial ability are found (Hier and Crowly, 1982). These studies support the hormonal hypothesis that differential exposure to androgens during human perinatal development may be one determinant of a masculine cognitive style.

Not all studies of hypogonadal men report diminished spatial function (Cappa et al., 1988). Conflicting evidence of organizational effects of androgens on cognitive behavior from studies of individuals with endocrine disorders may result from undocumented differences in androgen exposure during prenatal periods critical for cognitive development. Lacking precise knowledge of androgen levels during perinatal development, researchers have argued that an understanding of organizational effects of gonadal hormones on human behavior must therefore be based on converging evidence from studies of individuals with a variety of relevant hormone disorders ( Collaer and Hines, 1994). Indirect evidence of organizational effects of androgens on human cognitive behavior comes from research indicating that visuospatial ability and verbal ability may be affected by differential levels of androgens in adulthood (Christiansen and Knussman, 1987). Presumably, these effects occur because gonadal hormones activate neural networks organized early on to show a masculine or feminine cognitive style.

Activational effects of androgens on cognitive behavior were first suggested by studies of T-replacement therapy for hypogonadal men showing that the hormone enhances "cognitive" aspects of sexual behavior. Although hypogonadal men have normal erections to externally produced erotic visual stimuli that are not further enhanced by T (Bancroft and Wu, 1983; Kwan et al., 1983), sexual desire, erotic thought, and imagery are low during placebo conditions and increase with doses of T that induce plasma levels that approach the normal range of values for men (Skakkeback et al., 1981; Salmimies et al., 1982; Bancroft and Wu, 1983; Kwan et al., 1983; O'Carroll et al., 1985; Gooren, 1987). Thus, one suggestion is that cognitive abilities relevant for sexual thought and fantasy, such as visuospatial ability, may be T-dependent.

In women, menstrual cycle studies (Hampson and Kimura, 1988; Hampson, 1990; Silverman and Phillips, 1993) and studies of hormone replacement in menopausal women (Phillips and Sherwin, 1992) suggest that variations in levels of estrogen may influence sex-typed cognitive abilities. In men, research of androgens and cognitive behavior suggests similar effects of T on spatial function. A positive linear relationship between plasma levels of T and visuospatial ability, and a negative linear relationship between T and verbal ability, are documented in studies of European men (Christiansen and Knussman, 1987) and African bushmen (Christiansen, 1993). Positive correlations between visuospatial ability and T levels in a control sample of healthy men, but not in a sample of alcoholic men, are also consistent with a linear relationship between androgens and cognitive behavior (Errico et al., 1992). Other researchers have postulated that high levels of T may have a negative influence on spatial ability and a positive influence on verbal ability in men (Petersen, 1976). This suggests a curvilinear relationship between T and a masculine cognitive style may exist, such that optimal expression of spatial function is possible with mid-level concentrations of T (Andrew, 1978). Recent data provide some support for this notion (Gouchie and Kimura, 1991). A curvilinear association between T and cognitive behavior has also been used to argue a causal relationship between seasonal changes in T (Reinbert and Lagoguey, 1978) and seasonal changes in spatial function (Kimura andToussaint, 1991).

Although there is disagreement regarding the properties of T-cognitive behavior relations, strong evidence supporting the general activational hypothesis comes from a placebo-controlled investigation showing that exogenous T administered to older men with very low endogenous levels of T enhanced performance on the Block Design subtest of the WAIS-R, a measure of visuospatial ability (Janowsky et al., 1994). The activational hypothesis is not consistent with a report that men with acquired hypogonadism have normal male levels of visuospatial ability that are not further enhanced by T (Hier and Crowly, 1982). However, in that study of hypogonadal men, the small number of subjects (n=5) and the use of insensitive measures of spatial ability may have obscured treatment effects (Hines and Green, 1991).

To evaluate hormonal hypotheses of T-cognitive behavior relations in men, we evaluated cognitive abilities in hypogonadal men and healthy men prior to and following administration of exogenous androgens (Alexander et al., 1995). By examining cognitive abilities in these individuals before and after T administration, we could evaluate the *general* proposal that fluctuations in androgen levels in men influence their performance on cognitive tasks (Kimura and Hampson, 1994). The inclusion of both hypogonadal and eugonadal men permitted an examination of the *specific* properties of this relation, namely that cognitive behavior is: (1) dependent on critical amounts of T in adulthood (threshold property); (2) enhanced by increasing concentrations of T (linear property), or (3) optimized at mid-levels of T (curvilinear property). All three proposed relations predict that T replacement therapy will enhance spatial function in hypogonadal men. However, the threshold property proposal predicts that there will be no behavioral changes following administration of T in eugonadal men. Improved and impaired behavioral functioning during T therapy in eugonadal men is predicted by the linear property and curvilinear property proposals, respectively. Regarding organizational effects of androgens on sex-typed cognitive behavior, our sample of hypogonadal men includes hypogonadotropic hypogonadal men and hypergonadotropic hypogonadal men. Reduced spatial function in hypogonadotropic hypogonadal men relative to other men in our study is predicted by current understandings of the organizational effects of hormones on spatial function based on animal and human research (Collaer and Hines, 1994). We also tested, as a comparison group, healthy men who did not receive hormone treatment.

Subjects in the study were recruited from two clinical investigations of the metabolic effects of T conducted at the Division of Endocrinology, (Male Reproductive Research Center), Harbor-UCLA Medical Center, Torrance, CA. In these studies, exogenous T was administered to eugonadal men as a contraceptive or to hypogonadal men as a form of hormone-replacement therapy. In all, 33 hypogonadal men from the hormone-replacement study, 10 healthy men from the contraceptive study, and 19 healthy men who received no hormone treatment completed behavioral testing on two occasions separated by a 6 week interval. A questionnaire battery composed of three types of paper and pencil cognitive measures were administered to men at each of the two sessions. The test battery included tests of visuospatial ability that show sex differences favoring males and tests of verbal ability and perceptual speed that show sex differences favoring females. Measures selected for use are reliable and show consistent sex differences (Linn and Petersen, 1985; Hyde and Linn, 1988; Ekstrom et al., 1976).

Results from the three groups of men did not support the general hypothesis that T may have activational effects on cognitive behavior (Alexander et al., 1995). Measures of perceptual speed did not differ across groups of hypogonadal and healthy men. Moreover, all men showed enhanced performance on perceptual speed tasks, consistent with practice effects. Compared to eugonadal men, hypogonadal men showed poorer performance on measures of visuospatial ability and on measures of verbal fluency. However, deficits in cognitive function were most notable on tasks of verbal fluency. This is consistent with the general conclusion that hormonal deficiencies associated with hypogonadism may contribute to cognitive deficits that are not limited to diminished visuospatial abilities (Collaer and Hines, 1994). Our general finding, that changes in sex-typed cognitive functioning were not associated with hormone treatment, suggests correlations between T and cognitive style may not reflect a causal relationship between hormones and cognitive behavior, as has been recently suggested (Kimura and Hampson, 1994).

One explanation of our results is that measures used in our study may not have been sufficiently sensitive to hormone treatment effects. However, as indicated earlier, measures were selected because they show reliable sex differences. A model of hormonal effects on sex-typed cognitive behavior based on differentiation of male and female phenotypes and of sexual behavior suggests that cognitive measures showing sex differences are likely to be androgen sensitive (Collaer and Hines, 1994). Consistent with this conclusion, hypogonadal men in our study showed deficiencies on measures of verbal ability and spatial ability. We also found that, compared to hypogonadal men with an exclusive heterosexual orientation, hypogonadal men with a bisexual or homosexual orientation performed better on tasks of verbal fluency and less well on tasks of spatial function (Alexander et al., 1995). This finding is consistent with previous reports of associations between spatial abilities and sexual orientation (Gladue, 1994) and with proposals that sex-typed behaviors, such as cognitive style and sexual orientation, are similarly affected by early hormone exposure (Collaer and Hines, 1994; Meyer-Bahlburg et al., 1995).

In sum, our recent study did not support the hypothesis that androgens may activate human cognitive behavior (Alexander et al., 1995). However, our results are consistent with the notion that early hormone exposure may play a role in the development of sex-typed behaviors.

## SUMMARY AND CONCLUSIONS

Animal and human research indicate that androgens may influence the expression of cognitive function. In animals, such as the rat, androgens appear to exert organizational effects on the development of spatial function by means of their conversion to estradiol (Williams and Meck, 1993). In humans, androgens appear to influence the development of sex-typed cognitive functions, including verbal ability and spatial ability; although some evidence suggests that early hormonal deficiencies may result in more general cognitive dysfunction (Collaer and Hines, 1995).

One interpretation of correlational investigations of hormone-cognitive behavior relations in humans is that peripheral levels of T in adulthood can influence performance on cognitive tasks (Kimura and Hampson, 1994). This hypothesis is supported by the finding that T administration to older men enhanced performance on a measure of spatial cognition (Janowsky et al., 1994). However, our recent study of the effects of exogenous T on men's cognitive performance is not consistent with androgens having effects on adult cognition (Alexander et al., 1995).

Our studies of T and learning in male rats (Alexander et al., 1994a; Alexander et al., 1995) suggest one explanation for these discrepant conclusions regarding the role of androgens in adult cognitive behavior. In that research, transient changes in hormone levels enhanced memory and learning. This suggests that cognitive function in humans may also be similarily influenced by changing levels of hormone. Although the cyclic nature of T administration in the study of older men is suggested to have weakened androgen's behavioral effects (Janowsky et al., 1994), our animal data suggest that it may have contributed to the observed changes in spatial function. Cyclicity of hormone release has been proposed to play an important role in the expression of female sexual behavior (Sherwin, 1988). It remains to be decided whether this property is the necessary and sufficient condition in androgen activation of human cognitive behavior.

# REFERENCES

Alexander GM, Packard MG, Hines M (1994a): Testosterone has rewarding affective properties in male rats: Implications for the biological basis of sexual motivation. Behav Neurosci 108: 424-428.

Alexander GM, Packard MG, Nores WL, Olson RD (1994b): Acute administration of estradiol enhances spatial memory in intact male rats. Soc Neurosci Abstr 18: 721.

Alexander GM, Bhasin S, Wang C, Swerdloff RS, Hines M (1995): Effects of exogenous testosterone on sex-typed behavior in eugonadal and hypogonadal men. (Manuscript in preparation)

Bancroft J, Wu FCW (1983): Changes in erectile responsiveness during androgen replacement therapy. Arch Sex Beh 12: 59-66.

Bancroft J (1988): Sexual desire and the brain. Sex Marital Ther 3:11-27.

Beatty WW (1984): Hormonal organization of sex differences in playfighting and spatial ability. Prog Brain Res 61:315-330.

Booth A, Shelley G, Mazur A, Tharp G, Kittok R (1989): Testosterone and winning and losing in human competition. Horm Behav 23: 556-571.

Cappa SF, Guariglia C, Papgno C, Pizzamiglio L, Vallar G, Zoccolotti R, Ambrosi B, Santiemma V (1988): Patterns of lateralization and performance levels for verbal and spatial tasks in congenital androgen deficiency. Beh Brain Res 31:177-183.

Carr GD, Fibiger HC, Phillips AG (1989): Conditioned place preference as a measure of drug reward. In Leiblman JM, Cooper SJ (eds.) "Oxford Reviews in Psychophmarmacology: Vol 1. Neuropharmacological Basis of Reward." New York: Oxford University Press, pp 265-319.

Christiansen K (1993): Sex hormone-related variations of cognitive performance in !Kung San Hunter-Gathers of Namibia. Biol Psychol 27:97-107.

Christiansen K, Knussman R (1987): Sex hormones and cognitive functioning in men. Neuropsychobiology 18:27-36.

Collaer ML, Hines M (1995): Human behavioral sex differences: a role for gonadal hormones during early development? Psychol Bull (in press).

Ekstrom RB, French JW, Harman HH (1976): "Kit of factor referenced cognitive tests". Princton, NJ: Educational Testing Service.

Errico AL, Parsons OA, Kling OR, King AC (1992): Investigation of the role of sex hormone in alcholics' visuospatial deficits. Neuropsychologia 31: 417-426 .

Gladue BA (1994): The biopsychology of sexual orientation. Amer Psychol Soc 3: 150-154.

Gooren LJG (1987): Androgen levels and sex functions in testosterone-treated hypogonadal men. Arch Sex Beh 16: 463-473.

Gouchie C, Kimura D (1991): The relationship between testoterone levels and cognitive ability patterns. Psychoneuroendocrinology 16:323-334

Hampson E (1990): Variations in sex-related cognitive abilities across the menstrual cycle. Brain Cog 14: 26-43.

Hampson E, Kimura D (1988): Reciprocal effects of hormonal fluctuations on human motor and perceptual-spatial skills. Behav Neurosci 102: 456- 459.

Harding CF (1981): Social modulation of circulating hormone levels in the male. Amer Zoo 21: 223-231.

Hier D, Crowly W (1982): Spatial ability in androgen-deficient men. New Engl J Med 306: 1202-1205.

Hines M, Green R (1991): Human hormonal and neural correlates of sex-typed behaviors. Ann Rev Psychiatry, Hyde JS, Linn MC (1988): Gender differences in verbal ability: A meta-anlayses. Psychol Bull 104: 53-69.

Janowsky JS, Oviatt SK, Orwoll ES (1994): Testosterone influences spatial cogntition in older men. Behav Neurosci 108: 325-332.

Kashkin KB, Kleber HB (1989): Hooked on hormones? An anabolic steroid addiction hypothesis. JAMA 262: 3166-3170.

Kimura D, Hampson E (1994): Cognitive pattern in men and women is influenced by fluctuations in sex hormones. Amer Psychol Soc 3:57-61.

Kimura D, Toussaint C (1991): Sex differences in cognitive function may vary with the season. Soc Neurosci Abstr 17: 868.

Kwan M, Greenleaf WJ, Mann J, Crapo L, Davidson JM (1983): The nature of an drogen action on male sexuality: A combined laboratory self-report study on hypogonadal men. J Clin Endocrin Metab 57: 557-562.

Linn MC, Petersen AC (1985): Emergence and characterization of sex differences in spatial ability: A meta-analyses. Child Devel 56: 1479-1498.

Maccoby EE, Jacklin CN (1974): "The Psychology of Sex Differences". Stanford: Stanford University Press.

Meyer-Bahlburg HFL, Ehrhardt AA, Rosen LR, Gruen RS, Veridiano NP, Vann FH, Neuwalder HF (1995): Prenatal estrogens and the development of homosexual orientation. Devel Psychol 31: 12-21.

O'Carroll R, Shapiro C, Bancroft J (1985): Androgens, behavior, and nocturnal erection in hypogonadal men: The effects of varying the replacement dose. Clin Endocrin 23: 527-238.

Petersen AC (1976): Physical androgny and cognitive functioning in adolescence. Devel Psychol 12: 524-533.

Phillips SM, Sherwin BB (1992): Effects of estrogen on memory function in surgically menopausal women. Psychoneuroendocrinology 17: 485-495.

Reicher MA, Holman EW (1977): Location preference and flavor aversion rein forced by amphetamine in rats. Anim Learn Behav 5: 343-346.

Reinberg A, Lagoguey M (1978): Circadian and circannual rhythms in sexual activity and plasma hormones (FSH, LH, testosterone) of five human males. Arch Sex Behav 7: 13-30/.

Resnick SM, Berenbaum SA, Gottesman II et al., (1986): Early hormonal influences on cognitive functioning in congenital andrenal hyperplasia. Devel Psychol 22:191-198.

Roof RL, Havens MD (1992): Testosterone improves maze performance and induces development of a male hippocampus in females. Brain Res 572: 310-313.

Salmimies P, Kockett G, Pirke KM, et al., (1982): Effects of testosterone replace ment on sexual behavior in hypogonadal men. Arch Sex Behav 11: 345-348.

Serbin LA, Connor JM (1979): Sex-typing of children's play preferences and patterns of cognitive performance. J Genetic Psychol 134: 1106-1109.

Skakkeback NE, Bancroft J, Davidson DN, Warner P (1981): Androgen replace ment with oral testosterone undecanoate in hypogonadal men: A double blind controlled study. Clin Endocrin 14: 49-61.

Sherwin BB (1988): A comparative analysis of the role of androgen in human male and female sexual behavior: behavioral specificity, critical thresholds, and sensitivity. Psychobiology 16: 416-425.

Silverman I, Phillips K (1993): Effects of estrogen changes during the menstrual cycle on spatial performance. Ethol Sociobiol 14: 257-270.

Taylor GT, Weiss J, Pitha J (1989): Testosterone in a cyclodextrin-containing for mulation: Behavioral and physiological effects of episode-like pulses in rats. Pharm Res 6: 641-646.

Williams CL, Barnett AM, Meck WH (1990): Organizational effects of early gonadal secretions on sexual differentiation in spatial memory. Behav Neurosci 104: 84-97.

Williams CL, Meck WH (1993): Organizational effects of gonadal hormones induce qualitative differences in visuospatial navigation. In M. Haug et al., (eds). "The Development of Sex Differences and Simlarities in Behavior." Netherlands: Kluwer Academic Publishers, pp. 175-189.

—

# 18

# TESTOSTERONE, AGGRESSION, AND DELINQUENCY

**James M. Dabbs, Jr.**

**Department of Psychology**
**Georgia State University**
**Atlanta, Georgia 30303**

## INTRODUCTION

Testosterone has been related to energy, libido, rambunctious activity, a confrontational manner, and generally delinquent and antisocial behavior. A number of these findings are reviewed below. There is a popular belief that testosterone leads directly to aggression, but studies with human subjects have seldom found this to be true (Albert et al., 1993). Aggression is only part of the overall picture relating testosterone to behavior. Connections between testosterone and aggression or other antisocial behavior are very much moderated by social forces.

## CRIMINAL VIOLENCE

Studies of testosterone among prison inmates began in the early 1970's with Kreuz and Rose (1972) and Ehrenkranz et al. (1974) and have continued to the present day (Dabbs et al., 1987, 1988, 1991, 1995). Both the type of crime committed and behavior in prison have been examined. The general conclusion is that higher testosterone individuals are more likely to commit violent crimes, be seen by others as dominant, and get into trouble for misbehavior in prison.

The largest study of criminal behavior included 692 adult male prison inmates (Dabbs et al., In press). Testosterone was assayed from saliva samples, and each inmate was classified as having committed a violent personal crime (mostly homicide, rape, child molestation, assault, robbery), or a nonviolent property crime (mostly theft, burglary, or a drug offense). Inmates were also classified as to whether they had violated prison rules. The bi-serial correlation between testosterone and violence of crime was $r = .17$, $df = 691$, $p < .001$). The bi-serial correlation between testosterone and prison rule violations was $r = .19$, $df = 691$, $p < .001$). Less information is available on female inmates, but the relationships appear to be similar (Dabbs et al., 1988). An unpublished study of 87 adult female inmates by Dabbs and Hargrove supports a structural equation model in which an effect of age is mediated by testosterone level, with higher testosterone individuals committing more violent crimes and being rated as more dominant in prison.

*Pharmacology, Biology, and Clinical Applications of Androgens*, edited by Shalender Bhasin et al.
ISBN 0-471-13320-5 © 1996 Wiley-Liss, Inc.

These findings refer only to criminals in prison. Those who committed violent crimes were, on the average, higher in testosterone than those who committed nonviolent crimes. We do not know whether criminals as a group outside of prison tend to be high in testosterone, although this is plausible however, based on a study of adult delinquents described below (Banks and Dabbs, 1995).

The above findings provide information about average testosterone levels among perpetrators of different kinds of crime. Not everyone who commits the same crime has the same testosterone level. Even if violent criminals are high in testosterone as a group, there will be variation among the individuals within the group. Some rapists are low in testosterone, and some burglars are high. We are examining in detail the parole board records of the circumstances of the crimes committed by the 692 inmates described above. This work is in progress, but initial findings suggest higher testosterone criminals more often know their victims, attack stronger victims, and use excessive violence.

## DELINQUENT AND UNRULY BEHAVIOR

Relatively few people out of the entire population engage in criminal behavior, regardless of their testosterone levels. But many people, with some regularity and frequency, do engage in milder forms of delinquency. Studies relating testosterone to delinquency have been carried out with adults, adolescents, and children.

The Centers for Disease Control (1988) obtained measures of delinquent and antisocial behavior on the 4,662 former U. S. military personnel as part of a study of the Vietnam military experience. The subjects were 33- to 45-year-old men who underwent extensive physical, psychological, neurological, and biochemical testing. Using these data, Dabbs and Morris (1990), and Booth and Osgood (1993), reported relationships between testosterone and delinquency. Higher testosterone men were more likely to have engaged in antisocial behavior, gone AWOL, used marijuana and abused alcohol and hard drugs, and encountered trouble with the law. They more often had tattoos and many sex partners. Risk-ratio analyses indicated these behaviors were 1 1/2 to 2 1/2 times as likely among subjects in the upper ten percent of the testosterone distribution as among the rest of the subjects. Behavior correlated with testosterone is sometimes useful in a military setting. Gimbel and Booth (1994) found higher testosterone soldiers were preferred by commanders for combat assignments.

Terry Banks and I compared testosterone levels in a group of delinquent male and female young urban adults with the levels in a group of college students of similar age (Banks and Dabbs, 1995). The delinquent subjects were a rough bunch. Most of them were frequently involved in fights, several had served prison terms, and at least two had killed someone. Mean testosterone level was higher for the delinquent subjects, males and females, than for the control group of college students.

Olweus and his colleagues found testosterone associated with misbehavior among 14-16 year old school boys, especially when the boys were provoked (Olweus et al., 1988). Udry (1988) found more status violations among boys of this age who were higher in testosterone. Status violations involve behavior in which children do things that are legal for adults but are not legal for children, such as staying out all night, smoking, drinking, and having sex. Booth and Osgood (1993), in an analysis of the backgrounds of veterans in the Vietnam Experience Study, concluded that testosterone at adolescence predicted later difficulties, including problems in school.

Even young children may be affected negatively by testosterone. Dabbs and Morris (1990) found higher testosterone men reported having more problems with conduct disorders when they were children. The presumption is that the men high in testosterone as adults were also high when they were boys, and the testosterone affected their behavior. Others have reported testosterone associated with problem behavior in pre-adolescent children. Kirpatrick et al. (1993) found more learning disabilities associated with testosterone in 6-10 year old children, both boys and girls. Scerbo and Kolko (1993) found similar results in a mixed group of adolescents and younger children. I once assayed salivary testosterone levels in a pair of two- and four-year-old brothers. The younger boy was more active and caused more trouble for his parents, and he was higher in testosterone.

Not all misbehavior rises to the level where it could be called delinquent. Some people are "rambunctious," which means high spirited, exuberant, unruly, or unmanageable. Among twelve fraternities on two university campuses, we found more rambunctious behavior in fraternities that were higher in testosterone (Dabbs, Hargrove and Heusel, 1993). Whether or not rambunctious fraternity men misbehaved to the point of delinquency seemed to depend upon the university at which they were located. In a fraternity, the high testosterone levels of a few members may affect everyone. The behavior of a few high testosterone members may set the overall tone of the group and cause others to behave differently than they would if no high testosterone members were present.

## MARITAL DISTURBANCE

Delinquency and rambunctiousness affects more than the isolated behavior of individuals. It affects their relationships with others, including their friends and family. Julian and McKenry (1989) found high testosterone men were not as close to their wives and children as low testosterone men. Booth and Dabbs (1993), in examining the veterans described above, found high testosterone was a risk factor for marital distress. Men with testosterone levels two standard deviations above the mean, in comparison with those whose levels were two standard deviations below the mean, were 2.0 times as likely to be divorced, 1.8 times as likely to have extramarital sex, and 1.3 times as likely to have physically abused their wives. Low testosterone men in the sample tended to have been married and stayed married, medium testosterone men never to have married at all, and high testosterone men to have married and become divorced. Lower testosterone men appear to be more docile and develop more stable communal relationships.

Testosterone levels are in turn affected by marital relationships. Mazur, in a study of Air Force officers (1994), found changes in testosterone levels followed changes in marital status. Testosterone levels dropped when men married and rose when they divorced. Gubernick et al. (in press) report testosterone levels dropping in men who become fathers, and studies of birds show testosterone levels high in males when they are competing for mates, and low when they need to support their nesting mates and feed their new offspring (Ketterson and Nolan, 1992).

## SMILES, FROWNS, AND ANGER

Short of being overtly antisocial or delinquent, higher testosterone individuals are less friendly and accommodating in their manner and appearance. The most immediate example of this is in smiling. I measured testosterone levels and took portrait photographs of 119 male and 114 female college students (Dabbs et al., 1992). Objective scoring of facial expressions in the photographs showed males who were higher in testosterone had smaller smiles, with less upward and outward movement of the corners of the lips and less crinkling around the corners of the eyes. Females showed no relationship between smiling and testosterone. However, in a more natural discussion group setting, Cashdan (1994) found that higher testosterone females smiled less often. In their study of fraternities, Dabbs et al. (1993) found less smiling in photographs of members of fraternities that had higher mean testosterone levels. Two-thirds of the members of the lowest testosterone fraternity were smiling, in contrast with one-third of the members of the highest testosterone fraternity. The meaning of a smile is ambiguous. More smiling may indicate more good humor and friendliness, but it may also indicate less dominance (Keating, 1985). Individuals who are more powerful and dominant have less need to be pleasant and ingratiate themselves to others. Smiles can let others know that lower status and more submissive individuals pose no threat, and that interactions with them will be friendly and pleasant.

Anger may be tied more closely to testosterone than aggression is. Van Goozen (1994) studied women taking testosterone in preparation for sex change operations. The women reported increased "anger-proneness," a readiness to describe feeling irritated and angry, after they read a vignette about injustice. Anger is more common than aggression, and often anger remains at a private level and is not transformed into aggressive behavior. Actual aggressive behavior is restrained more by learning and by sanctions from others than anger is. Because anger is more common than aggression, there is more of it available to be affected by testosterone. Perhaps high testosterone individuals are not especially aggressive on the average, but they readily become aggressive when the proper circumstances arise. Perhaps they find it easy to be pleasant and relaxed under normal conditions, but find it hard to resist reacting when something irritates them. This would be a pattern reminiscent of the behavior of a high testosterone student who worked for me. He became so angry when he watched the movie, "Natural Born Killers," that he lost his temper and shouted both at his girlfriend and at a panhandler outside the theater.

## AGONISTIC ENCOUNTERS

"Agonistic" referred to athletic contests in ancient Greece. It now refers to any behavior, whether fighting, fleeing, or giving up, that is associated with competition between individuals. Testosterone seems closely linked to agonistic encounters. Testosterone levels are higher in males than females, which suggests these levels evolved out of sexual selection, the process of adapting to reproductive pressures unique to each sex. It is likely that evolutionary pressures included more competition for mates among males (in contrast to competition for resources among females), with higher testosterone males winning out over their competitors. Characteristics that would bring advantage in this arena of competition should include strength, assertiveness, a willingness to fight, persistence, skill at navigating and hunting, and a cognitive style of focused attention on the task at hand.

Testosterone levels rise and fall with success and failure in agonistic encounters. Winners increase in their testosterone levels, and losers decrease (Mazur, 1985). This has been observed in nonhuman primates (Bernstein et al., 1974), in hampsters (Huhman et al., 1991), and in competitors engaged in wrestling matches (Elias, 1981), tennis tournaments (Booth et al., 1989), and chess tournaments (Mazur et al., 1992). It has also been observed in spectators watching their favorite basketball teams win or lose (Berhnardt et al., 1995). It has been observed in Brazilian and Italian fans who watched their countries' teams win and lose, respectively, the 1994 World Cup soccer championship (Fielden et al., 1995). Testosterone levels drop when officers first enter military training boot camp, where their status is suddenly reduced; toward the end of boot camp the testosterone rises back to its pre-camp levels (Kreuz et al., 1971). The same initial drop and subsequent recovery in testosterone has been observed among criminal inmates in a "boot camp" type of prison (Thompson et al., 1990).

We are not sure what function is served by these changes in testosterone around agonistic encounters. It is plausible that higher testosterone resulting from winning will increase the likelihood of winning in the future, and lower testosterone resulting from losing will make one avoid fights in the future. Presumably anger-proneness or readiness for aggression changes along with the changes in testosterone. However, there have been no studies showing that changes in testosterone among human subjects carry over to affect their behavior.

In addition to the effect of winning, the mere present of a threat may increase testosterone levels. Wingfield proposed a "challenge hypothesis" to explain why male birds in the mating season increase more in testosterone when there are other male birds around than when they are alone (Wingfield et al., 1987). Kemper (1990) proposed a similar effect of fighting that would explain why blue collar workers have higher mean testosterone levels than white collar workers, as reported by Dabbs (1992). There are no direct data on this notion from human subjects, although Booth et al. (1989) found testosterone levels increased in competitors just before a tennis tournament.

## SOCIAL INTEGRATION AND CONTROL

Changes in testosterone function as part of a bio-social system. Testosterone is an individual characteristic, but it affects social behavior, and its levels are affected by the outcome of social encounters. Social forces go beyond just changing the level of testosterone; they can amplify, reduce, or modify the effects testosterone has on social behavior. It is a common view among sociologists, going back to Durkheim (1951), that misbehavior is the natural state of human beings, and that social forces restrain this natural tendency and promote good behavior. Studies of both adults and children support this view that social forces play a critical role in moderating the effects of testosterone.

Dabbs and Morris (1990) divided their sample of military veterans into groups low or high in socioeconomic status (SES). They defined high SES as being above the median in both income and education and low SES as being below the median in both income and education. Testosterone predicted delinquency more strongly in the low than in the high SES group. Both Booth and Osgood (1993) and Udry (1988) have found the controlling effects of education are more important for higher testosterone individuals. Low testosterone individuals tend to behave regardless of whether or not social controls are present. High testosterone individuals tend to behave only when these controls are present.

Social controls include all the things that civilize a person, integrating and enmeshing that person into the lives and concerns of others. Sociologists such as Booth et al. (1991) emphasize marital status, job stability, and membership in social organizations that meet regularly. Psychologists such as Kohlberg (1981) emphasize moral development, which is encouraged by a stable family and community. Sociologists and psychologists agree on the importance of child rearing and parental attention. Social forces are more powerful than testosterone. The greater peacefulness of Amish or Quaker communities, in contrast to war-torn communities throughout the world, is probably due to culture more than hormones. Communities that are well integrated and smoothly functioning will restrain disruptive effects of testosterone, and such communities may even direct high testosterone individuals along prosocial courses of development. Communities that are disturbed and disordered will allow more delinquent behavior, and in these communities high testosterone individuals will likely be among those who misbehave first and most. A recent review of intervention programs similar to Headstart (Zigler et al., 1992) suggests they bring more benefit to the social behavior of children than to their intellectual development. Children participating in such programs are less likely to develop behavior problems and run afoul of the law. No study on the topic has been done on the topic, but I suspect high testosterone children benefit more than low testosterone from such programs.

Considering the role of social forces leads to the conclusion that while testosterone may have bad effects, these bad effects are more potential than real. High levels of testosterone do not directly cause misbehavior, although they are risk factors for misbehavior. If we have a high level of testosterone, it helps to have something, either in our conscience or in the community around us, keeping an eye on how we act.

## TESTOSTERONE TREATMENT

Effects of testosterone on behavior are of practical concern to those who would administer testosterone to individuals. Most of the studies reviewed above are correlational ones, dealing with endogenous levels of testosterone, and these studies give us no certain answer about how testosterone treatments might change behavior. Endocrinologists who administer testosterone to patients generally report an increase in libido and sexual activity, sometimes along with increased energy and a more positive mood. However, such observations are usually based on small samples, and the subjects are medical patients rather than randomly selected individuals.

Experimental studies in which normal human subjects are randomly assigned to receive testosterone treatments have been rare. Early studies reported little more than an increase in activity level (Klaiber et al., 1971; McAdoo et al., 1978). Such studies are increasing now, as testosterone therapy increases (Janowsky et al., 1991), and we can expect more and larger studies in the future.

Based on findings reviewed here, we would expect individuals receiving testosterone to feel more energetic. We might also expect them to become a little less docile and manageable and a little more rambunctious. At the extreme, we might expect them to become unfriendly, unruly, or even engage in antisocial behavior. They might show the increase in the anger-proneness reported by van Goozen (1994), with the anger bringing an increased readiness to act and a preference for direct confrontation.

How people respond to testosterone treatments will be affected by the magnitude of the treatments and how long they last. Their responses will also undoubtedly be affected by their personality predispositions and the social forces surrounding them. Because most treatments are relatively brief, in comparison with each individual's years of exposure to endogenous testosterone levels, effects may be smaller than indicated by the correlational studies reviewed here. Because most subjects will not represent the most unruly and delinquent portions of society, the social forces that restrain misbehavior in their everyday lives will continue to restrain misbehavior when they receive testosterone.

Because effects are likely to be small in size, we will need large samples of experimental and control subjects to specify them exactly. Because the exact nature of the effects remains unclear for now, we need to continue developing measures and indicators to quantify them. The measures to be used will emerge as studies progress, and there is no point in trying to make an exhaustive list now, but questionnaires, free-response reports, and behavioral monitoring should be included. Measures of mood and anger-proneness should be used, along with behavioral check lists. Cognitive and neuropsychological tests should also be used, though there has been only limited use of such tests to date in research on testosterone. Cognitive and nouropsychological tests should include measures of spatial and verbal skills, persistence, and divided attention. It would be especially useful to develop measures that can be administered to subjects by mail, phone, or through telecommunication links such as the Internet.

## EFFECT SIZES

The matter of effect size deserves attention. The correlations between testosterone and behavior reviewed here are not high. Most of the correlations are on the order of about $r = .15$ to $r = .20$. The first point to be considered is that correlations are always attenuated by the unreliability of measurements, such that underlying true correlations is always higher than the observed correlations. For example, the true correlation between testosterone and criminal violence will be attenuated by unreliability of single samples of testosterone and single samples of criminal behavior. The reliability of testosterone measurements on the same individuals from day to day is about $r$ = .64 (Dabbs, 1990). The reliability of measurements of criminal behavior is unknown, but it is likely to be even lower. Attenuation of the true correlation is proportional to the square root of the reliability of the two measurements involved, such that in the present case true $r_{12}$ = observed $r_{12}$ / (SQRT ($r_{11}$) * SQRT ($r_{22}$)), where $r_{11}$ is the reliability of the testosterone measurement and $r_{22}$ is the reliability of the measurement of criminal behavior. Adjusting only for unreliability in the testosterone measurement, and ignoring unreliability in the behavioral measurement, an observed correlation of $r$ = .20 reflects an estimated true correlation of $r$ = .26.

A second point is that a correlation of $r$ = .26 explains more behavior than most investigators realize. The usual approach is to take $r^2$ as an index of the percent of variance accounted for, which in the case of $r$ = .26 is less than 7%. A different approach is to use Rosenthal's Binomial Effect Size Display (Rosenthal and Rubin, 1982), which would equate $r$ to the difference in the rate at which high or low testosterone individuals commit violent or nonviolent crimes. Where violent and nonviolent crimes are equal in number, an $r$ of .26 is equivalent to having 63% of the individuals above the median in testosterone and 37% of the individuals below the median in testosterone committing violent crimes. The difference between 63% and 37% is significant by any standard.

A final point is that testosterone is like a batting average. It is only useful in predicting over the long run. We may know that one player has a higher batting average than another. But at any one time at bat, given the vagaries of luck and the nature of the pitcher, game, crowd, sun, wind, and noise, knowing the batting average will not tell us much about whether the batter will hit the ball (Abelson, 1985). Only over the season as a whole will these factors will average out, allowing us to see the true difference between the two players. Something similar holds true with testosterone. Testosterone treatment at a single moment may have little effect, but if we continue the treatment and watch it over time, a picture of its effects will emerge.

## REFERENCES

Abelson RP (1985): A variance explanation paradox: When a little is a lot. Psychological Bulletin 97:129-133 .

Albert DJ, Walsh ML, Jonik RH (1993): Aggression in humans: What is its biological foundation? Neurosci Biobehav Rev 17:405-425.

Banks T, Dabbs JM, Jr (1995): Salivary testosterone and cortisol in a deviant and violent urban subculture. Unpublished manuscript, Georgia State University.

Bernhardt PC, Dabbs JM, Jr., Turner CW, Fielden JA, Lutter C (1995): Testosterone changes during vicarious experiences of victory and defeat in spectators of sporting events. Unpublished manuscript, University of Utah.

Bernstein IS, Rose RM, Gordon TP (1974): Behavioral and environmental events influencing primate testosterone levels. J Hum Evol 3:517-525.

Booth A, Dabbs JM, Jr (1993): Testosterone and men's marriages. Soc Forces 72:463-477.

Booth A, Edwards JN, Johnson DR (1991): Social integration and power. Soc Forces 70:207-224 .

Booth A, Osgood DW (1993): The influence of testosterone on deviance in adulthood: Assessing and explaining the relationship. Criminol 31:93-117.

Booth A, Shelley G, Mazur A, Tharp G, Kittok R (1989): Testosterone, and winning and losing in human competition. Horm Behav 23:555-571.

Cashdan E (1994): Hormones, sex, and status in women. Unpublished manuscript, University of Utah.

Centers for Disease Control (1988): Health status of Vietnam veterans. J Am Med Assn 259:2701-2719.

Dabbs JM, Jr (1990): Salivary testosterone measurements: Reliability across hours, days, and weeks. Physiol Behav 48: 83-86.

Dabbs JM, Jr (1992): Testosterone and occupational achievement. Soc Forces 70:813-824.

Dabbs JM, Jr., Carr TS, Frady RL, Riad JK (In press): Testosterone, crime, and misbehavior among 692 male prison inmates. Pers Indiv Diff.

Dabbs JM, Jr., Frady RL, Carr TS, Besch NF (1987): Saliva testosterone and criminal violence in young adult prison inmates. Psychosom Med 49:174-182.

Dabbs JM, Jr., Hargrove MF, Heusel C (1993): Testosterone differences among college fraternities: Well-behaved vs. rambunctious. Unpublished manuscript, Georgia State University.

Dabbs JM, Jr., Jurkovic GL, Frady RL (1991): Saliva testosterone and cortisol among late adolescent juvenile offenders. J Abnorm Child Psychol 19:469-478.

Dabbs JM, Jr., Morris R (1990): Testosterone, social class, and antisocial behavior in a sample of 4,462 men. Psychol Sci 1:209-211.

Dabbs JM, Jr., Riad JK, Lathangue LA (1992): The harsh facial regard of high estoterone males. Poster presented at American Psychological Association annual convention.

Dabbs JM, Jr., Ruback RB, Frady RL, Hopper CH, Sgoutas DS (1988): Saliva estoterone and criminal violence among women. Pers Indiv Diff 9:269-275.

Durkheim E. (1951): Suicide. Spaulding JA, Simpson, G (trans), New York: Free Press.

Ehrenkranz J, Bliss E, Sheard MH (1974): Plasma testosterone: Correlation with aggressive behavior and social dominance in man. Psychosom Med 36:469-475.

Elias M (1981): Serum cortisol, testosterone, and testosterone-binding globulin responses to competitive fighting in human males. Aggr Behav 7:215-224.

Fielden JA, Lutter C, Dabbs JM, Jr (1995): Basking in glory: Testosterone changes in World Cup soccer fans. Unpublished manuscript, Georgia State University.

Gimbel C, Booth A (1994): Who fought in Vietnam? Unpublished manuscript, Pennsylvania State University.

Gubernick DJ, Worthman CM, Stallings JF (In press): Hormonal correlates of fatherhood in men. Ethol Socio.

Huhman KL, Moore TO, Ferris CF, Mougey EH, Meyerhoff JL (1991): Acute and repeated exposure to social conflict in male golden hampsters: Increases in Plasma POMC-peptides and cortisol and decreases in plasma testosterone. Horm Behav 25:206-221.

Janowsky JS, Oviatt SK, Carpenter JS, Orwoll ES (1991): Testosterone administration enhances spatial cognition in older men. Soc Neurosci Abs 17:340.12.

Julian T, McKenry PC (1989): Relationship of testosterone to men's family functioning at mid-life: A research note. Aggr Behav 15:281-289.

Keating CF (1985): Human dominance signals: The primate in us. In Ellyson SL, Dovidio JF (eds): Power, dominance, and nonverbal behavior. New York: Springer-Verlag.

Kemper TD (1990): Social structure and testosterone: Explorations of the socio-bio-social chain. New Brunswick, NJ: Rutgers.

Ketterson ED, Nolan V, Jr (1992): Hormones and life histories: An integrative approach. Am Nat 140:S1-S62.

Kirkpatrick SW, Campbell PS, Wharry RE, Robinson SL (1993): Saliva testosterone in children with and without learning disabilities. Physiol Behav 53:583-586.

Klaiber EL, Broverman DM, Vogel W, Abraham GE, Cone FL (1971): Effects of infused testosterone on mental performances and serum LH. J Clini Endocrin 32:341-349.

Kohlberg L (1981): The meaning and measurement of moral development. Worcester, MA: Clark University Press.

Kreuz LE, Rose RM (1972): Assessment of aggressive behavior and plasma testosterone in a young criminal population. Psychosom Med 34:321-332.

Kreuz LE, Rose RM, Jennings R (1971): Suppression of plasma testosterone levels and psychological stress. Arch General Psychiat 26:479-482.

Mazur A (1985): A biosocial model of status in face-to-face primate groups. Soc Forces 64:377-402.

Mazur A (1994): The relationship of testosterone and thyroxin to divorce, felony arrest, and alcoholism in a panel study of male Air Force veterans. Unpublished manuscript, Syracuse University.

Mazur A, Booth A, Dabbs JM,Jr (1992): Testosterone and chess competition. Soc Psychol Quar 55:70-77.

McAdoo BC, Doering CH, Dessert N, Brodie HKH, Hamburg DA (1978): A study of the effects of gonadotropin-releasing hormone on human mood and behavior. Psychosom Med 40:199-209.

Olweus D, Mattesson A, Schalling D, Low H (1988): Circulating testosterone levels and aggression in adolescent males: A causal analysis. Psychosom Med 50:261-272.

Rosenthal R, Rubin DB (1982): A simple, general purpose display of magnitude of experimental effect. J Ed Psychol 74:166-169.

Scerbo AS, Kolko DJ (1993): Salivary testosterone and cortisol in disruptive children: Relationship to aggressive, hyperactive, and internalizing behaviors. J Am Acad Child and Adoles Psychol 33:1174-1184.

Thompson WM, Dabbs JM,Jr, Frady RL (1990): Changes in saliva testosterone levels during a 90-day shock incarceration program. Crim Just Behav 17:246-252.

Udry JR (1988): Biological predispositions and social control in adolescent sexual behavior. Am Sociol Rev 53: 709-722.

van Goozen S (1994): Male and female: Effects of sex hormones on aggression, cognition, and sexual motivation. Unpublished doctoral dissertation, University of Amsterdam.

Wingfield JC, Ball GF, Dufty AM,Jr., Hegner RE, Ramenofsky M (1987): Testosterone and aggression in birds. Am Sci 75: 602-608.

Zigler E, Taussig C, Black K (1992): Early childhood intervention: A promising preventative for juvenile delinquency. Am Psychol 47:997-1006.

# 19

# ANDROGEN AND MALE SEXUAL FUNCTION

**F.C.W. Wu**

**Department of Medicine**
**University of Manchester**
**Manchester Royal Infirmary**
**Manchester, England**

## MAJOR ELEMENTS OF HUMAN MALE SEXUAL FUNCTION

Human sexual experience involves a complex series of psychosomatic processes which are inter-linked within a functional cycle. The spontaneous occurrence of sexual thoughts, the awareness of a desire to initiate sexual activity, and the recognition and seeking out of sexual cues, together, determine an individual's readiness to become sexually aroused. This neurophysiological state of central arousability (involving the limbic system) is responsive to, and interacts with, cognitive processes which focus on and translate the sexual meaning of external stimuli (e.g., visual, tactile, and smell) or internal imagery (e.g., sexual fantasies).

As the level of central arousal increases, the peripheral sexual responses are activated via the spinal cord and the autonomic and somatic outflow tracts giving rise to penile erection and other non-genital manifestations of sexual excitement, such as increased blood pressure, heart rate, and skin blood flow. Perception and awareness of these peripheral responses and sexual activity (if it takes place) continue to reinforce the degree of central arousal, culminating in orgasm (an acute increase of erotic sensation accompanied by widespread involuntary muscle contraction) and ejaculation.

## ANDROGENS AND HUMAN MALE SEXUAL FUNCTION

Androgens play a key role in most, if not all, the major elements of male sexuality. Leaving the organizational and development aspects aside in this paper, recent advances in our understanding of the relationship between androgens and the activation of male sexual function can best be addressed through asking the following questions:

*Pharmacology, Biology, and Clinical Applications of Androgens*, edited by Shalender Bhasin et al.
ISBN 0-471-13320-5 © 1996 Wiley-Liss, Inc.

1.    Which components of sexual function are androgen dependent?

2.    How much androgen is required for normal sexual function?

3.    Which androgen is the most important?

4.    Where and how do androgens work in the relevant areas of the brain?

## WHICH COMPONENTS OF SEXUAL FUNCTION ARE ANDROGEN DEPENDENT?

### Sexual Desire

At the last androgen workshop, Julian Davidson reviewed the data from several groups studying the effects of androgen replacement under placebo-controlled conditions in hypogonadal men. He concluded that testosterone is necessary though not sufficient for normal sexual desire in men. There is a robust and consistent dose-response relationship between androgen replacement and increased sexual interest in hypogonadal men. However, it is not clear whether there is a threshold beyond which increased amounts of T will have no effect on sexuality or whether such threshold levels (if they exist) are within or outside the normal physiological range.

### Erectile Function

The relationship between androgens and erectile function is more complex. Spontaneous erections, best illustrated by nocturnal penile tumescence (NPT), are androgen dependent. They are impaired in hypogonadism and improve with androgen replacement. NPT is also impaired in men with low sexual interest. It is therefore thought that measurement of NPT provides a window into the neuro-physiological substrate of central arousal which relates both to spontaneous erectile responsiveness and sexual appetite. In contrast, erectile response to visual erotic stimuli (VES) are not androgen dependent. Normal responses to such stimuli is preserved in hypogonadal men and are not affected by androgen replacement. This led to a convenient conceptual distinction between androgen-dependent and -independent erectile responsiveness with NPT being a measure of spontaneous sexual appetite which is androgen sensitive and VES-evoked response involving a separate androgen insensitive system. However, it now looks as though this distinction between the two erectile response systems is an oversimplification based on earlier studies in which the only parameter of erectile response measured was maximal increase in penile circumference (see below). Recent data obtained by using the rigis-can suggests that in terms of the rigidity, duration of erection, and speed of detumescence, VES-evoked erections are also androgen-responsive, though to a lesser extent than NPT (Carani et al., 1992). Nevertheless, the differences between hypogonadal and eugonadal men and the effects of androgen replacement, were clearly much greater with NPT than with the response to VES. Thus, the distinction between NPT and VES response remain useful conceptually. NPT is unequivocally androgen dependent while VES-evoked erections are mush less so with some parameters, but not others, being influenced by androgens.

## Ejaculation and Orgasm

Ejaculation is androgen dependent because seminal fluid production is androgen sensitive. It is not clear whether androgen is required for normal orgasmic capacity.

## HOW MUCH ANDROGEN IS REQUIRED FOR NORMAL SEXUAL FUNCTION?

Bagatell et al. (1994) studied 10 subjects who were rendered acutely hypogonadal by daily injections of the GnRH antagonist, Nal Glu 75µg/Kg/day. They were compared with the other groups receiving Nal Glu with T enanthate replacement at a physiological (100 mg/week) and subphysiological dose (50 mg/week), and an additional group with T enanthate and the aromatase inhibitor, Testlac. The frequency of sexual desire and fantasy declined significantly by week 4 of GnRH antagonist treatment. T replacement at both doses were able to maintain sexual function and this effect was not affected by the aromatase inhibitor. These results showed that mean plasma T levels of around 9nmol/L (just below the lower limit of normal) were adequate in maintaining normal sexual behavior in acute experimentally-induced hypogonadism. This is in agreement with our previous finding in chronically hypogonadal men (Wu et al., 1982). Moreover, circulating oestradiol appears to have a limited role in the regulation of sexual function in men. Unfortunately, there was no information on NPT or VES-evoked erections in this study.

We have investigated the possible effects of increasing the levels of testosterone on sexual behavior in a placebo-controlled study (Anderson et al., 1991). 32 healthy adult men recruited into a male contraceptive trial were randomized into two groups after a baseline period of observation. 16 subjects received testosterone enanthate 200 mg weekly im for 8 consecutive weeks, while the other 16 were given a placebo injection weekly for the first 4 weeks, followed by TE 200 mg weekly for the next 4 weeks. Testosterone treatment induced a significant increase in sexual arousal compared to baseline and placebo administration. The mean reported frequency of masturbation, intercourse, full spontaneous erections, spontaneous erections, were not affected by testosterone treatment which increased plasma T by at least 2-fold and apparently stimulated sexual interest. These findings suggest that (1) physiological levels of testosterone do not provide a maximal stimulus for sexual interest. (2) While supraphysiological levels of testosterone *can* promote some aspects of sexual arousability, this was not accompanied by changes in overt sexual behavior in eugonadal men in stable heterosexual relationships. Perhaps in this situation, social and relationship factors tend to obscure or restrict the hormone effect.

Patients with 5-αreductase deficiency have normal sexual interest and erection. The use of 5-αreductase inhibitors in men with prostatic cancer causes only a low incidence of sexual dysfunction. These observations suggest that DHT may not play a major role in human sexual function. Although DHT replacement in castrated male monkeys can restore sexual behavior to some extent, similar studies have not been performed in hypogonadal men. The role of DHT in human sexuality, if any, remains unclear at present.

## WHERE AND HOW DO ANDROGENS WORK IN THE RELEVANT AREAS OF THE BRAIN?

Lesions in the medial preoptic area of the anterior hypothalamus (mPOA/AH) of the rat brain produce remarkably consistent deficits in coordinated sexual activity without affecting appetitive or motivational behaviors. In contrast, lesions of the basolateral ventral striatum or basolateral amygdala primarily affect appetitive or instrumental behavior without influencing copulatory activity. There is good experimental evidence in the rat that dopaminergic transmission is critical to these neural circuits connecting basolateral amygdala to the ventral striatum, relaying emotional information to recruit voluntary motor responses. This limbic-motor interphase is therefore important in linking cognitive processes to sexual response and arousal (Everitt and Bancroft, 1991).

In the early 1980s, a series of studies in intact rats clearly demonstrated the sexually enhancing effects of yohimbine, an alpha-2 adrenergic antagonists acting presynaptically (Clark et al., 1984). Yohimbine reduced ejaculatory latency, inter-copulatory interval and post-ejaculatory interval. This enhanced sexual motivation appears to be independent of erection, leading the authors to conclude that alpha-2 adrenergic blockade increases the state of arousal in the intact male rat. Yohimbine also increased dramatically the percentage of male rats displaying mounting and intromissive patterns up to 91 days after castration without any testosterone replacement (Clark et al., 1985). In addition, latencies to mount and intromission were decreased and frequency of copulatory acts increased with yohimbine. These results raised the possibility that androgen effects on sexual behavior could be mediated by specific neurotransmitters, such as noradrenaline. It is interesting to note that yohimbine has been used clinically since the 1920s for treatment of impotence. Results of several recent placebo-controlled studies were consistent in showing modest benefits in subgroups of men with sexual dysfunction (Reid et al., 1987; Sonda et al., 1990). However the etiologies of sexual dysfunction in the study subjects were usually mixed and improvements were based on self-reporting only. Although the results of these studies individually were inconclusive, together they built up a reasonably convincing trend which is compatible with the rodent data. Furthermore, the lack of side effects of yohimbine in men contrasts favorably with the dopaminergic or serotonergic agents.

The question of noradrenergic mediation of androgen action was recently investigated in men using short term IV infusion of a new highly selective alpha-2 antagonist (RS15385) at a low and a high dose to establish plasma concentrations of 50 and 150 ng/ml respectively (Munoz et al., 1994). Instead of using self reporting endpoints, the two distinct systems of VES-evoked and spontaneous erections were monitored in the laboratory under controlled conditions.  It was hypothesized that the antagonist will enhance the androgen-dependent erections i.e., NPT, but not, or to a lesser extent, those evoked by VES. The higher dose infusion increased spontaneous erections before the erotic film presentation.  The duration and rigidity, but not the maximal erectile response to erotic film in 12 normal men, were significantly increased by the drug but only at the high dose.  Sexual arousal before the exposure to the test film was increased by the high dose infusion, but there was no difference in arousal during or at the end of the test.  The effect of the alpha-2 antagonist on NPT was even more complex notwithstanding the drug's influence on sleep directly (Bancroft et al., 1995).  In brief, the low dose infusion increased erections, but only during non REM sleep (which is not usually associated with sleep erections), while the high dose unexpectedly reduced erection, but only during REM sleep.  The only positive effect of the high dose was an increase in spontaneous erection before sleep onset.  Although results obtained in the waking state were generally consistent with the hypothesis, the NPT data showed that spontaneous erections during sleep is probably much more complex than we have envisaged and possibly involve at least two separate noradrenergically mediated systems revealed by the pharmacological challenge at low and high doses (biphasic bell-shaped dose response).  The question of noradrenergic mediation of androgen effects on sexual function at present remains unresolved but the hypothesis certainly has not been rejected.

## CONCLUSIONS

We have advanced from the purely descriptive studies to define aspects of human sexuality influenced by androgens, although there are still unanswered questions, such as the role of DHT and the androgen dependency of orgasm.  Androgen effects on the CNS are manifested mainly as increased arousability across different species.  But in the human, we have the unique opportunity to measure spontaneous arousability by recording NPT, although some of our previous conceptual modeling seems to be an over-simplification.  The comparison (commonality as well as the differences) between animal and human data have already stimulated fruitful investigations, and future studies, especially in the primate, should be useful in testing hypothesis generated in the clinical situation, particularly in anatomical localization and causative relationships.  Conversely, design in human studies should take cognizance of animal data which so clearly distinguished between instrumental and consummatory behaviors.  One obvious experimental paradigm which can be directly translated from animal studies, is to see which aspect of sexual function in hypogonadal men can be restored by neurotransmitter analogues.  This will be very useful in dissecting out the different central response pathways which may have different neurochemical basis.  The availability of new alpha-2 antagonists and the new generation of dopamine agonists will make these neuropharmacological studies of the human sexual response much more accessible.  Technical improvements have provided the clinical investigator now with the instruments to directly measure specific aspects of sexual responsiveness in the laboratory under controlled conditions rather than relying purely on self reporting.  Perhaps in the next androgen workshop, we will be able to address the neurobiological basis of androgen action of the human sexual response.

## ACKNOWLEDGMENT

The author is grateful for helpful discussions with and data made available by Dr. John Bancroft, Kinsey Institute of Sexual Medicine, Bloomington, Indiana, USA. The support of the UNDP/UNFPA/WHO/World Bank Special Program of Research, Development and Research Training in Human Reproduction is also gratefully acknowledged.

## REFERENCES

Anderson RA, Bancroft, Wu FCW (1992): The effects of exogenous testosterone on sexuality and mood of normal men. J Clin Endocrinol Metab 75: 1503-1507.

Bagatell CJ, Heiman JT, Rifier JE, Bremner WJ (1994): Effects of endogenous testosterone and estradiol on sexual behavior in normal young men. J. Clin Endocrinol Metab 78: 711-716.

Bancroft J, Munoz M, Beard M, Shapiro C (1995): The effects of a new alpha-2 adrenergic antagonist on sleep and nocturnal penile tumescence in normal male volunteers and men with erectile dysfunction. Psychosomatic Medicine, in press.

Bancroft J (1989): The biological basis of human sexuality, in Human sexuality and its problems. 2nd ed Churchill Livingstone, Edinburgh pp12-145.

Carani C, Bancroft J, Granata A, Del Rio G, Marrama P (1992): Testosterone and erectile function, nocturnal penile tumescence and rigidity, and erectile response to visual erotic stimuli in hypogonadal and eugonadal men. Psychoneuroendocrinology 17:647-654.

Clark JT, Smith ER, Davidson JM (1984): Enhancement of sexual motivation in male rats by yohimbine. Science 225:847-849.

Clark JT, Smith ER, Davidson JM (1985): Testosterone is not required for the enhancement of sexual motivation by yohimbine. Physiol Behav 35:517-521.

Everitt BJ, Bancroft J (1991): Of rats and men: the comparative approach to male sexuality. Ann Rev Sex Res 2:77-118.

Munoz M, Bancroft J, Turner M (1994): Evaluating the effects of an alpha-2 adrenergic antagonist on erectile function in the human male. 1 The erectile response to erotic stimuli in volunteers. Psychopharmacology 115:463-470.

Reid K, Surridge DHC, Morales A et al. (1987): Double-blind trial of yohimbine hydrochloride in the treatment of psychogenic impotence. Lancet ii: 421-423.

Sonda LP, Mazo R, Chancellor MB (1990): The role of yohimbine for the treatment of erectile impotence. J Sex Marital Ther 16:15-21.

Wu FCW, Bancroft J, Davidson DW, Nicol K (1982): The behavioral effects of testosterone undecanoate in hypogonadal men: a double blind controlled study. Clin Endocrinol 14:49-61.

# PART IV: EFFECTS ON METABOLISM

# 20

# ANDROGEN EFFECTS ON METABOLISM: OVERVIEW

**Shalender Bhasin**

**King-Drew Medical Center**
**Los Angeles, California**

The goal of testosterone replacement therapy is to correct or restore the physiological derangement that results from testosterone deficiency. This metabolic derangement involves many more organ systems than just the changes in serum testosterone levels, changes in gonadotropins concentrations, and sexual dysfunction. In the context of contraceptive regimens that employ testosterone alone or in combination with other gonadotropin inhibitors, a minimal objective is not to perturb the prevailing eumetabolic state. We clearly have not achieved these therapeutic objectives for several complex reasons. First and foremost, testosterone is an important hormone that affects a number of organ systems. In fact, there are few organs that have been shown not to be affected by androgens. Second, testosterone effects on many of these organ systems remain poorly understood and quite controversial. The data are quite conflicting with regard to the testosterone effects on plasma lipids, carbohydrate metabolism, protein metabolism, and coagulation cascade. Third, the methods for quantitating many of these androgen-dependent physiological processes are quite cumbersome and not well standardized or validated. Therefore, these measures have not been widely incorporated into our clinical assessment of the adequacy of replacement therapy.

Testosterone dose dependency of androgen-dependent metabolic processes remains unknown. In the context of testosterone replacement therapy for example, we do not know what serum levels of testosterone we should aim for. In the context of contraceptive regimens that employ testosterone, we remain concerned and uncertain whether testosterone levels required to produce consistent suppression of sperm production will increase or decrease the risk of heart disease through its effects on plasma lipids, insulin sensitivity, and coagulation system. It is also conceivable that these regimens might confer additional benefits in terms of salutary effects on bone mineral metabolism, fat-free mass, and protein synthesis. Data on testosterone effects on plasm lipids derived from experimental trials are in conflict with those derived form epidemiologic data. Undoubtedly, androgen effects on lipids depend on the type of androgen used, whether the androgen is aromatizable or not, the route of administration (oral versus parenteral), the study paradigm and many other factors. In general, the clinical trials show that increasing serum testosterone levels lowers plasma HDL concentrations. It is also clear that very high testosterone levels, such as those in athletes abusing androgens, markedly decrease plasma HDL concentrations. On the other hand, epidemiological data suggest that serum testosterone levels are positively associated with plasma HDL concentrations and inversely with visceral fat. Thus it remains unclear whether testosterone levels in the range desired for male contraception will increase or decrease the cardiovascular risk.

Testosterone effects on coagulation system also remain somewhat uncertain. Testosterone increases red cell mass by effects on erythropoietin and stem cell production. There are a number of case reports of sudden death in athletes abusing androgens. In animal studies, exogenous testosterone augments platelet aggregation and accelerates activation of hemostasis. On the other hand, fibrinogen and TPA concentrations negatively correlate with endogenous testosterone. Thus, it is not clear whether testosterone in the range required for suppression of spermatogenesis will increase the risk of thrombotic events.

Testosterone effects on protein metabolism have been extensively reviewed. It is quite clear that increasing serum testosterone concentrations from hypogonadal to eugonadal range increases lean body mass. Data from our laboratory suggest that varying serum testosterone concentrations in the normal range does not change measures of protein synthesis. However, the data remain inconclusive on whether increasing plasma concentrations into the supraphysiological range will further increase protein synthesis and fat-free mass. Therefore, we do not know whether there is a linear dose-response curve as has been proposed, or two separate dose-response curves, one in the hypogonadal range and a second on in the supraphysiolgical range. We have recently completed a study on the effects of pharmacologic doses of testosterone on body composition (see Chapter 27). Androgen abuse by athletes has reached epidemic proportions mainly because of perceptions that pharmacologic doses of testosterone increase muscle size and strength in eugonadal men.

In summary, testosterone effects on cardiovascular risk, thrombotic events, and body composition remain controversial and will be the subject of discussion this morning.

# 21

# ANDROGENS AND HEMOPOIESIS, COAGULATION AND THE VASCULAR SYSTEM

**Gary Stephen Ferenchick**

**Department of Medicine**
**Michigan State University**
**East Lansing, Michigan 48824-1315**

## INTRODUCTION

Review of past investigations suggests an inverse relationship between **endogenous** testosterone and hemostatic risk factors for ischemic heart disease (IHD). However, the effect of **exogenous** androgens on IHD risk in humans has largely gone unstudied.

Thrombotic events, as well as sudden death, are documented in athletes using illicit androgens. Occlusive vascular events are also associated with medically administered androgens (Tables 1 and 4). Given the multiple uncontrolled variables present in case reports, precise cause-and-effect relationships are difficult to ascertain; but the occurrence of such events in young persons with few traditional risk factors for thrombosis, suggests a possible etiological role for **exogenous** androgens.

Significant advances in our understanding of the relationship between occlusive vascular disease and hemostatic function have occurred in the past several years. For example, there is little doubt about the significance of thrombus formation in the development of acute IHD. However, the extent to which hemostatic factors are *primary* mediators of IHD remains to be delineated.

Among the data supporting a primary role for hemostatic factors in the genesis of IHD include; the relatively poor predictive value of traditional risk factors for identifying those who will ultimately experience ischemic events (Heller et al., 1984); the lack of identifiable plaque rupture in up to 25% of individuals experiencing sudden death in the setting of acute myocardial infarction (AMI); the well described clinical scenario of AMI in the face of angiographically normal coronary arteries (Rapold et al., 1989); the importance of antiplatelet drugs in the treatment of IHD; the identified association between the soluble factors fibrinogen, plasminogen activator inhibitor (PAI), and Factor VII with the presence of IHD (Yarnell et al., 1993; Caron et al., 1989; Phillips et al., 1994; Glueck et al., 1993; Yang et al., 1993); and, the identification of enhanced platelet aggregation as a risk factor for subsequent IHD death (Trip et al., 1990). Such existing data is consistent

**Table 1. Thrombosis Associated with Therapeutic Uses of Androgenic Steroids**

| Age/Sex | Condition | Use Hx | Androgenic Steroid Used | Event | Author/Year |
|---------|-----------|--------|-------------------------|-------|-------------|
| 28 M    | Oligospermia | 3 M | | | |
| 34 M    | Oligospermia | 1 M | Mesterolone | DVT | Lowe 1979 |
| 27 M    | Oligospermia | ? | | | |
| 52 F    | Hypoplastic Anemia | 8 M | Fluoxymesterone | SSST/DVT | |
| 39 M    | Hypoplastic Anemia | 4 M | Fluoxymesterone | | Shiozawa 1982 |
| 26 F    | Hypoplastic Anemia | 6 W | Methenolone | SSST | |
|         |            |        |             | SSST | |
| 21 M    | Hypogonadism | 8 M | Testosterone | CVA | Nagelberg 1986 |
| 61 M    | Aplastic Anemia | 2 M | Methenolone | MI | Toyama 1994 |
| 59 F    | Aplastic Anemia | 13 Y | Oxymetholone | MI | |

Abbreviations:DVT = Deep Venous Thrombosis; SSST = Superior Sagittal Sinus Thrombosis; CVA = Cerebral Vascular Accident; MI = Myocardial Infarction; NA = not addressed; M = months; Y = years; W = weeks; Hx = history

with the notion that a primary hypercoagulable state may exist which favors the formation of thrombus.

Unfortunately, much is yet to be learned about the extent to which androgens impact hemostatic function. Among the issues requiring further delineation include: the relative effect of endogenous vs exogenous androgens; the synergistic effect of nonandrogen factors, such as exercise or concomitant vascular disease; the effect of route of administration, dose utilized, or the specific indication; the simultaneous use of single vs multiple androgens; continuous vs intermittent androgen use; age, amount, and location of atherosclerotic vessels.

## HEMOPOIESIS

Pharmacologic doses of testosterone increase RBC mass. Testosterone likely has an effect on erythropoiesis through more than one mechanism (Besa, 1994). Androgens stimulate an increase in levels of erythropoietin, possibly through a direct effect on renal biosynthesis. Androgens also directly effect erythropoiesis at the level of the bone marrow by increasing erythroid precursors from the pluripotent stem cell. In a study reported by Weber et al., (1991), castrate levels of serum testosterone achieved by inhibiting the pituitary release of LHRH, was associated with a mean decrease in hemoglobin of 1.1 grams, which returned to pretreatment levels after restoration of normal testosterone levels. Serum erythropoietin (EPO) levels remained unchanged during this study. A significant correlation was noted between serum testosterone and hemoglobin, whereas no interaction was noted between testosterone and EPO, or EPO and hemoglobin. Therefore, testosterone likely exerts a direct effect on erythropoiesis, independent of EPO. A postulated testosterone-induced increase in whole blood viscosity leading to CVA, has been reported (Krauss, 1991).

# ENDOGENOUS ANDROGENS AND HEMOSTATIC FACTORS

The relationship between endogenous testosterone and hemostatic risk factors for IHD has been directly evaluated in 5 recent studies (Table 2). Fibrinogen, PAI, and tissue plasminogen activator (tPA) were shown to negatively correlate with endogenous testosterone, whereas no apparent interaction was noted between Factor VII and testosterone. Additionally, both tPA and PAI were noted to correlate with other IHD risk factors, including triglycerides and body mass index, whereas PAI was found to be negatively associated with HDL-C. Fibrinogen correlated with glucose, cholesterol/HDL, age, and triglycerides. Yang (1993) noted no correlation between dehydroepiandrosterone sulfate (DHEAS) and tPA, PAI or fibrinogen. There appears to be no other studies evaluating the association between DHEAS and hemostatic risk factors.

This data suggests that endogenous testosterone, corrected for body mass index, is negatively correlated with many of the hemostatic risk factors for IHD, and that these factors themselves are positively correlated with many of the more traditional IHD risk factors, suggesting that endogenous testosterone is negatively associated with risk of IHD. Whether this association represents a direct cause and effect association or is a manifestation of a broader metabolic abnormality, remains to be determined.

## EXOGENOUS ANDROGENS

Testosterone administration has been shown to augment thrombosis in several animal-based studies. Animals pretreated with testosterone exhibit higher mortality rates, greater clot size and lower vessel occlusion times in response to the same thrombotic stimuli than non-treated controls: an effect blocked by estrogen and antiandrogens (Uzonova et al., 1978). These findings have been replicated in several other studies using both mechanical and chemical thrombotic stimuli (Uzonova et al., 1978; Uzonova et al., 1975b; Penhos et al., 1981; Myers et al., 1982). For androgens to have an etiologic role in the development of thrombus, an effect on circulating platelets, humoral coagulation/fibrinolytic proteins, and/or the structure or function of the vascular system would appear necessary.

## PLATELETS

Previously published biochemical, clinical and pathological studies have linked platelets to acute cardiovascular disease. The thesis that androgens may modify platelet function is supported by several lines of evidence, including experimental animal thrombosis models, *in vitro* platelet function testing of animals pretreated with androgens, and incubation of human platelet rich plasma (PRP) with testosterone (Ferenchick, 1991). The effect of testosterone as measured in the animal thrombosis models is attenuated by aspirin, suggesting that its prothrombotic effect may be mediated through a platelet sensitizing effect. Interestingly, in several studies on the prevention of thromboembolism, anti-platelet prophylaxis was found to be more efficacious in males than females (Spranger et al., 1989). Escholar has

**Table 2. Correlation of Endogenous Testosterone with Hemostatic Factors**

| Study | Year | N | tPA-Ag | Fibrinogen | PAI | Factor VII |
|-------|------|-----|--------|-----------|-------|-----------|
| Phillips | 1994 | 34 | - | -.46* | -.42* | -.18 |
| Yarnell | 1993 | 134 | - | -.07* | - | - |
| Glueck | 1993 | 55 | -.43* | -.39* | -.33* | - |
| Yang | 1993 | 30 | - | -.30 | -.49* | -.10 |
| Caron | 1989 | 54 | -.13 | - | -.39* | - |

\* = Statistical significance per authors

determined that platelet subendothelial interaction is greater in males than females and is antagonized to a greater extent in males than females.

Testosterone and dihydrotestosterone administration have been shown to increase the speed of platelet aggregation at the site of endothelial trauma and be associated with a greater consumption of platelets after a thrombotic challenge than that seen in control animals (Rosenblum et al., 1987). Pre-treatment of animals with testosterone enhances platelet aggregation in vitro, an effect not seen with pretreatment with progesterone, estrogen or glucocorticoid (Johnson et al., 1977).

*In vitro*, studies have demonstrated dose response relationship between the platelet sensitizing effect of androgen and the concentration and potency of the specific androgen used (Johnson et al., 1977). Mechanistically, testosterone is associated with an increased synthesis of platelet-derived thromboxane A2 (a potent platelet aggregator), and decreases the endothelial production of prostacyclin I2, which is an inhibitor of platelet aggregation (Pilo et al., 1981; Nako et al., 1981). Spranger has suggested that platelet surface characteristics may be altered by androgen exposure as well. Human platelets have been identified as an extraglandular source of androgen metabolism (Milewich et al., 1982). An age-dependent effect on *in vitro* platelet aggregation in androgen-using athletes has been reported (Ferenchick et al., 1992).

The only data on the influence of androgens on the platelet numbers comes from therapeutic trials where danazol increases the platelet count in patients with idiopathic thrombocytopenic purpura.

Enhanced platelet aggregation provides a biologically plausible link between exogenous androgen use and acute vascular events.

## COAGULANT/FIBRINOLYTIC FACTORS

Numerous plasma proteins are influenced by the 17 α-alkylated androgens. Such agents have been evaluated for possible therapeutic benefit on both the coagulation and fibrinolytic systems. For example, danazol has procoagulant activity in patients with hemophilia A and B, where increases of 100-240% in factors VII and IX have been reported (Gralnick et al., 1983). Other androgens have been reported to stimulate synthesis of procoagulant factors (Karacharov, 1971). Although isolated reports have suggested that increased coagulation factors may predispose to thrombosis, it is questionable whether increased concentrations of these factors by themselves are prethrombotic. It is interesting to note that disseminated intravascular coagulation (DIC) and thrombosis have been reported in male cancer patients after androgen stimulation. Additionally, DIC has been successfully reversed with an anti-androgen in two reports of patients with prostatic carcinoma (Martinez et al., 1988).

The antithrombin III (AT-III), protein C (PRC), and protein S (PRS) systems function as inhibitors of thrombin formation. AT-III neutralizes all serine proteases generated during clotting. Such enzymes are complexed with AT-III, neutralized and eliminated by the reticuloendothelial system. Depressed levels of AT-III, PRC and PRS predispose to thrombosis. Several 17 $\alpha$-alkylated androgens have been shown to actually increase plasminogen activator activity, and serum levels of plasminogen, PRC and AT III (Kluft et al., 1984a and 1984b). These changes suggest that these androgens may actually protect from thrombosis, however no prophylactic benefit has been reported with their use in controlled trials in surgical and other high risk patients (Blamey et al., 1985).

Stanozolol, known to increase plasminogen activator concentrations in humans, has been widely evaluated in Europe to enhance the fibrinolytic process. However, the value of stanozolol therapy for fibrinolytic enhancement in patients at heightened risk for thrombosis has yet to be demonstrated (Ferenchick, 1991).

Androgenic steroid use in weightlifters may be associated with accelerated activation of the hemostatic system. In one study of confirmed users, significant increases in D-dimer (D-di), the prothrombin activation fragment 1+2 (F1+2), and thrombin-antithrombin III (TAT) complexes. D-dimer is a fibrin split product. Elevated levels of D-dimer, F1+2 and TAT complexes are consistent with increased *in vivo* thrombin generation. This finding, coupled with decreases in t-PA antigen and PAI-1, were concluded to reflect increased activation of humoral coagulation (Ferenchick, 1993). Another smaller study of nonconfirmed androgen-using weightlifters failed to demonstrate changes consistent with a hypercoagulable state (Ansell, 1994). Given the generally illicit nature of androgen use for ergogenic purposes, studies designed to evaluate the synergistic effect of exercise, the simultaneous use of several different androgens, and the relative importance of intermittent use on hemostatic changes, is difficult to ascertain.

## VASCULAR SYSTEM

Androgens likely effect the structure and function of vascular tissues. Structurally, androgens decrease elastin and increase collagen, and other fibrous proteins, in arterial vascular tissue and skin (Cembrano et al., 1960; Wolinsky, 1972). Functionally, androgens have been linked with an enhancement of vascular reactivity and a decrease in aortic smooth muscle prostaglandin I2 (Greenberg et al., 1973). Consistent with these findings has been the identification of specific androgen receptors in the vascular tissues, and myocardium of several animal species (McGill et al., 1980). Several cases of cardiomyopathy have been associated

**Table 4. Thrombosis Associated with Recreational Uses of Androgenic Steroids**

| Age | Lifetime Use | | Event | Angiograph Results | History | Author/Year |
|---|---|---|---|---|---|---|
| | Steroid Used | Recent Use | | | Other | |
| 34 | NA | 8 wks | CVA | Thrombosis MCA | No Risk Factors<br>↓ HDL | Frankle 1988 |
| 22 | Various<br>Methandrostenolone | 6 wks | MI | No ASCVD | No Risk Factors<br>↑ Platelet Activity<br>↓ HDL, ↑ LDL | McNutt 1988 |
| 23 | NA<br>NA | 5 wks | MI | ASCVD | No Risk Factors<br>↓ HDL, ↑ LDL | Bowman 1989 |
| 22 | NA | | MI | Thrombosis ASCVD* | NA<br>Cardiomegaly LVH* | Ferenchick 1990 |

| | | | | | |
|---|---|---|---|---|---|
| 28 | Stanozolol, Oxandrolone, Nandrolone, Trembolone | CVA LE Art Thrombus | Thrombus No ASCVD | No Risk Factors | Laroche 1990 |
| 29 | Testosterone – – – NA | Portal Vein Thrombosis | NA | NA | Wilson 1990 (Pers Comm) |
| 28 | NA | MI | ASCVD* | NA | Lyngberg 1991 |
| 37 | Nandrolone, Testosterone, Stanozolol, Oxandrolone Boldenone – – – 16 wks | MI | No ASCVD | Fam Hx CVA ASA Use | Ferenchick 1992 |
| 36 | NA | *PE | | DM-II | Montine 1992 |
| 25 | Nandrolone | MI | Thrombus, No ASCVD | Remote Fam Hx MI | Huie 1994 |

Abbreviations: See table 1; PE = pulmonary embolism; * = On postmortem examination with androgen use in athletes (Ferenchick et al., 1992). Dilated cardiomyopathy is a known risk factor for thromboembolic phenomenon.

## CONCLUSION

Detectable plasma concentrations of protein activation factors, such as F1+2, TAT and D-dimer, suggests that low-grade ongoing coagulation activity exceeds the inhibitory ability of the endogenous anticoagulants system in most people. A hypercoagulable state likely exists between the extremes of this normal basal state and overt thrombosis (Meade et al., 1992). A variety of factors are known to be associated with a hypercoagulable state. Whether androgens will be found among them remains to be determined.

To date, attempts to understand the association between androgens and the development of vascular disease have been considered almost exclusively in terms of lipid metabolism and other more traditional risk factors for IHD. Evidence suggests that both endogenous and exogenous androgens are associated with significant changes in hemostatic function; some changes theoretically favoring a hypercoagulable state (i.e. platelet and vascular function), whereas, other changes theoretically favoring the opposite (increased AT-III and PRC). Therefore, no unifying data currently exists to link androgens with either thrombosis formation or its prevention. The hemostatic effect of androgens may differ with different classes of androgens as has been shown with androgenic influence on lipid profiles. Additionally, the relative importance of the aromatization of testosterone to estradiol and its impact on hemostatic function has yet to be fully clarified, as does the issues of dose, route of administration, and duration of androgen use. Patient-related characteristics, such as degree of atherogenesis, familial traits, such as pre-existing hypercoagulable abnormalities, and simultaneous use of other medications, are also likely to influence androgenic influence on the hemostatic balance. Further research is required to address these issues.

**Table 3. Effect of 17-α Alkylated Androgens on Hemostatic Parameters**

| Study | Year | ATIII | Plasminogen | Fibrinogen | PRC | FDP's |
|-------|------|-------|-------------|------------|-----|-------|
| Laurell | 1979 | ↑ | ↑ | NA | NA | |
| Preston | 1981 | ↔ | ↑ | ↓ | NA | ↔ |
| Small | 1982 | ↔ | ↑ | ↔ | NA | ↔ |
| Kluft | 1984 | NA | ↑ | ↓ | ↑ | ↔ |
| Kluft | 1984b | NA | NA | NA | ↑ | NA |

Abbreviations: ATIII = antithrombin III; PRC = protein C; FDP = fibrin degradation products. ↑ = increased; ↔ = no change; ↓ = decreased; NA = not assessed

# REFERENCES

Ahn YS, Harrington WJ, Simon SR, et al. (1983): Danazol for the treatment of idiopathic thrombocytopenic purpura. NEJM 308:1396-1399.

Al-Mondhiry H, Manni A, Owen J, Gordon R (1989): Hemostatic effects of hormonal stimulation in patients with metastatic cancer. Am J Hematol 28:141-145.

Ansell JE, Tiarks C, Fairchild VK (1993) Coagulation abnormalities associated with the use of anabolic steroids. Am Heart J 125:367-371.

Barbarosa J, Seal US, Doe RP (1971) Effects of anabolic steroids on haptoglobin, orosomucoid, plasminogen, fibrinogen, transferrin ceruloplasmin, alpha-antitrypsin, beta-glucuronidase and total serum proteins. J Clin Endocr 33:338-398.

Besa E (1994): Hematologic effects of androgens revisited:An alternative therapy in various hematologic conditions. Semin Hematol 31:134-145.

Blamey SL, McArdel BM, Burns P, Carter DC, Lowe GDO, Forbes CD (1984): A double-blind trial of intramuscular stanozolol in the prevention of postoperative deep vein thrombosis following elective abdominal surgery. Thromb Haemostas 51:71-74.

Blamey SL, Lowe DO, Bertina M, Kluft C, et al. (1985): Protein C antigen levels in major abdominal surgery: relationships to deep venous thrombosis, malignancy and treatment with stanozolol. Thromb Haemostas 54:622-625.

Bowman SJ, Tanna S, Fernando S, Ayodeji A, Wetherstone RM (1989): Anabolic steroids and infarction. Br Med J 299:632.

Capezzuto A, Achilli A, Suran N (1989): Myocardial infarction in a 21-year-old bodybuilder. Am J Cardiol 63:1539.

Cembrano J, Lillo M, Val J, Mardones J (1960): Influence of sex differences and hormones on elastin and collagen in the aorta of chickens. Circ Res 8:527-529.

Caron P, et al. (1989): Plasminogen activator inhibitor in plasma is related to testosterone in men. Metabolism 38:1010-1015.

Duarte APT, Ramwell P, Myers A (1986): Sex differences in mouse platelet aggregation. Thromb Res 43:33-39.

El-Maraghi N, Genton E (1980): The relevance of platelet and fibrin thromboembolism of the coronary microcirculation, with special reference to sudden cardiac death. Circulation 62:936-944.

Elwood PC, Beswick AD, Sharp DS, Yarnell JWG, Rogers S, Renaud S (1990): Whole blood impedance platelet aggregometry and ischemic heart disease: The Caerphilly Collaborative Heart Disease Study. Arteriosclerosis 10:1032-1036.

Elwood PC, Renaud S, Sharp DS, Beswick AD, O'Brien JR, Yarnell JW (1991): Ischemic heart disease and platelet aggregation: The Caerphilly Collaborative Heart Disease Study. Circ 83:38-44.

Escolar G, et al. (1986): Sex-related differences in the effects of aspirin on the interaction of platelets with the subendothelium. Thromb Res 44:837-847.

Ferenchick GS (1990): Are androgenic steroids thrombogenic? NEJM 322;476.

Ferenchick GS (1991): Anabolic-androgenic steroids abuse and thrombosis: is there a connection? Med Hypotheses 35:27-31.

Ferenchick GS, Potts R, Kirlin P (1991): Steroids and cardiomyopathy: How strong a connection. Phys Sportsmed 19:107-108.

Ferenchick GS, Adelman S (1992): Myocardial infarction associated with anabolic steroid use in a previously healthy 37-year-old weightlifter. Am Heart J 124: 507-508.

Ferenchick GS, Schwartz D, Ball M, Schwartz K (1992): Androgenic-anabolic steroid abuse and platelet aggregation: a pilot study in weightlifters. Am J Med Sci 303:78-82.

Ferenchick GS, Hirokawa S, Mammen E, Schwartz K (1993): Anabolic-androgenic steroid abuse in weightlifters:Evidence for activation of the hemostatic system. Clin Res 41:364A.

Fischer GM, Swain ML (1977): Effect of sex hormones on blood pressure and vascular connective tissue in castrated and noncastrated male rats. A J Physiol 2 32:H616-H621.

Frankle MA, Eichberg R, Zachariah S (1988): Anabolic-androgenic steroids and a stroke in an athlete: Case report. Arch Phys Med Rehabil 69:632-633.

Gaynor E (1975): Effect of sex hormones on rabbit arterial subendothelial connective tissue. Blood Vessels 12:161-165.

Glazer G (1991): Atherogenic effects of anabolic steroids on serum lipid levels: A literature review. Arch Int Med 151:1925-1933.

Glueck CJ, et al (1993): Endogenous testosterone, fibrinolysis and coronary heart disease risk in hyperlipidemic men. J Lab Clin Med 122:412-420.

Gralnick HR, Rick ME (1983): Danazol increases factor VII and factor IX in classic hemophilia and christmas disease. NEJM 308:1393-1395.

Greenberg S, George WR, Kaclowitz PJ, Wilson WR (1973): Androgen induced enhancement of vascular reactivity. Can J Physiol Pharmacol 52:14-22.

Heller RF, et al. (1984): How well can we predict coronary heart disease? Findings in the United Kingdom Heart Disease Prevention Project. Br Med J 288:1409-1411.

Horowitz KB, Horowitz L (1982): Canine vascular tissues are targets for androgens, estrogens, progestins and glucocorticoids. J Clin Invest 69:750-758.

Johnson M, Ramey ER, Ramwell PW (1975): Sex and age differences in human platelet aggregation. Nature 253:355-357.

Johnson M, Ramey E, Ramwell PW (1977): Androgen-mediated sensitivity in platelet aggregation. Am J Physiol 232:H381-H385.

Karacharov AT (1971): Effect of anabolic steroid preparations on the blood coagula· tion processes. Klin Med 40:131-134.

Kitchens CS (1985): Concepts of hypercoagulability: a review of its development, clinical application and recent progress. Semin Thromb Hemost 11:293-315.

Kluft C, Bertina RM, Preston FE, Malia RG, Blamey SL, Lowe GDO, Forbes CD (1984): Protein C, an anticoagulant protein, in increased in healthy volunteers and surgical patients after treatment with stanozolol. Thromb Res 33:297-304.

Kluft C, Preston FE, Malia RG, Bertina RM, et al. (1984): Stanozolol-induced changes in fibrinolysis and coagulation in healthy adults. Thromb Haemostas 54:622-625.

Krauss DJ, Taub HA, Lantinga LJ, Dunsky MH, Kelly CM (1991): Risks of blood volume changes in hypogonadal men treated with testosterone enanthate for erectile impotence. J Urology 146:1566-1570.

Kreig M, Smith K, Bartsch W (1978): Demonstration of a specific androgen receptor in rat heart muscle: relationship between binding, metabolism and tissue levels of androgen. Endocrinology 103:1686-1694.

Laroche GP (1990): Steroid anabolic drugs and arterial complications in an athlete-- a case history. Angiology 41:964-969.

Laurell CB, Ranneuk G (1979): A comparison of plasma protein changes induced by danazol, pregnancy, and estrogens. J Clin Endo Metab 49:719-725.

Litt MR, Bella R, Lepor HA (1987): Disseminated intravascular coagulation in prostatic carcinoma reversed by ketoconazole. JAMA 258:1361-1362.

Lowe GDO, Thompson JE, et al. (1979): Mesterolone: thrombosis during treatment and a study of its prothrombotic effects. Br J Clin Pharm 7:107-109.

Luke JL, Fard A, Virmani R, Sample PHB (1990): Sudden cardiac death during exercise in a weightlifter using anabolic-androgenic steroids: pathologic and toxicologic findings. J Forensic Sci 35:1441-1447.

Lyngberg KK (1991): A case of fatal myocardial infarction in a bodybuilder treated with anabolic steroids. Ugeskr Laeger 153:587-588.

Martine TJ, Gaedes T (1992): Massive pulmonary embolism and anabolic steroid abuse. JAMA 267:2328-2329.

Martinez JFT, Redondo MDT, Silva IA, Borrasca AL (1988): Disseminated intravascular coagulation reversed by anti-androgen therapy. JAMA 260:2507.

McGill HC, Anselmo VC, Buchanan JM, Sheridan PJ (1980): The heart is a target organ for androgen. Science 207:775-777.

McGill HC, Sheridan PJ (1981): Nuclear uptake of sex steroid hormones in the cardiovascular system of the baboon. Circ Res 48:238-244.

McNutt RA, Ferenchick GS, Kirlin PA, Hamlin NJ (1988): Acute myocardial infarction in a 22-year-old world class weightlifter using anabolic steroids. Am J Cardiol 62:164

Meade TW, North WRS, et al. (1980): Haemostatic function and cardiovascular death: early results of a prospective study. Lancet 1:1050-1054.

Meade TW, et al. (1991): Characteristics associated with the risk of arterial thrombosis and the prethrombotic state. In: Fuster V, Verstraete M, eds., Thrombosis in cardio vascular disorders. WB saunders Co. 79-98.

Milewich L, Whisenart MG (1982): Metabolism of androstenedione by human platelets: a source of potent androgens. J Clin Endocrinol Metab 54:969-974.

Mochizuki RM, Richter KJ (1988): Cardiomyopathy and cerebrovascular accident associated with anabolic-androgenic steroid use. Phys Sports Med 16:109-114.

Myers A, Papadopoulos D, et al. (1982): Sexual differentiation of arachidonate toxicity in mice. J Pharm Exper Ther 222:315-318.

Nagleberg SB, Lave L, Loriaux DL, Liu L, Sherins RJ (1986): Cerebrovascular accident associated with testosterone therapy in a 21-year-old hypogonadal man. NEJM 314:645-650.

Nako J et al. (1981): Testosterone inhibits prostocyclin production by rat aortic smooth muscle cells in culture. Atherosclerosis 39:203-209.

Penhos JC, Rabbani F, Myers A, Ramwell P (1981): The role of gonadal steroids in arachidonate-induced mortality in mice. Proc Soc Exp Biol Med 167:98-100.

Phillips GB et al. (1994): The association of hypotestosteronemia with coronary artery disease in men. Arterioscler Thromb 14:701-706.

Pilo R, Aharony L, Raz A (1981): Testosterone potentiation of ionophore and ADP induced platelet aggregation: relationship to arachidonic acid metabolism. Thrombos Haemostas 46:538-542.

Rapold HJ et al. (1989): Fibrin formation and platelet activation in patients with myocardial infarction and normal coronary arteries. Eur Heart J 10:323-333.

Rosenblum WI, El-Sabban F, Nelson GH, Allison TB (1987): Effects in mice of testosterone and dihydrotestosterone on platelet aggregation in injured arterioles and ex vivo. Thromb Res 45:719-728.

Rubenstein D, Wall RT, Baim DS, Harrison (1981): Platelet activation in clinical coronary artery disease and spasm. Am Heart J 102:363-367.

Schafer AI (1985): The hypercoagulable states. Ann Int Med 102:814-828.

Shiozawa Z, Yamada H, Mabuchi C, Hotta T, et al. (1982): Superior sagittal sinus thrombosis associated with androgen therapy for hypoplastic anemia. Ann Neurol 12:578-580.

Small M, McLean JA, McArdle BM, Bertina RM, Lowe GDO, Forbes CD (1984): Hemostatic effects of stanozolol in elderly medical patients. Thromb Res 35:353-358.

Small M, McCardle BM, Lowe GDO, Forbes CD, Prentice CRM (1982): The effect of intramuscular stanozolol on fibrinolysis and blood lipids. Thromb Res 28:27-36.

Spranger M, Aspey BS, Harrison MJ (1989): Sex difference in antithrombotic effect of aspirin. Stroke 20:34-7.

Tofler GH, Brezinski D, Schafer AI, et al. (1987): Concurrent morning increase in platelet aggregibility and the risk of myocardial infarction and sudden death. NEJM 75:505-513.

Toyama M, Watanabe S, Kobayashi T, et al. (1994): Two cases of acute myocardial infarction associated with aplastic anemia during treatment with anabolic steroids. Jpn Heart J 35:369-73.

Trip MD, Cats VM, vanCapelle FJL, Vreeken J (1990): Platelet hyperactivity and prognosis in survivors of myocardial infarction. NEJM 322:1549-1554.

Uzunova AD, Ramey ER, Ramwell PW (1975): Sex and age differences in human platelet aggregation. Nature 253:355-357.

Uzunova AD, Ramey ER, Ramwell PW (1975): Effect of testosterone, sex and age on experimentally induced arterial thrombosis. Nature 261:712-713.

Uzonova AD, Ramey ER, Ramwell PW (1977): Arachidonate-induced thrombosis in mice:effects of gender or testosterone and estradiol administration. Prostaglandins 13:995-1002.

Uzonova AD, Ramey ER, Ramwell PW (1978): Gonadal hormones and pathogenesis of occlusive arterial thrombosis. Am J Physiol 234:H454-H459.

Weber J, Walsh PC, Peters CA, Spivak JL (1991): Effect of reversible androgen deprivation on hemoglobin and serum immunoreactive erythropoietin in men. Amj Hematol 36:190-194.

Wolinsky H (1972): Effects of androgen treatment on the male rat aorta. J Clin Invest 51:2252-2555.

Yarnell JWG, et al. (1993): Endogenous sex hormones and ischemic heart disease in men. The Caerphilly Prospective Study. Arterio Thromb 13:517-520.

Yang XC, et al. (1993): Relation of hemostatic risk factors to other risk factors for coronary heart disease and to sex hormones in men. Arterioscler Thromb 13:467 -471.

# 22

# TESTOSTERONE, HDL-CHOLESTEROL, AND CARDIOVASCULAR DISEASE IN MEN

Elizabeth Barrett-Connor

Department of Family and Preventive Medicine
University of California, San Diego
La Jolla, California 92093

## ABSTRACT

For years it has been assumed that male testosterone levels play a central role in men's less favorable lipoproteins and greater susceptibility to ischemic heart disease. The evidence for this thesis is contradictory, however. Most clinical trials of quasi-physiologic doses of intramuscular testosterone in older men show no effect on high density lipoprotein (HDL)-cholesterol, while cross-sectional epidemiologic studies almost uniformly find that endogenous testosterone levels are positively associated with HDL-cholesterol levels. Further work is necessary to determine whether and why physiologic testosterone levels in the *high* normal range appear to represent optimal cardiovascular health for adult men.

## INTRODUCTION

By the mid-1980s it was axiomatic that testosterone and other androgenic steroids worsened lipoprotein patterns in adult men, and were probably responsible for their higher risk of heart disease. Only recently was attention paid to the possibility that the observed lipoprotein changes could have been caused by the use of androgens modified for oral administration, by the use of pharmacologic rather than physiologic doses, or by differences in age, obesity, or baseline testosterone levels of the treated men.

The recent history of androgens and lipoproteins in men can be neatly divided into clinical trials and cross-sectional observational studies. The former design has the advantage of randomization (not used in all reported trials), blinding (unsuccessful in the several trials that described this), and the ability to study mechanisms and direction of the association ("causality"). The latter design has the advantage of studying physiologic hormone levels and adjusting for possible confounding due to other common factors which also alter lipoproteins, such as cigarette smoking, alcohol intake, exercise, and obesity.  Unfortunately, these two designs have not yielded entirely consistent effects or conclusions, as reviewed here.

## CLINICAL TRIALS

In 1989, Thompson et al., compared an oral anabolic 17-alpha alkylated steroid (stanozolol) with supraphysiologic doses of parenteral testosterone enthanate in male weight lifters.  Over a six-week period of treatment, stanolozol, but not testosterone, caused a striking reduction in $HDL_2$-cholesterol and apolipoprotein A-1, and a striking increase in low density lipoprotein (LDL)-cholesterol and apolipo-protein B.  Stanozolol increased postheparin hepatic triglyceride lipase activity by 123%, compared to a (nonsignificant) 25% increase with testosterone. Because the androgenic potency of the dose of parenteral testosterone was higher than that of the dose of stanolozol used in this experiment, these results suggest that androgenicity per se was not responsible for the unfavorable lipoprotein changes observed when anabolic steroids are given orally.

In a study designed to determine whether these differences were due to the route of administration or the effect of alkylation, Friedl et al. (1990) compared oral methyltestosterone with parenteral testosterone given alone or in combination with testolactone, an aromatase inhibitor.  Within two weeks, posthepatic triglyceride lipase activity had increased by 102% in methyltestosterone-treated men, by 55% in men treated with both  testosterone and testolactone, and was unchanged in men treated with testosterone only.  By four weeks HDL-cholesterol had decreased significantly in men treated with methyltestosterone or testosterone plus testolactone, but not in men who received only intramuscular testosterone. LDL-cholesterol rose only in the men treated with methyltestosterone.  The men treated with parenteral testosterone without testolactone achieved 17ß estradiol levels comparable to those seen in premenopausal women; in contrast, methyltestosterone was not aromatized to any potent estrogen.  The authors concluded that estrogen modified the expected in-duction of hepatic triglyceride lipase activity by high dose testosterone, and speculated that the beneficial effect of testosterone was a function of its metabolism to estradiol.

More recently, Zmuda et al., (1993) reported that 200 mg of intramuscular testosterone enthanate in combination with testolactone, but not when given alone, increased lipoprotein lipase activity.  These investigators concluded that the usual aromatization of exogenous testosterone to estradiol may inhibit a testosterone-mediated increase in hepatic triglyceride lipase activity and reduction in $HDL_2$-cholesterol.  They also concluded that the estrogen effect was too small to completely explain the different effects of oral versus intramuscular testosterone.

Two small trials using relatively low dose intramuscular testosterone enanthate in older men found a decrease in total or LDL-cholesterol with no significant effect on HDL-cholesterol.  Thus Tenover (1992) treated 13 healthy older men with testosterone enthanate  (100 mg weekly) and found no significant change in HDL-cholesterol, but a significant decrease in total and LDL-cholesterol.  Morely et al. (1993) gave eight elderly men 200 mg of testosterone enthanate every other week and reported no change in HDL-cholesterol and a decrease in total cholesterol (most probably reflecting a decrease in LDL-cholesterol which was not measured directly). In contrast, higher doses of intramuscular estrogen given to younger men appear to lower HDL-cholesterol without effect on LDL-cholesterol. Thus, Bagatell and colleagues (1994) treated 19 men less than 45 years of age with 200 mg weekly of testosterone enthanate, and found a 13% fall in HDL-cholesterol, a 19% fall in $HDL_2$-cholesterol, and a nonsignificant fall in LDL-cholesterol. Interestingly, these unfavorable changes occurred despite a doubling of serum estradiol levels.

Overall, as summarized in Table 1, all clinical studies of 100 mg of intramuscular testosterone enthanate showed no significant decrease in HDL-cholesterol levels. This suggests that either the modification of androgenic steroids (designed to be taken orally) or supraphysiological doses of parenteral testosterone can cause an unfavorable change in lipoproteins, and challenges the thesis that more physiologic doses of testosterone are harmful.

Other evidence that endogenous testosterone is responsible for men's unfavorable lipoprotein pattern comes from studies which suppressed endogenous testosterone to castrate levels using a gonadotropin-releasing hormone analog (Goldberg et al., 1985) or antagonist (Bagatell et al., 1992). Thus, Goldberg and colleagues (1985) reported that testosterone suppression caused prompt increases in total cholesterol, HDL-cholesterol, and apo A-1 and B lipoprotein, despite a significant reduction in plasma estradiol levels; these changes were not observed in a separate group of men given both gonadotropin-releasing hormone analog and testosterone enthanate, although this combination also significantly reduced plasma-estradiol. Bagatell and colleagues (1992) also reported that testosterone suppression substantially increased HDL-cholesterol, particularly $HDL_2$ and apo A-1 concentrations, with no significant effect on LDL or triglyceride levels, an effect that was masked when the hormone antagonist was given with testosterone. The rise in HDL-cholesterol following extreme and abrupt reduction in testosterone supports an untoward effect of testosterone on lipoprotein levels. The relevance of this observation to a gradual decline in testosterone with aging, or with regard to replacement testosterone for elderly men, however, is uncertain.

Table 1. Effect of intramuscular testosterone enanthate on
HDL-cholesterol levels in healthy adult men

| First Author (yr) | Number | Age | Dose/wk | HDL |
|---|---|---|---|---|
| Goldberg (1985) | 6 | 26-42 | 100mg | increase |
| Thompson (1989) | 11 | 23±3 | 200mg | decrease |
| Friedl (1990) | 6 | 20-33 | 200mg | no change |
| Bagatell (1992)[1] | 5 | 20-36 | 100mg | no change |
| Tenover (1992) | 13 | 57-76 | 100mg | no change |
| Morley (1993) | 8 | 69-89 | 100mg[2] | no change |
| Zmuda (1993) | 14 | 27±7 | 200mg | decrease |
| Bagatell (1994) | 19 | 19-42 | 200mg | decrease |

[1]Given with a gonadotrophin-releasing hormone antagonist or analog
[2]Given as 200 mg every other week

## ENDOGENOUS TESTOSTERONE

Boys and girls have similar levels of HDL-cholesterol until puberty. Then male HDL-cholesterol levels fall, concordant with a rise in testosterone (Kirkland et al., 1987). This observation has been taken as evidence that endogenous testosterone lowers HDL-cholesterol and explains the sex differences in this lipoprotein. It is still possible that other factors are explanatory, such as changes in other hormones, an increase in body size, or the loss of subcutaneous fat occurring during this transition period (Solyom, 1972). Further, this pattern is not observed in all adolescents; for example, African-American boys do not show the same quantitative or temporal change in HDL-cholesterol (although they tend to have higher testosterone levels) than North American boys of European ancestry (Berenson et al., 1981).

Vermuelen (1980; Vermuelen and Deslypere, 1985) and others (Simon et al., 1992a) have shown that testosterone levels fall with age. This decrease often begins before age 30 in apparently healthy men (Simon et al., 1992a; Freedman et al., 1991). If high endogenous testosterone levels explain men's low HDL-cholesterol levels, one might expect to see a decrease in HDL-cholesterol with age. Instead, the level of HDL-cholesterol in men is fairly constant over each decade of adult life, at least until very old age (Kannel, 1988).

Ten of thirteen studies of adult men reviewed elsewhere (Barrett-Connor, 1992) found that total testosterone levels in adult men were significantly and *positively* correlated with HDL-cholesterol--the exact opposite of what would be expected if testosterone depressed HDL levels. Endogenous testosterone was not consistently associated with LDL or triglyceride levels in these cross-sectional studies.

An updated summary, revised to include only population-based studies with at least 100 men, is shown in Table 2 (Gutai et al., 1981; Lindholm et al., 1982; Heller et al., 1983; Dai et al., 1984; Miller et al., 1985; Abbott et al., 1987; Khaw and Barrett-Connor, 1991). All studies found a positive association between testosterone and HDL-cholesterol that usually persisted after adjusting for major covariates. This positive association does not seem to be explained by the conversion of testosterone to circulating estradiol, because levels of endogenous estrogen in men have not been found to be positively associated with HDL-cholesterol levels in epidemiologic studies.

Few studies have been conducted of dihydrotestosterone or of bioavailable testosterone. One study found a stronger positive association between HDL-cholesterol and 5α-dihydrostestosterone than the correlation between HDL-cholesterol and testosterone, and a somewhat weaker association between HDL-cholesterol and bioavailable testosterone (Hämäläinen et al., 1986).

## OTHER COVARIATES

A number of factors that affect HDL-cholesterol levels (Heiss et al., 1980) are also associated with endogenous testosterone levels. Because factors that adversely affect HDL-cholesterol may also suppress circulating testosterone levels, it

Table 2. Correlation of plasma testosterone with HDL-cholesterol in community-based studies of adult men.

| First Author (yr) | Number | Statistically Significant Correlation | |
| --- | --- | --- | --- |
| | | Unadjusted | Adjusted* |
| Gutai (1981) | 247 | + | + |
| Lindholm (1982) | 443 | + | Not significant |
| Heller (1983) | 295 | + | + |
| Dai (1984) | 225 | + | + |
| Miller (1985) | 113 | + | + |
| Lichtenstein (1987) | 2512 | + | Not done |
| Khaw (1991) | 391 | + | + |
| Freedman (1991) | 3562 | + | + |
| Haffner (1993) | 178 | + | + |

*Adjusted for covariates such as obesity, cigarette and alcohol consumption, and exercise.

has been suggested that these covariates explain the positive testosterone--HDL association observed in populations (Bagatell et al., 1992). The positive association between testosterone and HDL-cholesterol persisted, however, after controlling for these potential confounders in the cross-sectional studies (Table 2). For example, men who are overweight have significantly lower levels of both HDL-cholesterol (Heiss et al., 1980) and endogenous (total and bioavailable) testosterone (Zumoff et al., 1990) than men who are lean. Adjusting for obesity reduces but does not obliterate the positive testosterone--HDL-cholesterol association (Freedman et al., 1991; Haffner et al., 1993).

　　Male pattern (upper body or central) obesity, a characteristic fat distribution in middle-aged men, is associated with dyslipidemia and with lower testosterone levels in men (Stefanick et al., 1987; Seidell et al., 1991; Pasquali et al., 1991; Phillips 1993; Haffner et al., 1993). In a community-based study of men followed prospectively, Khaw and Barrett-Connor (1992) found that low plasma testosterone was predictive of a higher waist-hip ratio 12 years later. In a double-blind trial, Marin et al. (1992a) randomly assigned 23 middle-aged men to placebo or 80 mg of testosterone undecanoate twice a day for eight months. Treatment was not associated with a significant change in body mass index or waist-hip ratio, but the sagittal diameter and CT scan (measures of visceral adiposity) both decreased significantly in the hormone-treated men. In another study by the same group (Marin et al., 1992b), testosterone-treated men had a decrease in waist-hip ratio without a change in body fat mass. These same studies found that intramuscular testosterone reduced blood glucose and improved insulin resistance measured by the euglycemic/hyperinsulinemic glucose clamp method. (In contrast, injection of very high doses of testosterone [500 mg] caused the opposite effect, worsening glucose tolerance [Marin et al., 1992b] and highlighting the importance of studying physiologic levels of testosterone.)

Several cross-sectional studies have also reported an inverse association between glucose and insulin concentrations and total or bioavailable testosterone in men (Seidell et al., 1991; Simon et al., 1992b; Pasquali et al., 1991; Phillips, 1993; Haffner et al., 1993). In both the Rancho Bernardo Study and in the San Antonio Heart Study, men with diabetes had significantly lower levels of testosterone than men with normal glucose tolerance (Barrett-Connor, 1992; Haffner et al., 1993). Similar findings have been reported from Finland (Andersson et al., 1994).

## CARDIOVASCULAR DISEASE

If higher testosterone levels (within the normal range) are associated with more favorable lipoproteins levels in men, then one might expect testosterone to be associated with a reduced risk of cardiovascular disease in men. Three prospective studies (Cauley et al., 1987; Phillips et al., 1988; Barrett-Connor and Khaw, 1988) found no association of total testosterone with subsequent cardiovascular disease in men. This could reflect the limitations of a single measure of total testosterone to characterize an individual man's future risk, but levels of circulating testosterone show relatively little intraindividual variation, and a single value should be able to characterize an individual for epidemiologic studies at least as well as single plasma cholesterol level does (Dai et al., 1981). Bioavailable testosterone has not been studied prospectively.

## CONCLUSION

Adult men with high normal levels of endogenous testosterone have more favorable levels of several major heart disease risk factors, including HDL-cholesterol, favorable fat pattern, and lower glucose and insulin levels, than men with low testosterone levels. Prospective studies show no association between a single baseline measure of testosterone and the risk of cardiovascular disease in men. Small clinical trials suggest that exogenous testosterone given parenterally in physiologic doses to middle-aged men does not lower HDL-cholesterol and may reduce visceral adiposity, glycemia, and insulin resistance.

Nearly all of these observations, the reverse of associations observed in women, support the concept that men should be men, hormonally speaking, for the prevention of heart disease. The epidemiologic data appear to negate the thesis that endogenous testosterone is a direct or intermediary risk factor for cardiovascular disease in men. They are reassuring in that physiologic levels appear to have no untoward effect on lipids and lipoproteins. Prospective studies with more than a single baseline measurement of bioavailable testosterone will be necessary to test the hypothesis that low levels of endogenous testosterone are associated with dys-lipidemia *and* an increased risk of cardiovascular disease.

# REFERENCES

Abbott WG, Lillioja S, Young AA, Zawadski JK, Yki-Jarvinen H, Christin L, Howard BV (1987): Relationships between plasma lipoprotein concentrations and insulin action in an obese hyperinsulinemic population. Diabetes 36:897-904.

Andersson B, Marin P, Lissner L, Vermeulen A, Bjorntorp P (1994): Testosterone concentrations in women and men with NIDDM. Diabetes Care 17:405-411.

Bagatell CJ, Heiman JR, Matsumoto AM, Rivier JE, Bremner WJ (1994): Metabolic and behavioral effects of high-dose, exogenous testosterone in healthy men. J Clin Endocrinol Metab 79:561-567.

Bagatell CJ, Knopp RH, Vale WW, Rivier JE, Bremner WJ (1992): Physiologic testosterone levels in normal men suppress high-density lipoprotein cholesterol levels. Ann Intern Med 116:967-973.

Barrett-Connor E (1992): Lower endogenous androgen levels and dyslipidemia in men with non-insulin-dependent diabetes mellitus. Ann Intern Med 117:807-811.

Barrett-Connor E, Khaw KT (1988): Endogenous sex hormones and cardiovascular disease in men: a prospective population-based study. Circulation 78:539-545.

Berenson GS, Srinivasan SR, Cresanta JL, Foster TA, Webber LS (1981): Dynamic changes of serum lipoproteins in children during adolescence and sexual maturation. Am J Epidemiol 113:157-170.

Cauley JA, Gutai JP, Kuller LH, Dai WS (1987): Usefulness of sex steroid hormone levels in predicting coronary artery disease in men. Am J Cardiol 60:771-777.

Dai WS, Gutai JP, Kuller LH, LaPorte RE, Falvo-Gerard L, Caggiula A (1984): Relation between plasma high-density lipoprotein cholesterol and sex hormone concentrations in men. Am J Cardiol 53:1259-1263.

Dai WS, Kuller LH, LaPorte RE, Gutai JP, Falvo-Gerard L, Caggiula A (1981): The epidemiology of plasma testosterone levels in middle-aged men. Am J Epidemiol 114:804-816.

Freedman DS, O'Brien TR, Flanders WD, DeStefano F, Barboriak JJ (1991): Relation of serum testosterone levels to high density lipoprotein cholesterol and other characteristics in men. Arteriosclerosis and Thrombosis 11:307-315.

Friedl KE, Hannan CJ, Jones RE, Plymate SR (1990): High-density lipoprotein cholesterol is not decreased if an aromatizable androgen is administered. Metabolism 39:69-74.

Goldberg RB, Rabin D, Alexander AN, Doelle GC, Getz GS (1985): Suppression of plasma testosterone leads to an increase in serum total and high density lipoprotein cholesterol and apoproteins A-1 and B. J Clin Endocrinol Metab 60:203-207.

Gutai J, LaPorte R, Kuller L, Dai W, Falvo-Gerard L, Caggiula A (1981): Plasma testosterone, high density lipoprotein cholesterol and other lipoprotein fractions. Am J Cardiol 48:897-902.

Haffner SM, Mykkanen L, Valdez RA, Katz MS (1993): Relationship of sex hormones to lipids and lipoproteins in nondiabetic men. J Clin Endocrinol Metab 77:1610-1615.

Hämäläinen E, Adlercreutz H, Ehnholm C, Puska P (1986): Relationships of serum lipoproteins and apoproteins to sex hormones and to the binding capacity of sex hormone binding globulin in healthy Finnish men. Metabolism 35:535-541.

Heiss G, Johnson NJ, Reiland S, Davis CE, Tyroler HA (1980): The epidemiology of plasma high-density lipoprotein cholesterol levels. The Lipid Research Clinics Program Prevalence Study. Circulation 62(IV):V116-V136.

Heller RF, Wheeler MJ, Micallef J, Miller NE, Lewis B (1983): Relationship of high density lipoprotein cholesterol with total and free testosterone and sex hormone-binding globulin. Acta Endocrinol 104:253-256.

Kannel WB (1988): Cholesterol and risk of coronary heart disease and mortality in mn. Clin Chem 34:B53-B59.

Khaw KT, Barrett-Connor E (1992): Lower endogenous androgens predict central adiposity in men. Ann Epi 2:675-682.

Khaw KT, Barrett-Connor E (1991): Endogenous sex hormones, high density lipoprotein cholesterol, and other lipoprotein fractions in men. Arteriosclerosis and Thrombosis 11:489-494.

Kirkland RT, Keenan BS, Probstfield JL, Patsch W, Lin TL, Clayton GW, Insull W (1987): Decrease in plasma high-density lipoprotein cholesterol levels at puberty in boys with delayed adolescence: correlation with plasma testosterone levels. JAMA 257:502-507.

Lichtenstein M, Yarnell JWG, Elwood PC, Beswick AD, Sweetnam PM, Marks V, Teale D, Riad-Fahmy D (1987): Sex hormones, insulin, lipids, and prevalent ischemic heart disease. Am J Epidemiol;126:647-657.

Lindholm J, Winkel P, Brodthagen U, Gyntelberg F (1982): Coronary risk factors and plasma sex hormones. Am J Med 73:648-651.

Marin P, Holmang S, Jonsson L, Sjostrom L, Kuist H, Holm G, Lindstedt G, Bjorntorp P (1992): The effect of testosterone treatment on body composition and metabolism in middle-aged obese men. Int J Obes 16:991-997.

Marin P, Krotkiewski M, Bjorntorp P (1992): Androgen treatment of obese, middle-aged men: effects on metabolism, muscle and adipose tissues. Eur J Med 1:329-336.

Miller GJ, Wheeler MJ, Price SG, Beckles GL, Kirkwood BR, Carson DC (1985): Serum high density lipoprotein subclasses, testosterone and sex-hormone-binding globulin in Trinidadian men of African and Indian descent. Atherosclerosis 55:251-258.

Morley JE, Perry III, MP, Kaiser FE, Kraenzle D, Jenser J, Houston K, Mattammal M, Perry HM (1993): Effects of testosterone replacement therapy in old hypogonadal males: a preliminary study. J Am Geriatr Soc 41:149-152.

Pasquali R, Casimirri F, Cantobelli S, Melchionda N, Morselli Labate AM, Fabbri R, Capelli M, Bortoluzzi L (1991): Effect of obesity and body fat distribution on sex hormones and insulin in men. Metabolism 40:101-104.

Phillips GB (1993): Relationship between serum sex hormones and the glucose-insulin-lipid defect in men with obesity. Metabolism 42:116-120.

Phillips GB, Yano K, Stemmermann GN (1988): Serum sex hormones and myocardial infarction in the Honolulu Heart Program: pitfalls in prospective studies on sex hormones. J Clin Epidemiol 41:1151-1156.

Seidell JC, Bjorntorp P, Sjostrom L, Kvist H, Sannerstedt R (1991): Visceral fat accumulation in men is positively associated with insulin, glucose and C-peptide levels, but negatively with testosterone levels. Metabolism 391:897-901.

Simon D, Preziosi P, Barrett-Connor E, Roger M, Saint-Paul M, Nahoul K, Papoz L (1992): The influence of aging on plasma sex hormones in men: the Telecom Study. Am J Epidemiol 135:783-791.

Simon D, Preziosi P, Barrett-Connor E, Roger M, Saint-Paul M, Nahoul K, Papoz L (1992): Interrelation between plasma testosterone and plasma insulin in healthy adult men: the Telcom Study. Diabetologia 35:173-177.

Solyom A (1972): Effect of androgens on serum lipids and lipoproteins. Lipids 7:100-105.

Stefanick ML, Williams PT, Krauss RM, Terry RB, Vranizan KM, Wood PD (1987): Relationships of plasma estradiol, testosterone, and sex hormone-binding globulin with lipoproteins, apolipoproteins and high density lipoprotein subfractions in men. J Clin Endocrinol Metab 64:723-729.

Tenover JS (1992): Effects of testosterone supplementation in the aging male. J Clin Endocrinol Metab 75:1092-1098.

Thompson PD, Cullinane EM, Sady SP, Chenevert C, Saritelli AL, Sady MA, Herbert PN (1989): Contrasting effects of testosterone and stanozolol on serum lipoprotein levels. JAMA 261:1165-1168.

Vermeulen A (1980): Sex hormone status of the postmenopausal women. Maturitas 2:81-88.

Vermeulen A, Deslypere JP (1985): Testicular endocrine function in the aging male. Maturitas 7:273-279.

Zmuda JM, Fahrenbach MC, Younkin BT, Bausserman LL, Terry RB, Catlin DH, Thompson PD (1993): The effect of testosterone aromatization on high-density lipoprotein cholesterol level and postheparin lipolytic activity. Metabolism 42:446-450.

Zumoff B, Strain GW, Miller LK, Rosner W, Senie R, Seres DS, Rosenfield RS (1990): Plasma free and non-sex-hormone-binding-globulin-bound testosterone are decreased in obese men in proportion to their degree of obesity. J Clin Endocrinol Metab 71:929-931.

# 23

# ANDROGEN EFFECTS ON PLASMA LIPIDS: EXPERIMENTAL EFFECTS OF DECREASED AND INCREASED ANDROGEN LEVELS

Carrie J. Bagatell
William J. Bremner

Department of Medicine
University of Washington
Medicine Service, Seattle Veterans
Affairs Medical Center
Seattle, Washington  98108

## INTRODUCTION

It is widely appreciated that premenopausal women have a lower risk for coronary artery disease (CAD) than do men, and that this risk increases in women after menopause (Castelli, 1984, Knopp, 1988). The effects of estrogens on plasma lipids and other factors affecting coronary risk have been studied extensively; however, contributions of androgens to coronary risk have received less attention. In this chapter we will review the effects of androgens on plasma lipids and relate these data to the increased coronary risk associated with male gender.

## SUPPRESSION OF ENDOGENOUS ANDROGENS IN MEN

Endogenous androgen production is markedly reduced by surgical castration or by hormonal suppression of testosterone production. Castrated men have higher levels of $\alpha$-lipoproteins and lower levels of $\beta$-lipoproteins than intact men of similar ages (Furman et al., 1956). More recently, the development of GnRH analogs has offered investigators a means to suppress androgens by less drastic means. GnRH agonists initially stimulate the pituitary secretion of FSH and LH, but after a period of days to weeks, downregulation of the receptors occurs, and gonadotropin secretion decreases to very low levels (Karten and Rivier, 1986). Because testicular production of T is dependent on LH stimulation, hypoandrogenism ensues after a few weeks of GnRH agonist administration. GnRH antagonists also suppress go-

*Pharmacology, Biology, and Clinical Applications of Androgens*, edited by Shalender Bhasin et al.
ISBN 0-471-13320-5 © 1996 Wiley-Liss, Inc.

nadotropin and T secretion. However, their effect is immediate, with complete T suppression occurring within a few days after the initiation of the antagonist (Karten and Rivier, 1986).

GnRH agonists are used clinically in the management of advanced prostate cancer and other hormone-dependent conditions. Moorjani (Moorjani et al., 1987) reported that in men with advanced prostate cancer, administration of GnRH agonist, together with an antiandrogen, resulted in a significant increase in HDL cholesterol, but no change in VLDL or LDL cholesterol. They later reported (Moorjani et al., 1988) that men who underwent orchiectomy for their disease showed no change in HDL cholesterol, while apoprotein B levels increased. They speculated that the more complete suppression of estradiol levels in the men who had orchiectomy accounted for the disparity in the lipid levels in the two groups.

The studies mentioned above were conducted in older men with a co-existing illness, and the results therefore might not be applicable to the male population in general. However, other studies, using healthy men as subjects, also suggest that suppression of endogenous androgens results in increased HDL cholesterol. Goldberg (Goldberg et al., 1985) reported that in volunteers receiving GnRH agonist with no androgen replacement, T levels fell profoundly during the 7-10 week treatment period. At the same time, HDL cholesterol, apo AI, and apo B levels increased, with no change in plasma triglycerides. All parameters returned to the baseline levels after drug administration ended. A second group of men in this study received agonist plus partial T replacement. In these men, T levels were maintained at approximately half the baseline level. Modest increases in HDL cholesterol were noted towards the end of the treatment period; during the recovery period, HDL levels returned to baseline. More recently, Byerley and co-workers used a GnRH agonist to suppress androgens in normal men and then administered T at doses resulting in serum T levels at the low and high ends of the normal male range (Byerley et al., 1993). Under this paradigm, plasma lipids were similar in the two groups of subjects, despite their differing T levels. These data suggest that the relationship between serum T levels and plasma HDL is not a linear one. That is, there may be a threshold below which serum T levels must fall in order to effect an increase in plasma HDL cholesterol.

We have used the GnRH antagonist, Nal-Glu, to study testosterone's effects on lipoproteins in healthy young men (Bagatell et al., 1992). Initially, we studied 15 healthy young men. During the 6-week treatment period, each man received either Nal-Glu SC daily, plus sesame oil placebo IM weekly (Nal-Glu alone); Nal-Glu SC daily, plus T enanthate, 100 mg IM weekly; or placebo SC and IM injections. Serum T and $E_2$ levels in men receiving Nal-Glu alone fell significantly within three days after the experimental regimen began; they reached the castrate range after one to two weeks and remained suppressed during the rest of the treatment period. In these men, mean HDL cholesterol concentrations increased by 26% during the treatment period ($p<0.05$) (Figure 1). Mean levels of $HDL_2$ and $HDL_3$ cholesterol increased by 63% and 17%, respectively, during the treatment period ($p<0.05$), and mean apo AI concentration increased by 17% ($p<0.05$) (Figure 2). In contrast, there were no significant changes in plasma lipids in the other treatment groups, although there was a slight decrease in HDL cholesterol in men who received Nal-Glu with T replacement.

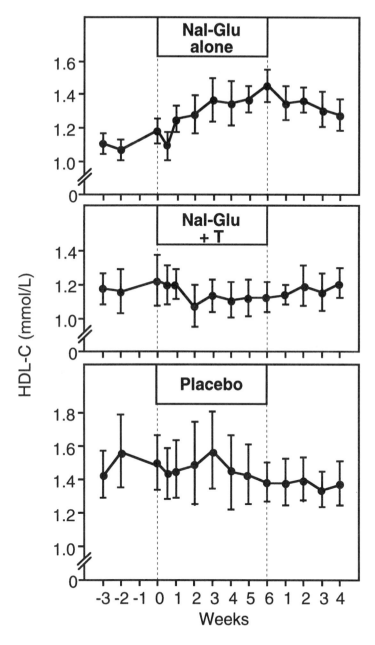

Figure 1. Mean (± SE) high-density lipoprotein cholesterol levels during baseline, treatment, and post-treatment periods. Top: Nal-Glu 75 μg/Kg body weight sc/wk. Middle: Nal-Glu 75 μg/Kg body weight sc/wk plus testosterone (T) 100 mg IM/wk. Bottom: Placebo control (n=5 in each group). HDL-C = high-density lipoprotein cholesterol; Nal-Glu = an antagonist of gonadotropin-releasing hormone. Reprinted with permission from Ann Int Med 116: 967-973, 1992.

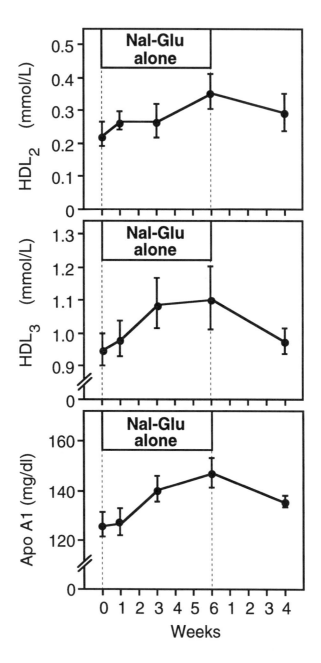

Figure 2. Mean (± SE) high-density lipoprotein-2 and -3 cholesterol and apoprotein A1 levels during the baseline, treatment, and post-treatment periods in men receiving Nal-Glu alone (n=5). Apo A1 = apoprotein A1; HDL = high density lipoprotein; Nal-Glu = an antagonist of gonadotropin-releasing hormone. Reprinted with permission from Ann Int Med 116: 967-973, 1992.

We later studied additional men in each of the treatment groups (for a total of 9 or 10 men per group); our results were very similar. We also found that administration of Nal-Glu, together with T, 50 mg/wk, resulted in no change in plasma lipoproteins . Pavlou (Pavlou et al., 1991) reported that administration of Nal-Glu, together with subphysiological T replacement (25 mg IM weekly), resulted in an increase in HDL cholesterol of approximately 25% after 20 weeks of drug administration.

We have also demonstrated that the small amount of circulating estradiol in men is important in maintaining HDL levels, particularly the $HDL_2$ subfraction, in normal men (Bagatell et al., 1994a). Using the same approach as described above, we administered Nal-Glu, together with T enanthate, 100 mg IM weekly, to healthy men for 6 weeks. Another group of men received Nal-Glu together with the same dosage of T; in addition, they were given testolactone orally. Testolactone is an aromatase inhibitor and inhibits the enzymatic conversion of T to $E_2$ in peripheral tissues. Thus, the men who received Teslac had normal T levels but markedly suppressed $E_2$ levels. After 6 weeks of treatment, plasma HDL, particularly the $HDL_2$ subfraction, was suppressed significantly in men who received Teslac, whereas these parameters were not suppressed significantly in the other men (Figure 3).

Could the physiological regulation of HDL cholesterol by androgens contribute to the difference in the incidence of CAD between men and pre-menopausal women? The magnitude of increase in HDL cholesterol, induced by androgen deficiency, is similar to the gender difference in HDL cholesterol levels between men and premenopausal women. In the Lipid Research Clinics Prevalence study (Lipid Research Clinics, 1980), HDL cholesterol levels at the 50th percentile were 22% (0.26 mmol/L) higher in women aged 30-34 than in men of the same age. In other studies (Manninen et al., 1988; Gordon et al., 1989), risk for coronary disease decreased by 2 to 3% for each increment in HDL cholesterol of 0.026 mmol/L. As noted above, there is a strong inverse relationship between plasma levels of HDL cholesterol and risk of CAD in epidemiological studies. It is therefore quite possible that suppression of HDL cholesterol, induced by physiologic levels of androgens, contributes to the known increased risk of coronary disease in men.

## ANDROGEN ADMINISTRATION IN DELAYED PUBERTY

Kirkland and colleagues (Kirkland et al., 1987) administered T enanthate to 14 boys, ages 13-16 years, with delayed puberty, for 3 months. Each boy received a 100 mg injection once during the first month and 200 mg injections monthly during the second and third months. Serum T levels reached the normal adult male range, and plasma HDL levels decreased by a mean of 7.4 mg/dL (0.2 mmol/L) after a 100 mg T injection, and by 13.7 mg/dL (0.35 mmol/L) after a 200 mg injection. These investigators also followed 12 of these boys during spontaneous puberty. As serum T levels increased to the adult range, plasma HDL levels decreased by a mean of 12.0 mg/dL (0.30 mmol/L). Thus, increasing T levels during puberty appear to be directly linked to the decrease in HDL cholesterol observed during the same time period. However, this association is likely complex, because increased androgen production is also associated with increases in body mass, body composition, and a variety of metabolic variables (Mooradian et al., 1987).

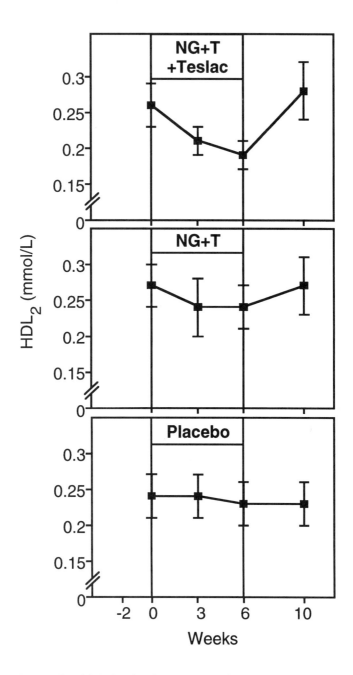

Figure 3. Mean (± SE) high-density lipoprotein-2 cholesterol levels during the study in men receiving Nal-Glu (NG) plus T plus Teslac (*top panel; n=10*), Nal-Glu plus T (*middle panel; n=10*), or placebo (*bottom panel; n=9*). Reprinted with permission from J Clin Endocrinol Metab 78: 855-61, 1994.

# ANDROGEN ADMINISTRATION IN HYPOGONADAL MEN

Androgens are used therapeutically in post-pubertal men with hypogonadism, and several groups have examined their effects on plasma lipids in hypogonadal men of varying ages. Sorva and co-workers (Sorva et al., 1988) studied 13 young men with hypopituitarism and severe androgen deficiency. These men were treated with T enanthate. Plasma lipids, post-heparin plasma hepatic lipase, and lipoprotein lipase activities were measured before and after one and 4 weeks of weekly T injections. After one week, serum T levels were within the normal male range. Plasma HDL and apoprotein AI levels had decreased, although not significantly. After 4 weeks, plasma HDL, LDL cholesterol, and apoprotein AI levels had decreased, although only the decrease in apo AI was statistically significant. Post-heparin plasma hepatic lipase and lipoprotein lipase activities were significantly increased after one week, although only hepatic lipase activity remained increased after 4 weeks. These findings support the data of Kirkland et al. (1987) and suggest that androgens may stimulate post-heparin plasma hepatic lipase activity, which in turn increases the catabolism of HDL cholesterol. In contrast, another group of investigators (Jones et al., 1989) studied 10 men with Klinefelter's syndrome who were receiving T ester implants. Blood samples were drawn 4-6 months after implantation of a capsule (baseline) and then, 1 and 4 weeks after insertion of a new capsule. Serum T levels increased from 18.4 ±4.0 nmol/L to 34.1 ±3.2 nmol/L after 4 weeks and a small increase in LDL cholesterol was observed, but HDL and apoproteins AI and AII did not change. However, plasma lipids in the hypogonadal state were not reported, and it is possible the pre- and post-injection values in these men were somewhat lower than the true baseline levels.

Although T levels do not decline uniformly with age in men, some elderly men do exhibit symptoms of hypogonadism. Recently, the possibility of androgen replacement in elderly men has been evaluated. In a double blind, cross-over study, Tenover (Tenover, 1992) administered T enanthate, 100 mg/wk, or placebo, for 3 months to 13 elderly men. Mean serum T levels increased from 11.6±0.4 nmol/L to 19.7±0.7 nmol/L during T administration. Mean plasma HDL levels and apo AI levels decreased from 49±3 mg/dL to 44±2 mg/dL and 135±6 to 118±6 mg/dL, respectively, and mean LDL levels decreased from 128±7 to 113±5 mg/dL (p<0.05). In contrast, other investigators (Morley et al., 1993) reported no change in plasma HDL levels in older, hypogonadal males who were treated with T enanthate, 200 mg every 2 weeks for 3 months. LDL levels were not reported, but total cholesterol levels fell significantly. These studies were small and of limited duration. Longer and larger studies will be needed to better evaluate the lipid-related effects of androgen replacement in the elderly. Cardiovascular disease is a major cause of morbidity and mortality in older men and these data will be important in evaluating the practicality of androgen replacement on a widespread basis.

## ANDROGEN SUPPLEMENTATION AND
## ANABOLIC STEROIDS

### Exogenous Testosterone

In addition to their use as replacement therapy in hypogonadism, androgens, particularly, T, are being explored as potential hormonal male contraceptive agents (Cummings and Bremner, 1994), T is being tested alone (Paulsen et al., 1982; Matsumoto, 1990; World Health Organization, 1990), or in combination with other hormonal agents (Pavlou et al., 1991; Paulsen et al., 1982; Bagatell et al., 1993; Tom et al., 1992). In order to be acceptable to a large number of men, a potential regimen must be highly effective, reversible, and it must also have no adverse effects on other physiological processes. Therefore, the metabolic effects of supplemental androgens are of considerable importance in this area. In addition, anabolic steroids are being used by large numbers of athletes, from high-school age to the professional level. The lipid effects of exogenous androgens are therefore of clinical importance as well.

The effects of exogenous androgens on plasma lipids vary considerably with type of androgen administered (aromatizable or non-aromatizable) and with the route of administration (oral vs. parenteral). The lipid responses to both T esters and alkylated androgens have been examined under a variety of experimental paradigms.

Three different groups of researchers (Friedl et al., 1990; Thompson et al., 1989; Zmuda et al., 1993) administered T enanthate (200-280 mg IM weekly) to normal men for 3-6 week periods. Friedl et al. (1990) reported that plasma HDL levels decreased by approximately 5%, and LDL levels did not change. Thompson et al. (1989) and Zmuda et al. (1993) reported decreases in plasma HDL of 9% and 16% ($p<0.05$ in each case), respectively. In the former study, LDL cholesterol levels decreased by 16% ($p<0.05$), with no change in plasma triglycerides.

We have administered T enanthate (200 mg IM weekly) to healthy men for up to 20 weeks (Bagatell et al., 1994b). We found that HDL cholesterol levels decreased significantly within the first 4 weeks of treatment. This suppression persisted until the period of T administration was completed (Figure 4); mean plasma HDL levels were 13% lower than baseline at the end of the treatment period. Apoprotein AI and the $HDL_2$ and $HDL_3$ subfractions were also significantly suppressed during T treatment; however, LDL cholesterol and triglycerides did not change. The decrease in plasma HDL cholesterol is maintained throughout periods of T administration lasting as long as one year (Meriggiola et al., 1994).

Although the reasons for the variability of HDL suppression under differing paradigms are unclear, it seems that the duration of treatment is not a major contributing variable. However, the subjects' baseline HDL levels may affect the degree of HDL suppression seen during T administration. In our study and in the study of Zmuda et al. (1993), baseline levels were somewhat higher than in the studies of Friedl et al. and Thompson et al. (1987), and the degree of HDL suppression was somewhat greater as well. The mechanisms underlying this effect are not known.

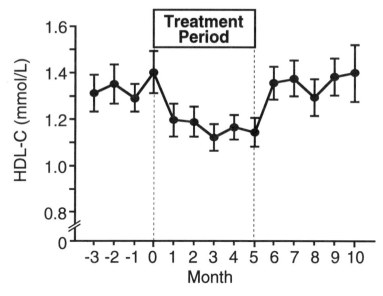

Figure 4. Mean ± SE plasma HDL cholesterol levels in the subjects during the course of the study (n=19 until month 7; n=8-15 thereafter). All data points during the treatment period (testosterone enanthate, 200 mg IM/wk) were significantly decreased (p<0.05) compared with the baseline and posttreatment values. Reprinted with permission from J Clin Endocrinol Metab 79: 561-67, 1994.

## Anabolic Steroids

In both males and females, anabolic steroids induce profound (>30%) decreases in HDL cholesterol, particularly the $HDL_2$ density fraction, and in apoproteins AI and AII (Friedl et al., 1990; Thompson et al., 1987; Alen at al., 1985; Kantor et al., 1985; Taggart et al., 1982). In addition, LDL levels increase by 30-40% during anabolic steroid usage (Thompson et al., 1987; Haffner et al., 1983; Taggart et al., 1982). In two recent studies (Friedl et al., 1990; Thompson et al., 1987), the effects of parenteral and anabolic agents were compared directly. The marked suppression of total HDL, $HDL_2$, and apoprotein AI, and the increase in plasma LDL observed with anabolic agents, contrasted sharply with the more moderate suppression of these parameters by testosterone enanthate in these studies.

Anabolic steroids may also decrease plasma triglycerides. This effect has been observed in normal men (Thompson et al., 1987) and in hyperlipidemic subjects (Hazzard, 1984; Gleuck, 1971).

A subpopulation of LDL particles is linked by a disulfide bond to apoprotein (a), forming Lp (a). Apo (a) has a high degree of homology to plasminogen, and it is thought that at least some isoforms of Lp (a) bind to the plasminogen receptor and interfere with fibrinolysis (Scanu and Fless, 1990). Lp(a) has been shown to be a risk factor for CAD in both cross-sectional (Murai et al., 1986) and longitudinal studies (Schaefer et al., 1994) although not all reports have agreed with these findings (Ridker et al., 1993; Gurewich and Mittleman, 1994). Interestingly, two groups have reported a 65-80% decrease in Lp(a) levels in women treated with danazol (Crook et al., 1992), or stanozolol (Albers et al., 1984), even in the face of elevated LDL levels. Preliminary observations from our own studies and those of others suggest that this phenomenon may also hold true for injectable, aromatizable androgens (Dioyssiou-Asteriou and Katimertzi, 1993 and unpublished data.) The clinical significance of decreased Lp(a) in the face of increased LDL and/or decreased HDL levels is unknown, however, especially in subjects whose baseline Lp(a) levels are low.

## MECHANISMS OF ACTION

The decreases in HDL cholesterol, $HDL_2$, and apoprotein AI induced by androgens appear to be mediated at least in part by hepatic lipase. This enzyme is in part responsible for the catabolism of HDL and for conversion of lipoprotein particles from the $HDL_2$ density fraction to the $HDL_3$ fraction (Eisenberg, 1984). Post-heparin plasma hepatic lipase activity increases during administration of both T enanthate administration and of nonaromatizable androgens (Friedl et al., 1990; Thompson et al., 1987; Kantor et al., 1985; Haffner et al., 1983; Hazzard et al., 1984), resulting in enhanced catabolism of HDL particles (Haffner et al, 1983). This increase is much more marked during administration of anabolic steroids than during T enanthate administration (Friedl et al., 1990; Thompson et al., 1987). With stanozolol, an increase in post-heparin plasma hepatic lipase activity precedes the decrease in $HDL_2$ cholesterol (Applebaum-Bowden et al., 1987), suggesting a causal relationship. A dose-response relationship between hepatic lipase activity and plasma $HDL_2$ during administration of the androgenic progestin, norgestrel, has also been reported (Colvin et al., 1991). The triglyceride-lowering effect of anabolic steroids may also be mediated by increased hepatic lipase activity, although in at least one study, the degree of stimulation of hepatic lipase activity did not correlate with the degree of decrease in triglycerides (Enholm et al., 1975). Although lipoprotein lipase may also contribute to HDL metabolism, only one group of investigators has reported stimulation of lipoprotein lipase activity during androgen administration (Thompson et al., 1987).

The factors underlying the differing effects of the two types of androgens on HDL and post-heparin plasma hepatic lipase activity have not been completely defined, but it is likely that differences in their routes of administration and their metabolic pathways contribute to the observed differences. Orally administered agents are absorbed into the portal circulation but are somewhat resistant to hepatic metabolism, resulting in high hepatic concentrations of androgen shortly after ingestion. Hepatic lipase is found in highest concentration in the liver, and it is likely that high local concentrations of androgens stimulate its activity. However, at present, there are no androgens available in both oral and injectable forms, and a direct test of the effects of route of administration has not been possible.

It is also clear that aromatization of T to $E_2$ accounts in part for the lesser suppression of HDL cholesterol by T enanthate, than by some other anabolic steroids. Estrogens, particularly oral estrogens, stimulate HDL cholesterol, particularly the HDL density fraction (Sacks and Walsh, 1990). In part, this stimulation is a result of estrogen's suppressive effect on hepatic lipase activity, resulting in decreased catabolism of HDL particles (Applebaum-Bowden et al., 1977). When aromatizable androgens such as T enanthate are administered, both androgens and estrogens are formed, and the net effect on post-heparin plasma hepatic lipase activity is a mild stimulation. The role of aromatization in the regulation of plasma HDL has been demonstrated in studies by Friedl et al. (1990) and Zmuda et al. (1993). These investigators administered T enanthate to healthy volunteers and monitored the resulting changes in plasma lipids over 3-12 weeks. At the same time, a separate group of volunteers received T enanthate at the same dosage, and they also received testolactone 4 times daily. Because testolactone inhibits conversion of T to $E_2$, $E_2$ levels in these men did not increase in response to T injection. In both studies, plasma HDL and apo AI levels were suppressed and post-heparin plasma hepatic lipase activity was stimulated to a greater extent in the men who received T together with testolactone, than in the men who received only T; although the magnitude of the differences was greater in the study of Friedl et al. (1990). Our own study of physiological levels of $E_2$ in the regulation of HDL cholesterol in men (Bagatell et al., 1994 a) also demonstrates the importance of aromatization in limiting the suppression of HDL, resulting from administration of T enanthate.

## SUMMARY AND CONCLUSIONS

Androgens are physiological regulators of plasma lipoproteins, particularly, the HDL density fraction. Their effects are modulated by the structure of each compound as well as by the route of administration. In males, both endogenous and exogenous androgens have a suppressive effect on plasma HDL cholesterol, with little effect on plasma LDL or triglyceride levels. Oral and non-aromatizable androgens have a greater suppressive effect on HDL, particularly $HDL_2$, than do aromatizable androgens.

The data we have reviewed suggest that endogenous androgens may contribute to the increased risk of cardiovascular disease in men, especially in comparison to premenopausal women. The data also suggest that the use of androgenic hormones may induce changes in plasma lipids that potentially alter risk factors for CAD. Regimens that include androgens should be evaluated carefully for their effects on plasma lipoproteins, and agents which have the fewest adverse effects on plasma lipoproteins should be used preferentially in most settings.

## REFERENCES

Albers JJ, Taggart HM, Applebaum-Bowden D, Haffner S, Chestnut CH, Hazzard WR (1984): Reduction of lecithin-cholesterol acyltransferase, apoprotein D and the Lp(a) lipoprotein with the anabolic steroid, stanozolol. Biochemical et Biophysica Acta 795:293-296.

Alen M, Rahlika P, Marniemi J (1985): Serum lipids in power athletes self administering testosterone and anabolic steroids. Int J Sports Med 6:139-144.

Applebaum-Bowden D, Goldberg AP, Pyalisto OJ, Brunzell JD, Hazzard WR (1977): Effect of estrogen on post-heparin hepatic lipase. J Clin Invest 59:601-608.

Applebaum-Bowden D, Haffner SM, Hazzard W (1987): The dyslipoproteinemia of anabolic steroid therapy: increase in hepatic triglyceride lipase precedes the decrease in high density lipoprotein2 cholesterol. Metabolism 36:949-952.

Bagatell CJ, Knopp RH, Vale WW, Rivier JE, Bremner WJ (1992): Physiologic levels of testosterone suppress HDL cholesterol levels in normal men. Ann Int Med 116: 967-973.

Bagatell CJ, Matsumoto AM, Christensen RB, Rivier JE, Bremner WJ (1993): Comparison of a gonadotropin releasing hormone antagonist plus testosterone (T) versus T alone as potential male contraceptive regimens. J Clin Endocrinol Metab 77:427-432.

Bagatell CJ, Knopp RH, Bremner WJ (1994 a): Physiological levels of estradiol stimulate plasma high density lipoprotein2 cholesterol levels in normal men. J Clin Endocrinol Metab 78: 855-861.

Bagatell CJ, Heiman JR, Matsumoto A, Rivier JE, Bremner WJ (1994b): Metabolic and behavioral effects of high dose, exogenous testosterone (T) in normal men. J Clin Endocrinol Metab 79: 561-567.

Byerley L, Lee WN, Swerdloff RS, Buena F, Nair SK, Buchanan TA, et al. (1993): Effect of modulating serum testosterone levels in the normal male range on protein, carbohydrate, and lipid metabolism in men: implications for testosterone replacement therapy. Endocrine Journal 1:253-262.

Castelli WP (1984): Epidemiology of coronary heart disease: the Framingham study. Am J Med 76A:4-12.

Colvin PL, Auerback BJ, Case LD, Hazzard WR, Applebaum-Bowden D (1991): A dose-response relationship between sex-hormone induced change in hepatic triglyceride lipase and high-density cholesterol in postmenopausal women. Metabolism 40: 1052-1056.

Crook D, Sidhu M, Seed M, O'Donnell MO, Stevenson JC (1992): Lipoprotein (a) levels are reduced by danazol, an anabolic steroid. Atherosclerosis 92:41-47.

Cummings DE, Bremner WS, (1994): Prospects for new hormonal male contraceptives. Endocrinology and Metabolism Clinics of North America 23: 893-922.

Dioyssiou-Asteriou A, Katimertzi M (1993): Endogenous testosterone and serum apolipoprotein (a) levels. Atherosclerosis 100:123-126. Eisenberg S (1984): High density lipoprotein metabolism. J Lipid Res 25:1017-1058.

Enholm C, Huttunen JK, Kinnunen PJ, Miettinen T, Nikkila EA (1975): Effect of oxandrolone treatment on the activity of lipoprotein lipase, hepatic lipase, and phospholipase A-I of human post-heparin plasma. N Engl J Med 292:1314-1317.

Friedl KE, Hannan CJ, Jones RE, Kettler TM, Plymate SR (1990): High-density lipoprotein is not decreased if an aromatizable androgen is administered. Metabolism 39:69-77.

Furman RH, Howard RP, Imagawa R (1956): Serum lipid and lipoprotein concentrations in castrate and noncastrate male subjects. Circulation 14:490.

Gleuck CJ, Swanson F, Fishbak J (1971): Effects of oxandrolone on plasma triglycerides and post-heparin lipolytic activity in patients with types II, IV, and V hyper lipoproteinemia. Metabolism 20:691-702.

Goldberg RB, Rabin D, Alexander A, Doelle N, Getz GS (1985): Suppression of plasma testosterone leads to an increase in serum total and high density lipoprotein cholesterol and apoproteins A1 and AII. J Clin Endocrinol Metab 60:203-207.

Gordon, DL, Probstfield, JL, Garrsion, RJ (1989): High-density lipoprotein cholesterol and cardiovascular disease: four prospective American studies. Circulation 79: 8-15.

Gurewich V, Mitteman M. (1994) Lipoprotein ($\alpha$) and coronary heart disease: is it a risk factor after all? J Am Med Assoc 271: 1025-26.

Haffner SM, Kushwaha RS, Foster DM, Applebaum-Bowden D, Hazzard W (1983): Studies on the metabolic mechanism of reduced high density lipoproteins during anabolic steroid therapy. Metabolism 32:413-420.

Hazzard WR, Haffner SM, Kushwaha RS, Applebaum-Bowden D, Foster DM (1984): Preliminary report: kinetic studies on the modulation of high-density lipoprotein, apolipoprotein, and subfraction metabolism by sex steroids in a post-menopausal woman. Metabolism 33:779-784.

Jones DB, Higgins B, Billet JS, Price WH, Edwards CRW, Beastall GH, et al (1989): The effect of testosterone replacement on plasma lipids and lipoproteins. European J Clin Invest 19:438-441.

Kantor MA, Bianchini A, Bernler D, Sady SP, Thompson PD (1985): Androgens reduce $HDL_2$-cholesterol and increase hepatic triglyceride lipase activity. Med Sci Sports Exerc 144:62-65.

Karten MJ, Rivier JE (1986): Gonadotropin releasing hormone analog design. Structure function studies toward the development of agonists and antagonists: rationale and perspective. Endocr Rev 7:44-66.

Kirkland RT, Keenan BS, Probstfield JL, Patsch W, Lin TL, Clayton GW, et al. (1987): Decrease in plasma high-density lipoprotein cholesterol levels at puberty in boys with delayed adolescence. JAMA 257:502-507.

Knopp RH (1988): The effects of postmenopausal estrogen therapy on the incidence of arteriosclerotic vascular disease in women. Obstet Gynecol 72:295-305.

Lipid Research Clinics (1980): "Population Studies Data Book : the Prevalence Study" (Vol 1). Dept. of Health and Human Services.

Manninen,V, Elo MO, Frick MH, Haapa K, Heinonen OP, Heinsalmi P et al (1988): Lipid alternations and the decline in the incidence of coronary heart disease in the Helsinki Heart Study. J Am Med Assoc. 260: 641-650.

Matsumoto A (1990): Effects of chronic testosterone administration in normal men: safety and efficacy of high-dosage testosterone and parallel dose-dependent suppression of luteinizing hormone, follicle-stimulating hormone, and sperm production. J Clin Endocrinol Metab 70:282-287.

Meriggiola, MC, Paulsen CA, Bremner WJ (1994): Effects of a 12 month 200 mg/week testosterone enanthate administration on lipoproteins in healthy men. Proceedings of the 76th Annual Meeting of the Endocrine Society, Anaheim, CA, p. 528.

Morley JE, Perry M, Kaiser FE, Kraenzle D, Jensen J, Houston K, et al. (1993): Effects of testosterone replacement therapy in older hypogonadal males: a preliminary study. J Am Geriatrics Soc 41:149-152.

Mooradian AD, Morley JE, Korenman SG (1987): Biological effects of androgens. Endocr Reviews 7:1-28.

Moorjani S, Dupont A, Labrie F, Lupien PJ, Brun D, Gagne C, et al. (1987): Increase in plasma high-density lipoprotein concentration following complete androgen blockage in men with prostatic carcinoma. Metabolism 36:244-250.

Moorjani S, Dupont A, Labrie F, Lupien PJ, Gagne C, Brun D, et al. (1988): Changes in plasma lipoproteins during various androgen suppression therapies in men with prostatic carcinoma: effects or orchiectomy, estrogen and combination treatment with luteinizing hormone-releasing hormone agonist and flutamide. J Clin Endocrinol Metab 66:614-621.

Murai A, Mihara T, Fujimoto T, Matsuda M, Kameyama M. (1986): Lp (a) as a risk factor for myocardial infarction. J Am Med Assoc 256: 2540-4.

Paulsen CA, Bremner WJ, Leonard JM (1982): Male contraception: clinical trials, In D.R. Mishell (ed): "Advances in Fertility Research." New York: Raven Press, pp 157-170.

Pavlou SN, Brewer K, Lindner J, Farley MG, Bastias C, Rogers BJ, et al. (1991): Combined administration of a gonadotropin releasing hormone antagonist and testosterone in men induces reversible azoospermia without loss of libido. J Clin Endocrinol Metab 73:1360-1369.

Ridker PM, Hennekens CH, Stampfer, MJ. (1993): A prospective study of lipoprotein (a) and the risk of myocardial infarction. J Am Med Assoc 270: 2195-2225.

Sacks FM, Walsh BW (1990): The effects of reproductive hormones on serum lipoproteins: unresolved issues in biology and clinical practice. Ann NY Acad Sci 592:273-285.

Scanu, AM and Fless GM (1990) Lipoprotein (a): heterogeneity and biological relevance. J Clin Invest 85: 1790-15.

Schaefer EJ, Lamon-Fava S, Jenner JL, McNamara JR, Ordovas JM, Davis CE, et al. (1994): Lipoprotein (a) levels and risk of coronary heart disease in men: the Lipid Research Coronary Primary Prevention Trial. J Am Med Assoc. 271: 994-1003.

Sorva R, Kuusi T, Taskinen M-R, Perheentupa J, Nikkila EA (1988): Testosterone substitution increases the activity of lipoprotein lipase and hepatic lipase in hypogonadal males. Atherosclerosis 69:191-197.

Taggart HM, Applebaum-Bowden D, Haffner S, Warnick GR, Cheung MC, Albers JJ, et al. (1982): Reduction in high density lipoproteins by anabolic steroid (stanozolol) therapy for postmenopausal osteoporosis. Metabolism 31:1147-1152.

Tenover JS (1992): Effects of testosterone supplementation in the aging male. J Clin Endocrinol Metab 75: 1092-1098.

Thompson PD, Cullinane EM, Sady SP, Chevenevert C, Saritelli AL, Sady MA, et al. (1989): Contrasting effects of testosterone and stanozolol on serum lipoprotein levels. JAMA 261: 1165-1168.

Tom L, Bhasin S, Salameh W, Steimer BS, Peterson M, Sokol RZ, et al. (1992): Induction of azoospermia in normal men with combined Nal-Glu gonadotropin releasing hormone antagonist and testosterone enanthate. J Clin Endocrinol Metab 75: 476-483.

World Health Organization Task Force on Male Fertility (1990): Contraceptive efficacy of testosterone-induced azoospermia in normal men. Lancet 336:955-959.

Zmuda JN, Fahrenbach MC, Younkin BT, Bausserman LL, Terry RB, Catlin DH, *et al.* (1993): The effect of testosterone aromatization on high-density lipoprotein cholesterol level and post-heparin lipolytic activity. Metabolism 42: 446-450.

# DISCUSSION: ANDROGEN EFFECTS ON METABOLISM
## Chairpersons: Shalender Bhasin, Jean Fourcroy

**Jean Fourcroy:** The only data we have on the use of anabolic steroids by athletes is purely anecdotal. It is very difficult to get that information reported to us in any meaningful way. Do you have any ideas how those data can be collected?

**Gary Ferenchick:** It is exceedingly difficult. The nonmedical use of these agents is largely illegal. I have gotten calls about unusual thrombotic outcomes in androgen-abusing athletes that never seem to make their way into the literature. In one of the cases that I know about, the pathologist who did an autopsy on a 21-year-old football athlete who was using androgens, didn't make the connection until the police presented to him a vial of testosterone.

**Jean Fourcroy:** It is a major problem internationally. We do have a system called Med-Watch for reporting such information.

**Elizabeth Barrett-Connor:** When men were given supraphysiologic doses of estrogen in the Coronary Drug Project, they died of heart attacks and those treatments were discontinued. It may be that supraphysiologic doses of all the sex-steroids have thrombotic qualities.

**C. Alvin Paulsen:** Since 1971, we have had approximately 400 normal men treated with androgens. Some of them have been on six different studies from 1971 to the present time. There was a 15% or 20% reduction in HDL levels but cholesterol and LDL levels did not increase. We did not include overweight people with cholesterol values that were extremely high. At this present time we are not aware of any vascular complications in these normal men.

**Victor Goh:** We have used a female transsexual model to study the effect of androgen on lipids. These are women who want to be men. They have been on long-term testosterone injections ranging from one to ten years. The levels of androgen attained in these women fall within the normal range of men. We have found in these androgenized women a definite lowering of HDL levels; the total cholesterol was not different from those in normal men. In addition, LDL levels were significantly increased as compared to those in normal women.

**Elizabeth Barrett-Connor:** I think it goes with my bottom line that men should be men and women should be women.

**William Bremner:** Dr. Goh's results are consistent with what we reported in hypogonadal men; raising serum testosterone levels to normal lowered their HDL levels. There were no changes in LDL or triglyceride levels.

**Joel Finkelstein:** As we consider the issue of the potential cardiovascular risks and androgen replacement, it is important that we not focus entirely on the changes in cholesterol. Although I do believe that changes occur and are likely to be important, it seems likely that androgens may have other effects that are important determinants of cardiovascular risk. If you examine the data from the Nurses Health Study, which has approximately 350,000 patient-years of follow-up, the cardioprotective effect of estrogens in women, is restricted to the women who are current users of estrogen. If the cardioprotective effect of estrogen was mediated by long-term lowering of cholesterol, I would have expected both current and former estrogen users to have a decreased risk of cardiac disease. Therefore, I think that immediate effects of gonadal steroids on vascular reactivity or hemostasis are likely to be extremely important. Recently, it was reported that administering sublingual estradiol to women with cardiovascular disease, improved their treadmill performance within about 15 minutes, suggesting that estrogens have rapid effects on vascular reactivity. Thus, as people investigate the potential cardiovascular risks of androgen therapy, I think we will need to pay attention to changes in vascular reactivity and other hemostatic factors in addition to assessing alterations in cholesterol profiles.

**Elizabeth Barrett-Connor:** You have made a case for outcome studies. We as clinical scientists always study the risk factors, but the bottom line is whether or not you have more disease or more death with a higher or lower level of "X". With new methods, we can determine within our own clinical lifetime, our own research lifetime, whether or not the treatments are useful or not. We need these trials.

**Joel Finkelstein:** I agree. The outcomes are the bottom line. There are plenty of examples where the intermediate end points that we measure to predict the outcome, does not determine the final outcome of the disease.

**Eric Orwoll:** How can you try to correlate peripheral testosterone concentrations with behavior without any good knowledge of CNS aromatase activities? Similarly, Dr. Barrett-Connor's attempt to look at the correlation between testosterone concentrations and lipid or mortality is made incredibly more difficult by our lack of understanding of aromatase activity. If you give supraphysiologic doses of testosterone to a normal man, do estradiol levels go up or down? You can imagine either one could happen and the direction would have some importance in understanding how androgens affect cholesterol concentration.

**William Bremner:** If you give supraphysiologic testosterone doses to men, estradiol goes up. The issue of central nervous system aromatization is very difficult to deal with particularly with regard to its effects on behavior in humans. We are not sure about the effects of testosterone on central nervous system estradiol levels.

**Elizabeth Barrett-Connor:** In general circulating endogenous estrogen is associated with less favorable levels of triglycerides and total cholesterol. In men, circulating endogenous estrogen is not cardioprotective either.

**David Handelsman:** I was very reassured to hear that death rates from cardiovascular disease were not changed by testosterone in the physiological range. That is very reassuring in many respects. Could you give us some idea of what you think are the explanations for the sexual dimorphism in cardiac death rates?

**Elizabeth Barrett-Connor:** I don't have an answer. The sex hormones are important but I think that the notion that female sex hormones would be good for males is just as absurd as the idea that male hormones would be good for women. I think we need to look within the sexes at the relationship of hormone levels to disease, in order to explain the sex differences. It may be that we are programmed from early life to handle lipid metabolism differently or to have more flexible blood vessels in response to sex hormones. It is one of the most interesting questions there is: Why do women live longer than men?

**J. Lisa Tenover:** Dr. Ferenchick, what happens to red blood cell mass is a function of how the androgens are administered or dosed. In elderly men, the increase in red blood cell mass doesn't seem to be related to the area under the dose curve (that is, total androgen) but more to peak androgen levels obtained. Men who use androgen patches don't seem to demonstrate the same magnitude of rise.

**Gary Ferenchick:** As a hypothesis, androgens may be synergistic, with say, hypoxemia and perhaps some other factors in terms of erythropoietin stimulation when they are given exogenously.

**Adrian Dobs:** We have been studying the non-scrotal patch and find that giving testosterone will decrease HDL, but that testosterone was directly correlated to HDL. We found that the big confounder here is obesity, that is, fatter men have lower testosterone and lower HDL levels. Are low testosterone levels part of the syndrome X, and if they are, are those low levels the cause or the result of obesity?

**Elizabeth Barrett-Connor:** Testosterone may be related to the insulin resistance syndrome. The best evidence that testosterone is important comes from the Marin study, where he was able to reduce visceral adiposity by replacing testosterone. Visceral adiposity is closely associated with the dyslipidemia and the hyperinsulinemia that characterize the insulin resistance syndrome.

**William Bremner:** Obesity, at least in most of the epidemiologic studies, has been reasonably subtracted out as a factor. Are there other intervening variables that may explain the positive correlations between testosterone and HDL in some normal population groups? It would be surprising if this dose-related effect of testosterone on HDL, that we have reported in the supraphysiologic and hypogonadal ranges of testosterone, doesn't apply to the people in the normal range as well.

**Hermann Behre:** There is a clear circadian variation of testosterone levels and testosterone levels can be quite low in the late evening. We have done a study with small doses of GnRH antagonists to lower testosterone levels in the low normal range and found increase in HDL cholesterol. Is there any implication of this circadian rhythm for the metabolic effects of androgens?

**Gary Ferenchick:** There is circadian variation to cardiovascular events. They seem to occur more in the morning. A biologically plausible link between the early morning increase in platelet activity and the heightened risk of thromboembolic events has been suggested. One could hypothesize that an early morning increase in testosterone may affect platelet aggregation. Some other hemostatic factors may have diurnal variation as well.

**William Bremner:** - I am not aware of any data that has clearly established a relationship between the circadian rhythm of testosterone and any biological end point.

**Christina Wang:** Could you clarify the thrombotic/thrombolytic factors that are associated with testosterone administration? When you administer testosterone, it increases the levels of thrombotic factors, but correlation studies show that increasing serum testosterone in fact decreases thrombosis?

**Gary Ferenchick:** It is incredibly complex array of factors that you are looking at. Many of the newer assays that assess for low grade ongoing *in vivo* thrombin formation and platelet activation have been correlated with other risk factors, but not with clinical outcome. We do not know if people who have higher levels of prothrombin activation fragments have worse outcomes than those who don't. Testosterone increases fibrinolysis but we do not know how this biochemical change correlates to the outcome. We also do not know how concomitant disease, exercise, and other well known endogenous risk factors for thrombosis affect the overall hemostatic balance. Protein C deficiency, at least in a heterozygous form, is known to occur in one in 300 people. So chances are somebody in this room is heterozygous for protein C deficiency. When you add androgen on top of that, what happens to the hemostatic balance? A new variant of factor 5, has recently been identified which has a hard time complexing with protein C. Preliminary data suggest that this is very common in people who have idiopathic thrombotic events. There are probably more factors operant here than just the effect of testosterone on basal hemostatic function.

**Ronald Swerdloff:** Many of us who want to utilize androgens for many new uses, including male contraception, have concerns about safety. We want to make sure that the overall balance is positive. In terms of the overall outlook for androgen influenced cardiovascular risk, the final answer may require the large scale prospective studies that had to be done with estrogens. There is increasing interest in nitric oxide synthase in the atherosclerotic and thrombogenic process. In the penile vascular level, testosterone seems to influence the nitric oxide system. Perhaps this will extend to the general vascular system.

The red cell mass is determined partly by the length of circulation of the red cells. Therefore, you have to have either a very long washout period or a naive group of hypogonadal men to properly assess the influence of testosterone treatment on changes in red cell mass.

**Elizabeth Barrett-Connor:** It is important to recognize that there are tremendous differences in cardiovascular disease rates in different countries, such that the absolute rates for men are much lower in some countries than they are in our country. When people move from high to low risk countries, as we heard yesterday about prostate cancer, they tend to assume a lower risk and vice versa, suggesting that this is not a genetic characteristic, but a lifestyle issue. I think men now are going to be very soon in the situation that women are, where they have to weigh their quality of life and the things that are important to them with unknown risk. Women are being prescribed estrogen in order to improve quality of life, and being told there is probably no increased risk of breast cancer. There are men for whom the quality of life will be improved by replacement testosterone, and this may override any potential life shortening that low dose testosterone might cause. There are lifestyle factors which appear to reduce those risks and at the same time that we give the testosterone we should be trying to get people to improve their diet and their lifestyles.

**Robert Lustig:** All of you have been measuring blood levels, but biological activity at the level of the cell maybe very different. Different estrogen preparations can be associated with different breast cancer risks. Can we equate all of the different androgen delivery systems, and do they actually have the same actions at the level of the cell?

**William Bremner:** Androgens differ in terms of their effects of lipids, depending on whether the steroid is administered orally and whether it is aromatizable. There is no good cell or molecular assay for androgen effects. I have come to believe that HDL and behavioral end points are not bad assessments of androgen effects in vivo in men.

**F. C. Wu:** We have studied 32 men in the WHO Male Contraceptive Trial in which they were given testosterone enanthate 200 mg weekly for a period of 12 months. The major findings are that fibrinogen decreased and antithrombin 3 increased. There was no change in D dimer or in platelet aggregation. There is no evidence using this particular dose of androgens that there is any increase in thrombogenesis in men. I think that we should not equate the use of testosterone as a male contraceptive with anabolic steroid abuse.

**Richard Clark:** Could you give us some better guidelines for assessing thrombotic risk in our patients, deciding how best to measure hematocrit and red blood cell mass and at what frequency and at what level should we be concerned about. Should we be considering more sophisticated measures?

**Gary Ferenchick:** A paper in the American Journal of Urology, 1991, identified baseline hematocrits greater than 48%, a change from baseline hematocrit of 15% or greater as being risk factors for hyperviscosity and possible thrombosis. I think if you use those as general guidelines, you may identify those at relative risk for thrombosis.

# 24

# ANDROGENS AND SKIN: 5α-REDUCTASE ACTIVITY IN SKIN AND ANDROGEN DEPENDENT SKIN DISORDERS

**Tehming Liang**

**Department of Dermatology**
**School of Medicine and VA Medical Center**
**Wright State University**
**Dayton, Ohio 45435**

## INTRODUCTION

Skin contains various androgen-responsive structures, such as hair follicles, sebaceous glands, and apocrine glands. Before puberty, the hair follicles, with the exception of the scalp, eyebrows, and eyelashes, are small, producing villus hair; the sebaceous glands and apocrine glands are small and non-functional. Under the influence of increased levels of androgen during and after puberty, terminal hair grows in the pubis and axilla of men and women. The sebaceous glands enlarge and produce sebum and the apocrine sweat glands, which are limited to the axilla and perineum, become functional.

In addition to affecting normal functions of the skin, androgens have been recognized as one of the pathogenic factors in certain skin diseases such as acne, female hirsutism, androgenetic alopecia (male-pattern baldness), and hidradenitis suppurativa. Current hormonal therapy for some of these androgen-dependent disorders include birth control pills, which reduce ovarian secretion of androgens, and anti-androgens, which block androgen binding to intracellular receptors. Androgen action in the skin, like in the prostate, requires the conversion of testosterone to a more active metabolite 5α-dihydrotestosterone. Finasteride, a 5α-reductase inhibitor, has been approved by the FDA for treating benign prostatic hyperplasia. Because treatment with a 5α-reductase inhibitor is expected to block the androgen actions mediated by 5α-dihydrotestosterone, but not those mediated by testosterone, such as sexual functions and masculinization, 5α-reductase inhibitors are also desirable for treating androgen-dependent skin disorders. The following is a review of selected articles on the characterization of human skin 5α-reductases and investigations with 5α-reductase inhibitors.

*Pharmacology, Biology, and Clinical Applications of Androgens*, edited by Shalender Bhasin et al.
ISBN 0-471-13320-5 © 1996 Wiley-Liss, Inc.

# CHARACTERIZATION OF SKIN 5α-REDUCTASES

## Tissue Distribution

5α-reductase (NADP$^+$:3-oxo-4-delta-steroid 5α-oxido-reductase, EC 1.3.99.5) activity has been demonstrated in skin specimens from various parts of the body. The levels of 5α-reductase activity are found to be higher in skin known to be more sensitive to androgens than the skin of less sensitive areas. For example, Wilson and Walker (1969) showed that 5α-reductase activity in the genital skin, such as the scrotum, prepuce, clitoris, and labia majora, were 6 to 12-fold higher than the non-genital skin, including the thigh, back, breast, inguinal area, sole of foot, abdomen, and chest. Hay and Hodgins (1978) reported that in the adult forehead skin, 40-66% of 5α-reductase activity was found in the sebaceous gland, whereas, in the axillary skin 50-70% of 5α-reductase activity was found in the sweat gland, especially the apocrine sweat gland. Takayasu et al. (1980) have measured 5 α-reductase activity in dissected skin specimens. The activity in de-creasing order is apocrine gland > sebaceous gland = eccrine gland > hair follicle > dermis > epidermis (Table 1). In hair follicles, 5α-reductase activity has been detected in both the epithelium (plucked hair root) (Schweikert and Wilson, 1974) and the dermal papilla (Itami et al., 1991).

## Increased Levels of 5α-Reductase Activity in Acne, Bald, and Hirsute Skin

Because acne, androgenetic alopecia, and idiopathic hirsutism develops in individuals with normal circulating levels of androgens, an increase of skin sensitivity to androgens in these individuals has been proposed. Several laboratories have investigated whether 5α-reductase activity is increased in the skin of the diseased individuals.

Table 1.  Distribution of 5α-Reductase Activity in Human Skin

| Tissue | 5α-Reductase activity (pmoL/mg tissue/h) |
|---|---|
| Apocrine gland | $388 \pm 15$ |
| Sebaceous gland | $152 \pm 55$ |
| Eccrine gland | $145 \pm 108$ |
| Hair follicle | $40 \pm 10$ |
| Dermis | $22 \pm 22$ |
| Epidermis | negligible |

Skin specimen from 7 men and 5 women (age 13 - 51): scalp, axilla, forehead, prepuce, chest, and back. (Adapted from Takayasu et al., 1980)

Sansone and Reisner (1971) compared 5α-reductase activity in acne-bearing skin with that of normal skin. In women, 5α-reductase activity was increased 5-20 fold in acne-bearing skin. In men, the 5α-reductase activity of normal skin was higher than that of women; acne bearing skin also had a higher 5α-reductase activity. Kuttenn et al. (1977) compared 5α-reductase activity in pubic skin biopsy specimens from normal and hirsute women. 5α-reductase activity was found to be 5 fold higher in the idiopathic hirsute than that of the non-hirsute women. Fibroblasts cultured from the pubic skin of hirsute women also had higher 5α-reductase activity than the fibroblasts cultured from that of normal women (3.3 ± 2.6 vs. 1.1 ± 0.6 fmol 5α-reduced metabolites/μg DNA/h, P < 0.05). Interestingly, the androgen receptor binding capacity of the fibroblasts were similar between those derived from the skin of the normal versus the hirsute women (411 ±171 vs, 313 ± 141 fmol/mg DNA) (Mowzowicz et al., 1983). The levels of 5α-reductase activity in the genital skin have been reported to be correlated with the degree of hirsutism measured by Ferrimen-Gallwey scores (r = 0.66) (Serafini & Lobo, 1985). Serum levels of 3α, 17β-androstandiol glucuronide, a metabolite of DHT, was found to be higher in hirsute women than those of normal women (604 ± 376 vs. 40 ± 10 ng.dl) and has been proposed as a marker for idiopathic hirsutism (Horton et al., 1982).

When comparing the hairy and bald areas of the scalp on the same individual, three out of four individuals showed a higher 5α-reductase activity in the bald area of the scalp (42%, 127%, and 134%) (Bingham and Shaw, 1973). Puerto and Mall (1990) confirmed this finding and they also found that sebaceous glands in the bald scalp were significantly larger than those of the hairy scalp. They attribute the higher levels of 5α-reductase activity in the balding scalp to a larger proportion of sebaceous glands in the tissues. Recently, Dallob et al. (1994) measured DHT levels in the balding and hairy scalps of 10 men and found a higher level in the balding area than the hairy area (7.37 ± 1.24 vs. 4.20 ± 0.65 pmol/g, P <0.01). Testosterone levels were similar with the balding and the hairy areas.

Schweikert and Wilson (1974) compared 5α-reductase activity in hair roots plucked from various areas of the scalp from balding and non-balding men. They found that in balding men, the hair root from the balding frontal area had a higher activity than those from the hairy occipital, temporal, and nuchal area. 5α-reductase activity of the corresponding areas was higher in the balding men than that in the non-balding men.

## Human 5α-Reductase Isozyme 1 and 2

Two human 5α-reductase isozymes, type 1 and 2, have been identified (Anderson & Russell, 1990; Anderson et al., 1991; Jenkins et al., 1991; Thigpen et al., 1992). Both consist of a single polypeptide, 259 amino acids for type 1, and 254 amino acids for type 2. The two isozymes have only 50% homology in their amino acid sequences. A major distinctive feature is that type 1 isozyme has a sharp pH optimum, around 5, whereas type 2 isozyme has a broad pH optimum, between 6.5 and 8. Type 1 isozyme has a slightly lower affinity than type 2 isozyme for both testosterone (Km 3.6 μM for type 1, 0.5-1 μM for type 2) and NADPH (29 μM for type 1 and 8-13 μM for type 2). The 5α-reductase inhibitor finasteride has Ki 230 nM for type 1 and 5 nM for type 2 isozyme. Mutations for type 2 isozymes have been found in male pseudohermaphroditism, whereas type 1 isozyme is normal in these patients. In addition, these two isozymes are encoded by genes in different chromosomes; chromosome 5 for type 1 and chromosome 2 for type 2.

Type 1 isozyme has been shown to be the major form of 5α-reductase in the human scalp (Harris et al., 1993). 5α-reductase activity in the human scalp has similar properties to cloned type 1 isozyme and is distinct from the human prostate which mainly contains the type 2 isozyme. The scalp 5α-reductase and the cloned type 1 isozyme both have a broad pH 6-8 optimum (5.5 for human prostate) and higher Kms for testosterone 7.7 μM (0.3 for prostate) and NADPH 26 μM (3.9 μM for the prostate). The rank order of potency of 5α-reductase inhibitors for the scalp enzyme activity is similar to that of the cloned type 1 isozyme and is quite different from that for the prostate 5α-reductase activity. The concentration of finasteride required to produce 50% inhibition (IC50) of the scalp (500 nM) was close to that for the cloned type 1 enzyme (1200 nM) and was 125-fold higher for the prostate enzyme (4.2 nM). On the other hand, 2',3' -tetrahydrofuran-2'-spiro-17-(4-methyl-4-aza-5α-androstane-3-one (compound 1e) had a higher affinity for the scalp enzyme (IC50 5 nM) than for the prostate enzyme (IC50 140 nM). Type 1 isozyme was detected in the sebaceous gland of human skin by immunohistochemical localization (Luu-The et al., 1994).

Thigpen et al. (1993) have investigated the expression of both type 1 and type 2 isozymes in skin extracts by immunobloting techniques using isozyme specific antibodies. In the chest and scalp skin, while both type 1 and type 2 isozymes were detected in the neonate, only type 1 was detected after puberty. When comparing the levels of type 1 isozyme in the bald and nonbald areas of the same individuals, there were no dramatic differences. Type 2 isozyme was not detected in the balding or hairy region of the scalp. The scalp of women also only contained type 1 isozyme.

# EFFECTS OF 4-AZASTEROIDAL 5α-REDUCTASE INHIBITORS ON HAIR GROWTH AND SEBUM SECRETION

## Effects of 4-MA and Finasteride in Monkey Model for Baldness

Rittmaster et al. (1987) reported the 5α-reductase inhibitor 4-MA applied topically prevented baldness in the stumptail macaque, a monkey model for male pattern baldness. In this investigation, 4-MA dissolved in dimethylsulfoxide was applied daily to the frontal scalp. The control group received the solvent alone. The treatments lasted for 27 months. The hair growth measured during the last 6 months was higher for the 4-MA treated group than the control group (38.4 ± 11.1 vs. 22.0 ± 4.7 mg). The scalp was biopsied before and after treatment periods and examined histologically. The control group showed a reduction in the percent of hair follicles in the growing phase (63 ± 9.8 vs. 25 ± 21%), whereas there was no change for the 4-MA treated group (46 ± 9.8 vs. 47 ±6%).

Diani et al. (1992) investigated oral finasteride (0.5 mg/day), topical minoxidil (2% daily), and a combination of both for their effects on the growth of hair in the stumptail macaque. Hair was collected from the balding frontal scalp at 4-week intervals for 20 weeks. They found oral finasteride was as effective as topical minoxidil in stimulating hair growth. The combination of finasteride and minoxidil produced an additive effect, consistent with the different mechanisms of action between finasteride and minoxidil.

## Finasteride Treatments Reduced DHT Concentrations in Human Scalp

In a double blind study, men with male pattern baldness were either treated with finasteride (5 mg/daily, orally, n=8) or with a  placebo (n = 9). Before treatment, the DHT contents in the bald scalp were similar between the placebo and the finasteride group (7.58 $\pm$ 1.34 vs. 6.40 $\pm$1.07 pmol/g tissue, mean $\pm$ sem). After 28 days of treatment, the DHT content in the finasteride treated group was reduced to 65.9 $\pm$ 9.9 % (p < 0.01) of the pretreatment level.  The placebo group did not change significantly.  The amount of testosterone was  not significantly changed before and after treatment in both the placebo and the finasteride groups.   The finasteride treatment reduced the serum levels of DHT to 34.9 $\pm$ 6.2 % (p < 0.01) of the pretreatment levels.  The serum levels of DHT did not change in the placebo group.  The serum level of T was not significantly changed in both groups (Dallob et al., 1994).

## Improvement of Female Hirsutism by Finasteride Treatments

Moghetti et al. (1994) treated 17 idiopathic hirsute women (age 24.0 $\pm$ 1.9 year) with finasteride at a daily oral dose of 5 mg for 6 months.  The degree of hirsutism was scored by a modified Ferriman-Gallwey method before and after treatments.  Finasteride treatments significantly reduced the hirsutism score (after 5.9 $\pm$ 0.6 vs. before 11.7 $\pm$ 1.3; p < 0.01).

Fruzzetti et al. (1994) treated 10 hirsute women, age 16-28, with finasteride (5 mg daily, orally).  After three months of treatment, the clinical improvement of the hirsutism was observed in 9 of 10 patients and the Ferriman-Gallwey score significantly decreased from 24.4 $\pm$ 3.9 to 17.6 $\pm$ 6.1 (p < 0.001).  The total serum testosterone was slightly increased (1.63 $\pm$ 0.59 vs. 2.18 $\pm$ 0.62 nmol/l; p < 0.01), whereas the free testosterone level was not changed (0.091 $\pm$ 0.043 vs. 0.098 $\pm$ 0.039 nmol/l).

Wong et al. compared the effectiveness by oral daily treatments between finasteride (5 mg, n=9) and spironolactone (100 mg, n=5), an antiandrogen, for their effects on women with moderate to severe hirsutism.  Hair diameters and Ferriman-Gallwey hirsutism scores were compared in the same group of patients before and after 6 months of treatment.  Both treatments produced a small but significant decrease in hair diameter: - 14.0 $\pm$6.7% (p < 0.05) for finasteride and - 13.4 $\pm$ 3.8% (p < 0.05) for spironolactone.  The Ferriman-Gallwey scores were reduced -2.1 $\pm$ 0.4 (p < 0.05) for finasteride and -2.5 $\pm$ 0.7 (p < 0.05) for spironolactone.

## No Effect of Finasteride Treatments on Sebum Secretion

Imperato-McGinley et al. (1993) investigated finasteride (5mg/day) in men (age 66 ± 4.7) for its effect on sebum secretion. They found that the finasteride treatment reduced the serum level of DHT by 82% measured at 6 months but did not reduce the rate of sebum secretion after 6 months and after 1 year. They found that male patients with hereditary 5α-reductase type 2 deficiency (age 19 to 40) have a rate of sebum secretion from the forehead similar to the normal adult male. These findings are consistent with type 1 but not type 2 isozyme in the sebaceous glands.

## ALIPHATIC UNSATURATED FATTY ACIDS AS INHIBITORS OF 5α-REDUCTASES

### *In Vitro* Studies

Liang and Liao (1992) have investigated selected tissues to determine whether they contain 5α-reductase inhibitor activity. We found that 5α-reductase inhibitor activity could be extracted from rat liver microsomes using organic solvents such as acetic acid or methylene chloride. Because of the lipid nature of the inhibitor substances, we tested various lipids for their ability to inhibit 5α-reductase activity in rat liver microsomes. We found that certain aliphatic polyunsaturated fatty acids could inhibit 5α-reductase activity at μM concentrations. Of the lipids tested, γ-linolenic acid (C18:3, cis-6,9,12) is the most potent. α-Linolenic acid (C18:3,cis-9,12,15), linoleic acid (C18:2,cis-9,12) and oleic acid (C18:1,cis-9) are less active, whereas stearic acid (C18:0) is inactive. γ-Linolenic acid inhibition of 5α-reductase is specific since it has no effect on other microsomal enzymes such as UDP-GA:DHT glucuronosyltransferase and NADH:menadione reductase, or other steroid metabolic enzymes such as 17 β-hydroysteroid dehydrogenase. When γ-linolenic acid was tested for inhibiting human 5α-reductases, γ-linolenic acid was found to inhibit 5α-reductase activity of the prostate and that of the liver. Hiipakka and Liao found that γ-linolenic acid was equally effective in inhibiting human type 1 and type 2, 5α-reductase isozymes (personal communication).

## γ-Linolenic Acid Inhibition of Testosterone-Stimulated Growth of the Hamster Flank Organ

We have investigated whether γ-linolenic acid can inhibit testosterone action in the hamster flank organ model. Immature male hamsters were castrated and divided into groups. The right flank organs of the animals in each group was treated topically once a day with a selected solution as shown in Table 2. The flank organ of the group treated with vehicle only did not grow. Testosterone treatments stimulated the growth of the flank organs to became darker and larger. The flank organs that were treated with testosterone plus γ-linolenic acid were lighter and smaller (-53%) than those treated with testosterone alone, indicating inhibition of testosterone action by γ-linolenic acid. In contrast, there were no significant differ-

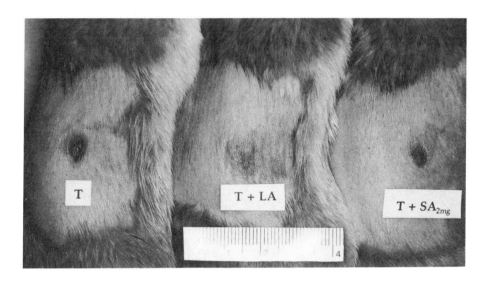

Fig. 1. Inhibition of testosterone(T)-stimulated growth of the hamster flank organ by γ-linolenic acid (LA), but not by stearic acid (SA). These animals shown are from Table 2. γ-Linolenic acid is known to be an inhibitor of 5α-reductases, whereas stearic acid is not a 5α-reductase inhibitor.

ences of the flank organs between those treated with testosterone plus stearic acid, which is not a 5α-reductase inhibitor, and those treated with testosterone alone. Treatments with stearic acid or γ-linolenic acid alone produced no significant effects when compared with the vehicle control. Figure 1 shows representative animals. The areas of the flank organs are shown in Table 1.

If γ-linolenic acid inhibits testosterone action by inhibition of 5α-reductases, γ-linolenic acid should not inhibit DHT stimulated growth of the flank organ. We compared the effect of γ-linolenic acid (0.2, 0.4, and 0.6 mg/flank organ/day) to inhibit T-(0.5 μg) and DHT-(0.5μg) stimulated growth of the flank organ in castrated hamsters. We found that γ-linolenic acid inhibited T- but not DHT-stimulated growth of the flank organ.

We investigated whether γ-linolenic acid inhibition of androgen action was only local or also systemic, γ-linolenic acid was applied daily to one of the flank organs of the immature intact male hamster and the contralateral flank organ received vehicle only. The control group received vehicle only on both flank organs. The flank organs of the control group grew darker and larger in area as the animal grew. γ-Linolenic acid treatments inhibited the growth of the flank organ of the treated side, but it had no effect on the untreated side. Thus, topical application of γ-linolenic acid inhibited androgen action locally without systemic effect.

Table 2. Effects of γ-linolenic acid (γ-LA) and stearic acid (SA) on T-stimulated growth of the flank organ of castrated hamsters. Immature male hamsters were castrated and were divided into 8 groups, 5 per group. The right flank organ of each hamster in a group received daily topical treatment with an ethanol solution (5 μl) containing the compound(s) shown. The left flank organ was not treated. The areas of the pigmented spot were determined after 18 days.

| Treatment | Pigmented Spot ($mm^2$) | |
| 5μl/day | Untreated (L) | Treated (R) |
| --- | --- | --- |
| T (0.5μg) | 3.6±0.5 | 32.7±9.2 |
| T +LA(1mg) | 4.1±0.3 | 15.3±3.9 (-53%)* |
| T +SA(1mg) | 4.3±0.6 | 27.7±4.4 (N.S.)# |
| T +SA(2mg) | 4.2±0.4 | 30.1±7.1 (N.S.)# |
| Vehicle (ethanol) | 5.1±1.9 | 4.2±0.5 |
| LA (1mg) | 4.2±0.6 | 4.1±0.3 |
| SA (1mg) | 4.4±0.4 | 4.9±0.9 |
| SA (2mg) | 4.6±1.4 | 5.0±0.8 |

*T vs. T + LA
#N.S = not significant: T vs. T + SA

## CONCLUSION

Important progress has been made in the characterization of 5α-reductases in human skin. Investigations with 5α-reductase inhibitors in animals and humans have produced encouraging results. Therapy of androgen-dependent skin disorders with 5α-reductase inhibitors may become a reality in the near future.

## REFERENCES

Andersson S, Berman DM, Jenkins EP, Russell DW (1991): Deletion of steroid 5 α-reductase 2 gene in male pseudohermaphroditism. Nature 354:159-161.

Anderson S, Russell DW (1990): Structural and biochemical properties of cloned and expressed human and rat steroid 5 α-reductases. Proc Natl Acad Sci USA 87:3640-3644.

Bingham KD, Shaw DA (1973): The metabolism of testosterone by human male scalp skin. J Endocr 57:111-121.

Diani AR, Mulholland MJ, Shull KL, Kubicek MF, Johnson GA, Schostarez HJ, Brunden MN, Buhl AE (1992): Hair growth effects of oral administration of finasteride, a steroid 5α-reductase inhibitor, alone and in combination with topical minoxidil in the balding stumptail macaque. J Clin Endocr Metab 74:345-350.

Fruzzetti F, De Lorenzo D, Parrini D, Ricci C (1994): Effects of finasteride, a 5α-reductase inhibitor, on circulating androgens and gonadotropin secretion in hirsute women. J Clin Endocrinol Metab 79:831-835.

Harris G, Azzolina B, Baginsky W, Cimis G, Rasmusson GH, Tolman RL, Raetz CR, Ellsworth K (1992): Identification and selective inhibition of an isozyme of steroid 5α-reductase in human scalp. Proc Natl Acad Sci USA 89:10787-10791.

Imperato-McGinley J, Gautier T, Cai L-Q, Yee B, Epstein J, Pochi P (1993): The androgen control of sebum production. Studies of subjects with dihydrostestosterone deficiency and complete androgen insensitivity. J Clin Endocrinol Metab 76:524-528.

Itami S, Kurata S, Sonoda T, Takayasu S (1991): Mechanism of action of androgen in dermal papilla cells. Ann. NY Acad Sci 642:385-395.

Jenkins EP, Hsieh CL, Milatovich A, Normington K, Berman DM, Francke U, Russell DW (1991): Characterization and chromosomal mapping of a human steroid 5α-reductase gene and pseudogene and mapping of the mouse homologue. Genomics 11:1102-1112.

Kuttenn F, Mowszowicz I, Schaison G, Mauvais-Javis P (1977): Androgen production and skin metabolism in hirsutism. J Endocr 75:83-91.

Luu-The V, Sugimoto Y, Puy L, Labrie Y, Lodet SI, Singh M, Labrie F (1994): Characterization, expression, and immunohistochemical localization of 5α-reductase in human skin. J Invest Dermatol 102:221-226.

Moghetti P, Castello R, Magnani CM, Tosi F, Negri C, Armanini D, Bellotti G, Muggeo M (1994): Clinical and hormonal effects of the 5α-reductase inhibitor finasteride in idiopathic hirsutism. J Clin Endocrinol Metab 79:1115-1121.

Mowszowicz I, Melanitou E, Doukani A, Wright F, Kutten F, Mauvais-Jarvis P (1983): Androgen binding capacity and 5α-reductase activity in pubic skin fibroblasts from hirsute patients. J Clin Endocrinol Metabol 56:1209-1213.

Puerto AM, Mallol J (1990): Regional scalp differences of the androgenic metabolic pattern in subjects affected by male pattern baldness. Revista Espanola de Fisiologica 46:289-296.

Rittmaster RS, Uno H, Povar ML, Mellin TN, Loriaux DL (1987): The effects of N,N-diethyl-4-methyl-3-oxo-4-aza-5α-androstane-17β-carboxamide,a5α-reductase inhibitor and antiandrogen, on the development of baldness in the stumptail macaque. J Clin Endocr Metab 65:188-193.

Sansone G, Reisner RM (1971): Differential rates of conversion of testosterone to dihydrotestosterone in acne and in normal human skin - a possible pathogenic factor in acne. J Invest Dermatol 56:366-372.

Serafini P, Lobo RA (1985): Increased 5α-reductase activity in idiopathic hirsutism. Fertility & Sterility 48:74-78.

Thigpen AE, Davis DL, Milatovich A, Mendonca BB, Imperato-McGinley J, Griffin JE, Francke U, Wilson JD, Russell DW (1992): Molecular genetics of steroid 5α-reductase 2 deficiency. J Clin Invest 92: 799-809.

Thigpen AE, Silver RI, Guileyardo JM, Casey ML, McConnell JD, Russell DW (1993): Tissue distribution and ontogeny of steroid 5α-reductase isozyme expression. J Clin Invest 93:903-910.

Wilson JD, Walker JD (1969): The conversion of testosterone to dihydrotestosterone by skin slices of man. J Clin Invest 48:371-379.

Wong IL, Morris RS, Chang L, Spahn MA, Stanczyk FZ, Lobo RA (1995): A
    prospective randomized trial comparing finasteride to spironolactone in the
    treatment of hirsute women.  J Clin Endocrinol Metabol 80: 233-238.

# DISCUSSION: ANDROGEN EFFECTS ON SKIN
## Chairpersons: Shalender Bhasin, Jean Fourcroy

**Richard Horton:** We have been able to block 5 alpha-reductase activity in human sexual skin fibroblasts with less than 5 nM finasteride, suggesting that in that skin area it's a type II enzyme. Is there current data on whether different regions of the skin express these two types of isoforms differently?

**Tehming Liang:** Judging from the acidic pH optimum, the genital skin appears to express type II isozyme. All these studies used neonatal foreskin. I don't know about the adult genital skin.

**Jean Fourcroy:** There has been such a rush of articles on the treatment of hirsutism in women. Flutamide really has no indication ever to be used in a women as an antiandrogen. We have had 21 deaths from liver disease, unexpected and not dose related. Finasteride is a good drug but one has to go back and look at the risks versus the benefits and include in the informed consent what finasteride might do to pregnant women.

**Tehming Liang:** I agree. When using medicine to treat skin diseases which are not life-threatening, the standard of safety has to be very high.

**W. A. Meikle:** We have observed in male twins that a substantial proportion of the apparent 5 alpha-reductase activity is determined by genetic factors or hereditary factors. My question is whether circulatory levels of some of these fatty acids that inhibit 5 alpha-reductase may alter the apparent enzyme activity in tissues.

**Tehming Liang:** There was a report by Morello, et al., (J. Invest. Dermatol. 66:319-323, 1976) which compared fatty acids in the skin surface of acne patients and normal subjects. They found a selective reduction of linoleic acid in the acne patients. I don't know whether a lower level of linoleic acid results in a higher 5 alpha-reductase activity in the skin.

**Somnath Roy:** A young man, age about 26 years, has normal testicular development and normal androgenic manifestations, but no beard growth. Could it be due to deficiency in 5 alpha-reductase or the androgen receptor locally? A second patient with mild hypoandrogenism had some pubic hair growth, very sparse body hair, and no beard. He was put on androgen therapy and after one year's treatment, he has developed facial acne, but no beard. Would you like to comment?

**Tehming Liang:** When one area of skin does not respond to androgen, a local 5 alpha-reductase deficiency certainly is a consideration, but there are many other possibilities, like androgen receptor defect, or defect in other steps of androgen action.

# 25

# MECHANISM OF ACTION OF ANDROGENS ON BONE CELLS

Jon E. Wergedal and  David J. Baylink

**Departments of Medicine and Biochemistry**
**Loma Linda University and**
**Jerry L. Pettis Medical Center**
**Loma Linda, California 92357**

## INTRODUCTION

Bone is a target organ of androgens, which not only affect bone maturation but also have profound effects on the homeostasis of mature bone. In 1941, Rubinstein and Salomon showed that small doses of androgens stimulate linear bone growth in the rat (Rubinstein and Salomon, 1941). Subsequently, androgens were also found to promote endochondral ossification and stimulate fracture healing (Clein and Kowalewski, 1962). These findings indicated a stimulatory effect of androgens on bone growth. More recently, clinical studies reported an increase in the serum level of the osteoblastic marker enzyme, alkaline phosphatase, by androgen treatments (Chestnut et al., 1983). Bone density has also been reported to be positively correlated to serum androgen levels in men and women. These observations suggest an important role of androgens in the regulation of bone formation. Consistent with this premise, human osteoblastic cells have been shown to possess androgen receptors (Orwoll et al., 1991). We have found direct stimulatory effects of androgens and anabolic steroids on human and murine osteoblastic cell proliferation and differentiation  (Kasperk et al.,  1989). Thus, the action of androgens to stimulate bone formation is due at least in part to direct actions of androgens on osteoblasts.

## ANDROGENS DIRECTLY STIMULATE OSTEOBLAST PROLIFERATION AND DIFFERENTIATION

### Proliferation

We have shown that a number of androgens can stimulate proliferation of mouse bone cells. Androgens tested, include testosterone, dihydrotestosterone, methenolone, nandrolone, and fluoxymesterone (Kasperk et al., 1989, Fitzsimmonds

*Pharmacology, Biology, and Clinical Applications of Androgens*, edited by Shalender Bhasin et al.
ISBN 0-471-13320-5 © 1996 Wiley-Liss, Inc.

et al., 1990). Stanozolol, an anabolic androgen, has also been shown to stimulate bone cell proliferation (Vaishnav et al., 1988). Proliferation was measured by both incorporation of [$^3$H]thymidine into DNA and by the increase in cell number with time. The stimulation of proliferation by DHT was dose dependent between the concentrations of $10^{-11}$ and $10^{-8}$M (Fig. 1). Stimulation of proliferation was not confined to mouse bone cells but was also evident when human bone cells were tested, including normal human bone cells, and TE89 osteosarcoma cells. The nonsteroidal antiandrogen hydroxyflutamide, as well as the steroidal antiandrogen cyproterone acetate, inhibit the proliferation response to either DHT or methenolone. This is consistent with the androgens exerting their effect through the androgen receptor.

The magnitude of the response to testosterone and DHT was similar even though the androgen receptor binds DHT more strongly than testosterone. This raises the possibility that testosterone might be converted into DHT in bone cells prior to stimulating cell proliferation. Bone cells have been shown to contain the $5\alpha$ reductase that converts testosterone to DHT. Whether the rate of conversion of testosterone to DHT is sufficient to account for the stimulation of proliferation is not known. In some tissues testosterone can also be converted to estrogens which are thought to play a role in controlling bone mass. Our observations that fluoxymesterone, a synthetic androgen, and DHT, neither of which can be metabolized to estrogens, increased mouse bone cell proliferation, argues against the possibility that testosterone was converted to estrogens by the bone cells and exerted its effect through the estrogen receptors which are present in human bone cells (Eriksen et al., 1988).

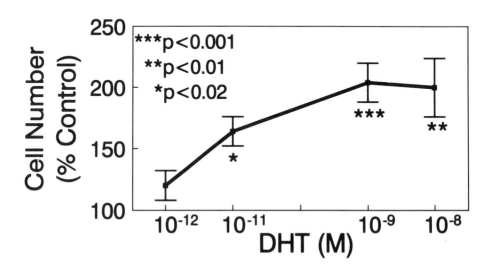

Figure 1. Treatment of mouse bone cells with DHT for 3 days increases cell number in a dose dependent manner.

## Stimulation of Osteoblastic Differentiation

Androgens also stimulated osteoblastic differentiation. In our studies of cultured bone cells, treatment with DHT not only increased the number of bone cells but also increased the % of cells that stained for the osteoblastic marker enzyme alkaline phosphatase. This increase in alkaline phosphatase positive cells could be blocked by the antiandrogen flutamide (Fig. 2) (Kasperk et al., 1989). Collagen production is another osteoblastic characteristic; and, testosterone and DHT have been shown to increase $\alpha 1$, type I procollagen mRNA expression in the human osteosarcoma cell line TE-85 (Benz et al., 1991) and collagen production in rat bone cells. These observations demonstrate that androgens stimulate osteoblastic differentiation.

## MECHANISM OF ACTION OF ANDROGENS ON BONE CELLS

### Androgens Act on Bone Cells by Increasing TGFβ Production

One of the major effects of androgens appears to be to increase production of TGFβ. DHT (1 nM) increased TGFβ production 2.6 fold after 24 hours in mouse bone cells (Kasperk et al., 1990) and increased TGFβ mRNA levels in the human osteosarcoma cells SaOS-2 (Benz, 1991). TGFβ is a differentiating agent known to stimulate alkaline phosphatase activity and collagen production (Wergedal et al., 1992). Therefore, the effects of testosterone and DHT to increase alkaline phosphatase activity and collagen production may be mediated by an increased production of TGFβ. The increased % of alkaline phosphatase positive cells could be due to a stimulation of the proliferation of alkaline phosphatase positive cells, or to increased conversion of alkaline phosphatase negative cells to alkaline phosphatase positive cells. Previous study of chick bone cells showed that TGFβ stimulates proliferation, primarily of the alkaline phosphatase negative cells (Lundy et al., 1991). Additionally TGFβ increases the % of alkaline phosphatase positive bone cells under conditions where little cell proliferation occurs (Wergedal et al., 1992). Thus, androgens may be increasing the % of alkaline phosphatase positive cells by stimulating the production of TGFβ which stimulates the conversion of alkaline phosphatase negative cells to the more differentiated alkaline phosphatase positive cells.

### Androgens Increase Proliferation of Bone Cells by Increasing the Response to Growth Factors

A major local regulatory control mechanism for bone cells is through the IGF system. Several aspects of this system have been investigated in androgen treated cells. To determine whether growth factor production is affected by androgens, the production of IGF-I and IGF II by bone cells were measured. However, the production of these two growth factors was not affected by treatment of bone cells

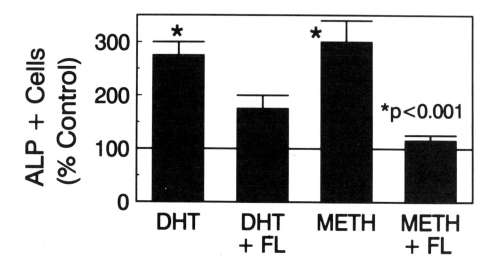

Figure 2.   Flutamide (10 nM) reduces the stimulation of alkaline phosphatase positive cells by DHT (1 nM) and methenolone (1 nM) in human bone cell cultures.

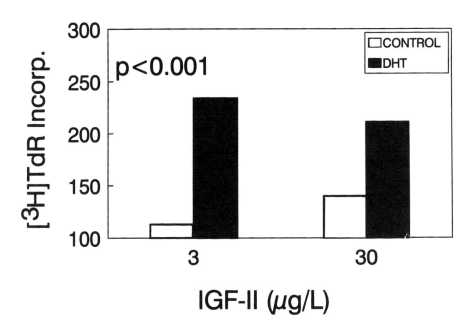

Figure 3.   Increased mitogenic response to IGF-II in mouse bonecells pretreated with DHT (1 nM) for 48 hours.

# SUMMARY

Clinical studies indicate that androgens are important regulators of bone formation. *In vitro* studies demonstrate that androgens can directly stimulate the proliferation and osteoblastic differentiation of bone cells from several species, including man. These *in vitro* actions are consistent with the possibility that the stimulation of bone formation *in vivo* is mediated by direct effects on bone osteoblasts. The presence of the androgen receptor in bone cells and the actions of antiandrogens are consistent with the mechanism where the androgen receptor mediates the actions of androgens on bone cells.

Androgens act on bone cells by altering several aspects of growth factor metabolism. They stimulate production of TGF$\beta$ by bone cells. Increased TGF$\beta$ production may be responsible for the stimulation of osteoblastic characteristics, including alkaline phosphatase activity and collagen production. Increased proliferation is associated with increased responsiveness to IGF-II and FGF. The increased responsiveness to IGF-II is due to increased IGF-II receptor levels and to increased production of IGFBP-5, a binding protein that enhances the action of IGF's on bone. Furthermore, there is an increased responsiveness to FGF by an undetermined mechanism. Thus the actions of androgens to increase proliferation and osteoblastic differentiation is due, at least in part, to alterations in the metabolism of TGF$\beta$, IGF-II and FGF.

# ACKNOWLEDGMENTS

This research was supported by the Veterans Administration and by Loma Linda University.

# REFERENCES

Benz DJ, Haussler MR, Thomas MA, Speelman B, Komm BS (1991): High-affinity androgen binding and androgenic regulation of $\alpha$1(I)-procollagen and transforming growth factor-$\beta$ steady state messenger ribonucleic acid levels in human osteoblast-like osteosarcoma cells. Endocrinology 128: 2723-2730.

Chestnut CH, Ivey JL, Gruber HE, et al (1983): Stanozolol in postmemopausal osteoporosis: therapeutic efficacy and possible mechanism of action. Metabolism 32:571-580.

Clein LJ, Kowalewski K (1962): Some effects of cortisone and anabolic steroid on healing fractures. Can J Surg 5:108-117.

Eriksen EF, Colvard DS, Berg NJ, Graham ML, Mann KG, Spelsberg TC, Riggs BL (1988) Evidence of estrogen receptors in normal human osteoblast-like cells. Science 241: 84-86.

Fitzsimmonds RJ, Wergedal JE, Kasperk C, Baylink DJ (1990): The effects of nandrolone on human bone cells, in vitro. Osteoporosis, 3rd International symposium on osteoporosis, Copenhagen, Denmark, pp 2012-2017.

Kasperk CH, Wergedal JE, Farley JR, Linkhart TA, Turner RT, Baylink DJ (1989):
    Androgens directly stimulate proliferation of bone cells *in vitro*. Endocrinology
    124:1576-1578.

Kasperk C, Fitzsimmons R, Strong D, Mohan S, Jennings J, Wergedal J, Baylink D
    (1990): Studies of the mechanism by which androgens enhance mitogenesis and
    differentiation in bone cells. J Clin Endocrinology Met 71:1322-1329.

Lundy MW, Hendrix T, Wergedal JE, Baylink DJ (1991): Growth factor-induced
    proliferation of osteoblasts measured by bromodeaxyuridine immunocyto-
    chemistry. Growth Factors 4:257-264.

Orwoll ES, Stribrska L, Ramsey EE, Keenan EJ (1991): Androgen receptors in
    osteoblast-like cell lines. Calcified Tissue International 49:183-187.

Rubinstein H, Salomon ML (1941): The growth depressing effect of large doses of
    testosterone propionate in the castrate albino rat. Endocrinology 28:310-318.

Vaishnav R, Beresford JN, Gallagher JA, et al. (1988): Effects of anabolic steroid,
    Stanozolol, on cells derived from human bone. Clin Sci 74:455-460.

Wergedal JE, Matsuyama T, Strong DO (1992): Differentiation of normal human
    bone cells by transforming growth factor-$\beta$ and $1,25(OH)_2$ vitamin $D_3$. Metabo-
    lism: Clinical and Experimental 41:42-48.

# 26

# ANDROGENS AND OSTEOPOROSIS: CLINICAL ASPECTS

Joel S. Finkelstein

Endocrine Unit
Department of Medicine
Massachusetts General Hospital
Boston, MA 02114

## INTRODUCTION

Osteoporosis is one of the leading causes of morbidity and mortality in the elderly. Osteoporosis affects 20 million Americans and leads to approximately 1.5 million fractures each year (Finkelstein, 1995). The annual cost of health care and lost productivity attributed to osteoporosis exceeds $10 billion in the United States. During the course of their lifetimes, women lose about 50% of their trabecular bone and 30% of the cortical bone while men lose about 30% of their trabecular bone and 20% of their cortical bone. Thus, even though osteoporosis is less common in men than in women, one fifth of all hip fractures occur in men and by the age of 90 one of every six men will have fractured their hip.

## EFFECTS OF ANDROGEN DEFICIENCY ON BONE MASS IN MEN

### Effects of Androgens in Normal Men

In adults, bone density at any point in time is determined both by the peak bone mass achieved during development and the subsequent amount of bone loss. Androgens, by affecting both of these processes, are an important determinant of bone mass in men. Both cortical and trabecular bone density increase dramatically during puberty in boys (Krabbe and Christiansen, 1984; Bonjour et al., 1991). The pubertal rise in testosterone is followed closely by an increase in serum alkaline phosphatase, a marker of osteoblast function, and subsequently bone density increases. These data strongly suggest that tes-tosterone, or one of its metabolites, is responsible for the puberty rise in bone mineral density. Peak trabecular bone density is usually achieved by the age of 18 years in males (Bonjour, 1991) though peak cortical bone density may not be reached for a few more years. Bone density then remains relatively stable in young adults males before it declines slowly in later life. Although several cross-sectional studies have suggested that a decline in gonadal function may be responsible for the decrease in bone density as men age, not all studies have been able to demonstrate a correlation between serum androgens and bone mass in aging men. Longitudinal studies of bone density in older adult men are needed to assess the relationship between changes in gonadal function and bone mass more precisely.

## Bone Density in Hypogonadal Men

The observation that androgen deficiency could produce osteoporosis in men was first made by Albright, who noted that eunuchs often developed osteoporosis. With the advent of improved methods for measuring bone density, most of the data examining the relationship between androgen deficiency and bone mass in men have been pub-lished in the last 15 years. A series of reports involving a small number of patients suggested that cortical bone density is decreased in men with Klinefelter's syndrome. However, it is difficult to determine whether the osteopenia of these men is due to their hypogonadism or is an independent effect related to their genetic defect. In a case control study of 105 men with osteoporotic fractures, hypogonadism was one of the most common underlying disorders (Seeman et al., 1983). Another case control study reported that hypogonadism was twice as common in men with recent minimal trauma hip fractures than in controls. Histomorphometric analyses of iliac crest bone biopsies from men with androgen deficiency have shown both decreased and increased bone formation. This variability may be due to patient heterogeneity, or to complex effects of androgens on bone turnover.

Comprehensive studies of the effects of androgen deficiency on bone mass in men have recently been reported in several groups of men: men with primary hypo-gonadism; men with several forms of secondary hypogonadism, and men with histories of constitutionally delayed puberty. These studies provide prospective data on the effects of androgens on bone mass in men and will be discussed in detail.

## Studies in Men with Primary Hypogonadism

In contrast to women, in whom there is a large amount of data relating primary hypogonadism to bone mass, little such data exist in men. Stepan et al. (1989) measured bone mineral density of the lumbar spine using dual photon absorptiometry in 12 men who had undergone bilateral orchiectomy because of sexual delinquency up to 11 years previously (mean 5.6 years). In 9 of these men, measurements were repeated 1 to 3 years later. As shown in Figure 1, bone density decreased progressively with increasing years since castration. Although it appeared that the rate of bone loss was greater in the first several years after orchiectomy, the number of observations was too small to demonstrate such a relationship conclusively. Biochemical indices of bone resorption and bone formation were increased compared to normal men and there was a significant association between urinary hydroxyproline excretion and the rate of bone loss. These findings suggest that gonadal steroid deficiency is associated with increased bone turnover. All of the

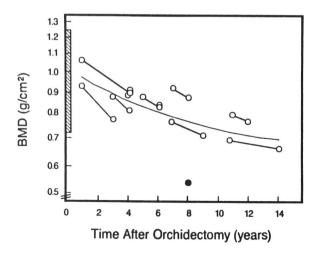

Figure 1. Scattergram of lumbar spinal bone mineral density (BMD) as a function of time after orchidectomy in 12 men. In 8 patients the measurement was repeated after 1-3 years. The hatched bar indicates the normal range for 20 men matched for age. The solid circle represents the value for one man who developed a hip fracture. (Reproduced with permission from Stepan et al., J Clin Endocrinol Metab 69:523-527, 1989.)

measured indices of bone turnover decreased during treatment with intranasal calcitonin, an agent that inhibits bone resorption.

Recently, we have investigated bone density and the effects of androgen replacement therapy in 29 men with acquired primary or secondary hypogonadism (Katznelson et al., 1994). Spinal bone density was measured using both dual energy x-ray absorptiometry (DXA), a technique that assesses both trabecular and cortical bone in the spine, and quantitative computed tomography (QCT), a technique that assesses exclusively trabecular bone. Spinal bone density was significantly lower than that of age-matched normal men using both techniques. Spinal bone density increased signi-ficantly (5% by DXA and 13% by QCT) during 12 to 18 months of androgen replace-ment therapy. Baseline lean body mass was decreased in the hypogonadal men. Lean body mass increased and the percent body fat decreased in response to testosterone replacement.

## Studies in Men with Hyperprolactinemic Hypogonadism

Greenspan et al. (1986) measured cortical bone density in the forearm by single photon absorptiometry (SPA) and trabecular bone density in the spine by QCT in 18 men between the ages of 30 and 79 with secondary hypogonadism caused by prolactin-secreting tumors. Five men had secondary hypothyroidism and/or secondary adrenal insufficiency and were receiving physiological hormone replacement. Both cortical (Figure 2a) and trabecular (Figure 2b) bone mineral

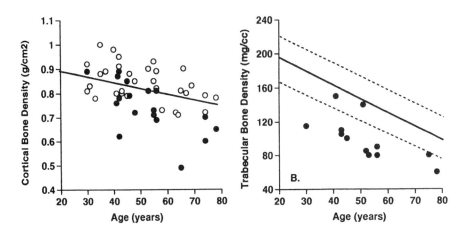

Figure 2. a. Cortical bone density of the radius in patients with hyperprolactinemia (solid circles) and controls (open circles) with the regression of cortical bone density with age in controls (broken line). b. Trabecular bone density of the lumbar spine in patients with hyperprolactinemia (solid circles). The solid line represents the expected mean normal bone density for age ($\pm$ SD). (Modified and reproduced with permission from Greenspan et al., Ann Intern Med 104:777-782, 1986.)

density were significantly decreased in the hyperprolactinemic men compared to age-matched controls. Cortical bone den-sity correlated with the duration of hyperprolactinemia. There was no significant correlation between cortical and trabecular bone density, suggesting that cortical and bone respond differently to androgen deficiency. These findings suggest that hypogonadism in hyper-prolactinemic men leads to osteopenia but do not rule out the possibility that other hormone deficiencies present in men with central hypogonadism may have an adverse effect on skeletal integrity.

To assess the effects of restoration of gonadal steroid secretion on bone density in men with hyperprolactinemic hypogonadism, Greenspan et al. (1989) performed serial measurements of bone density for 6 to 48 months in 20 such men who were treated with bromocriptine, transsphenoidal surgery, and/or cranial radiation. In those men whose serum testosterone levels normalized (Group I), cortical bone density increased significantly (Figure 3a) and there was a significant correlation between the change in serum testosterone levels and the change in bone density. In the men who remained hypogonadal (Group II), cortical bone density did not change (Figure 3a). Trabecular bone density of the lumbar spine did not change significantly in either group (Figure 3b).

## Studies in Men Receiving Long-Acting GnRH Analog Therapy

The effects of secondary hypogonadism on bone mass have also been studied by examining the effects of daily administration of a long-acting GnRH analog to men with benign prostatic hyperplasia (Goldray et al., 1993). GnRH

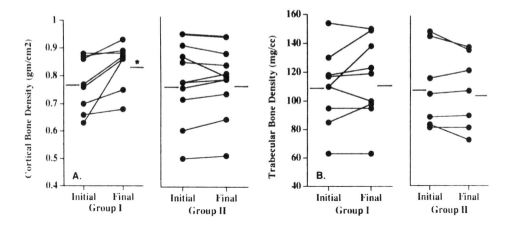

Figure 3. Initial and final cortical and trabecular bone densities in men with hyperprolactinemia who had normalization of their gonadal status (Group I) or who remained hypogonadal (Group II). Horizontal bars represent the mean bone density. * denotes P<0.05 vs initial value. (Modified and reproduced with permission from Greenspan et al., Ann Intern Med 120:526-531, 1989.)

analog therapy produced severe testosterone deficiency in all men. In 10 of 17 men, bone density of the lumbar spine decreased significantly over a period of 6 to 12 months (Figure 4). Serum alkaline phosphatase and osteocalcin levels increased significantly, suggesting that bone turnover was increased. Serum levels of calcium, vitamin D metabolites, and parathyroid hormone did not change significantly. In general, the effects of GnRH analog administration on bone metabolism in men were similar to those previously described in women.

## Studies in Men with Idiopathic Hypogonadotropic Hypogonadism

Men with idiopathic hypogonadotropic hypogonadism (IHH) are hypogonadal due to an isolated absence of hypothalamic gonadotropin-releasing hormone (GnRH) secretion. Otherwise, pituitary function is intact in these men. Thus, they provide a useful model to examine the effects of complete, isolated gonadal steroid deficiency on bone mass in men.

Furthermore, because IHH is almost always a congenital abnormality, men with IHH provide a valuable model to assess the effects of gonadal steroid deficiency on pubertal bone development (i.e. the attainment of peak bone mass). We measured cortical bone density by SPA and trabecular bone density by QCT in 23 young men with IHH (Finkelstein et al., 1987). Because bone density increases dramatically during puberty, patients with open epiphyses were compared to adolescent controls matched for bone age whereas patients with fused epiphyses were compared to age-matched adult men. Both cortical (Figure 5) and trabecular (Figure 6) bone mineral density were markedly decreased in IHH men and the

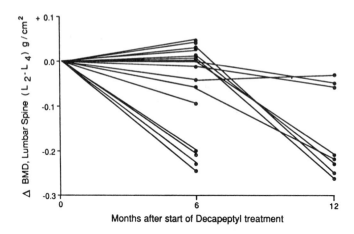

Figure 4. Individual changes (D) in lumbar BMD during 6-12 months of GnRH analog therapy. (Reproduced with permission from Goldray et al., J Clin Endocrinol Metab 76:288-90, 1993.)

osteoporosis was equally severe in the men with open and fused epiphyses. In 8 men, trabecular bone density was below the fracture threshold despite their young age (Figure 6). As in the men with hyperprolactinemic hypogonadism, there was no association between cortical and trabecular bone density. These data demonstrate that GnRH-deficient men have severe osteopenia affecting both cortical and trabecular bone. Because severe osteopenia was already present in men who were skeletally immature, these data suggest that the osteopenia of IHH men is due to inadequate pubertal bone accretion rather than post-maturity adult bone loss.

To assess the effects of androgen replacement on bone mass in IHH men, we made longitudinal measurements of cortical and trabecular bone density in 21 of these 23 men while serum testosterone levels were maintained in the normal range with either pulsatile GnRH, human chorionic gonadotropin, or intramuscular testosterone therapy for an average of 2 years (Finkelstein et al., 1989). In the men who were initially skeletally mature (Group I), there was a small but significant increase in cortical bone density (Figure 7a) whereas trabecular bone density did not change (Figure 7b). These responses are similar to those described above for adult men with hyperprolactinemic hypogonadism. In the men who were still skeletally immature at the beginning of the study (Group II), both cortical and trabecular bone density increased significantly (Figure 7 a and b). Furthermore, cortical bone density increased more in the skeletally immature men, suggesting that much of the increase in bone density in men with open epiphyses is due to a completion of the process of pubertal bone accretion. Despite these increases, bone density remained well below the levels of normal men. This finding suggests either that factors other than gonadal steroid deficiency are involved in the pathogenesis

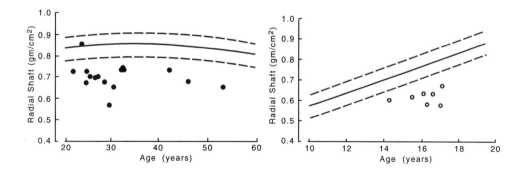

Figure 5. a. Radial (cortical) bone density compared with age in 16 men with idiopethic hypogonadotropic hypogonadism (IHH) with fused epiphyses. The lines indicate the mean ($\pm$ 1 SD) radial bone density in normal men. b. Radial bone density compared with bone age in 7 IHH men with open epiphyses. (Modified and reproduced with permission from Finkelstein et al., Ann Intern Med 106:354-361, 1987.)

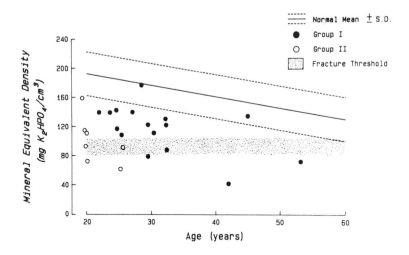

Figure 6. Spinal (trabecular) bone density compared with age in 23 IHH men. Closed circles refer to patients in Group I (fused epiphyses), and open circles refer to patients in Group II (open epiphyses). The lines indicate the mean ($\pm$ 1 SD) spinal bone density in normal adult men. The stippled bar indicates the fracture threshold (Reproduced with permission from Finkelstein et al., Ann Intern Med 106:354-361, 1987.)

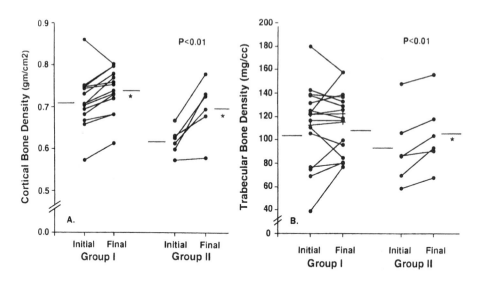

Figure 7. Initial and final cortical (panel a) and trabecular (panel b) bone densities after treatment of IHH men who initially had fused epiphyses (Group I) or open epiphyses (Group II). Solid lines represent the mean bone density. (Modified and reproduced with permission from Finkelstein et al., J Clin Endocrinol Metab 69:776-783, 1989.)

of the osteopenia of IHH men or that there may be a critical period in development when gonadal steroid secretion must be normal in order to achieve a normal peak bone density.

## Studies in Adult Men with Histories of Constitutionally Delayed Puberty

As noted above, the observation that bone density failed to normalize during prolonged gonadal steroid replacement in IHH men suggested that there may be a critical period in development during which puberty must occur in order to achieve a normal peak bone mineral density. To test this hypothesis, we measured radial bone mineral density using SPA and spinal bone mineral density using DXA in 23 adult men with histories of constitutionally delayed puberty and compared their values with a well-matched group of normal men (Finkelstein et al., 1992). Both radial and spinal bone mineral density were significantly lower in men with histories of delayed puberty than in normal controls (Figure 8 a and b). In fact, radial bone density was at least 1 standard deviation (SD) below the mean in 15 of the 23 men and at least 2 SD below the normal mean in 8 men. Spinal bone density was at least 1 SD below the normal mean in 10 of the 23 men. These findings demonstrate that men with histories of constitutionally delayed puberty have

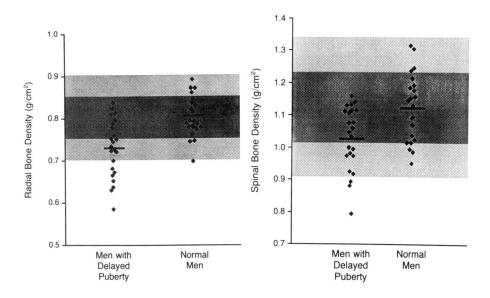

Figure 8. Radial bone density (panel a) and spinal bone density (panel b) in 23 men with histories of delayed puberty and 21 normal controls. The horizontal lines indicate the group means, and the shaded areas the mean $\pm$ 1 SD and $\pm$ 2 SD for the normal men. (Reproduced with permission from Finkelstein et al., N Engl J Med 326:600-604, 1992.)

decreased radial and spinal bone mineral density and suggest that the timing of puberty is an important determinant of peak bone mass. Because the peak bone density achieved during development is an important determinant of bone density in later life, men with histories of delayed puberty may be at increased risk for osteoporotic fractures. Finally, a history of delayed puberty may be an important clue to the etiology of low bone density in men with "idiopathic" osteoporosis.

## AREAS FOR FUTURE INVESTIGATION

### Mechanism of Action of Androgens on Bone

The mechanism(s) whereby androgens affect bone density is still unclear. Data suggest that androgens may stimulate bone formation directly. Several observations are consistent with this notion. First, androgen receptors have been found on osteoblasts. Second, both aromatizable and non-aromatizable androgens stimulate proliferation of human osteoblasts *in vitro*, as indicated by enhanced uptake of [$^3$H]thymidine. Androgens also stimulate collagen production *in vitro*. Third, androgens stimulate osteoblast differentiation *in vitro*, as indicated by an increase in the percentage of cells that stain for alkaline phosphatase (Kasperk et al., 1989). The effect of androgens on osteoblast proliferation and differentiation might be due to increased local production of TGF-β or increased sensitivity to the effects of fibroblast growth factor and IGF-II. Finally, androgens inhibit PTH-stimulated accumulation of cAMP by osteoblasts *in vitro*.

Androgens have also been shown to affect bone formation in humans, though it is not clear if the effects result from a direct action on osteoblasts or through an indirect mechanism. Data dervied primarily from using surrogate markers of bone formation indicate that androgens may stimulate osteoblast function. For example, some investigators have reported that serum osteocalcin levels increase when androgens are administered to men (Young et al., 1993) though others have not detected a significant change (Tenover, 1992).

Although it appears likely that androgens stimulate osteoblast activity, this finding does not explain the increase in bone resorption that is seen both in animals and men after orchiectomy. Biochemical markers of bone turnover (serum osteocalcin levels and urinary hydroxyproline excretion) increase in men after castration (Stepan et al., 1989). Testosterone administration reduces urinary hydroxyproline excretion in men with borderline low serum testosterone levels (Tenover, 1992). Both osteoclast number and the extent of osteoclast-covered bone surfaces increase after orchiectomy and these effects can be prevented by administration of testosterone or dihydrotestosterone. The mechanism by which androgens inhibit the up regulation of osteoclastogenesis that follows orchiectomy may involve effects on local production of cytokines in bone. For example, it has been reported that androgens inhibit the transcription of interleukin-6 (IL-6) and that interleukin-1 (IL-1) production was increased in a hypogonadal male. Because these cytokines promote osteoclast activation and differentiation, increased local production of IL-1, IL-6, or other osteoclast-stimulating cytokines may be the mechanism whereby androgen deficiency stimulates bone resorption.

Androgens may also affect bone metabolism by effects on calcium regulatory hormones. It has been reported that serum calcitonin levels are lower in hypogonadal men than in normal men; that testosterone administration increases calcitonin levels in hypogonadal men; and that testosterone administration enhances the hypocalcemic effect of calcitonin in orchiectomized rats. One group of investigators reported that testosterone replacement increases serum 1,25-(OH)$_2$ vitamin D levels in hypogonadal men (Francis et al., 1986). However, we did not detect any change in 1,25-(OH)$_2$ vita-in D levels in GnRH-deficient men before and after androgen replacement (Finkelstein et al., 1989) and no changes were observed in 1,25-(OH)$_2$ vitamin D levels of older men with borderline low serum testosterone levels during testosterone therapy (Tenover, 1992). Furthermore, no changes in serum 25-OH vitamin D, 1,25-(OH)$_2$ vitamin D, or PTH levels occur during GnRH analog-induced hypogonadism in men (Goldray et al., 1993).

It is still unclear whether the ability of testosterone to stimulate bone formation and inhibit bone resorption is due to testosterone itself or one of its metabolites such as estradiol or dihydrotestosterone. It has been demonstrated that testosterone can be converted to dihydrotestosterone by human bone *in vitro*. Nonetheless, inhibition of dihydrotestosterone formation by administration of an inhibitor of 5α-reductase has no effect on bone mass in humans (Matzkin et al., 1992) or rats. Several observations suggest that aromatization of testosterone into estrogens is crucial for many of the effects of testosterone on bone. First, estrogen receptors have been demonstrated in human osteoblasts. Second, estrogens can maintain bone mass in castrated male-to-female transsexuals. Third, and most important, it has recently been reported that a male with complete estrogen resistance due to a genetic defect in the estrogen receptor has severe osteopenia despite normal testosterone levels and complete virilization (Smith et al., 1994). This finding provides the most compelling evidence to date that estrogens are required for a normal peak bone mass in men. However, because cortical bone mineral density is higher in normal men than in women (Bonjour et al., 1991), it appears likely that androgens have an independent effect on peak bone mass. Further studies are needed to assess the relative roles of androgens and estrogens in bone metabolism in men.

## Therapy of Androgen-Deficiency Bone Loss

As noted above, several studies have demonstrated increases in bone density in hypogonadal men receiving androgen replacement therapy, particularly in those men who are still skeletally immature (Finkelstein et al., 1989; Greenspan et al., 1989). However, the degree of androgen deficiency needed to produce osteoporosis in men is currently unknown. This issue is of considerable clinical importance because many men are seen with mildly decreased or low normal levels of testosterone and it is not clear whether these men are at risk for developing osteoporosis that might be preventable with testosterone therapy. There are also no data comparing different modes of androgen replacement (e.g. parenteral vs topical) on bone density. Finally, the use of non-androgenic agents such to prevent bone loss in hypogonadal men with contraindications to testosterone therapy (e.g. men with prostate cancer receiving GnRH analog therapy or after surgical castration) has not been examined. Because bone resorption is increased in such men, anti-resorptive therapy would seem to be logical. In addition, we have recently demonstrated that daily parathyroid hormone administration, an agent that stimulates bone formation, prevents GnRH analog-induced bone loss in women with endometriosis, in whom estrogen therapy may be contraindicated (Finkelstein et al., 1994). Thus, it seems likely that parathyroid hormone might also prevent GnRH analog-induced bone loss in men. The use of anabolic agents like parathyroid hormone, or antiresorptive agents, such as bisphosphonates or calcitonin, to prevent bone loss in hypogonadal men with contraindications to testosterone therapy needs further evaluation.

# REFERENCES

Bonjour J-P, Theintz G, Buchs B, Slosman D, Rizzoli R (1991): Critical years and stages of puberty for spinal and femoral bone mass accumulation during adolescence. J Clin Endocrinol Metab 73:555-563.

Finkelstein JS, Klibanski A, Neer RM, Greenspan SL, Rosenthal DI, Crowley WF (1987): Osteoporosis in men with idiopathic hypogonadotropic hypogonadism. Ann Intern Med 106:354-461.

Finkelstein JS, Klibanski A, Neer RM, Doppelt SH, Rosenthal DI, Segre GV, Crowley WF (1989): Increases in bone density during treatment of men with idiopathic hypogonadotropic hypogonadism. J Clin Endocrinol Metab 69:776-783.

Finkelstein JS, Neer RM, Biller BMK, Crawford JD, Klibanski A (1992): Osteopenia in adult men with a history of delayed puberty. N Engl J Med 326:600-604.

Finkelstein JS, Klibanski A, Schaefer EH, Hornstein MD, Schiff I, Neer RM (1994): Parathyroid hormone for the prevention of bone loss induced by estrogen deficiency. N Engl J Med 331:1618-1623.

Finkelstein JS (1995): Osteoporosis. In Bennett JC, Plum F (eds.): "Cecil Textbook of Medicine." Philadelphia: W.B. Saunders, (in press).

Francis RM, Peacock M, Aaron JE, Selby PL, Taylor GA, Thompson J, Marshall DH, Horsman A (1986): Osteoporosis in hypogonadal men: role of decreased plasma 1,25-dihydroxyvitamin D, calcium malabsorption, and low bone formation. Bone 7:261-268.

Goldray D, Weisman Y, Jaccard N, Merdler C, Chen J, Matzkin H (1993): Decreased bone density in elderly men treated with the gonadotropin-releasing hormone agonist decapeptyl (D-Trp6-GnRH). J Clin Endocrinol Metab 76:288-290.

Greenspan SL, Neer RM, Ridgway EC, Klibanski A (1986): Osteoporosis in men with hyperprolactinemic hypogonadism. Ann Intern Med 104:777-782.

Greenspan SL, Oppenheim DS, Klibanski A (1989): Importance of gonadal steroids to bone mass in men with hyperprolactinemic hypogonadism. Ann Intern Med 110:526-531.

Kasperk CH, Wergedal JE, Farley JR, Linkhart TA, Turner RT, Baylink DJ (1989): Androgens directly stimulate proliferation of bone cells in vitro. Endocrinology 124:1576-1578.

Katznelson L, Finkelstein J, Baressi C, Klibanski A (1994): Increase in trabecular bone density and altered body composition in androgen replaced hypogonadal men. The Endocrine Society. 76th Annual Meeting 581 (abstract #1524).

Krabbe S, Christiansen C (1984): Longitudinal study of calcium metabolism in male puberty. I. Bone mineral content, and serum levels of alkaline phosphatase, phosphate and calcium. Acta Paediatr Scand 73:745-749.

Matzkin H, Chen J, Welsman Y, Goldray D, Pappas F, Jaccard N, Braf Z (1992): Prolonged treatment with finasteride (a 5α-reductase inhibitor) does not affect bone density and metabolism. Clin Endocrinol 37:432-436.

Seeman E, Melton LJ, O'Fallon WM, Riggs BL (1983): Risk factors for spinal osteoporosis in men. Am J Med 75:977-983.

Smith EP, Boyd J, Frank GR, Takahashi H, Cohen RM, Specker B, Williams TC, Lubahn DB, Korach KS (1994): Estrogen resistance caused by a mutation in the estrogen-receptor gene in a man. N Engl J Med 331:1056-1061.

Stepan JJ, Lachman M, Zverina J, Pacovsky V, Baylink DJ (1989): Castrated men exhibit bone loss: effect of calcitonin treatment on biochemical indices of bone remodeling. J Clin Endocrinol Metab 69:523-527.

Tenover JS (1992): Effects of testosterone supplementation in the aging male. J Clin Endocrinol Metab 75:1092-1098.

Young NR, Baker HWG, Liu G, Seeman E (1993): Body composition and muscle strength in healthy men receiving testosterone enanthate for contraception. J Clin Endocrinol Metab 77:1028-1032.

## DISCUSSION: ANDROGENS AND BONE
## Chairpersons:  Eric Orwoll, Lisa Tenover

**Robert Lustig:**  I was wondering if the use of growth hormone, or measuring the levels of endogenous growth hormones, makes any difference in terms of bone mineralization.  Your data would suggest that we ought to be giving androgen therapy much earlier in children with delayed puberty or panhypopituitarism.  Usually, we give it much later because we are trying to maximize final height.  Does the mineralization in some way obviate this decision?

**Joel Finkelstein:**  The only information we have on the growth hormone status and bone mass in men with histories of delayed puberty is on IGF-1 levels measured during the two year follow-up visits.  Although IGF-1 levels in these men are within the normal range, the levels were about 40% lower than those of control men.  This finding raises the question whether or not constitutional delay is merely a shift in the timing that people go through puberty or whether or not these individuals may have permanent defects in their growth hormone-IGF axis.  The next question is whether the observation that men with histories of constitutional delays have osteopenia indicates that early intervention in these men, or in men with disorders that lead to puberty, will improve their peak bone mass.  Those are two separate questions.  Delayed puberty is associated with decreased bone density, but it remains to be shown that early treatment of these boys will improve their peak bone density.

**Robert Lustig:**  Androgen increases 24-hour integrated growth hormone concentration.  Could it be that decreased 24-hour GH secretion rather than androgen is the basis of decreased bone density?

**Joel Finkelstein:**  The implication of the data on IGF is that the osteopenia of men with delayed puberty may be related to the effects of diminished growth hormone secretion rather than to a critical period in development during which the skeleton must be exposed to pubertal sex steroid secretion.

**Todd Nippoldt:**  Is there a threshold of serum testosterone level  below which osteoporosis is likely to develop in a man?

**Joel Finkelstein:**  I do not know of any information regarding this issue.  It is generally difficult to demonstrate a significant correlation between serum testosterone levels and bone density in normal men.  We know that hypogonadal men are at risk for osteoporosis.  What is unclear is the degree of testosterone deficiency that leads to osteoporosis.

**Richard Horton:**  While osteoblasts have been reported to convert testosterone to dihydrotestosterone, patients with type II 5 alpha-reductase deficiency have normal bone density.  The four year report on finasteride in men with BPH has not demonstrated altered bone density.  This suggests that bone is responding to testosterone directly.  Have you done any experiments with 5 alpha-reductase blocker inhibitor and testosterone?.

**Jon Wergedel:**  No, we have not looked at the possibility of whether or not testosterone has been metabolized in the bone cells.  I would expect that this is a direct effect of testosterone, but we have not studied the inhibitors.

**Joel Finkelstein:** It is unclear whether finasteride gets into bone tissue as effectively as it gets into other tissues. Furthermore, finasteride may only be blocking 5 alpha-reductase type II, though at high doses it may block both forms of the enzymes. This negative experiment, using a 5 alpha-reductase blocker, does not necessarily rule out the possibility that there may be an effect of DHT in bone.

**Jon Wergedel:** In studies in castrated animals, DHT seems to be as effective as testosterone in maintaining bone remodeling.

**Dirk Vanderschueren:** I agree with you that androgens are very important for the development in bone, the modeling of bone, and for maintaining normal male bone density. We do not know whether or not androgen replacement prevents bone loss at later age. In that sense, we should study osteoclasts not osteoblasts. Today we only discussed effects on osteoblasts. Stefan, who did a study in men castrated after puberty, showed that there is an increase in both resorption by osteoclasts, and secondarily, an increase in bone formation. Androgen effects on osteoclast function have not been well studied. Do you think that for the maintenance of the bone density in men, there may be a role for estrogens?

**Richard Horton:** If you block resorption or reduce resorption that impact has only a limited effect on the net amount of bone (approximately 10%). If you stimulate formation, you can increase the amount of bone several fold.

**Dirk Vanderschueren:** When hypogonadal men who develop androgen deficiency before puberty receive androgen, there is stabilization of the bone density and not a gain of bone density. Another issue that remains unclear is whether or not androgen stabilizes bone density in men becoming hypogonadal after puberty.

**Joel Finkelstein:** There is clearly a gain in bone density in the GnRH-deficient men who are still skeletally immature when treated, and a smaller increase in cortical bone density in the GnRH-deficient men who were skeletally mature. It appears that the major effect of androgens in skeletally mature men is to stabilize bone mass.

When male animals are castrated, osteoclastogenesis increases, and this increase can be prevented with androgen replacement. The mechanism whereby androgens inhibit osteoclast activity may be related to its effects on local production of cytokines in bone. Androgens inhibit transcription of interleukin-6, a factor that stimulates differentiation of osteoclast precursors. Androgen deficiency may also lead to increased production of interleukin-1, another substance that stimulates osteoclast differentiation and activity. The effects of androgen deficiency and replacement on bone cytokines, that are related to osteoclast function, appears to be similar to the effects of estrogens on these bone cytokines.

**Carrie Bagatell:** I have a question regarding osteoporosis and androgens in women. Since the data clearly show that androgens have effects on bone that are independent of aromatization to estradiol, I am wondering about potential use of small amounts of androgen in women. Are there studies in women who are taking a combination of estrogen and androgen? Is this potentially a worthwhile strategy to undertake in certain subsets of women, particularly those who are taking prednisone and are postmenopausal, or have had an organ transplant and are taking cyclosporine and therefore are not candidates for etidronate?

**Joel Finkelstein:**  First, in postmenopausal women one can completely prevent bone loss with estrogen replacement alone.  Thus, there is no clear mandate, from the standpoint of prevention of bone loss, for adding androgens to estrogens in postmenopausal women.  There are several published studies in which pharmacological doses of anabolic steroids have been given to women with postmenopausal osteoporosis.  These studies reported that bone density increases between 3 and 20%.  I am not aware of any published data concerning the skeletal effects of estratest.

**Barbara Sherwin:**  I just want to tell you that there are data and I will be presenting them.

**Eric Orwoll:**  In correlational studies, Charlie Slemenda showed that the rate of bone loss during early menopause is positively correlated with androgens as it is with estrogens.  Bone density of androgenized women is actually higher than that of nonandrogenized women (for instance, congenital adrenal hyperplasia, or idiopathic hirsutism).

**Joel Finkelstein:**  It is clear that pathological states of androgen excess in women are associated with higher bone mass.  However, those findings do not prove that physiological levels of androgens have important effects on the skeleton in women.

**William Bremner:**  Are there any changes in calcium, PTH, vitamin D, or any other vital humor that is related to bone when you give androgens in any of those hypogonadal states?  When we carried out the studies of supraphysiological doses of testosterone (200 mg TE/wk) it did cause a slight decrease in calcium levels and a fairly impressive increase in PTH levels.

**Joel Finkelstein:**  In most of the studies of androgen treatment in hypogonadal men, there have not been any changes in calcium regulatory hormones.  One small study reported an increase in 1,25- dihydroxyvitamin D levels in androgen-treated hypogonadal men.  The finding that pharmacological doses of testosterone are associated with slightly diminished calcium levels and increased PTH levels could be explained on the basis of elevated estrogen levels because estrogen administration is well known to have these effects in postmenopausal women.

**William Bremner:**  What is the effect in that setting of estrogens on vitamin D levels?

**Joel Finkelstein:**  I am not aware of any clear effects of estrogen on vitamin D levels, other than an increase in vitamin D binding protein.  We have made several measurements of 25-hydroxyvitamin D and 1.25-dihydroxyvitamin D in women rendered estrogen-deficient with a long-acting GnRH analog and have not observed any change in total vitamin D levels.  *In vitro*, estrogen has no direct effect on 1.25-dihydroxyvitamin D formation.  *In vivo*, however, estrogen administration may lower serum calcium levels leading to increased PTH secretion which may then increase 1.25-dihydroxyvitamin D formation.  Furthermore, the effects of estrogen replacement on vitamin D levels in postmenopausal women appears to depend on the mode of delivery.  Oral estrogens may increase total and free 1.25- dihydroxyvitamin D levels, whereas transdermal estrogen has no such effect.  Although the reason for this differential effect, based on the mode of estrogen delivery is not well known, it may be related to the ability of oral estrogen to lower plasma phosphorus, which is a known stimulus for 1.25-dihydroxyvitamin D formation.

**Adrian Dobs:** There was a fascinating recent article about a man with an estrogen receptor defect who presented with tall stature. He had not closed his epiphyses, which suggested that estrogen rather than testosterone was required to close epiphyses.

**Joel Finkelstein:** That is a fascinating report. Not only does this man have open epiphyses and tall stature, he has marked osteopenia. These findings suggest that estrogens are important both for epiphysial closure and for maintenance or achievement of peak bone density in men. Yesterday, data were presented in the poster session evaluating the effects of aromatization blockade on bone metabolism in adult male rats which demonstrated that aromatization blockade increased bone resorption and caused bone loss. Therefore, estrogens probably have important effects on skeletal integrity in males. However, the observation that cortical bone density is clearly higher in normal men than in normal women suggests that androgens are also important determinants of peak bone mass. The relative importance of estrogens and androgens in the determination of peak bone mass and the maintenance of normal bone density is still unclear.

**Eric Orwoll:** Studies in animals examining the effectiveness of DHT in the prevention of bone loss following orchiectomy show that DHT is as effective as testosterone; not more effective, but equally effective. In the reported man with estrogen receptor defect, spinal bone density was dramatically decreased, but cortical bone density was decreased to a lesser degree. This raises the issue of the dichotomy between trabecular and cortical bone regulation.

**Ronald Swerdloff:** Do we have data to suggest that there are organizational differences in the bone cells in males versus females?

**Jon Wergedel:** There are some data which suggest that there are differences in responses of bone cells from males and females to the steroid hormones.

**Eric Orwoll:** In trabecular bone, the remodeling response to estrogen or androgen exposure appears very similar. In periosteal bone, there are some interesting discrepancies. If you castrate a male animal, periosteal bone formation goes down. If you castrate a female animal, it goes up. We know very little about periosteal bone regulation, but it is interesting that it is in cortical bone mass where the sexual dichotomy is most marked. Prepubertally, boys and girls have a very similar cortical bone mass. In girls, bone density begins to increase at an earlier age, but by the time peak bone mass is achieved, cortical bone mass is higher in boys. Joel, could you speculate about the determinants of lumbar spine bone density in patients with androgen insensitivity?

**Joel Finkelstein:** There are several possible explanations why women with androgen insensitivity syndrome have osteopenia in the lumbar spine. Their gonadal steroid milieu is not normal when compared to that of normal women. These patients do not have cyclic estrogen secretion, they have lower levels of estrogen secretion and they do not have progesterone secretion. In addition, they are not sensitive to adrenal androgens. Finally, these women are castrated and then put on androgen replacement therapy. Their osteopenia could be related to failure to comply completely with their replacement program.

# 27

# ANDROGEN EFFECTS ON BODY COMPOSITION AND MUSCLE PERFORMANCE

**[1]Richard Casaburi, [2]Thomas Storer, and [3]Shalender Bhasin**

**[1]Division of Respiratory and
Critical Care Physiology and Medicine
Harbor-UCLA Medical Center
Torrance, California 90509
[2]Laboratory of Exercise Sciences, El Camino College
Torrance, California 90506
[3]Division of Endocrinology
King-Drew Medical Center
Los Angeles, California 90059**

## INTRODUCTION

Programs of resistive exercise training have been shown capable of inducing increases in muscle strength. Changes in cellular morphometry and biochemistry accompany, and presumably mediate, these improvements in muscle function. Yet, we remain essentially ignorant about the specific cellular triggers that connect exercise training to cellular remodeling (Casaburi, 1994). This makes it difficult to rationally predict whether a given training intervention or pharmacologic agent will improve muscle performance. Clinical trials are required to evaluate such drugs.

Based principally on empiric observations, androgenic steroids have received much attention (and widespread use) for their perceived ergogenic properties. There is little question that androgynic steroid administration to castrated animals, hypogonadal men, boys before puberty, and women, results in increased nitrogen retention and increased muscle mass. To this point, we recently examined the effects of 10 weeks of weekly intramuscular injections of 100 mg of testosterone enanthate on five hypogonadal men (Bhasin et al., 1994). Despite being maintained on a eumetabolic diet, lean body mass (as assessed by both underwater weighing and deuterium water) increased significantly (by an average of 11%). Further, muscle cross-sectional area of both the non-dominant upper arm and thigh muscles (as assessed by magnetic resonance imaging) also increased significantly (by an average of 21% and 12%, respectively).

*Pharmacology, Biology, and Clinical Applications of Androgens,* edited by Shalender Bhasin et al.
ISBN 0-471-13320-5 © 1996 Wiley-Liss, Inc.

However, extrapolation of these data to suggest that supraphysiologic doses of androgens will lead to increases in muscle mass or strength in healthy engonadal men seems unwise. In healthy men, the androgen receptors in most tissues are either fully saturated, or even down regulated by the prevailing androgen levels (Wilson and Griffin, 1980; Wilson, 1988). It seems likely that, if supraphysiologic doses of androgen are effective in healthy men, it must involve mechanisms independent of androgen receptors with a separate dose-response relationship. To date, no such separate mechanisms have been defined with certainty (though some have been speculated on, e.g. the antiglucocorticoid pathway).

Despite roughly 50 years of worldwide experience in the athletic community, it still remains unclear whether androgynic steroids increase muscle mass and strength in healthy men. Though condemned for the serious side effects they bring, anabolic steroid use is widespread in virtually all competitive events requiring muscle strength or bulk. It is difficult for the scientific community to evaluate this extensive experience, since the endeavor, for the most part, has been driven underground.

A large number of scientific investigations have been conducted whose goal has been to evaluate the effectiveness of androgynic steroids in inducing body composition and muscle strength improvements in healthy subjects. Roughly a dozen studies are considered sufficiently well-designed (e.g. randomized, controlled trials) so that their results can be evaluated. Most of these studies were performed in the 1970's and a surprisingly large number of reviews have appeared in the intervening years whose major focus has been to distill the message these investigations give us as to the effectiveness of androgynic steroids (Wilson and Griffin, 1980; Wilson, 1988; Wright, 1980; Ryan, 1981; Haupt, Rovere, 1984; Lamb, 1984; American College of Sports Medicine, 1987; Elashoff et al., 1991; Strauss and Yesalis, 1991).

It is the consensus of these reviews that androgynic steroids improve athletic performance only in limited circumstances. First of all, there is no convincing evidence that performance of endurance activities improves: aerobic capacity (e.g., maximal oxygen uptake) does not increase. The effects on muscle strength gleaned from these studies are not clear and are the subject of considerable controversy. Approximately half of the blinded placebo controlled studies have found an increase in strength; the other half have failed to show a significant increase. Some reviewers believe there is a pattern among experimental protocols that distinguish those studies that have detected strength increases as a result of androgynic steroids, from those that have not. The studies in which a beneficial effect has been observed are often characterized by:

1. Use of athletes who had experience with weight lifting training.
2. Consumption of a protein-supplemented diet during the study.
3. Use of higher doses of androgynic steroid.

It is important to stress that the doses of androgynic steroids used in studies to date have been relatively low, considering that (1) all the testosterone derivatives are less potent than testosterone itself; (2) the daily production rate of testosterone in healthy men is on the order of 7 mg/day; (3) the absorption after oral administration is erratic and incomplete; (4) a portion of the orally administered steroid is metabolized in the liver during its first pass through the portal circulation. In view of these facts, it would not be surprising if no effects were seen at oral doses of 10 mg/day or less. Yet, many of the trials reported to date used doses this low.

The answer to one key question remains hotly disputed. Do androgynic steroids help athletes to enhance the effectiveness of strength and body building programs? Perusal of the aforementioned reviews of the androgynic steroid literature reveal fundamental differences of opinion about the conclusions that can be reached from the studies performed to date. Authors have stated that the weight of evidence indicates that androgynic steroids are probably effective (Wright, 1980; Haupt and Rovere, 1984; American College of Sports Medicine, 1987; Strauss and Yesalis, 1991), probably ineffective (Wilson, 1988; Ryan, 1981), or that no firm conclusion can be reached (Wilson and Griffin, 1980; Lamb, 1984; Elashoff et al., 1991).

Two quotations will serve to make the contrast of opinions clear:

"Anabolic-androgynic steroids in the presence of an adequate diet can contribute to increases in body weight, often in the lean mass compartment...The gains in muscular strength achieved through high-intensity exercise and proper diet can be increased by the use of anabolic-androgynic steroids in some individuals." American College of Sports Medicine Position Stand (1987)*

"...neither enhancement of weight nor improvement in strength can be demonstrated consistently when androgens are administered double blind to athletes" (Wilson, 1988).

It is our conclusion that a major reason for this disagreement is that the experimental design of the studies performed to date has been flawed. A number of problems can be identified.

## Drug Doses Too Low

It is widely believed that users of androgynic steroids often employ very high doses and utilize combinations of drugs. In contrast, largely for ethical reasons, most scientific investigations of the effects of anabolic steroids have utilized relatively low doses of single agents. Since we are uncertain as to the dose-response relationships involved, it is certainly conceivable that higher doses might yield larger effects.

## Poorly Controlled Training Stimulus

It has been argued that androgynic steroids have a range of psychologic effects (Pope and Katz, 1992), among them increased aggression. While the effects of androgynic steroids on human aggression continue to be debated, it is quite plausible that athletes taking androgynic steroids may train more vigorously and, thereby, obtain an enhanced training effect. If the physiologic effects of anabolic steroids are to be isolated, it becomes imperative to control the exercise training stimulus. A fixed schedule of training, with a specifically prescribed exercise regimen, is a necessary feature of experimental design.

---

*It is of interest that the ACSM Position Stand of 1977 (American College of Sports Medicine, 1977) concluded that anabolic steroids were probably ineffective.

## Effort Dependent Strength Measures

Psychologic factors may also corrupt the assessment of strength gains. Increased aggression may improve effort and result in better performance on tests involving maximal efforts. The 1-repetition maximum of a weight lifting exercise, the most widely used measure of strength gains in studies of androgynic steroids, is clearly effort dependent. Are there well-established non-effort dependent measures of strength? Surprisingly, the answer is no. This is in contrast to the assessment of exercise *endurance*, where several non-effort dependent measures are available (e.g., blood lactate level in response to a given level of heavy intensity constant work rate exercise) (Casaburi, 1994).

## Inadequate Body Composition Measures

In studies of androgynic steroids performed to date, changes in body composition have been modest. There seems to be little justification for using indirect or imprecise measures, such as body weight, skinfold thickness, limb circumference, or bioelectrical impedance, as primary outcome measures. Further, since androgens often engender sodium and water retention, it is important to be able to distinguish gains in lean muscle mass from increase in water mass. Newer techniques of measuring body composition can be used to advantage. Magnetic resonance imaging allows measurement of cross-sectional area increase of specific muscle groups (e.g., trained vs. untrained). Dual energy x-ray absorptometry (DEXA) allows non-invasive, precise, *regional* measurement of fat, bone and non-fat, non-bone (i.e., lean) body mass. Deuterium water ingestion yields accurate total body water measurement. Further, stable isotope infusion techniques can be used to detect increases in protein synthesis.

## Variable Nutritional Status

An anabolic response is dependent on adequate nutrition. Yet allowing ad lib access to food may bias study results if those taking the active drug consume more food. Nutritional intake should be controlled and geared to the intensity of the training program.

## Unsuitable Study Groups

Appropriate study design requires a control group (ideally *both* a group training but taking no androgens, and a group neither training nor taking androgens). Double blinded trails are clearly desirable, though minor side effects (e.g., acne) often preclude true blinding even when placebo drug administration is employed. Finally, study groups have likely been too small to detect modest drug effects. Formal power analyses have seldom been utilized in the design of these studies.

We have just completed a 3-year study to determine whether high dose androgynic steroids are capable of increasing lean body mass, muscle size, and strength of eugonadal men. We will be able to present the results in the near future. In this study, we randomized 40 healthy young men to a 10 week intervention. There were 4 groups who received placebo or testosterone injections intramuscularly every week and who participated in a strength training program or were limited to a sedentary life style.

A number of the experimental design features were employed to overcome the deficiencies of previous studies.

1. We specifically chose subjects who were athletes with prior experience in non-competition weight lifting activities.
2. Both we and the athletes were blinded to whether they received testosterone or placebo.
3. We administered a dose of 600 mg of testosterone enanthate per week, several times higher than had previously been used in similar investigations.
4. Dietary intake was strictly regulated and monitored.
5. Subjects randomized to the exercise groups performed weight lifting exercise of the arms and legs. Importantly, the intensity and number of lifts as well as the frequency of the training sessions and duration of the training program were strictly controlled.
   To define the results of this intervention, we assessed a range of outcome measures.

1. Lean body mass was assessed by deuterium water dilution and by underwater weighing.
2. Muscle size was assessed by obtaining upper arm and thigh cross sections by magnetic resonance imaging. This allowed us to assess muscle groups directly involved in the training exercise, specifically the triceps and quadriceps.
3. Protein metabolism was assessed by nitrogen balance on a fixed dietary intake. We also utilized stable isotope leucine infusion to assess protein turnover of the whole body and also, through muscle biopsy, of the quadriceps muscle.
4. Muscle strength of the arms and legs was measured in two ways. We performed 1-repetition maximum measurements for both the bench press and squat. We also performed an effort independent test first suggested by Moritani and DeVries (1979): force-EMG analysis. The electromyogram was recorded during standardized lifts. If the muscle became stronger, a given lift should be accomplished with activation of fewer motor units, and thus with lower electromyographic activity.

While the experimental design improvements will allow a clearer definition of the physiologic effects of androgynic steroids, we hasten to add that, whatever the results of this study, the findings will in no way justify high-dose, long-term abuse of androgynic steroids by athletes; both on ethical and medical grounds.

## REFERENCES

American College of Sports Medicine (1977): Position statement on the use and abuse of anabolic-androgenic steroids in sports. Med Sci Sports Exerc 9(4):xi-xiii.

American College of Sports Medicine (1987): Position stand on the use of anabolic-androgenic steroids in sports. Med Sci Sports Exerc 19:534-539.

Bhasin S, Storer T, Strakova J, Phillips J, Phillips C, Berman N, Bunnell T, Casaburi R (1994): Testosterone increases lean body mass, muscle size and strength in hypogonadal men. Clin Res 42(1):74A.

Casaburi R (1994): Physiologic responses to training. Clin Chest Med 15:215-227.

Elashoff JD, Jacknow AD, Shain SG, Braunstein GD (1991): Effects of anabolic-androgenic steroids on muscular strength. Annals Intern Med 115:387-393.

Haupt HA, Rovere GD (1984): Anabolic steroids: A review of the literature. Amer J Sports Med 12:469-484.

Lamb DR (1984): Anabolic steroids in athletics: How well do they work and how dangerous are they? Amer J Sports Med 12:31-38.

Moritani T, DeVries HA (1979): Neural factors versus hypertrophy in the time course of muscle strength gain. Am J Phys Med 58:115-130.

Pope HG, Katz DL (1992): Psychiatric effects of anabolic steroids. Psych Ann 22:24-29.

Ryan AJ (1981): Anabolic steroids are fool's gold. Federation Proc 40:2682-2688.

Strauss RH, Yesalis CE (1991): Anabolic steroids in the athlete. Annu Rev Med 42:449-457.

Wilson JD, Griffin JE (1980): The use and misuse of androgens. Metabolism 29:1278-1295.

Wilson JD (1988): Androgen abuse by athletes. Endocrine Rev 9:181-199.

Wright JE (1980): Anabolic steroids and athletics. Exerc Sport Sci Rev 8:149-202.

# 28

# ANDROGEN ABUSE BY ATHLETES

Don H. Catlin

Departments of Medicine and
Molecular and Medical Pharmacology
University of California
Los Angeles, California 90024

## BACKGROUND

Anabolic androgenic steroids (AAS) are banned by the International Olympic Committee (IOC) and all other sport organizations that engage in urine testing (Catlin and Hatton, 1990). The ban is enforced by identifying the steroid, its metabolites, or both by gas chromatography-mass spectrometry (GC-MS).

Although anecdotal reports of AAS use first appeared in the nineteen-fifties, it was not until the Olympics in 1976 that an immunoassay was available to screen urines for AAS, and GC-MS was sufficiently developed to confirm the immunoassay findings. There are no data available on the testing at the 1980 Olympics in Moscow. By 1984 it was possible to screen all samples directly by GC-MS and the testosterone/epitestosterone (T/E) ratio was introduced as a test for T administration (Catlin et al., 1987; Donike et al., 1982).

## SUMMARY OF URINE TESTING RESULTS

Over the past decade, testing methods rapidly improved and the number of laboratories certified by the IOC grew from 5 to 24. Figure 1 summarizes the number of tests conducted by these laboratories in the past eight years and gives the percent of the samples positive for AAS. Of the total number of samples tested in any year, the US accounts for about one third and about 90 percent of these are divided between the National Collegiate Athletic Association, the United States Olympic Committee, and the National Football League. The remaining 10 percent come from the universities, US military and forensic investigations. Although national surveys indicate that about 6 percent of high school males have used AAS, and we receive inquiries for testing information from high schools, the high cost (approximately $100.00 per sample) and legal constraints have deterred testing in this population.

The distribution of AAS detected by all IOC laboratories for 1988 and 1993 is shown in Table 1 with the steroids sorted by percent for 1993. It can be seen that

*Pharmacology, Biology, and Clinical Applications of Androgens,* edited by Shalender Bhasin et al.
ISBN 0-471-13320-5 © 1996 Wiley-Liss, Inc.

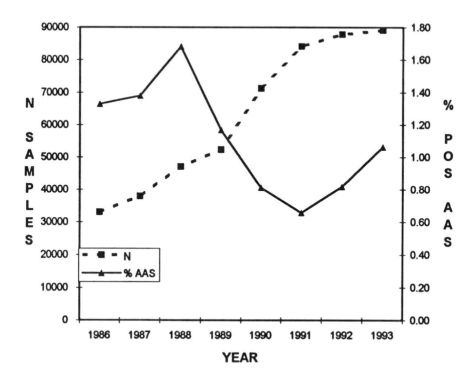

Figure 1. Number of samples tested in IOC accredited laboratories and percent positive for AAS.

over half of the cases are due to nandrolone plus T/E with methandienone plus stanozolol accounting for another ~20 percent. It is noteworthy that T/E cases increased from 1988 to 1993, while nandrolone decreased. Dihydrotestosterone (DHT) was first reported in 1993, although no details are available on the criteria for detection on this case. The 1994 summary, which is still in the process of being compiled, will show at least 13 cases due to DHT. It is difficult to obtain an accurate breakdown of the summary by country, although it is evident that T/E now accounts for the majority of the US cases, whereas in the early eighties nandrolone accounted for ~75 percent of US positives.

## FACTORS AFFECTING SUMMARY STATISTICS

The data in table 1 do not reflect the true incidence of use of any of the AAS because the table does not take into account crucial variables, such as the formulation and pharmacokinetics of the AAS, the type of competition, the sophistication of the AAS using population, the experience of the laboratory performing the analysis, and the degree of advance warning that the athlete received about the testing occasion. For example, metabolites of nandrolone are detectable for ~ 6 weeks after a single 25 mg IM dose of nandrolone decanoate in oil (Bjorkhem and Ek, 1982); these are detectable for several months after multiple doses have been taken over several weeks. Conversely, stanozolol is detectable for ~3 days after a single oral 10 mg dose (Bjorkhem et al., 1980), and probably for no more than 7-10 days after multiple doses. Anecdotal reports indicate that oxandrolone is widely used, yet very few cases are reported. This is probably due to rapid urinary clearance, together with a relatively high degree of difficulty in detecting oxandrolone by GC-MS.

Gradually, sport authorities have recognized that scheduled, advance-notice testing has reached a plateau with respect to its ability to curtail AAS abuse. Short-notice, or so-called out-of-competition testing, is replacing scheduled testing;

Table 1  Anabolic steroids identified by IOC accredited laboratories for 1988 and 1993.

| ANABOLIC STEROID | 1988 N | % | 1993 N | % |
|---|---|---|---|---|
| T/E | 155 | 19.6 | 308 | 32.5 |
| NANDROLONE | 304 | 38.4 | 227 | 23.9 |
| STANOZOLOL | 89 | 11.3 | 108 | 11.4 |
| METANDIENONE | 54 | 6.8 | 101 | 10.7 |
| METENOLONE | 60 | 7.6 | 73 | 7.7 |
| MESTEROLONE | 11 | 1.4 | 31 | 3.3 |
| METHYLTESTOSTERONE | 33 | 4.2 | 23 | 2.4 |
| BOLDENONE | 19 | 2.4 | 17 | 1.8 |
| CLOSTEBOL | 6 | 0.8 | 12 | 1.3 |
| OXANDROLONE | 22 | 2.8 | 11 | 1.2 |
| OXYMETHOLONE | 12 | 1.5 | 10 | 1.1 |
| DROSTANOLONE | 4 | 0.5 | 9 | 0.9 |
| FLUOXYMESTERONE | 1 | 0.1 | 5 | 0.5 |
| DEHYDROCHLORMETHYLTESTOST. | 16 | 2.0 | 4 | 0.4 |
| FORMEBOLONE | 2 | 0.3 | 3 | 0.3 |
| DANABOL | 0 | 0.0 | 2 | 0.2 |
| DANAZOL | 0 | 0.0 | 1 | 0.1 |
| DIHYDROTESTOSTERONE | 0 | 0.0 | 1 | 0.1 |
| OXYMESTERONE | 0 | 0.0 | 1 | 0.1 |
| TRENBOLONE | 1 | 0.1 | 1 | 0.1 |
| METHANDRIOL | 1 | 0.1 | 0 | 0.0 |
| NORETHANDROLONE | 0 | 0.0 | 0 | 0.0 |
| TOTAL SAMPLES | 47098 | | 89166 | |
| TOTAL STEROIDS | 790 | | 948 | |

however, it is considerably more expensive and difficult to administer. The most difficult doping problem facing sports today is the increasing incidence of doping with testosterone and other endogenous androgens. The chemical methods for detecting xenobiotic androgens are reasonably well developed, and once properly identified by GC-MS, with few exceptions (Debruyckere et al., 1992), the conclusion is that deliberate doping took place.

## TESTOSTERONE ADMINISTRATION

Detection of T administration differs because natural or endogenously produced T is present in all urine, and GC-MS, as it is employed in routine urine testing, cannot distinguish between endogenous T and exogenous or synthetic T. Detection of exogenous T is based on measurement of the T to E ratio in urine (Donike et al., 1992). According to a 1982 IOC recommendation, a urine with a T/E ratio greater than six is considered to indicate T administration.

Support for the use of the T/E ratio to detect T administration is based on metabolic studies and review of frequency distributions of T/E in populations not exposed to T. Several reports confirm that T administration increases urine T/E (Kicman et al., 1993; Dehennin and Matsumoto, 1993). The administration of $^{14}$C- or $^2$D$_2$- labelled T (Tamm et al., 1966), or $^{14}$C-androstenedione (Korenman et al., 1964), does not result in labeled E in urine. Therefore, E does not appear to be a metabolite of T. Furthermore, it is now known that the elevated T/E is the result of both an increase in T and a decrease in E (Dehennin and Matsumoto, 1993).

### NATURALLY ELEVATED T/E

Recently, several case reports have described males with T/E > 6 and no evidence of T administration (Dehennin and Matsumoto, 1993; Kicman et al., 1993). This has led to additional tests that might distinguish between elevated T/E ratios due to natural causes and elevations due to T administration (Catlin and Cowan, 1992). These include the urine ratio of T/LH, the ratio of 17-hydroxyprogesterone to T in serum, and administration of ketoconazole, followed by measurement of urine T/E ratios (Kicman et al., 1993). Sport authorities in the US are hesitant to recommend blood tests and even more reluctant to suggest pharmacological challenges, e.g., the ketoconazole test. At the level of the Olympic Games, blood testing was permitted for the first time in 1994, but only for serological tests for blood doping. Given the difficulties in detecting T adminis-tration and recent evidence of doping with DHT, international authorities are discussing testing blood and probably would approve it if a fully validated blood test for T administration were available.

## CARBON ISOTOPE RATIO

A novel approach, and one that has the advantage of utilizing urine, is the measurement of the ratio of $^{13}$C to $^{12}$C in T (Becchi, et al., 1994). The T molecule includes 19 carbon (C) atoms. Most carbon atoms are carbon twelve ($^{12}$C);

however, a few are carbon thirteen ($^{13}$C).  The carbon isotope ratio can be determined with a gas chromatograph connected to an isotope ratio mass spectrometer, via a combustion interface.  The source of the carbon used to synthesize pharmaceutical T is vegetable, whereas endogenous T is synthesized biochemically from the body pool of carbon.  From related studies, these two sources of carbon are known to differ in their carbon isotope ratio, thus measurement of this ratio may indicate the source of the T.

## LONGITUDINAL T/E PROFILES

Currently, the most practical means of suspecting that T was administered is to follow the urine T/E over time - "longitudinal steroid profiling."  Figure 2 shows the urine T/E of a healthy male over ten years.  In this case the baseline T/E is about 0.7 and the graph shows little variability (+/-25%) over the entire period.  If this individual had taken enough T to elevate the ratio above 6, the disruption in the pattern would be quite obvious.  In fact, if the ratio rose to 2.5, T administration would be suspected.  Other normal controls show a similar pattern, i.e., remarkable stability of the T/E over months. Many elite athletes have 4-10 tests per year, thus longitudinal monitoring of various elements of a urine steroid profile is an approach that merits further investigation and validation.

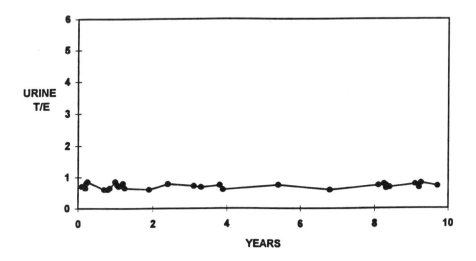

Figure 2.  Urine T/Es over ten years for a healthy non-steroid-using subject.  Each circle represents one urine sample.

## EPITESTOSTERONE ADMINISTRATION

Another recent development is the use of epitestosterone (E) as an emergency measure to rapidly lower the T/E ratio. Apparently, sophisticated athletes have obtained E from chemical companies and developed a dosing regimen - possibly by the cutaneous route of administration. In the event they are doping with T and asked to comply with a short-notice test, the E will rapidly lower the T/E. The IOC has attempted to thwart this maneuver by imposing a quantitative limit on urine E at 200 ng/ml. In our experience, with nearly 500 urines from normal non drug-using males, the maximum E was ~220 ng/ml. In the context of testing athletes, we have encountered urines with E levels in excess of 1000 ng/ml.

## DIHYDROTESTOSTERONE ADMINISTRATION

The most recent addition to the doping armamentarium is DHT. Although the details are sketchy, an IOC accredited laboratory recently reported 11 cases of DHT doping, stemming from a short-notice testing occasion. All the athletes were from one country; 5 were women, and at least one of these was a world record holder. The analysis was based on elevated levels of DHT, and elevated ratios of androsterone to etiocholanolone, and $3\alpha,5\alpha$-androstan-$17\beta$-diol to $3\alpha,5\beta$-androstan-$17\beta$-diol. These abnormalities are expected given that DHT can only be metabolized to other $5\alpha$ reduced compounds. No information is available on the source of the DHT or the infrastructure behind the affair.

## ACKNOWLEDGMENTS

The author thanks the National Collegiate Athletic Association, the United States Olympic Committee, and the National Football League, for their continual support.

## REFERENCES

Becchi M, Aguilera R, Farizon Y, Flament MM, Casabianca H, James P (1994): Gas chromatography/combustion/isotope-ratio mass spectrometry analysis of urinary steroids to detect misuse of testosterone in sport. Rapid Comm Mass Spect: 8:304-308

Bjorkhem I and Ek H (1982): Detection and quantitation of 19-norandrosterone in urine by isotope dilution-mass spectrometry. J Steroid Bioche: 17:447-451.

Bjorkhem I, Lantto O, Lof A (1980): Detection and quantitation of methandienone (Dianabol) in urine by isotope dilution-mass fragmentography. J Steroid Biochem: 13:169-175.

Catlin DH and Cowan DA (1992): Detecting testosterone administration. Clin Chem: 38:1685-1686.

Catlin DH and Hatton CK (1991): Use and abuse of anabolic and other drugs for athletic enhancement. Adv Int Med 36: 399-424.

Catlin DH, Kammerer RC, Hatton CK et al.(1987): Analytical chemistry at the games of the XXIIIrd Olympiad in Los Angeles Clin Chem 1987; 33:319-327.

Debruyckere G, de Sagher R, van Peteghem V (1992): Clostebol-positive urine after consumption of contaminated meat. Clin Chem: 38:1869-1873.

Dehennin L, Matsumoto AM (1993) Long-term administration of testosterone enanthate to normal men: alterations of the urinary profile of androgen metabolites potentially useful for detection of testosterone misuse in sport. J Steroid Biochem Molec Biol:44:179-189.

Donike M, Barwald KR, Klostermann K, et al (1982): Nachweis von exogenem Testosteron (The Detection of Exogenous Testosterone), in Heck H, Hollmann W, Liesen H et al. (eds): Sport: Leistung und Gesundheit. Koln, Kongressbd. Dtsch. Sportarztekongress pp 293-298.

Kicman AT, Oftebro H, Walker C, Norman N, Cowan DA (1993): Potential use of ketoconazole in a dynamic endocrine test to differentiate between biological outliers and testosterone use by athletes. Clin Chem: 39:1798-1803.

Korenman SG, Wilson H, Lipsett MB (1964): Isolation of 17-alpha-hydroxyandrost-4-en-3-one (epitestosterone) from human urine. J Biol Chem:239:1004-1006.

Tamm J, Volkwein U, Starcevic Z (1966): The urinary excretion of epitestosterone, testosterone, and androstenedione following intravenous infusions of high doses of these steroids in human subjects. Steroids: 8:659-669.

# DISCUSSION: ANDROGENS, BODY COMPOSITION, AND ABUSE
## Chairpersons: Eric Orwell, Lisa Tenover

**Jean Wilson:** I think the androgen study by Drs. Casaburi and Bhasin is a very impressive study that can make enormous impact in the field. I know how difficult it was to do and I congratulate you on the overall design. It is really a validation, I think, of what Gilbert Forbes has been maintaining for several years, i.e., if you take an enormous amount of androgen, it does have profound effect on body composition and this is the first real objective test of his thesis, because everything he has done up until now has been uncontrolled. I calculated the total dose of androgen that your people received; it is astonishingly close to the 20 gram figure that he came up with. If you remember that his deduction from that meta-analysis was that in order to have a significant effect on body composition, you had to virtually double the amount of androgen required to carry a boy through puberty which is approximately 20 grams from the age of 11 to 18. The testes put out about 20 grams of testosterone and he came up with that figure from analysis and that is close to what your people were getting.

**Richard Casaburi:** I think the total dose was about 6 grams. It is still a substantial dose.

**Jean Wilson:** In going over the protocol in my own mind, I cannot think of any objection to it. I really like the design, but I want to ask you one question. What made you think it was blinded? Everybody else has said that at these doses, blinding is not possible. That would not influence the left hand wing of the study, but if it were not blinded, according to the publish, it would have an enormous impact on the exercise half of the study.

**Shalender Bhasin:** I do not know if the study was entirely blinded. The investigators were blinded, the design was blinded, but we do not entirely know whether the subjects were blinded. There were three or four people who had fairly significant acne form eruptions. We do not know which groups they were in.

**Richard Casaburi:** We tried to get around that by using controlled training stimulus and effort independent measures of muscle performance. We did not use competitive athletes, because we could not control their training. They were very closely supervised and we have every reason to believe that we were successful in controlling the training stimulus.

**Avraam Grinvald:** What kind of side effects did you observe in those patients receiving supraphysiological doses of androgenic steroids?

**Shalender Bhasin:** One of the most striking thing was the lack of effect on transaminases. The safety parameters were very closely monitored. In some of the subjects, plasma HDL concentrations declined very markedly. We do not have the analyses of those data yet. PSA levels have not yet been measured completely in all the subjects.

**Ralph Hall:** I was one of the authors of the American Colleges of Sports Medicine Physician Paper. We only found one paper that we really felt was worthwhile. Peaks at the University of New Mexico did a study very similar to the one Drs. Casaburi and Bhasin have done. He used cybex machine-like apparatus, and he blinded how much the athletes were really moving. When they were on the testosterone they thought they were moving much more than they actually were. When they were off testosterone, their power movements were identical on and off testosterone. So there was no difference in their performance, but they thought it was a lot better when they were on testosterone.

**Richard Casaburi:** It is interesting and instructive that the ACSM essentially has two positions, one in '77 and one in '87 and with fairly diametrically opposite conclusions.

**Ralph Hall:** Since NCAA started doing the testing for anabolic steroids on and off season basis and in a very unexpected way within 24-36 hours, the incidence of drug abuse has really dropped dramatically.

**Carlos Callegari:** Are there any long-term effects of taking steroids or exercise training? If so, how long do these effects last? Has Ben Johnson, performed the same way after he stopped taking the medication?

**Don Catlin:** It goes to the issue of once you do build yourself up and set a record, can you maintain that indefinitely. Nobody has done a controlled study of the turn off rate or the decline in performance. Ben Johnson was monitored very closely for two or three years and his performance went way down. He competed four years later in Barcelona and came in miserably last. In the next few weeks, his time started to come down again. His body started to change, and he was caught again, this time on testosterone. The effects do go away, but the rate is dependent mainly on the particular drug that they are using and if it is long lasting nandrolone, it will probably take some months to go away because the drug is still there.

**Adrian Dobs:** What do you think about legalizing these drugs? The short-term complications are nil, it looks like just acne, we are not so sure of the long-term side effects and perhaps we should not be so concerned about it with the athletic population.

**Don Catlin:** There is not a day that goes by that I do not ponder this, because I can get fairly frustrated with the sport's authorities. The reality is that as long as the drugs are perceived to have such a dramatic effect on performance, there will be abuse. If you do stop the screening process, the use of these drugs will increase and the records are going to fall again. The game would be played only by those who take drugs.

**Richard Casaburi:** This is not only a slippery slope, it is a cliff. Once we start, we will never be able to stop.

**Todd Nippoldt:** Dr. Catlin, how do you monitor GH abuse by athletes?

**Don Catlin:** We have no way of testing for GH abuse. Nor do we have a way of testing for erythropoietin. My own bias is that it does not work nearly as well as testosterone, so why bother if you can take testosterone.

# PART V: ANDROGEN THERAPY

# 29

# GROWTH AT PUBERTY: THE ANDROGEN CONNECTION

Alan D. Rogol

**Departments of Pediatrics and Pharmacology**
**University of Virginia School of Medicine**
**Charlottesville, Virginia 22908**

## GROWTH AT PUBERTY

Puberty is characterized normally by the onset of development of the se-secondary sexual characteristics and an impressive acceleration of linear growth in mid-to-late adolescence. The secondary sexual characteristics are a result of androgen production from the adrenals in both sexes (adrenarche); testosterone from the testes in the male and estrogens from the ovaries in females (gonadarche). Although the rapid growth spurt had previously been attributed directly to the rising concentrations of gonadal steroid hormones, an indirect effect mediated through altered growth hormone release and insulin-like growth factor I (IGF-I) is now considered to predominate.

During early childhood, linear growth velocity steadily decreases from its initially rapid rate to reach a steady state of approximately 5.5 cm/year at 3 to 5 years of age. As puberty approaches, the rate of growth slows slightly before its sudden acceleration to reach a peak during mid-adolescence (later in the process of development in boys than in girls) and then diminishes toward zero as epiphyseal fusion approaches. At the peak of the pubertal growth spurt, the growth velocity often rises to rates greater than at any other time since early infancy. There appears to be little doubt that the neuroendocrine axis for growth hormone (GH) plays a pivotal role, for an adequate pubertal growth spurt cannot occur without sufficient quantities of GH. However, GH alone is apparently not sufficient, since an important physiological synergism exits between the gonadal and somatotropic axes co-incident with normal pubertal development. Thus, the combined growth-promoting effects of the concerted activation of these axes is required for pubertal development to proceed adequately.

When one determines the appropriateness of a subject's growth velocity, one must consider the state of biological development. Skeletal, or pubertal maturation, may be used to assess a child's degree of biological development. The most commonly used method for bone age determination is that of Greulich and Pyle, which utilizes a single radiograph of the left hand and wrist, and comparison is

*Pharmacology, Biology, and Clinical Applications of Androgens*, edited by Shalender Bhasin et al.
ISBN 0-471-13320-5 © 1996 Wiley-Liss, Inc.

made with standard photos in an atlas. Pubertal maturation status is derived from the development of pubic hair and the genitals (boys), or breast and pubic hair development (girls). Both the timing and *tempo* of pubertal development are variable and partly genetically determined. Although there is great variability in these parameters, the peak height velocity is tightly correlated to the rising testosterone levels in boys.

# HORMONAL CONTROL OF GROWTH AT PUBERTY

## Gonadotropins

The secretion of the gonadotropins is pulsatile at virtually all ages studied, especially since the newer and more sensitive third generation immunoradiometric assays have been used. Because of the very long circulating half-life of FSH, it has been difficult to quantitate pulsatile FSH release. On the other hand, new information is evolving for the pubertal onset of higher amplitude and diurnal fluctuations in circulating LH concentrations. The mean LH level increases much more than that for FSH in boys as they prepare to attain early pubertal changes in genital development (Dunkel et al., 1992). The increase is most notable at night, in early and mid-puberty, giving rise to the previously described unbalanced 24-h LH secretion (diurnal variation). The important physiological message is that there is a re-awakening of the quantitative neurosecretory events for pulsatile GnRH (hence, LH) release before the more reliable external signs of pubertal development are evident. The surges in release of LH are biologically relevant. In boys testosterone concentrations are high after the initial nighttime augmentation in pulsatile LH release. The higher circulating testosterone levels fall to much lower levels in the late afternoon and evening because the feedback sensitivity of the GnRH neurons to testosterone is still very high, permitting the raised (for prepubertal boys) levels of this androgen to inhibit higher amplitude GnRH (and LH) release.

## Gonadal Steroid Hormones

The gonadal steroid hormones affect the ultimate height of children by promoting epiphyseal closure. However, certain "experiments of nature" can give us several clues toward mechanistic insights. Uriarte and co-workers (Uriarte et al., 1992) studied 41 men with isolated hypogonadotropic hypogonadism, that is, they had an intact growth hormone axis. The subjects had greater adult height than expected based on (1) historical controls; (2) concurrent young adult controls; and (3) their genetic height potential based on their sex-adjusted midparental target height. Very recent data based on a mutant aromatase enzyme (P450 aromatase) (Conte et al., 1994) and a mutated estrogen receptor gene (Smith et al., 1994) indicate that in both sexes, it is an estrogen, and not an androgen-dependent mechanism that accomplishes epiphyseal closure. The obverse also indicates direct effects of the gonadal steroid hormones on the epiphyseal growth plate. Sexual precocity of virtually any cause will accelerate epiphyseal closure more rapidly than it will the growth rate.  Such children of both sexes are usually tall and rapidly growing as young children, but become shorter than predicted adults, based on early growth plate fusion.

## GROWTH HORMONE PHYSIOLOGY (HUMAN)

Growth hormone is produced in, and released from, the pituitary somatotropes under the influence of two hypothalamic hypophysiotropic factors, GH releasing hormone (GHRH), and GH release inhibiting hormone (somatostatin).  It is released in an episodic, burst-like (pulsatile) manner throughout the day, but especially during deep (stages 3 and 4) sleep.  Additional control points include brain neurotransmitters and neuropeptides, insulin-like growth factor I [IGF-I (long-loop feedback)], GH itself (short-loop feedback), and the hypophysiotropic peptides noted above (ultra short-loop feedback).  Moreover, metabolic substrates such as carbohydrates and free fatty acids take part in the regulation of GH secretion.  It is the qualitative and quantitative aspects of the GH secretory pattern that ultimately permit growth, although nutritional, genetic and disease factors may obscure any direct relationship between the circulating GH pattern and linear growth rate.

Growth hormone circulates in both a bound and a "free" form.  The bound hormone is complexed to small and large serum binding proteins.  The smaller protein with its characteristic high affinity, is precisely the extracellular domain of the cellular GH receptor.  Signal transduction occurs at the cellular level by GH acting as a 2 epitope bridge between receptor molecules.  Levels of the binding protein increase slowly during late childhood and adolescence with peak values attained in the early third decade.  Approximately one-half of the circulating concentration of GH is bound, yielding a half-life much longer than that for free GH. The bound form may act as a reservoir for GH action, since free GH can be released to its proper tissue sites over a prolonged period of time.  Regulation of GHBP levels is by both GH and gonadal steroid hormone concentrations.  The sex steroid hormones exert their influence over GH secretion at multiple sites of the somatotropic axis; the most profound of which is to augment the GH secretory rate 2-to-3 fold during late mid-puberty in boys (Martha et al., 1989; Kerrigan and Rogol, 1992).  Androgens have been considered facilitory and estrogens both facilitory (very low dose) and inhibitory (higher dose), to the functioning of the somatotropes.

A number of recent studies however, have cast doubt upon a mechanism that functions through the androgen receptor (see below).  Androgen and estrogen receptor antagonists, as well as non-aromatizable androgens, such as oxandrolone and dehydrotestosterone (DHT), have been used to buttress the conclusion that the effects of sex-steroid hormones to augment GH release are limited to estrogen receptor-mediated actions.  In fact, androgen receptor-mediated effects may be inhibitory.  Both hypothalamic (dominant) and hypophyseal mechanism may be important.

Rising and falling in concert with altered GH release at puberty are two GH-dependent proteins, IGF-I and IGFBP-3, the latter is the major circulating binding protein for the IGFs.  Although there are log-order increases in the circulating levels of both androgens and estrogens during pubertal maturation in all children, there is no significant decline in the levels of sex steroids as there is for GH and IGF-I.

## CLINICAL OBSERVATIONS AND CORRELATIVE STUDIES

In a carefully controlled study of adult men over a large age range plasma, IGF-I and 24 hour mean GH levels correlated directly with free serum estradiol levels, but not with free testosterone levels (Ho et al., 1987). Children who have excess amounts of sex steroid hormones (e.g., precocious puberty or adrenal hyperplasia) have an accelerated growth rate. Treatment of the primary disease yields lower levels of sex steroid hormones and a slower growth rate. Subjects with delayed growth and adolescence have decreased mean GH, IGF-I and sex steroid hormone concentrations. Therapy with *aromatizable* androgens augments GH release and the growth velocity; however, the growth velocity, but not growth hormone secretion, is increased by non-aromatizable androgens, indicating a more complex pattern of augmented growth than merely mediated by increased GH release. A direct epiphyseal growth plate mechanism, perhaps mediated by increased *local* IGF-I production underlies this non GH-dependent growth mechanism. Girls with complete androgen insensitivity are a natural model to study the effects of specific gonadal hormones on the functioning of the GH axis. Affected phenotypic females (karyotype 46,XY) have their adolescent growth spurt at the same time, but have an intermediate mean adult height between normal men and women. Plasma estradiol and IGF-I levels are directly correlated and gonadectomy is followed by an immediate decrement in circulating levels of GH, IGF-I, testosterone and estradiol, suggesting that androgens are not critical for the adolescent growth spurt, if estrogens are available. Although both estrogen insensitivity and partial aromatase deficiency have now been described, there are no proper studies of GH release. Both patients were tall for age, the man with estrogen insensitivity reaching more than 200 cm, more likely because of an increased growth period than by a short-term burst of augmented GH secretion.

## EFFECTS OF EXOGENOUS GONADAL STEROID HORMONES ON GH SECRETION

### Testosterone

Intermediate and long-acting testosterone esters have been administered to boys with delayed puberty and hypogonadal men. Virtually all have shown an increased growth rate and augmented GH release, but the mechanism through which this effect occurs, androgen or estrogen, could not be determined (see below for studies with the non-aromatizable androgens or with androgen receptor blockade).

## Estrogens

Oral estrogen therapy may be complicated by hepatic transformation, especially for the conjugated forms. Most studies with oral estradiol have shown that extraordinarily small doses (less than 100 ng/kg body weight) can permit augmented GH release in hypogonadal girls. In fact, pre-treatment with estrogens is a standard practice in some pediatric endocrine clinics when evaluating GH release in short children of either gender. Both puberty and estrogen administration (40 micrograms/m$^2$/day, given as ethynyl estradiol) significantly increased the peak GH response to standardized tests: exercise, arginine or insulin-induced hypoglycemia in normal children and young adults (Marin et al., 1994).

## NON-AROMATIZABLE ANDROGENS

## Oxandrolone

There have been a number of investigations to show the growth-augmenting effects of oxandrolone. Fewer studies have been done to evaluate the effect of this synthetic androgen on GH release. Although there have been a few studies to the contrary, the consensus is that there is no effect of oxandrolone to augment 24 hour mean serum GH, the frequency or amplitude of pulsatile GH release, or plasma IGF-I levels in pre- and early pubertal boys (Metzger et al., 1994).

## Dihydrotestosterone

Keenan and co-workers (Keenan et al., 1993) compared testosterone and dehydrotestosterone in therapeutic doses (for growth) for the ability to raise circulating GH levels in boys with constitutional delay of growth and adolescence. Testosterone not only induced a growth spurt, but also raised mean GH and IGF-I levels and decreased the LH response to exogenous GnRH. On the other hand, those treated with DHT had lower mean levels of GH and IGF-I, but the LH response to GnRH decreased showing the androgenic effect of the DHT preparation. A second group of boys, those with gynecomastia, were treated with DHT. As noted previously, the mean GH level decreased, although there was no change in IGF-I level.

Taken together, these data suggest that the marked increase in mean and pulsatile GH level at puberty is due to an estrogen-receptor dependent mechanism. Further studies with receptor-blocking agents, described below, have confirmed these findings.

## ANDROGEN RECEPTOR BLOCKADE

Flutamide, a non-steroidal antagonist of the androgen receptor, administered in an amount large enough to increase the serum LH, free testosterone and estradiol levels, in normal, late pubertal boys, was associated with an increase in

24 hour mean serum GH concentration and 24 hour GH production rate (Metzger and Kerrigan, 1993a).

## ESTROGEN RECEPTOR BLOCKADE

Tamoxifen, a non-steroidal antagonist of the estrogen receptor, administered in an amount large enough to augment circulating LH levels in late pubertal boys, was associated with decreased 24 hour mean GH and IGF-I levels (Metzger and Kerrigan, 1994). This finding, precisely the converse of that noted for the studies with flutamide in a similar set of late pubertal boys, strongly suggests that the stimulatory effect of testosterone on the GH axis is mediated indirectly through estrogen sensitive mechanisms.

## SUMMARY

Androgens and estrogens exert profound effects on growth and adolescent development. In the human, although the precise neuroendocrine mechanisms cannot be easily delineated, it appears that profound neurosecretory influences, predominantly at the hypothalamus, alter circulating GH concentrations. Studies using sex-steroid hormone agonists, as well as androgen and estrogen receptor antagonists, are concordant. They strongly suggest that the alterations in GH secretion, most notably during mid-to-late puberty, depend to a large extent on estrogen-receptor mechanism.

## ACKNOWLEDGMENTS

I wish to acknowledge a number of our pediatric endocrine fellows whose ideas and studies have given rise to this research effort: Drs. Mark Parker, Kathleen Link, Nelly Mauras, Paul Martha, Jr., James Kerrigan, Francisco Nieves-Rivera, Nancy Wright and especially Daniel Metzger. My long term colleagues at the University of Virginia, Drs. Robert Blizzard and Johannes Veldhuis are gratefully acknowledged for their many helpful suggestions as this line of research was being developed. Finally, none of the studies carried out at the University of Virginia could have been done without the superb patient care given by Ms. Sandra Jackson and her staff of nurses at the General Clinical Research Center.

Partially supported by RR 00847 (to the General Clinical Research Center) and the NSF Center for Biological Timing at the University of Virginia.

## REFERENCES

Conte FA, Brumback MM, Ito Y, Fisher CR , Simpson ER (1994): A syndrome of female pseudohermaphroditism, hypergonadotropic hypogonadism, and multicystic ovaries, associated with missense mutations in the gene encoding aromatase (P450 aromatase). J Clin Endocrinol Metab 78: 1287-1292.

Dunkel L, Alfthan H, Stenman U-H, Selstam G, Rosberg S, Albertsson-Wikland K (1992): developmental changes in 24-hour profiles of luteinizing hormone and follicle stimulating hormone from prepuberty to midstages of puberty in boys. J Clin Endocrinol Metab 74: 890-897.

Ho KY, Evans WS, Wcna WS, Blizzard RM, Veldhuis DJ, Merrian GR, Samojlik E, Furlanetto R, Rogol AD, Kaiser DL, Thorner MO (1987): Effects of sex and age on the 24-h secretory profile of GH secretion in man: importance of endogenous estradiol concentrations. J Clin Endocrinol Metab 64: 51-58.

Keenan BS, Richards GE, Ponder SW, Dallas JS, Nagamani M, Smith ER (1993) Androgen-stimulated pubertal growth: the effects of testosterone and dihydrotestosterone on growth hormone and insulin-like growth factor-I in the treatment of short stature and delayed puberty. J Clin Endocrinol Metab 76: 996-1001.

Kerrigan JR, Rogol AD (1992): The impact of gonadal steroid hormone action on growth hormone secretion during childhood and adolescence. Endocr Rev 13: 281-298.

Marin G, Domené M, Barnes KM, Blackwell BJ, Cassorola FG, Cutler GB, Jr., (1994): The effect of estrogen priming and puberty on the growth hormone response to standardized treadmill, exercise, and arginine-insulin in normal girls and boys. J Clin Endocrinol Metab 79:37-541.

Martha PM, JR. Rogol AD, Veldhuis JD, Kerrigan JR, Goodman DW, Blizzard RM (1989): Alterations in the pulsatile properties of circulating growth hormone concentrations during puberty in boys. J Clin Endocrinol Metab 69: 563-567.

Metzger DL, Kerrigan JR (1994): Estrogen receptor blockade with Tamoxifen diminishes growth hormone secretion in boys: evidence for a stimulatory role of endogenous estrogens during male adolescence. J Clin Endocrinol Metab. 79:513-518.

Metzger DE, Kerrigan JR (1993): Androgen receptor blockade with flutamide enhances growth hormone secretion in late pubertal males: evidence for independent actions of estrogen and androgen. J Clin Endocrinol Metab. 76: 1147-1152.

Metzger DL, Kerrigan JR, Rogol AD (1994): Gonadal steroid hormone regulation of the somatotropic axis during puberty in humans: mechanisms of androgen and estrogen action. Trends Endocrinol Metab 5:290-296.

Smith EP, Boyd J, Frank GR, Takahashi H, Cohen RM, Specker B, Williams TC, Labahn DB, Korach KS (1994): Estrogen resistance caused by a mutation in the estrogen -receptor gene in a man. New Engl J Med 331: 1056-1061.

Uriarte MM, Baron J, Garcia HB, Barnes KM, Loriaux DL, Cutler GB, Jr. (1992): The effect of pubertal delay on adult height in men with isolated hypogonadotropic hypogonadism. J Clin Endocrinol Metab. 74: 436-440.

# 30

# ANDROGEN THERAPY IN AGING MEN

**J. Lisa Tenover**

**Department of Medicine**
**Emory University**
**Wesley Woods Hospital**
**Atlanta, Georgia 30329-5102**

## TESTOSTERONE AND NORMAL MALE AGING

A decline in the serum level of testosterone accompanies normal aging in men. Although there is not universal agreement in this literature in this regard, the majority of studies (21 of 25 articles published between 1980 and 1993) have supported this age-associated decrease in testosterone. Some of the discrepancy in reported testosterone levels with age can be explained by variability in health of the individuals studied and by the failure to recognize that there is a circadian rhythm in blood levels of testosterone, making the time of day when blood is sampled an important factor. While there is little argument that testosterone levels decline in healthy men as they age, the physiological and clinical impacts of this decline are still in question.

Total serum testosterone is composed of three components (Figure 1): that which is not bound to any protein ("free" testosterone), that which is bound to albumin, and that which is bound to sex hormone-binding globulin (SHBG-bound testosterone). Testosterone has a relatively high binding affinity for SHBG and some investigators have defined "bioavailable" testosterone as the non-SHBG-bound portion. As more data become available, it appears that this single definition for "bioavailable" testosterone may be simplistic. The portion of serum testosterone available to a particular tissue may vary and depends on the characteristics of the tissue and its blood supply.

Regardless of which component of serum testosterone is measured, most data suggest that all portions of serum testosterone decrease as men age. In a num-

$$\text{Total T} = \text{Free T} + \text{Albumin-T} + \text{SHBG-T}$$
$$[\text{--"Bioavailable" T-}]$$

Figure 1. The components of serum total testosterone

*Pharmacology, Biology, and Clinical Applications of Androgens*, edited by Shalender Bhasin et al.
ISBN 0-471-13320-5 © 1996 Wiley-Liss, Inc.

ber of studies, non-SHBG-bound testosterone levels have been shown to decrease to an even greater extent with age than total testosterone levels. Consequently, a number of investigators who study testosterone replacement therapy use serum non-SBHG-bound testosterone levels as a measurement criteria for therapy.

The normal range for serum testosterone for young adult men depends on the laboratory doing the measurement and the population being assessed. Most laboratories use 10.4 to 12.1 nmol/L (300 to 350 ng/dL) as the lower limit of normal for serum testosterone in healthy young adult men; but the defined normal range for serum non-SHBG-bound testosterone may be extremely variable. Even when defining 'hypogonadism" as a serum total or non-SHBG-bound testosterone level consistently below the lower limit of normal; it is not possible from the data in the literature to extract an estimated prevalence for "hypogonadism" in aging men. Clearly, unlike females who uniformly become hypogonadal with menopause, not all men will develop "hypogonadal" androgen levels. However, the number of older men with a low serum testosterone level is not insignificant. Table 1 lists the prevalence of low serum total testosterone levels in healthy older Caucasian men from two data sets: one generated in Seattle, Washington from 1985 through 1990; and one generated in Atlanta, Georgia from 1992 through 1994.

Serum gonadotrophin levels are generally not helpful in defining an older man as being hypogonadal, unless the values are clearly very high or very low. Many older men who have low serum testosterone levels have gonadotrophins within the normal reference range and blunted gonadotrophin responses to GnRH administration.

## HYPOGONADISM AND THE AGING MAN

Unfortunately, there is no single measure of clinically significant hypogonadism. Therefore, it is as yet unknown whether older men who have serum testosterone levels below the normal range established in young adult men are truly physiologically hypogonadal. Data suggesting that older men with low serum testosterone levels may be hypogonadal fall into three categories: (1) descriptions of age-related changes in androgen target organs, such as bone and muscle, and comparisons of these changes with similar target organ findings in young hypogonadal men; (2) evaluation of the effects of androgen replacement therapy on

Table 1. Prevalence of Low Serum Total Testosterone (TT) in Healthy Older
        Caucasian Men in Two Geographical Areas

|  | Age (years) | Total Studied | TT<350 ng/dL | TT<300ng/dL |
|---|---|---|---|---|
| Seattle, WA | 60-80 | 96 | 28 (29.2%) | 19 (19.7%) |
| Atlanta, GA | 65-83 | 283 | 110 (38.8) | 54 (19.1%) |

various androgen target organs in young hypogonadal men; and (3) evaluation of androgen replacement therapy in older hypogonadal men. The purpose of this brief review is to highlight what is known about androgen replacement therapy in older men.

Although androgens have important physiological actions in a large number of tissues, their effects in the older male have focused on those listed in Table 2. Age-related decrements in the function of muscle, bone, and the central nervous system are a part of normal aging, and testosterone (and other androgens) are under evaluation as potential "trophic factors" that might either slow or partially reverse some of these decrements. Of course, any discussion of the use of androgens as a possible trophic factor to prevent frailty or disability in the aging male must also consider the possible risks of testosterone supplementation in this age group. Possible detrimental effects of androgens would include, (1) changes in the cardiovascular system through effects on lipoproteins or through other mechanisms; (2) effects on the prostate, resulting in promotion of benign hyperplasia or pre-existent prostate cancer; (3) exacerbation of sleep apnea; (4) effects on hematopoiesis (development of polycythemia) and hemostatis; and (5) fluid retention resulting in elevation in blood pressure, edema, or exacerbation of congestive heart failure.

## STUDIES OF ANDROGEN REPLACEMENT IN OLDER MEN

Until recently, results of androgen therapy in older men have been published only in sporadic case reports or as a small subset of adult men studied in androgen replacement trials. Within the past several years, however, there have been several studies, reported in articles or as abstracts, that have directly addressed the effects of androgen therapy in the older man. Categorized by the specific target organs evaluated, the findings of these studies will be reviewed.

### Androgens and Body Composition

Since normal aging results in an increase in upper and central body fat, a decrease in muscle mass, and a decline in some aspects of muscle strength, androgens, long noted for their anabolic effects, have begun to be evaluated as a modality for improving body composition and strength in the elderly. In one study, (Tenover, 1992a) thirteen men, mean age 67.5 years, who had serum testosterone

Table 2. Tissues of Interest for Androgen Therapy in the Aging Man

| Body Composition: | Bone |
|---|---|
| Muscle | Hematopoiesis/hemostatis |
| Fat | Brain: |
| Prostate | Cognition |
| Cardiovascular | Mood |
| Lipoproteins | Sleep |
| Sexual Function | Fluid volume |

levels equal to or below 400 ng/dL (13.9 nmol/L), were treated in a double-blind, placebo-controlled crossover study with testosterone enanthate (100 mg/week) or placebo, for three months each. Body composition was measured by hydrostatic weighing. At the end of the testosterone treatment phase, there was an increase in body weight (an average increase of 1.5 kg over that during placebo treatment or baseline), an increase in lean body mass (1.8 kg over than during placebo treatment or baseline), and a tendency for a decrease in total body fat (27.9% during testosterone treatment, compared to 28.8% at baseline or 28.9% during placebo therapy). Body circumference measurements and grip strength were not noted to change with androgen therapy in this study.

Another study (Morley et al., 1993) involved fourteen men, ages 69 to 89 years, with bioavailable testosterone less that 70 ng/dL. Eight of these men received testosterone enanthate (200 mg every two weeks) for three months, and six men received no treatment. In this study, handgrip strength increased with the androgen therapy, compared to the non treatment group. These results were confirmed by the same group in a larger cohort of men (n=23; Sih et al., 1994). Another group has reported that in eight men with baseline serum testosterone levels of less than 250 ng/dL, some of whom ere in the older age range, testosterone therapy for six months with the scrotal patch resulted in a 2% decrease in body fat and a 3% increase in lean body mass, as determined by dual energy X-ray absorptometry (Haddad, et al., 1994). Strength, as measured by dynamometry, also increased with testosterone therapy.

A study in obese men over the age of 40 (mean age 56.7 years) who were treated with testosterone for nine months, demonstrated a decline in visceral fat, as measured by CT scan, without a change in overall lean body mass (Marin et al., 1993). Katznelson et al. (1994) have reported that in men up to age 69 years, eighteen months of testosterone ester therapy at 100 mg/week resulted in a 20% decline in body fat, and a 5% increase in lean body mass. A summary of the results from all these studies is presented in Table 3.

In summary, there are data that demonstrate a decrease in body fat, increase in lean body mass, and perhaps a change in some aspects of muscle strength with short-term testosterone therapy in older men. It will be important, however, for longer term and larger studies to collaborate this data, to determine if effects are sustained, and to elucidate if the increase in muscle strength with testosterone will be of such magnitude as to have clinically meaningful impact on function. There are a number of studies of testosterone therapy in older men currently in progress that may add some information in this regard.

## Androgens and Bone

As men live longer, the loss of bone mass with age becomes more clinically significant. Osteoporosis and hip and vertebral fractures all become more prevalent as men age, resulting in increased morbidity and mortality. Hypogonadism is a risk factor for minimal trauma hip fracture in the elderly male, and treatment of older men with a GnRH analog or castration can lead to a rapid decline in vertebral bone density and a rapid rise in bone turnover. For these reasons, and because of the

Table 3. Summary of Body Composition Results for Studies Involving Testosterone Therapy to Older Men.

| Study (Ref) | Age (yrs) | Length of Treatment (months) | Treatment Type | Fat Mass | Lean Body Mass | Strength |
|---|---|---|---|---|---|---|
| A | 67.5 (mean) | 3 | TE* | NC+ | ⇑ | NC |
| B | 69-89 | 3 | TE | — | — | ⇑ |
| C | various | 6 | S Patch# | ⇓ | ⇑ | ⇑ |
| D | 56.7 (mean) | 9 | Gel prep | ⇓ | NC | — |
| E | 50-90 | 3 | TE | — | — | ⇑ |
| F | 22-69 | 18 | TE | ⇓ | ⇑ | — |

*TE = testosterone ester; #S Patch = scrotal patch; +NC = no change; ⇑ = increase; ⇓ = decrease; Ref A = Tenover, 1992a; Ref B = Morley et al., 1993; Ref C = Haddad et al., 1994; Ref D = Marin et al., 1993; Ref E = Sih et al., 1994; Ref F = Katznelson et al., 1994.

effects of androgen therapy on bone in hypogonadal young men, the effect of testosterone supplementation on bone density and bone turnover in older men has begun to be studied. As long ago as 1948 , Albright reported that testosterone given to a 72 year-old man with osteoporosis resulted in a decline in total calcium excretion. Lafferty, in 1964 reported similar results in a 75 year-old osteopenic male. Oppenheim and co-workers gave testosterone for six to eight months to 6 older (mean age 61 years) hypogonadal (mean testosterone = 144 ng/dL) men with spinal bone densities below those of age-matched controls. Spinal bone densities were reported to increase in all six men (Tenover, 1994).

Several recent studies have evaluated the effect of testosterone on parameters of bone turnover and/or bone density in older men. In two studies previously cited (Tenover, 1992a; Morley et al., 1993), a significant decline in urinary excretion of hydroxyproline, or an increase in serum osteocalcin, were reported in men after three months of testosterone therapy. After eighteen months of testosterone therapy in twelve older men, another study (Katznelson et al., 1994) noted a 5-13% increase in trabecular bone density, depending on modality of measurement used. Finally, a study in four hypogonadal men (ages 38-74 years), given one year of testosterone enanthate therapy (200 mg every 2 weeks), reported a 23% increase in lumbar bone mineral density at one year (Tomasic et al., 1994).

In summary, there are data that androgen therapy may affect bone density and bone turnover in elderly men. Again, more and longer term data are needed to confirm that testosterone therapy can sustain a stabilization or reversal of bone loss in most hypogonadal elderly men.

## Androgens and Mood, Cognition, and Sexual Behavior

Measures of sexual function, such as potency, orgasmic frequency and quality, sexual thoughts, and sexual enjoyment have been reported to decline with age. Data to support a relationship between androgen levels and these age-related declines in sexual function are scarce, difficult to obtain, and often contradictory. Studies of androgen replacement in hypogonadal young men have shown that some testosterone is necessary for normal libido, ejaculation, and spontaneous erections. Studies in older men have shown a mild correlation between serum testosterone levels and sexual activity.

Data on the relationship of androgens and mood or cognition are limited, but studies in hypogonadal young men have shown an overall improvement in mood and sense of well-being, as well as a decline in anxiety, with testosterone therapy. Studies in young hypogonadal men have shown a correlation of testosterone level with spatial ability and an increase in concentration with testosterone replacement.

In elderly men, the effects of testosterone therapy on mood, aspects of cognition, and sexual behavior, have not been extensively evaluated. Several studies have shown improvement in spatial cognition with androgen therapy (Janowsky et al., 1991; Orwoll et al., 1992), while others have reported improvement in sense of well-being (Tenover, 1992a; Ellyin, 1994; Marin et al., 1993) and/or an increase in libido (Ellyin, 1994; Tenover, 1992b) with testosterone. Impotence in older men is often multifactorial and testosterone therapy usually has not been beneficial.

## The Potential Risks of Androgen Therapy, Especially in Older Men

As noted previously, androgen supplementation carries some potential risks, especially in the older man, who may have certain co-existent medical problems. Among the specific risks that need to be considered are water retention, development of polycythemia, hepatotoxicity, exacerbation of sleep apnea, development of detrimental effects on the cardiovascular system, and exacerbation of pre-existent benign or malignant prostate disease.

## Water Retention

Water retention is known to occur with androgen therapy and it is possible that testosterone supplementation in older men could lead to hypertension, peripheral edema, or exacerbation of congestive heart failure. In the four studies of androgen therapy in older men that have reported on fluid status (Tenover, 1992a; Morley et al., 1993; Marin et al., 1993; Sih et al., 1994) a total of 52 men received androgens from three to nine months and no man was reported to have developed hypertension, edema, or congestive heart failure. However, some of the increased weight noted in two of the studies (Tenover, 1992a; Morley et al., 1993) was thought to have been due to water retention. One ongoing study of 70 men over the age of 65 years, with baseline testosterone levels below 350 ng/dL, has men receiving testosterone replacement (200mg of testosterone enanthate every two weeks). At the current time, the men collectively have received over 500 months of testosterone therapy and no peripheral edema or congestive heart failure has been noted. However, five men with pre-existing hypertension, have developed an elevation in their blood pressure.

## Erythropoiesis

The stimulatory effects of androgens on erythropoiesis are well documented. Studies in which young hypogonadal or eugonadal men have been supplemented with testosterone have shown an increase in hematocrit with treatment. Similar results have been reported in the studies of androgen therapy in older men (Table 4). Because healthy older men tend to have slightly lower hematocrits and hemoglobin levels than do young adult men, except in those men with other clinical causes that could elevate hemoglobin levels, the erythropoietic effects of testosterone in the older age group may only rarely lead to problems with polycythemia. Furthermore, the method and extent of testosterone replacement may impact the effects on erythropoiesis with presumably less of an effect being seen with lower, more frequent doses of testosterone esters or with the scrotal or transdermal patch.

## Hepatotoxicity

Although hepatotoxicity has been reported with administration of some oral androgens, it is not usually seen with non-oral forms of testosterone supplementation in young adult men. There have been no reports of hepatotoxicity (abnormal liver enzyme blood tests) in any of the studies of testosterone therapy in older men.

Table 4. Hematocrit Changes in Elderly Men with Testosterone (T) Supplementation.

| Study (Ref) | Treatment Type | Treatment Dose | Mean Change in Hematocrit |
|---|---|---|---|
| A | TE | 100mg/wk X 3 mth | +3.6 |
| B | TE | 200mg/2 wks X 3 mths | +7.0 |
| C | TE | 200mg/2 wks X 3 mths | +4.7 |
| D | TC | 25-50mg/2 wks X 12 mths | no change |

TE = testosterone enanthate; TC = testosterone cypionate; Ref A = Tenover, 1992a; Ref B = Morley et al., 1993; Ref C = Sih et al., 1994; Ref D = Marin et al., 1993.

## Sleep Apnea

Testosterone administration has been reported to exacerbate pre-existing sleep apnea, but none of the reports of testosterone therapy in older men has noted the development of sleep apnea. However, several of the studies have prescreened study participants for sleep apnea, a procedure that would seem prudent if androgen therapy is considered.

## Lipoproteins

A portion of the increase in mortality attributed to cardiovascular disease in men, compared with premenopausal women, may be the result of androgens. Some of this increased risk may be mediated through androgen effects on serum lipoprotein levels, or through other factors, such as, modulation of plasma levels of the vasoconstrictor endothelin or effects on hemostasis.

The data on effects of testosterone therapy on serum lipids in older men are summarized in Table 5. Overall, the changes in cholesterol levels with testosterone therapy have been modest and the ultimate impact on cardiovascular risk is unclear. Effects of testosterone therapy on other factors affecting cardiovascular risk have not been reported in the elderly.

## Prostate

Benign prostatic hyperplasia (BPH) and prostate cancer are diseases of the aging male. Androgens appear to have a role in promotion of both BPH and prostate cancer, and androgen deprivation therapy has been used as a treatment modality in both processes. The role of androgen supplementation as a potentiator of prostate disease in the older male is based largely on theoretical grounds at this point; but it is one of the areas of highest concern in regards to the long term safety of testosterone therapy. Many of the studies of testosterone replacement in older

Table 5. Effect of Testosterone Therapy on Serum Cholesterol in Older Men.

| Study | N | Treatment Duration (months) | Average Percent Change | | |
|-------|---|------------------------------|-------------|----------|----------|
|       |   |                              | Total Chol | HDL-Chol | LDL-Chol |
| A | 20 | 9 | ⇓11.7% | NC | ___ |
| B | 8 | 3 | ⇓ 9% | NC |  |
| C | 13 | 3 | ⇓11.0% | NC | ⇓ 11.2% |
| D | 10 | 12 | ⇓ * | NC | ⇓ * |

Chol = cholesterol; ⇓ = decrease; NC = no change; * exact change not stated; Ref A = Marin et al., 1993; Ref B = Morley et al., 1993; Ref C = Tenover, 1992a; Ref D = Ellyin, 1994.

men have monitored the effect of therapy on prostate specific antigen (PSA) levels, prostate size, and/or prostatic symptoms. Of the five testosterone studies in older men that have monitored for prostate changes (Tenover, 1992a; Morley et al., 1993; Marin et al., 1993; Sih et al., 1994; Ellyin, 1994), only one has noted any significant change with therapy, a 21% increase in serum PSA from baseline values (a mean change from 2.1 ng/dL to 2.7 ng/dL; Tenover, 1992a). However, all these studies were of relatively short duration, which could limit the detection of any augmentation of benign or malignant prostate growth. Clearly, further data in regards to the long-term effects of testosterone therapy on the prostate in older men need to be generated before the relative risk of such therapy can be fully evaluated.

## CONCLUSION

Several short-term studies involving small numbers of subjects suggest that older men, with serum testosterone levels that are near or below the lower end of the normal range for young adult men, may be a group in whom testosterone replacement therapy might benefit bone, muscle, and psychosexual functions. These studies also have demonstrated that, in the short term and with adequate prescreening and monitoring, significant adverse effects can be averted. However, results from longer term and larger studies are needed before testosterone therapy in hypogonadal older men can be considered in a general clinical setting.

## REFERENCES

Ellyin FM (1994): The beneficial effects of low dose testosterone treatment in the aging male. 76th Endocrine Society Annual Meeting, Abstract #1299, p 525.

Haddad G, Peachey H, Slipman C, and Snyder PJ (1994): Testosterone treatment improves body composition and muscle strength in hypogonadal men. 76th Endocrine Society Annual Meeting, Abstract #1302, p 506.

Janowsky JS, Oviatt SK, Carpenter JS, et al. (1991): Testosterone administration enhances spatial cognition in older men. Society for Neurosciences Annual Meeting, Abstract #340.12, p 868.

Katznelson L, Finkelstein J, Baressi C, and Klibanski A (1994): Increase in trabecular bone density and altered body composition in androgen replaced hypogonadal men. 76th Endocrine Society Annual Meeting, Abstract #1524, p 581.

Marin P, Holmang S, Gustafsson C, et al. (1993): Androgen treatment of abdominally obese men. Obesity Res 1:245-251.

Morley JE, Perry HM, Kaiser FE, et al. (1993): Effects of testosterone replacement therapy in old hypogonadal males: a preliminary study. J Am Geriatr Soc 41:149-152.

Orwoll E, Oviatt S, Biddle J, et al. (1992): Transdermal testosterone supplementation in normal older men. 74th Endocrine Society Annual Meeting, Abstract #1071, p 319.

Sih R, Kaiser FE, Morley JE, et al. (1994): Testosterone increases strength in older hypogonadal men. 31st American Geriatrics Society Meeting, Abstract #A25, p SA7.

Tenover JS (1994): Androgen administration to aging men. Endocrinol Metab Clin N Am 23:877-892.

Tenover JS (1992a): Effects of testosterone supplementation in the aging male. J Clin Endocrinol Metab 75:1092-8.

Tenover JS (1992b). Effect of testosterone (T) and 5α-reductase inhibitor (5-ARI) administration on responses to a sexual function questionnaire in older men. 17th Annual Meeting of the American Society of Andrology, Abstract #129, p 50.

Tomasic PV, Sollock RL, Armstrong DW, and Shakir KMM (1994): Osteoporosis in men with borderline idiopathic hypogonadotrophic hypogonadism. 76th Endocrine Society Annual Meeting, Abstract #1043, p 461.

# 31

# ANDROGEN USE IN WOMEN

Barbara B. Sherwin

Department of Psychology and
Obstetrics - Gynaecology
McGill University
Montreal Quebec
Canada H3 A 1B1

## INTRODUCTION

The increase in female life expectancy in industrialised societies, coupled with the profusion of evidence demonstrating an estrogenic protective effect vis-à-vis osteoporosis and coronary heart disease, have led to an increase in the use of estrogen replacement therapy in postmenopausal women. Although the ovarian production of androgens is also decreased after menopause, until recently, few have questioned the possible functional significance of androgens in women. Not surprisingly, the addition of androgen to an estrogen replacement therapy regimen for the treatment of postmenopausal women has remained an unconventional practice.

## FEMALE ANDROGEN PRODUCTION

In women, both the adrenal and the ovary contain the biosynthetic pathways necessary for androgen synthesis and secretion. It has been estimated that in premenopausal women, 49% of testosterone, the most potent androgen, is of adrenal origin, 17% arises from peripheral conversion of other steroid precursors, and 33% is produced by the ovary (Longcope, 1986). The ovary also produces approximately 60% of androstenedione and 20% of dehydroepiandrosterone (DHEA). After the menopause, the ovarian production of androstenedione decreases profoundly and secretion of testosterone declines as well, due to atrophy of ovarian stromal tissue (Longcope, 1986). The fall in the secretion of androstenedione, a major source of testosterone, results in a further decline in circulating testosterone in most postmenopausal women.

## NEUROBIOLOGICAL EFFECTS OF ANDROGENS

Autoradiographic studies have demonstrated that neurons containing specific receptors for testosterone are predominantly found in the preoptic area of the

*Pharmacology, Biology, and Clinical Applications of Androgens*, edited by Shalender Bhasin et al.
ISBN 0-471-13320-5 © 1996 Wiley-Liss, Inc.

hypothalamus, with smaller concentrations in the limbic system (amygdala and hippocampus) and in the cerebral cortex (McEwen, 1980).

In male rats, there is evidence that serotonin receptor subtypes mediate androgen effects on sexual behavior. The type of androgen treatment which induces male sexual behavior increases 5HT1A receptor binding in the preoptic area and decreases 5HT3 receptors in the amygdala (Mendelson and McEwen, 1990). No such studies have been undertaken in female rats whose sexual behavior is largely under the control of estrogen and progesterone acting on the ventromedial nucleus. On the other hand, effects of testosterone on various components of mating behavior have been studied intensively in female nonhuman primates. On the whole, these studies show that the administration of testosterone to ovariectomized rhesus monkeys increased perceptive behavior (i.e., increased attempts to solicit mounts from the male). Implantation of minute amounts of testosterone into the anterior hypothalamus of estrogen-treated ovariectomized and adrenalectomized unreceptive female rhesus monkeys also resulted in restoration of their perceptivity without affecting other aspects of sexual behavior, such as attractivity (Everitt and Herbert, 1975).

These studies on testosterone and sexual behavior in female nonhuman primates serve to underline two points. One, is that there is a specificity of action of testosterone on components of sexual behavior such that it enhances proceptivity (the animal's motivation to engage in sexual behavior), but has no effect on its attractivity or receptivity to males. Second, the efficacy of the very small dose of testosterone implanted into the hypothalamus, in the Everitt and Herbert (1975) study, suggests that testosterone exerts its effect on sexual desire in female rhesus via a direct effect on the brain and not by an influence on peripheral tissues.

## ANDROGENS AND SEXUALITY IN POSTMENOPAUSAL WOMEN

Survey data on the frequency of sexual dysfunctions in the postmenopause generally show that from one-third to two-thirds of women experience a decrease in sexual interest around the time of menopause, while fewer complain of decreases in frequencies of coitus and/or orgasm around this time (Sherwin, 1988). However, none of these epidemiological studies empirically assessed the relationship between circulating levels of the sex hormones and the reported changes in sexual behavior.

The paradigm that is perhaps most powerful for the study of specificity of the sex steroids on female sexuality involves administering hormone replacement therapy to women who have just undergone total abdominal hysterectomy (TAH) and bilateral salpingo-oophorectomy (BSO). When both ovaries are removed from premenopausal women, circulating testosterone levels decrease significantly within the first 24-48 hours postoperatively (Longcope et al., 1986). The fact that these women are deprived of ovarian androgen production following this surgical procedure has provided a rationale for administering both estrogen and androgen as replacement therapy.

In Britain and Australia, subcutaneous implantation of pellets containing estradiol and testosterone has been used as a treatment for menopausal symptoms for several decades. This route of sex-steroid administration results in a slow constant release of the sex hormones over a period of at least six months. Women complaining of decreased libido, despite treatment with estrogen, received subcutaneous implants of 40 mg estradiol and 100 mg testosterone (Burger et al., 1984). Patients reported a significant increase in libido by the third postimplantation month. These findings gained support from a double-blind study of women complaining of loss of libido during treatment with oral estrogens (Burger et al., 1987). They randomly received a subcutaneous implant containing either estrogen-alone or estrogen plus testosterone. After six weeks, the loss of libido in the single implant group remained, whereas the combined group showed significant symptomatic relief.

During the past decade, several prospective, controlled studies of general and sexual effects of combined estrogen-androgen parenteral preparations in surgically menopausal women were carried out. These studies have shown that the addition of testosterone to an estrogen replacement regimen induces a greater sense of energy level and well-being and is associated with fewer somatic and psychological symptoms compared to the administration of estrogen alone (Sherwin, 1985; Sherwin and Gelfand, 1984, 1985). Furthermore, the intramuscular administration of testosterone, either alone or in combination with estradiol, increased motivational aspects of sexual behavior (such as desire and fantasies), compared with the administration of estrogen alone or a placebo (Sherwin et al, 1985). Levels of sexual desire and interest covaried with plasma T level throughout the treatment month as the intramuscular drug was being metabolised (Sherwin, 1985). The androgynic enhancement of sexual motivation in women treated with the combined intramuscular drug has been shown to persist with long-term chronic administration of monthly injections that cause an initial surge in testosterone levels followed by gradual decline over a period of several weeks (Sherwin and Gelfand, 1987).

In a recent prospective study, premenopausal women underwent TAH and BSO and received either esterified estrogens 0.625 mg/day orally, or a combined tablet containing esterified estrogens 0.625 mg and methyltestosterone 1.25 mg/day for four months (Sherwin et al., 1993). Women who received the estrogen-androgen combined drug reported a significant increase in the number of times they left the house for work or social reasons (taken to be an index of physical activity), compared to those given estrogen-alone. Also, patients in the combined group experienced increased sexual arousal after the sixth postoperative month, whereas the estrogen-only treated women's sexual arousal was unchanged.

Taken together, the findings from the subcutaneous implant pellet studies and the prospective studies on oophorectomized women, provide compelling evidence that testosterone acts to increase overall energy level and also to enhance sexual desire and arousal in women, while frequency of sexual activity and of orgasm are unaffected. These findings allow the conclusion that in women, just as in men (Bancroft and Wu, 1983), testosterone has its major impact on the cognitive, motivational, or libidinal aspects of sexual behavior, such as desire and fantasies, and not on physiological responses. Moreover, studies of nonhuman primates suggest the likelihood that testosterone exerts this effect on sexual desire via mechanisms that impact directly on the brain rather than by any effect on peripheral tissues (Everitt and Herbert, 1975).

## POSSIBLE ADVERSE EFFECTS

### Hirsutism

Empirical data from controlled studies on the incidence of hirsutism in postmenopausal women treated with combined estrogen-androgen preparations could not be located. However, our own extensive clinical experience suggests that approximately 20% of women who receive 150 mg testosterone enanthate intramuscularly every four weeks, along with estrogen, will develop mild hirsutism manifested by an increased growth of hair on the chin and/or upper lip. When the dose is reduced to 75 mg testosterone enanthate per month, less that 5% of women have any increased hair growth. Moreover, hair growth decreases or, usually, stops entirely when the patient is switched to treatment with estrogen-alone.

### Lipoprotein Lipids

It has been well established that orally administered estrogens provide protection against coronary heart disease in postmenopausal women. A portion of this cardioprotective effect is due to the estrogenic increase of high-density lipoprotein cholesterol (HDL) and its ability to decrease low-density lipoprotein cholesterol (LDL). On the other hand, male athletes who self-administer large doses of anabolic-androgenic steroids, experience a significant decrease in HDL and an increase in LDL (Webb et al., 1984).

Several studies have reported on effects of combined estrogen-androgen preparations on lipid fractions in postmenopausal women. Teran and Gambrell (1988) treated women with subcutaneous implants of pellets containing 25 mg estradiol and 150 mg testosterone. After 12 months of treatment, there were no changes in total cholesterol, HDL, LDL or in VLDL, compared to preimplantation values. In oophorectomized women who had been receiving a combined intramuscular estrogen-androgen preparation chronically for four years, total cholesterol, LDL and HDL values were not different from oophorectomized women treated with intramuscular estrogen-alone, or from those who had remained untreated since their bilateral oophorectomy four years earlier (Sherwin et al., 1987). These findings are not surprising in view of the fact that parenteral routes of administration of the sex hormones bypasses the so-called "first-pass hepatic effect". Since sex steroid influences on lipoprotein fractions occur in the liver, they are largely attenuated by parenteral routes of hormone administration.

Recently, effects of an oral-combined regimen on lipoprotein lipids was tested in postmenopausal women (Hickok et al., 1993). Subjects randomly received either esterified estrogen 0.625 mg alone, or esterified estrogen 0.625 mg and methyltestosterone 1.25 mg, daily. Following six months of continuous treatment, there was a significant decrease in cholesterol, HDL, $HDL_2$, $HDL_3$ and apolipoproteins A1, compared to baseline in the group that received esterified estrogens plus methyltestosterone. Low-density lipoprotein cholesterol decreased in both treatment groups. However, there were no adverse effects of low-dose androgen on other parameters of hepatic function, such as total bilirubin, or gamma-glutamyl transferase, with combined therapy.

There is still a paucity of well-controlled studies on psychological and biological effects of combined estrogen-androgen replacement in postmenopausal women. However, the consistencies among available studies allow several conclusions. First, testosterone administered along with estrogen to surgically menopausal women, increases energy-level and general well-being over and above estrogen alone. Second, testosterone has its major impact on libido or sexual desire and interest in women, just as it does in men. Finally, adverse effects of exogenous testosterone on hair growth and on lipoprotein lipids are not only dose-dependent in women, but are also related to route of administration. There is evidence to show that such adverse effects are attenuated, or possibly even precluded, by parenteral routes of administration. Given the steady increase in female life expectancy over the past century, these findings suggest that combined estrogen-androgen replacement regiments for the treatment of postmenopausal women may enhance the quality of life for a significant segment of the population.

## REFERENCES

Bancroft J, Wu FCW (1983): Changes in erectile responsiveness during androgen replacement therapy. Arch Sex Behav 12:59-66.

Burger HG, Hailes J, Menelaus M, Nelson J, Hudson B, Balazs N (1984): The management of persistent menopausal symptoms with oestradioltestosterone implants: Clinical, lipid and hormonal results. Maturitas, 6, 351-358.

Burger HG, Hailes J, Nelson J, Menelaus M (1987): Effects of combined implants of oestradiol and testosterone on libido in postmenopausal women. Lancet 294, 936-937.

Everitt BJ, Herbert J (1975): The effects of implanting testosterone propionate in the central nervous system on the sexual behavior of the female rhesus monkey. Brain Res 86:109-120.

Hickok LR et al. (1993): A comparison of esterified estrogens with and without methyltestosterone: effects on endometrial histology and serum lipoproteins in post-menopausal women. Obstet Gynecol 82:919-924.

Longcope C (1986): Adrenal and gonadal androgen secretion in normal females Clin Endocrinol Metab 15:213-228.

Longcope C, et al. (1986): Steroid and gonadotropin levels in women during their peri-menopausal years. Maturitas 8:189-196.

McEwen BS (1980): The brain as a target organ of endocrine hormones. In Kreiger DT, Hughes JS (eds.): "Neuroendocrinology" Sunderland, MA: Sinauer Assoc., pp 33-42.

Mendelson S, McEwen BS (1990): Testosterone increases the concentration of ($^3$H 8-Hydroxy-2-di-n-propylamine) tetialin binding at 5-HTA receptors in the medial preoptic nucleus of the castrated male rat. Eur J Pharmac 181:329-331.

Sherwin BB, Gelfand MM (1984): Effects of parenteral administration of estrogen and androgen on plasma hormone levels and hot flushes in surgical menopause. Am J Obstet & Gynecol 148:552-557.

Sherwin BB, Gelfand MM (1985): Differential symptom response to parenteral estrogen and/or androgen administration in the surgical menopause. Am J Obstet & Gynecol 151:153-160.

Sherwin BB, Gelfand MM (1987): The role of androgen in the maintenance of sexual functioning in oophorectomized women. Psychosom Med 49:397-409.

Sherwin BB et al. (1993): Effects of a combined estrogen-androgen preparation on sexual behavior and lipid metabolism in surgically menopausal women. Proceedings of the 4th Annual Meeting of the North American Menopausal Society, Washington, DC (Abstr. 5-10).

Sherwin BB et al. (1985): Androgen enhances sexual motivation in females: A Prospective cross-over study of sex steroid administration in the surgical menopause. Psychosom Med 7:339-351.

Sherwin BB et al. (1987): Postmenopausal estrogen and androgen replacement and lipoprotein lipid concentrations. Am J Obstet Gynecol 156:414-419.

Teran AZ, Gambrell RD Jr. (1988): Androgens in clinical practice. In Speroff L (ed.): "Androgens in the Menopause." New York: McGraw Hill, pp 14-22.

Webb OL, Laskarzewski PM, Glueck CJ (1984): Severe depression of high-density lipoprotein cholesterol levels in weight lifters and body builders by self-administered exogenous testosterone and anabolic-androgenic steroids. Metabolism: 33:971.

## DISCUSSION: ANDROGEN THERAPY
## Chairpersons: Peter Snyder and Joel Finkelstein

**Richard Horton:** Dr. Tenover mentioned a controversy about the changes in testosterone levels in aging men. This controversy seems to have a life of its own. First, there are a number of studies on aging men that free testosterone levels progressively fall significantly from age 55 on to 90+. We have compared free testosterone with bioavailable testosterone in about 200 unselected samples coming into a reference lab in men. The correlation coefficient between those two methods is essentially one; there is really no difference between measuring it in either way, which is logical because the only thing that would really change the bioavailable from the free testosterone is a very major change in albumin levels. Another parameter is production rates. The metabolic clearance rate of testosterone also falls with age. It is actually only about half of that of young men, so that even in aging men that have a plasma testosterone within the normal range, the production rate of such an individual is reduced about 50%.

**J. Lisa Tenover:** The issue about which testosterone component one should measure will probably not be solved until we have a better handle on how to interpret androgen levels in relation to target organ response. The issue of testosterone production and metabolism rate is important because, in terms of replacing androgens in older men, you usually need lower doses than in younger men. The amount of testosterone I give my 25-year-old hypogonadal men, I rarely use in older men, at least when giving testosterone by injection.

**Todd Nippoldt:** For Dr. Sherwin. The data you showed, I believe, was all on surgically menopausal women. Can that data be extrapolated to women undergoing natural menopause?

**Barbara Sherwin:** Yes, the controlled studies I presented were undertaken on surgically menopausal women because they present such a neat experimental paradigm. We do treat naturally post menopausal women with the combined preparation. In fact, we regularly measure free T in our menopause clinic and I would absolutely disagree with the literature which says that in 50% of women the ovarian stroma goes on producing testosterone. I see that happen in about 10 to 20% in women.

**Participant:** Dr. Sherwin, you have shown us bone density data with estrogen alone or estrogen plus androgen and showed that the estrogen plus androgen was superior. Those data were reminiscent of the types of differences one might get if one gave estrogen plus progestins to women undergoing the natural menopause in which the addition of a progestin does appear to have a slight enhancement on bone mass. Have you compared the results of your two regimens to more conventional estrogen plus progestin replacement therapy in terms of its effects on the bone?

**Barbara Sherwin:** A very good point. It is reminiscent of those other graphs, but these were surgically menopausal women. There are a lot of reasons for not wanting to give women progestins. The absence of a uterus markedly reduces progestin use with estrogen therapy.

**Participant:** Another way of putting the question is whether one would extrapolate the potential benefit from estratest given to surgically postmenopausal women, to those women who have an intact uterus and are getting estrogen and progestins for benefits on bone.

**David Handelsman:** A question for Dr. Rogol. I noticed that in your list of problems with oxandrolone you didn't mention liver dysfunction. Oxandrolone is a 17 alpha alkylated androgen, which is in a class of anabolic androgens believed to be capable of hepatotoxicity and may produce liver tumors. Could you give us some idea of what kind of systematic testing you do for liver function and what proportions of subjects/patients have abnormal liver function tests?

**Alan Rogol:** With the doses of oxandrolone that we use (0.1 mg/kg) we checked liver function tests and found virtually no abnormalities in liver function tests.

**David Handelsman:** You don't do any monitoring now?

**Alan Rogol:** No, as we have very few kids receiving oxandrolone and the kids are often on the medication for less than a year.

**Ronald Swerdloff:** First, I might say something to David Handelsman. There seems to be something special about oxandrolone amongst the alkylated androgens with regard to liver dysfunction. In fact, oxandrolone has been reported to be advantageous in the management of patients with moderately severe alcoholic liver disease. The exact reason for the benignity is unclear to me.

**David Handelsman:** I think oxandrolone (like many other drugs) will always look more benign if its hazards are not looked at.

**Ronald Swerdloff:** These are not my data, but it has also been looked at in the oxandrolone clinical trials for delayed sexual maturation with a good safety profile. I want to ask Dr. Sherwin a question. You are talking about the use of androgens in post menopausal women and much of the positive effects have to do with psychosexual benefits and effects on bone. I wondered if you could report to us on the partner satisfaction. You are dealing with several issues. One is the increase in hirsutism which might be perceived as a negative effect and the increase in libido and well being which could be considered by some partners as positive effects. Did you get an inventory of partner responses? Secondly, I might say that the dosage of testosterone you are using is quite impressive for women since the threshold for CNS effects of androgen in men seems to be lower than many of the other metabolic effects. You may have an opportunity to go down the scale of treatment dosage further; it certainly would be worth investigating.

**Barbara Sherwin:** Let me try and answer some of that. First of all, perhaps I should say that I don't consider the combined estrogen testosterone drug for post menopausal women first-line treatment. Mostly, I think, its place is in the case where a woman is on estrogen alone and is reporting these residuals symptoms that are not alleviated by estrogen alone, and that I know are alleviated by adding some testosterone to the estrogen. So its use is indicated only in those cases. I don't think anyone thinks that we ought to be treating a low blood level of free T when the patient is asymptomatic. With respect to partner satisfaction, I have two kinds of anecdotes. Usually, the woman who complains of loss of libido is one who is in a good marriage or relationship and is unhappy about her lack of sexual interest. They are the people who spontaneously come forth seeking treatment. We have had cases, and you will probably chuckle, like everyone else has, when we put the woman on the combined drug and then get a phone call from her husband who will say, "I don't know what you have my wife on, but take her off of it", because the increase in her sexual appetite was not pleasing to him. I think it is the same reason why you often don't see increases in frequency of sexual activity with testosterone therapy. You don't see it with hypogonadal men and you don't see it with treated women, because it is a social issue, it is a relationship issue and that is often not modified by hormones.

**Somnath Roy:** Dr. Sherwin, you have just now commented on the problem when you were treating the wife with estrogen plus androgen, and the husband had some problem. When I was in the VA Hospital at Seattle with Dr. Paulsen and Dr. Jack Bakke in 1960-1961, one gentleman was being treated with testosterone at the age of 62 years because of signs of hypogonadism. One day we got a frantic phone call from his wife and everybody was looking for me in the hospital; she wanted to meet me urgently. She came and asked, "Doctor, what have you done to my husband? His sex desire has suddenly very much increased, and my life has been made miserable". So my question to Dr. Tenover is, do you also counsel the wife, because you said about counseling the husband. Simultaneous counseling of the wife while providing androgen therapy to aging men would be important.

**J. Lisa Tenover:** Almost all the older men I treat are in studies, and in this context, they *do* get counseled; we talk about the issue that increased sexual desire may be an adverse effect, depending on their situation. In the younger men that I treat, decreased libido is usually one of the reasons why they come to me for treatment in the first place, and in this situation I don't usually counsel the wife. In a couple of cases, when men have been on testosterone therapy in the past and their wives haven't liked the previous therapy because of the "ups and downs" in libido and mood, I have also involved the wife in therapy counseling. Otherwise I generally don't counsel spouses.

**Somnath Roy:** One short question to Dr. Sherwin. What are the relative roles of androgen and estrogen in maintaining the normal sexual function in women? The reason I am asking this is because in the early 1960's when I was with Dr. R. B. Greenblatt at Augusta, I got the impression that adrenal androgen was the main component which maintained libido and sexual function in women. But from your data, it seems that androgen, as well as estrogen, probably play a role.

**Barbara Sherwin:** Undoubtedly, estrogen is necessary to maintain the integrity of reproductive tissues. With low levels of estrogen, the vaginal epithelium becomes thin and there are all kinds of mechanical problems, apart from the fact that it is simply uncomfortable. You would absolutely need to replace the estrogen and that would be first-line treatment when someone walks in with a sexual problem who is not estrogen treated. There is little doubt in my mind that some minimal dose of testosterone within the normal female range is important for female libido.

**Richard Spark:** Dr. Tenover, I would like to apologize. I was one of the individuals who was frequently and relentlessly interviewed by Gail Sheehy for that article and I tried to explain to her that aging is not an equal opportunity affliction and she would not buy this. Basically the issue that she could not deal with was the fact

that she had responded so well to hormone replacement during her menopausal epi-
sode and had written an entire book about this; she was recruited by Esquire to do
this particular article. Indeed, I tried to explain to her the difference between primary and secondary gonadal failure and it fell on deaf ears. I have subsequently
heard from other reporters about this matter and from a variety of different individuals, who are for the most part largely female, who are convinced that this is an
issue that deserves attention. In the Scientific American article that was quoted, it
indicates that there are physicians in England running what they call Andropause
Clinics, and it was the reported experiences in those clinics that she used to show
the value of continued androgen supplementation in the aging men. I agree with
you, we don't know what is normal for a man as he ages. Dr. Horton points out the
fact that there is a lowering of level of free T due to decreased production, but a simultaneous decline in metabolic rate, so I think this has to be addressed appropri-
ately. The key is, it is not a menopausal state because there is incomplete gonadal
failure. Whether there is any benefit to androgen supplementation, I think it is
something that has to come out over the long run. This is going to be an issue that
will not go away unless we sort it out and get together to make some decision on
how to present this to the media, because the media has their own agenda on how
they want to deal with what they perceive as the "male menopause" controversy.

**J. Lisa Tenover:** I wholeheartedly agree. The words "menopause", "male cli-
macteric" or "andropause" look exciting in the headlines, so they are used. As men
age, you *do* actually see primary gonadal decline, but there is not a total loss of gonadal function and it is *not* a "menopause". The real issue is, and we talked about
this yesterday, that we need some way of finding an androgen end organ response
that one could measure and use as a yardstick to define a man as being
"hypogonadal".

**C. Alvin Paulsen:** I would like to emphasize the point on the genetic influence
that Dr. Rogol mentioned. We don't see this quite as much, but it used to be that
physicians would delay administering androgens or estrogens to hypogonadal boys
or girls because they were concerned that the epiphysis would close prematurely if
they were given sex steroid therapy. Their frame of reference was males with congenital adrenal hyperplasia, who were very short, but they had been exposed to androgens even in utero. In two situations the genetic influence plays a part. In the
Pygmy, for example, there is no decrease in linear height until the onset of puberty,
then the genetic influence inhibits any further linear growth that you would ordinarily see during puberty due to sex steroid secretion. Second, patients with idiopathic
hypogonadotrophic hypogonadism lack GnRH. If they are ages 13 to 15 and their
peers are going through sexual maturation, if you treat them with testosterone there
is no adverse impact on their eventual height. I can remember one such patient who
was treated adequately at age 15 and achieved a foot and a half of linear growth
during the time of androgen therapy. I believe that physicians should not be reluctant to treat these patients at the appropriate time when their peers are undergoing
sexual maturation.

**Alan Rogol:** I have just three very short comments. I think with testosterone and
the doses that are usually used, there are enough data in the literature to show that if
you start at a bone age of at least 11 years or above, you won't take inches or centi-

meters off the final height. With IHH, especially if it is familial with anosmia, where you do have an external marker of the hypogonadal state, should be treated to allow puberty to take place at an age when their peers are going through spontaneous puberty.

**C. Alvin Paulsen:**  I have two questions for Dr. Sherwin. In your studies of combined androgen and estrogen, I certainly agree with you in terms of the menorrhagia or the intermittent menstrual disorders. When you treat women with androgens, for example, the female to male transsexual before they have had a hysterectomy, you will see many instances of bleeding problems in these patients. My question to you is, what is your "dropout" rate with the women receiving combined androgen/estrogen therapy? I am concerned about the initiation of hirsutism, regardless of how small an incidence it is.

**Barbara Sherwin:**  We have a very low dropout rate in our research studies. First of all they don't go on for long enough. It takes a while for hirsutism to became manifest, if indeed its going to occur. Usually it doesn't happen within the time course of a given research study. In actual clinical practice, at least in our hands, hirsutism is reversible when you take them off testosterone and put them on estrogen alone.

**Alan Rogol:**  May I make a follow-up to one of your points, Dr. Paulsen, regarding the height in the people with constitutional delay? There may be another reason for treating them. Our data show, and I think at least two or three other groups have published data, that people with constitutional delay actually may end up with compromised adult height. They are about 5 cm or so shorter than their target, which is the difference between being in the 50th percentile for height and being in the 30th percentile. It is unknown whether or not intervening will "add" that height back. One can clearly show that they are about 5 cm less than their genetic potential based on their parent's heights. It is unclear whether or not treatment will correct that.

**F. C. Wu:**  I have a short comment for Dr. Sherwin and a question for Dr. Tenover. We have just finished a study on 24 women with premenstrual tension in which they have received testosterone implants at 100 mg every six months for three years or more and they were compared with a control group, also with the premenstrual syndrome, which did not receive any testosterone. We have found the HDL cholesterol and ApoA proteins in the treated group have decreased and the LDL and ApoB have increased. I think, therefore, that the systemic route of T administration is not entirely free from lipid effects.

**Barbara Sherwin:**  We used the combined drug containing 150 mg of testosterone enanthate in addition to estrogen, and we have had a large number of patients on that for up to 20 years. That specific drug doesn't affect lipids at that dose, but other compounds containing testosterone alone will when they are given to eugonadal women.

**F. C. Wu:**  My question to Dr. Tenover is that we have heard earlier that the effect on lipids between exogenous and endogenous testosterone may be very different. When you are giving testosterone to the older men who still produce their own testosterone, how do you choose the right dose and how do you know that their circulating testosterone is exogenous or endogenous? I think Dr. Nieschlag has some data that if you give testosterone to eugonadal men, you may actually reduce the level of testosterone.

**J. Lisa Tenover:** It is often "trial and error", but it is based on some background data. Prior to my first testosterone replacement studies in older men, I did a pilot study in six men using a number of testosterone dosing regimens. This was to evaluate which schedule would be most acceptable and also would keep the serum testosterone levels within the mid range of normal for young men. I tried testosterone enanthate at 50 mg twice a week, 50 mg once a week, 100 mg every week, and 200 mg every two weeks. In general, 100 mg every week gave the best results but the ideal dose can vary a good deal from individual to individual. During treatment, I usually measure serum T nadir and peak levels and use those to adjust the dose. In terms of exogenous vs. endogenous testosterone, in the studies where we have looked at that, the gentlemen on testosterone have no detectable serum LH or FSH. I assume that we have basically turned off all endogenous testosterone production by the exogenous testosterone administration.

**Barbara Sherwin:** Dr. Wu, can I ask whether your subjects with premenstrual tension getting 100 mg of testosterone were given estrogen as well?

**F. C. Wu:** No, these are premenopausal women because they have the premenstrual syndrome and they are all cycling normally.

**Barbara Sherwin:** I want to make the point, though it doesn't apply to your women, that giving testosterone in combination with estrogen is very different from giving testosterone alone. Estrogen increases SHBG and testosterone reduces it. SHBG remains stable with combined therapy in the doses we administer; it is not the same as giving an equivalent amount of testosterone alone.

**F. C. Wu:** I guess we are talking about the differences between endogenous and exogenous sex steroids in the female.

**Alvin Matsumoto:** Dr. Tenover, your study of testosterone replacement in elderly men is the best design in terms of its double-blind, placebo-controlled crossover-design, albeit in smaller numbers of men and preliminary in nature. I found it remarkable that 12 out of 13 men could tell when they were on testosterone in terms of the way they were feeling. Even though it is not hard data and did not use instruments that are validated for psychological testing, I thought this finding was quite remarkable. In terms of the studies that have been performed, administering testosterone to elderly men, most of them have selected men that are relatively healthy and some healthier than others. I would like to emphasize that as men get older they also get sick and also have illnesses and medications that tend to impact on testosterone negatively. When considering unselected elderly men, not just selected healthy men, the overall incidence of low testosterone levels might be much greater. Certainly if you look at a nursing home population or elderly patients that have functional disabilities, testosterone levels are lower than healthy men. Thirdly, many of us have had experience in treating older men with testosterone. These are older men that have, for example, pituitary tumors or that have had hypophysectomies or that have acquired gonadal disorders and have testosterone levels that are extremely low and are symptomatically androgen deficient. After doing a rectal exam and clinical evaluation, I generally institute therapy in these men. We have been treating these individuals for quite a while and I dare say that there are no reports of any problems in treating very blatantly hypogonadal men with testosterone. There is some historical data on treating elderly men with testosterone.

**J. Lisa Tenover:** During my training in Seattle, Dr. Paulsen used to tell me the same thing you have just said; that is, testosterone has been given for years to older men and major problems have not been obvious. Part of this may be that if you don't look, you don't see, but it is also probably true that we may not be creating major problems by giving testosterone in physiological doses to older men. However, I still worry about this and at this stage in studies, we need to monitor things carefully.

**Margaret Wierman:** Dr. Sherwin, the oral compounds that you used, Estratest and Estratab, are esterified estrogens and have a different pharmacology than the conjugated estrogens that are used more frequently in the United States. They have not been, to my knowledge, studied in large numbers of women long-term for their effects on either bone or cardiovascular system. Thus, there may be a potential problem in the dose equivalencies of these compounds. Since only a subset of women have libido problems at the time of menopause on physiologic hormone replacement, it raises the issue whether the women that have these symptoms actually may be rapid metabolizers of estrogen. When you use the conjugated estrogens in experimental protocols, one other possibility is that in the combination of the estrogen plus the testosterone, the benefit that you are getting is from some conversion of testosterone to estrogen. Those kinds of issues have not been addressed in the literature. I would urge you or someone to do those kinds of studies. I don't feel that the data are clear that androgens alone control libido in women independently or more importantly than estrogen.

**Barbara Sherwin:** First, let me just tell you that Estratest and Estratab, which contain esterified estrogens, are not available in Canada and are only available in the United States and actually I had to do that study in the United States. Secondly, you raised an absolutely legitimate point; how do we know that it is not estrogen affecting sexuality and maybe patients are not getting enough estrogen or they are metabolizing estrogen differently. I can tell you that there are some really elegant animal studies, particularly one in rhesus monkeys done at Cambridge in which minute amounts of testosterone were infused into the hypothalamus of animals who had no perceptive sexual behavior after oophorectomy and estrogen replacement, and it had a dramatic effect in restoring their sexual behavior.

**Margaret Wierman:** We know that aromatase activity in the hypothalamus is quite high. Testosterone administration would not answer the question of the role of androgen versus estrogen in libido.

**Barbara Sherwin:** Well, I thought it was a good study. There are lots of animal studies that make the point well.

**Bernard Robaire:** I would like to get back to the endogenous/exogenous issue. The question is for Dr. Tenover. Do you have any data to indicate that older men will not respond like young men to feedback loops; in other words when giving the same amount of testosterone to an older man, is the ability of that dose to inhibit LH secretion and therefore inhibit endogenous testicular production of testosterone reduced in the older individual?

**Stephen Winters:** Thank you, Dr. Robaire, for raising this issue. About ten years ago we were interested in why LH concentrations fail to rise although testosterone levels are reduced in elderly men. We induced T, DHT, or E2 continuously intravenously for 4 days and matched serum steroid levels produced by the infusion in groups of young and elderly men. We found that DHT was a more effective inhibitor of gonadotropin concentrations in older men than in young men. Testosterone was slightly more effective in older men whereas estradiol was equipotent in the two groups. We concluded that there is an increased responsiveness to testosterone negative feedback with aging. Others have subsequently found that LH pulse amplitude is less in older men. Thus, there is a double defect in testicular function with age, a major abnormality at the level of the testis such that FSH levels rise and a second abnormality in the hypothalamic pituitary unit perhaps due to increased negative feedback.

**J. Lisa Tenover:** Steve, do you know of any study in older men where testosterone levels have been lowered acutely and gonadotropin levels assessed? In your studies, you raised androgen levels and looked at it, thus, the opposite study design would be of interest.

**Stephen Winters:** Yes, such a study was conducted with flutamide; but I think the sample was small, and results have not been consistent.

**Bernard Robaire:** The second part of the question is if you drive testes with hCG, is the amount of testosterone production decreasing with age? I believe it is.

**J. Lisa Tenover:** You are correct. The testosterone response to hCG is lower in older men compared to younger men. Also, if you block steroid negative feedback to the hypothalamus, an older man does not have as vigorous a gonadotropin response as a younger man does.

**Stephen Winters:** Dr. Tenover, you said that about 7% of your men had total testosterone levels of less than 250 ng/dl. How many of the older men that you screened and found to have low testosterone levels proved to have clearly definable anatomical disorders?

**J. Lisa Tenover:** For my current testosterone study, I screened all the older men, who had testosterone levels less than 350 ng/dl by getting TSH and prolactin levels. I found 2 out of about 100 men I screened had prolactinomas. That is not a high prevalence, but I think the screening was worthwhile to do and I'm glad I did it.

# PART VI: ANDROGENS AND MALE CONTRACEPTION

# 32

# THE NEED FOR MALE NONBARRIER CONTRACEPTION METHODS

## C. ALVIN PAULSEN

## University of Washington
## School of Medicine
## Seattle, Washington 98195

The development of new and effective male contraceptive methods presents investigators and health care workers with complex challenges that extend beyond the gender issues involved. Society in general has a large vested interest in the problem. (Table 1)

Since some women experience adverse reactions to one or more of the female contraceptive methods, these reactions impact on continuance rates. (Table 2) Furthermore, the awareness of these potential reactions undoubtedly influences women/couples in deciding whether to use any female contraceptive method. Then, they are presented with current male methods, i.e., condoms, vasectomy or interrupted coitus. Each of these methods are associated with disadvantages (Table 3) that compound the problem of optimal contraception.

Table 1

**Society's Interest**

Men
- Share responsibility for family planning
- Obtain control over their fertility
- Concern for partner's health

Women
- Adverse reactions with present methods
- Reversible, safe, effective male method
- Shared male responsibility

*Pharmacology, Biology, and Clinical Applications of Androgens*, edited by Shalender Bhasin et al.
ISBN 0-471-13320-5 © 1996 Wiley-Liss, Inc.

Table 2

**Rationale for Developing New Male Methods**

Variable and unsatisfactory continuance rate for
female methods

- O.C's                25-80%
- I.U.D's              40-92%
- Injectables          22-63%
- Norplant 2 year      67- ? %

In the early 1970's several organizations recognized the need to expand the available menu of methods for male contraception. A consensus was reached to (1) evaluate various hormonal preparations known to inhibit gonadotropin secretion which would lead to the suppression of spermatogenesis and also (2) encourage basic research to fill in the gaps of knowledge with respect to the mechanisms controlling the male reproductive system.

In terms of the former strategy, the Male Task Force of the World Health Organization, the Contraceptive Development Branch of NICHD, the Ford Foundation, The Rockefeller Foundation, the Population Council and others supported a series of small, well-monitored clinical trials that studied the effect of testosterone alone or in combination with various progestational agents or impeded androgens, e.g., danazol to determine which agent or combination of compounds would suppress spermatogenesis most efficiently without significant adverse reactions. In addition, there was the need to demonstrate reversibility of spermatogenesis and a return to a normal hormonal environment.

The results of these small clinical trials indicated that the use of testosterone enanthate alone was the best candidate to use in an actual field trial to assess the actual efficacy in the administration of testosterone to induce a state of temporary infertility and evaluate whether the concept that a steroid such as testosterone could be used in some fashion as an effective male contraceptive agent.

These clinical trials involved ten centers in seven countries. Each of the 271 men enlisted in this first protocol received 200 mg of testosterone enanthate intramuscularly each week. One hundred fifty-seven (157) became azoospermic within 6 months, then these men who had become azoospermic and their partners relied only on the testosterone injections for their contraception method for an additional twelve months. Those men who did not develop azoospermia within 6 months were dropped from the study and did not participate in the efficacy phase. There was one pregnancy, or 0.8 conceptions, per 100 person years.

A second multicenter clinical trial using weekly injections of testosterone enanthate to assess the contraceptive efficacy of both severe oligospermia (<3.0 million/ml) and azoospermia has just been completed. The pregnancy rate of 1.4

Table 3

**Target Population**

---

Couples in a stable monogamous union

Couples desiring:
- Spacing method
- Delay of family

---

per 100 person years observed in both groups of men remained well below condom failure rate.

Thus it appears that the concept has been established that testosterone suppressed spermatogenesis could prove to be an effective male contraceptive method. Other agents with similar actions on the hypothalamic pituitary testicular axis could be used in conjunction with testosterone administration to improve the suppression of spermatogenesis.

Several points with respect to the use of a hormonal method for fertility regulation, require improvement. For example, if the goal is induction of azoospermia in virtually all men receiving such preparations, then testosterone administration will have to be coupled with agents like the GnRH analogues or a

Table 4

**If Hormonal Method Is Testosterone Based**

---

- Long term experience human exposure > 40 years

- Mechanism of action known

- Well-tolerated <10-15% dropout rate in clinical trials to date

- Probable less time to market

- Demonstrated efficacy

- Diminish the decrease in HDL-C as a potential health problem

- Otherwise acceptable human toxicological profile

---

Table 5

**Viable Alternative Hormonal Approaches**

---

Testosterone/progestogens
- TE + Levonorgestrel
- TE + Cyproterone acetate

GnRH analogues/testosterone

---

progestational preparation. Furthermore, a longer acting form of testosterone, e.g., the buciclate ester, or a different delivery system will be required to increase the interval between testosterone injections to once every two to three months instead of once weekly since weekly injections would be acceptable to only highly motivated men. Also, whichever combination of agents is considered, sustained azoospermia should be induced within four to six weeks of drug exposure.

Finally, if society accepts a failure rate of 2 - 3% per 100 person years then a hormonal regimen should induce severe oligospermia ($\leq 3$ million/ml), or azoospermia in virtually 100% of men, would be an acceptable contraceptive method.

Critics of the use of hormonal methods state that such an approach is associated with an excessive delay in achieving the desired suppression of spermatogenesis which makes it unsatisfactory. But if one focuses on the main features of our target population (Table 4) this problem should disappear when appropriate communication exists between the partners.

In summary, a testosterone based hormonal method appears to be the most likely for further consideration. (Table 5) Other viable possibilities have been studied to varying degrees but require further investigation before actual field trials can be conducted. (Table 6)

# REFERENCES

Andersch B, Milsom I (1992): Contraception and Pregnancy among Young Women in an Urban Swedish Population: Contraception 26 (3) 211-219.

Bebb RA, Anawalt BD, Christensen RB, Paulsen CA, Bremner WJ, Matsumoto AM (1995): Combined Administration of Levonorgestrel and Testosterone Induces more Rapid and Effective Suppression of Spermatogenesis than Testosterone Alone: A Promising Male Contraceptive Approach. (In Press) Journ Clin Endo and Metab.

Bauman KE, Varavej P (1972): Reason for Contracepting and Choice Between IUD and Pill - Implications for the Difference in Continuation Rates: Social Biology 19 292-296.

Bisset AM, Dingwall-Fordyce I, Hamilton MIK (1992): The Progestogen Only Pill: Acceptability and Continuation Rates: BR J Fam Plann 18 47-49.

Bounds W, Guillebaud J, Newman GB: Female Condom (Femidom) (1992): A Clinical Study of its Use-Effectiveness and Patient Acceptability: BR J Fam Plann 18 36-41.

Cummings DE, Bremner WJ (1994): Prospects for New Hormonal Male Contraceptives: Endocrinol and Metabol. Clinics of North America 23 (4): 893-922.

Diaz S, Pavez M, Miranda P, Robertson DN, et al. (1982): A Five-Year Clinical Trial of Levonorgestrel Silastic Implants (Norplant TM): Contraception 25 (5) 447-456.

Forrest JD, Fordyce RR (1993): Women's Contraceptive Attitudes and Use in 1992: Fam Plann Perspect 24/4 175-179.

Gui-yuan Z, Guo-zhu L, Wu FCW, Baker HWG, Xing-hai W, Soufir JC, Huhtaniemi I, Paulsen CA, Gottlieb C, Handelsman DJ, Farley TMM, Waites GMH (1990): Contraceptive Efficacy of Testosterone-induced Azoospermia in Normal Men. Lancet 336:955-959.

Hammerslough CR (1984): Characteristics of Women Who Stop Using Contraceptives: Fam Plann Perspect 16(1) 14-18.

Leonard JM and Paulsen CA (1978): Contraceptive Development Studies for Males: Oral and Parenteral Steroid Hormone Administration. In: D.J. Patanelle (ed.) Hormonal Control of Male Fertility, US Dept. of Health, Education and Welfare, Pub. No. (NIH) 78-1097.

Lodewijckx E (1987): Attitudes Towards Contraception and Some Reasons for Discontinuation: Contracept Fertil Sex BA#85052523 15(11) 1025-1030.

Mansour D (1994): Long-Acting, Reversible Methods of Contraception: Contemp Rev Obstet Gynaecol 6/2 89-94.

Mbizvo MT, Adamchak DJ (1992): Male Fertility Regulation - A Study on Acceptance Among Men In Zimbabwe: Cent Afr J Med 38 (2) 52-57.

Narkavonnakit T, Bennett T, Balakrishnan TR (1982): Continuation of Injectable Contraceptives in Thailand: Stud Fam Plann BA#75005504 13 (4) 99-105.

Paulsen CA (1977): Regulation of Male Fertility. In: R.O. Greep and M.S. Koblinsky (eds.) Frontiers in Reproduction and Fertility Control: Part 2. Cambridge, Mass., MIT Press, pp. 458-465.

Paulsen CA, Leonard JM, Burgess EC, Ospina LF (1978): Male Contraceptive Development: Re-Examination of Testosterone Enanthate as an Effective Single Entity Agent. In: D.J. Patanelli (ed.) Hormonal Control of Male Fertility, US Dept. of Health, Education and Welfare, publication No. (NIH) 78-1097.

Paulsen CA, Leonard JM, Bremner WJ (1980): The Use of Androgens, Androgen-Danazol or Androgen-Progestogen Combinations for the Regulation of Male Fertility. Proceedings of the VI International Congress of Endocrinology, Melbourne, Australia. Australian Academy of Science, Canberra. Griffin Press Limited, Netley, South Australia. pp. 516-519.

Paulsen CA, Bremner WJ, Leonard JM (1982): Male Contraception: Special Emphasis on Clinical Trials Using Steroid Hormones. In: Advances in Fertility Research, D. Mishell (Ed.) Raven Press, New York, pp. 157-170.

Singh K, Viegas OAC, Ratnam SS (1992): Acceptability of Norplant-2 Rods as a Method of Family Planning: Contraception 45 (5) 453-461.

Spinelli A, Grandolfo M, Donati S, Medda E (1993): Family Planning in Italy: Adv Contracept 9(2) 153-160.

Sunyavivat S, Chumnijarakij T, Onthuam Y, Mehyar AH, et al. (1983): Reasons for Discontinuing Contraception Among Women in Bangkok: Bull WHO 61(5) 861-865.

WHO Task Force (1995): Contraceptive Efficacy of Testosterone-Induced Azoospermia and Oligozoospermia in Normal Men: New Eng J of Med (submitted).

Weist WM, Webster PC (1988): Effects of a Contraceptive Hormone, Danazol, On Male Sexual Functioning: Journ of Sex Research: Vol. 24 170-177.

# DISCUSSION: ANDROGENS AND MALE CONTRACEPTION
## Chairpersons: Henry Gabelnick, Ronald Swerdloff

**Anita Nelson:**  When I was being interviewed on the 30th birthday of the birth control pill, the first question that was always asked was: "How do we feel being responsible for the sexual revolution?" The second question was: "Why is it that women must bear the burden of birth control? Why is it that we do not have a method for men?" The answer to that is that it is a little bit more difficult to come up with a male pill. One woman raised an interesting issue. She said, "Regardless of how the method lowers sperm count, I want it to make his left ear lobe turn blue so that I would know it was working." Do you have those issues raised?

**Henry Gabelnick:**  We have heard over and over again concerns about relying on the partner because it is the woman who becomes pregnant. Many of the systems that are being discussed rely on delivery systems that do not require daily compliance. Being able to palpate the device subcutaneously or going as partners to the clinic and seeing that the male partner gets a three month injection is the equivalent of having the blue earlobe.

**Somnath Roy:**  I would like to share with you the experience that we have had in family planning in India. At the present time the contraceptive prevalence rate in India is about 43%. Out of the 43% of couples that are practicing contraception, 33% are covered by sterilization. If you take the sterilization figures to date, only 5% are due to vasectomy and 95% are due to female sterilization. In 1978, about 80-85% of sterilization acceptors had vasectomies. One needs to look into why this is happening. Some studies on the knowledge, perception, attitude, practice and the decision making processes are being undertaken. We have very few methods for the male. Therefore, it is necessary to have a wider choice of reversible contraceptives for the male.

**C. Alvin Paulsen:**  I believe that the sharp decrease in vasectomies in India was based on the political approach to the vasectomy, at least at the time that I visited in 1974. It may be different now. I would like to comment on an issue that Dr. Nelson raised. None of our volunteers in the last 17 years (Circa, 500 couples), have been referred by OB-GYN doctors or the Planned Parenthood Organization. There needs to be a better relationship between the approaches for family planning by those care givers and society's interest.

**Anita Nelson:**  I sometimes feel a little foolish when a woman gets sent to the clinic to take care of this problem, her problem, when we realize that it is a couple's issue. I would much prefer talking with couples and finding a method that would work best with them.

**Somnath Roy:**  Regarding Dr. Paulsen's remark, I would like to point out that only for a short period there were some instances of forced vasectomies, many years ago. Later on, many other factors have contributed. After the setback, the family planning program in India gradually picked up momentum because of increasing female participation as they are the real sufferers. In recent years, there has been a tremendous amount of pressure from the women's activist group who are demanding gender equity and more male participation in all family life responsibilities including family planning. In the last International Conference on Population and Development (Cairo, 1994), this particular point was also strongly emphasized. Hence, there is urgency for development of new reversible male methods of contraception.

**Karin Ringheim:** The onset of sexual activity occurs at about age 15 for many women and continues until menopause. This means that a woman faces perhaps 25 or 30 years of using a contraceptive method. The demographic and health surveys have shown that in developing countries 50% of pill discontinuation occurs because of side effects. Women do not have any ideal contraceptive methods and couples really want to share the burden particularly where there are problems. Increasingly, this is going to become a gender issue where women's health advocates are going to be more and more demanding about the rights of men to have some opportunity for noncoital reversible methods.

**Avraam Grinvald:** Dr. Nelson, what is your opinion about female condoms as compared with male condoms?

**Anita Nelson:** The female condom has an inferior design to the male condom, the label even tells us that. The clinical trials went on for six months, not 12 months. We had a 12.5% use failure rate in 6 months. They rounded that out and doubled it, so on the average it is between 25 and 26% failure. It is very difficult to get women to use the condom for very much longer than six months. Another issue that comes up is noise. You can place it ahead of time, but it sounds like polyurethane as you walk and during coitus. It comes in a starter kit with more lubricant if you want to dampen that noise.

**Henry Gabelnick:** In a small number of women there is a noise and a lubricant issue. The CONRAD Program did that study on the female condom. It was designed for six months because the statistics clearly demonstrate that you do not need to go any longer than six months to get efficacy rates. The numbers were somewhat small. The device has a long way to go because aesthetically there are problems, but it is an important method.

**Anita Nelson:** The female condom fills an important niche. It is meeting a need where women cannot get their partners to use more effective latex condoms. We are also advocating it for the reduction of the STD risk.

**Henry Gabelnick:** The failure rate for perfect use is 2.6% at six months.

**Eberhard Nieschlag:** Dr. Nelson, the target group for which a male hormonal contraceptive is being developed includes couples in stable relationships and not the promiscuous young people. You are emphasizing the problems of the USA with a large group of promiscuous young people who practice sex without proper education. In the Netherlands, we have the most liberal laws concerning abortion and it is the very country with the lowest abortion rate in the world! Why?. Because together with liberal abortion laws, they have very good sex education and contraceptive services. People in Holland and in many other European countries are well educated and they know what to do to prevent a pregnancy. I am not saying unwanted pregnancies are not a problem in Europe and not in Holland, but the problem is of much smaller magnitude than in this country. The key to the solution of this issue is not male contraception but education. People in stable relationships need more contraceptive methods. They need a wider array of methods to be available for them. I think it is our obligation to develop a male method based on hormones or on other pharmacological entities.

**Anita Nelson:** Before developing new products, we need to think about where these products will fit in any given society. It sounds as if they might fit very well into Holland. But if we are talking about NIH money from the US, we have to anticipate how that might occur here and what the cost would be.

**Gabriel Bialy:** I should like to remind people that coitus interruptus has had a profound effect on the demographic transition in many countries. Secondarily, we do have spermicides that are good virucides. Maybe what we should be doing is not so much emphasizing the failure rates, but improve the products so that failure rates will be much, much less.

**Henry Gabelnick:** It is only fair to have balance and expand the opportunities for males to exercise their responsibilities as well as women.

# 33

# CONTRACEPTIVE EFFICACY OF HORMONAL SUPPRESSION OF SPERMATOGENESIS

## Geoffrey M. H. Waites and Timothy M. M. Farley

**UNDP/UNFPA/WHO/World Bank Special Program of Research, Development, and Research Training in Human Reproduction World Health Organization 1211 Geneva 27, Switzerland**

## SUMMARY

Two large clinical studies were conducted by the World Health Organization in the period 1986-1995 to examine the contraceptive efficacy of hormonally induced suppression to azoospermia or severe oligozoospermia. A total of 670 couples from 16 centers in 10 countries participated in the studies that required weekly intramuscular injections of 200 mg testosterone enanthate (TE). Although this regimen is impractical as a contraceptive method for widespread use, it was chosen because of its previously demonstrated efficacy in suppressing sperm production with minimal side effects. The main reasons given by couples for volunteering to take part in the studies was dissatisfaction with the currently available contraceptive methods. During the 6-month suppression phase, a greater proportion of men from the Asian centers suppressed to consistent azoospermia, compared to men from the non-Asian centers, but over 97% of men from both population groups suppressed to severe oligozoospermia (defined as a sperm concentration $\leq 3$ million/mL). Escape from spermatogenic suppression was rare. The first study showed that azoospermia, assessed by analysis of monthly semen samples, equated with high contraceptive efficacy. However 30% of men did not qualify for the efficacy phase in this study since they failed to suppress to azoospermia; the second study, therefore, addressed the contraceptive efficacy of suppression to oligozoospermic levels. During the 12 month efficacy phase, during which the TE injections were the sole form of contraception, the overall failure rate attributable to all men with sperm concentrations in the range 0 - 3.0 million/mL was comparable with typical first year failure rates of modern, reversible female methods. Recovery of sperm output occurred in those men who were followed after stopping injections and all term deliveries of pregnancies that occurred, while men were partially suppressed, resulted in healthy infants of normal weight. There was high compliance and acceptance of the hormonal regimen, although the requirement for weekly injections was a significant factor leading to discontinuation. Thus, spermatogenic suppression to sustained severe oligozoospermia can be achieved by an androgen-alone regimen with an acceptably high contraceptive efficacy. The results and experience from these studies will provide a stimulus to the development of second generation hormonal contraceptive methods for men that can be administered at longer intervals.

## INTRODUCTION

A reversible contraceptive method for men would provide them with an additional means of sharing the burdens and benefits of family planning. Such a method would need to consistently reduce the output of fertile spermatozoa sufficiently to prevent conception reliably. In principle, this could be accomplished by reducing sperm numbers, sperm function, or both. In addition, to broaden the options from vasectomy, the only reliable method currently available, the effect would need to be reversible. The level to which sperm output must be reduced to ensure adequate contraceptive efficacy has not been established, and an expert consultation in 1977 was divided whether azoospermia or severe oligozoospermia would be necessary (Patanelli, 1978). This uncertainty provided the motivation for the World Health Organization to conduct two major clinical studies to examine the contraceptive efficacy achieved by men suppressed to azoospermia or severe oligozoospermia by an androgen-alone regimen, based on weekly intramuscular injections of testosterone enanthate (TE). In spite of its inconvenience and impracticability as a contraceptive method for widespread use, this regimen was chosen because of its well documented efficacy in reversibly suppressing sperm output with few side effects (Patanelli, 1978).

The first study using this prototype hormonal regimen was conducted in 7 countries between 1986 and 1990. It demonstrated that testosterone-induced azoospermia yielded high efficacy with a pregnancy rate of 0.8 per 100 person-years (WHO, 1990). In that study, however, efficacy was not tested among the 30% of men who failed to achieve consistent azoospermia. Subsequently, a second study was undertaken between 1990 and 1994 in 9 countries to explore the level of fertility of normal men rendered azoospermic or severely oligozoospermic over a 12-month period. During this time, weekly intramuscular injections of TE were again the only form of contraception. Although these trials have added considerable data on safety (Wu et al., 1995) and provided unique experience in the conduct and management of such studies, they were not planned as an investigation of weekly testosterone injections as a contraceptive method. Their aim was to establish the pregnancy rates in the oligozoospermic and azoospermic subgroups (WHO, 1995b) and the rates of spermatogenic suppression in different populations (Handelsman et al., 1995; WHO, 1995a). In addition, they provided an opportunity to explore the motivations for men to enter such studies, to assess the reactions of couples to the treatment, and to develop and test acceptability protocols.

These studies and their significance are reviewed in this paper. They provide a basis for the conduct of future male contraceptive efficacy trials and a stimulus for the accelerated development of the next generation of contraceptive drugs for men.

# SPERMATOGENIC SUPPRESSION BY
# ANDROGENS ALONE

The first study using weekly injections of 200 mg TE (WHO, 1990) was conducted in 10 centers in 7 countries and involved 271 volunteers, 82 of whom were from China. A total of 225 men completed the six month suppression phase, of whom 70% achieved consistent azoospermia (defined as three consecutive azoospermic semen samples provided 2 weeks apart). The mean minimum sperm concentration among the 30% of men who failed to suppress to azoospermia was 3.0 million/mL (SD 5.8 million/mL). The mean time to the third consecutive azoospermic sample was 120 days since starting injections. An unexpected observation was that 91% of men from the Chinese centers became azoospermic, compared to only 60% of men from the non-Chinese centers ($P < 0.001$). This difference in suppression rates had not been previously reported and could not be explained by differences in physical characteristics or by the routine clinical chemistry screening, hormonal or semen profiles, prior to starting injections (Handelsman et al., 1995). The observation of possibly different androgen responses between population groups was supported by the results from another study using a different hormonal regimen (depot-medroxyprogesterone acetate for gonadotropin suppression and TE for androgen replacement) conducted among men in Indonesia (WHO, 1993) which showed higher rates of suppression to azoospermia than previously reported with the same regimen from other countries.

The second study, primarily designed to establish the fertility of the 30% of men whose sperm output was only partially suppressed, allowed population differences in response to be studied in more detail. This study was conducted in a total of 15 centers in 9 countries and involved 399 volunteers. Only 8 (2.2%) of 357 men who completed the suppression phase had to stop injections because they did not suppress to severe oligozoospermia. However, 86% of the men from the six Asian centers (China, 4; Singapore, 1; Thailand, 1) were azoospermic within six months of starting injections, compared to 68% of the men from the other centers (Australia, 2; Europe 5; USA, 2) ($P < 0.001$). This tended to confirm the differential responses previously noted, but when the suppression target was raised from azoospermia to severe oligozoospermia, the differences became less marked (Table 1).

Table 1. Proportions of Men with at Least One Semen Sample Below Different Thresholds within 6 Months of Starting Injections (Cumulative Life Table Rates)

| Suppression Target | Asian Men (123) | Non-Asian Men (276) |
|---|---|---|
| ≤5.0 million/mL | 100% | 98% |
| ≤3.0 million/mL | 98% | 95% |
| ≤1.0 million/mL | 92% | 90% |
| Azoospermia | 86% | 68% |

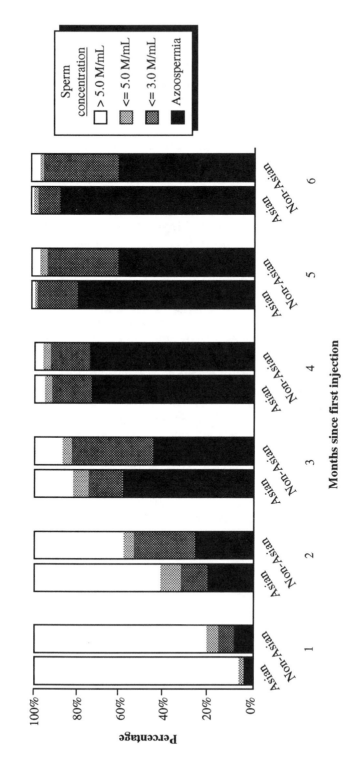

## Distribution of sperm concentration by population group

**Sperm concentration**
- ☐ > 5.0 M/mL
- ▨ <= 5.0 M/mL
- ▨ <= 3.0 M/mL
- ■ Azoospermia

**Percentage** (axis: 0%, 20%, 40%, 60%, 80%, 100%)

**Months since first injection** (1, 2, 3, 4, 5, 6; each with Asian / Non-Asian pair)

Figure 1. Distribution of sperm concentrations by time since first injection for Asian men (left bar of pair) and non-Asian men (right bar of pair) (cumulative lifetable estimates of the percentage of men with at least one sample below threshold). (Source: WHO 1995a)

However, an analysis of the dynamics of sperm suppression from the two studies (WHO, 1995a) showed that they were more complex; men from the non-Asian centers appeared to suppress faster, but were subsequently overtaken by the men from the Asian centers (Fig. 1). The mean times to suppress to sperm concentrations of 5 or 3 million/mL or azoospermia were 75, 81 and 101 days, respectively, in the men from the Asian centers, and 64, 70 and 119 days, respectively, in the men from the other centers. No physical, behavioral, or laboratory differences between the men from the different types of center have been identified to account for the different patterns of sperm suppression (WHO, 1995a).

While the times taken to suppress to azoospermia or severe oligozoospermia are critical, it is also important to know whether men remain suppressed while receiving weekly TE injections. In the first study (WHO, 1990), among men who had qualified for the efficacy phase by achieving consistent azoospermia, sperm were detected in only 21 of 1515 semen samples (1.4%) and no men had to stop injections for spermatogenic rebound (two consecutive non-azoospermic samples). In the second WHO study, escape from suppression of sperm output after reaching the oligozoospermic threshold for the efficacy phase, led to the discontinuation of 4 men, and escape from spermatogenic suppression was rare among the remaining men.

Thus, regular testosterone injections can suppress spermatogenesis to azoospermia or severe oligozoospermia in 97% of men, regardless of their population group, with little risk of spermatogenic rebound.

# CONTRACEPTIVE EFFICACY OF AZOOSPERMIA

The first study demonstrated that, from 157 men who became azoospermic, only one pregnancy occurred during 1486 months (124 years) of the efficacy phase, equivalent to a pregnancy rate of 0.8 (95% confidence interval 0.02-4.5) per 100 person-years. The second study also underlined that the laboratory diagnosis of azoospermia equates with high contraceptive efficacy (WHO, 1995b).

# CONTRACEPTIVE EFFICACY OF OLIGOZOOSPERMIA

In the second study, couples stopped using their usual or barrier contraceptive method once they had suppressed to severe-oligozoospermia and relied on TE suppression alone during the 12-month efficacy phase. Pregnancy rate was strongly related to sperm concentration. The overall pregnancy rate attributable to all men with a sperm concentration of 0 - 3.0 million/mL was comparable with typical first year failure rates of modern, reversible female methods. No pregnancies occurred among the Asian couples, but these couples contributed only 15% of the non-azoospermia exposure to the risk of pregnancy. The more effective suppression to azoospermia among men from the Asian centers would make an androgen-alone method highly effective in this population.

## SUBJECTS AND REASONS FOR DISCONTINUATION

In both studies the men from the Asian centers were on average shorter and lighter than those from the other centers. Their mean age was 34.2 years compared to 30.4 years and that of their partner was 31.1 compared to 27.2 years, respectively. Fertility had been demonstrated by 84% and 86% of the volunteers in the two studies, respectively, with a median of 2 pregnancies and intervals of 24 and 27 months since the last pregnancy, respectively. At entry, 97% of the couples in the second study were using a contraceptive method (barrier, 48%; oral contraceptive, 27%; IUD, 12%; other methods, 10%), closely similar to the first study where the percentages were 43%, 23%, 22% and 13%, respectively. Dissatisfaction with their current contraceptive method (83%) was the main reason for participating.

The patterns of discontinuation and adverse events were similar in the two studies. The main reasons for stopping injections were personal reasons, medical reasons, injection problems, or pregnancy. Some volunteers did not adhere strictly to the instruction to use other forms of contraception during the suppression phase, and a number of pregnancies occurred during this time. Only in the first study was failure to suppress an important reason for stopping injections. The majority of the men who stopped injections for personal reasons did so because they had no further need for contraception (41%), were moving away from the study site (24%), or were unwilling to continue (21%). Eight couples stopped because they desired a pregnancy. The most common 'other medical' discontinuations were acne (27%) and psychological changes (23%), which included changes of mood, behavior or libido.

The patterns of discontinuations and adverse events in the two clinical studies confirms the overall safety of TE for use for up to 18 months. Clearly, more research is needed to provide reassurance that male contraceptive methods based on androgens not only provide acceptable levels of contraceptive efficacy for the couple but also are safe for long-term use. They may even have potential beneficial effects on bone, muscle and other androgen-responsive tissues. Already there is evidence that exogenous androgen, even when provided by the imperfect pharmacokinetic profile of TE, has minimal short-term effects on the prostate of healthy or hypogonadal men (see Wu et al., 1995). Although the administration of TE to normal men lowers, or leaves unchanged, high-density lipoprotein with minimal changes in total and low-density lipoprotein cholesterol levels, the influence of androgens on the evolution of cardiovascular disease remains controversial (Plymate and Swerdloff, 1992).

## RECOVERY AND OUTCOME OF PREGNANCY

Most men recovered to their baseline sperm concentration in a median time of 201 days (6-7 months), and the remainder to normal levels (> 20 million/mL) by 112 days (3-4 months). There were no differences in times to recover between men who were consistently, never, or intermittently azoospermic in the efficacy phase. Some couples planned pregnancies after completion of the studies and all term pregnancies have resulted in healthy infants of normal weight.

# RELEVANCE FOR OTHER HORMONAL METHODS

These pioneering male contraceptive efficacy studies using a prototype hormonal regimen have provided the basis for the future development of second generation hormonal contraceptive drugs. The likely contraceptive efficacy of such drugs may be predicted from the degree to which they are able to suppress spermatogenesis and the pregnancy rates at different levels of sperm suppression. Other hormonal regimens, such as lower dose androgens combined with progestogens, may be more effective than androgen alone if they additionally render residual sperm infertile due to metabolites in the semen. However these results give an upper limit on the pregnancy rates to be expected from the use of such drugs and can therefore be used to plan and conduct further efficacy studies of hormonal regimens that are more practical to deliver, and hence more acceptable.

# POPULATION AND INDIVIDUAL DIFFERENCES IN RESPONSE

The non-uniformity of suppression to azoospermia in the first study was not due to anthropometric or population differences, to variations in androgen effects, or poor compliance with treatment. It was considered to be more consistent with quantitative differences in the hormonal regulation of spermatogenesis in the two groups of Asian and non-Asian men (Handelsman *et al.*, 1995). The high rate of suppression to azoospermia among the Asian, largely Chinese, populations in the WHO studies, together with the high rate of suppression to azoospermia achieved in Indonesian men by androgen alone (Arsyad, 1993), and by DMPA and an androgen (WHO, 1993), has encouraged investigators in China, India, and Indonesia to plan multicenter efficacy studies to start in 1995.

# SOCIO-BEHAVIORAL ASPECTS

Couples were asked to keep a diary of menstrual bleeding and sexual activity. Questionnaires (designed by Dr. K. Ringheim, now at USAID, Washington) exploring acceptability of the method, including behavioral aspects, were administered and focus group discussions with the volunteers were conducted in some centers.

Despite the high degree of compliance and acceptance of the injection schedule among this motivated population, the requirement for weekly injections was a significant factor leading to discontinuation. The low incidence of psychological reactions is consistent with the lack of behavioral changes observed in a small placebo-controlled study of normal men given injections of TE (Anderson et al., 1992). About three-quarters of the female partners of men who completed the trial in one center would have been happy for their partner to continue with the treatment had it been available, most indicating that they had experienced an increase in enjoyment of intercourse as a result of confidence in the method and of being given temporary respite from the responsibility for contraception (K. Ringheim, personal communication). The advent of long-acting depot androgen preparations, which would allow administration at intervals of three or four months or longer, would provide more acceptable and practical family planning options (Ringheim, 1993). Preparations, such as testosterone buciclate (Behre and Nieschlag, 1992; Behre et al., 1995), testosterone microspheres (Bhasin et al., 1992) and implants (Handelsman et al., 1992) are in advanced stages of clinical development. These preparations provide more uniform androgen release and there is some evidence that they have fewer metabolic side-effects than TE and that suppression may be more uniform. Longer-acting preparations with these characteristics may make it less necessary to monitor sperm output when they are used for contraception.

## CONCLUSIONS

In conclusion, it is suggested that the findings in the WHO studies reviewed here enhance the feasibility of developing a hormonal contraceptive method for men suitable for widespread use. It is likely that similar contraceptive efficacy could be expected for other hormonal regimens which suppress spermatogenesis by inhibiting gonadotropin secretion. Combinations of lower dose androgens with GnRH antagonists or progestogens, even if they do not achieve azoospermia in all men, can readily achieve the levels of oligozoospermia shown here to equate with an acceptable level of contraceptive efficacy. The intention of three large developing countries to conduct multicenter efficacy studies to start in 1995 is a clear signal of confidence in the potential of male hormonal methods. However, the choice of drugs for such studies remains limited. The need for the rapid development of the next generation of contraceptive drugs for men poses an urgent challenge to funding agencies and the clinical scientific community. Moreover, rapid progress in all aspects of the field and growing awareness of mens' responsibilities in reproductive health should also serve to rekindle the interest of the pharmaceutical industry.

## ACKNOWLEDGMENTS

Financial support to the two US centers was provided by USAID through the CONRAD Program and to the remaining centers by the UNDP/UNFPA/-WHO/World Bank Special Program of Research, Development and Research Training in Human Reproduction. The guidance of the Steering Committee and of the chairpersons, Dr. E. Nieschlag and Dr. C. Wang, of the WHO Task Force on Methods for the Regulation of Male Fertility during the period 1985-1995 are gratefully acknowledged, as is the professional competence of the clinical investigators and their colleagues in the 16 centers. WHO also wishes to express appreciation to the volunteers and their partners for participating in the demanding protocols.

## REFERENCES

Anderson RA, Bancroft J, Wu FCW (1992): The effects of exogenous testosterone on sexuality and mood of normal men. J Clin Endocrinol Metab 75: 1503-1507.

Arsyad KM (1993): Sperm function in Indonesian men treated with testosterone enanthate. Int J Androl 16:355:361.

Behre HM, Nieschlag E (1992): Testosterone buciclate (20 Aet-1) in hypogonadal men: pharmacokinetics and pharmacodynamics of the new long-acting androgen ester. J Clin endocrinol Metab 75:1204-1210.

Behre HM, Baus S, Kliesch S, Keck C, Simon M, Nieschlag E (1995): Potential of testosterone buciclate for male contraception: endocrinological differences between responders and non-responders. J Clin Endocrinol Metab (in press).

Bhasin S, Swerdloff RS, Steiner B, et al., (1992): A biodegradable testosterone microcapsule formulation provides uniform eugonadal levels of testosterone for 10-11 weeks in hypogonadal men. J Clin Endocrinol Metab 74:75-83.

Handelsman DJ, Conway AJ, Boylan LM (1992): Suppression of human spermatogenesis by testosterone implants. J Clin Endocrinol Metab 75:1326-1332.

Handelsman DJ, Farley TMM, Peregoudov A, Waites GMH (1995): Factors in the non-uniform induction of azoospermia by testosterone enanthate in normal men. Fertil Steril 63: 125-133.

Patanelli DJ (ed.) (1978): "Hormonal Control of Male Fertility." Washington: US Department of Health Education and Welfare, Publication number (NIH) 78-1097.

Plymate SR, Swerdloff RS (1992): Androgens, lipids and cardiovascular risk. Ann Intern Med 117: 871-872.

Ringheim K (1993): Factors that determine prevalence of use of contraceptive methods for men. Stud Fam Planning 24: 87-99.

World Health Organization Task Force on Methods for the Regulation of Male Fertility (1990): Contraceptive efficacy of testosterone-induced azoospermia in normal men. Lancet 336: 955-959.

World Health Organization Task Force on Methods for the Regulation of Male Fertility (1993): Comparison of two androgens plus depot-medroxyprogesterone acetate for suppression to azoospermia in Indonesian men. Fertil Steril 60: 1062-8.

World Health Organization Task Force on Methods for the Regulation of Male Fertility (1995a): Rates of testosterone suppression to severe oligozoospermia or azoospermia in two multinational clinical studies. Int J Androl (in press).

World Health Organization Task Force on Methods for the Regulation of Male Fertility (1995b): Contraceptive efficacy of testosterone-induced oligozoospermia in normal men. (Submitted for publication).

Wu FCW, Farley TMM, Peregoudov A, Waites GMH (1995): Effects of testosterone enanthate in normal men: experience from a multicenter contraceptive efficacy study. (Submitted for publication).

# 34

# GnRH ANALOGUES AND MALE CONTRACEPTION

Ronald Swerdloff, Barbara Steiner,
Carlos Callegari, Shalender Bhasin

Harbor-UCLA Medical Center
Torrance, California 90502

## INTRODUCTION

GnRH analogues are classified as either agonists or antagonists based on their acute response. The agonists were initially developed as therapeutic agents to stimulate LH and FSH and therefore treat GnRH deficiency (hypogonadotropic hypogonadism). Early experimental studies demonstrated that GnRH agonists, when given in repeated doses, had interesting paradoxical effects on gonadotropin secretion and even more striking inhibition of testosterone secretion and intratesticular content (Heber et al., 1982; Heber and Swerdloff, 1980). The mechanisms by which GnRH agonists down regulate the reproductive system are complex, but for the purpose of this discussion can be thought of as initially stimulatory, and later inhibiting the pituitary's secretion of biologically active gonadotropins. This results in testosterone deficiency and decreased spermatogenesis.

This paradoxical inhibitory action of GnRH agonists has been utilized to treat a number of endocrine responsive conditions. These include: true precocious puberty, prostate cancer, BPH, endometriosis, polycystic ovarian disease, and their consideration as potential male contraceptive agents.

## GnRH AGONISTS AS EXPERIMENTAL MALE CONTRACEPTIVES

In the 1970's, a number of investigators explored the use of testosterone as a reversible hormonal contraceptive approach for men (Cunningham et al., 1977; Paulson et al., 1982; Rowley and Heller, 1977; Steinberger and Smith, 1977; Swerdloff et al., 1979). The results of these studies were encouraging in that they demonstrated the ability of testosterone when given for 3 to 6 months duration, to inhibit LH and FSH secretion and suppress sperm counts to low levels, but disappointing in their failure to induce azoospermia in more than about half of the subjects. Follow-up studies on steroid approaches were delayed for a number of years as

*Pharmacology, Biology, and Clinical Applications of Androgens*, edited by Shalender Bhasin et al.
ISBN 0-471-13320-5 © 1996 Wiley-Liss, Inc.

the few investigators actively involved in this area turned their attention to potential application of the new class of GnRH agonists for suppression of spermatogenesis. Since early studies demonstrated that they predictably suppressed serum testosterone to very low levels, testosterone replacement therapy was added in varying doses to the GnRH agonist treatment to prevent androgen deficiency and maintain libido and erectile function.

GnRH agonist preparations have been tested by at least 12 investigators studying the effects on 106 volunteer subjects. The overall results were summarized recently (Cummings and Bremner, 1994). They indicated that about 20% of men became azoospermic; an additional third developed severe oligospermia (less than 5 x 10 6/cc), and the remainder had lesser degrees of sperm suppression. (Table 1) Since the dosages and durations of treatment were highly variable, lumping these studies together is not totally revealing, but the results of even the best studies were disappointing for their failure to suppress sperm counts to lower levels than seen using testosterone alone. Several explanations exist for the limited success of GnRH agonist and androgen combinations. These include: inadequate dose; suboptimal route and frequency of administration; and interference of analogue effect by combined androgen therapy.

Since hypophysectomy produces azoospermia and GnRH antagonists in experimental animals will duplicate the effects of hypophysectomy on quantitative intratesticular spermatogenesis and sperm counts (Sinha-Hikim and Swerdloff, 1993), the most likely reason for incomplete suppression of spermatogenesis in clinical trials with GnRH agonists and testosterone combinations is the inability to completely inhibit LH and FSH secretion. The reasons that combined GnRH agonist and testosterone treatment fails to completely turn off gonadotropins has been a topic of major speculation by many investigators.

In general, the poorest results were seen in the earlier trials in which the doses were low. Progressively increasing the doses gave improved suppression of sperm counts, but azoospermia was inconsistently produced. It should be noted that even the largest doses were much lower than those used in subsequent antagonist trials (Bagatell et al., 1993; Pavlou et al., 1991; Tom et al., 1992) and many were a log unit less than those predicted to be optimally effective by non-human primate studies. Higher dose human studies will be required to resolve the question whether these agonists are inherently incapable of producing complete inhibition of LH and FSH (thereby failing to induce azoospermia in all men), or the doses were simply sub-optimal.

The route of administration, nature of formulation and pharmacokinetics of parenterally administered GnRH agonists are important factors in analyzing the results of GnRH agonist trials. Since subcutaneous daily dosing with GnRH agonists were adequate to lower serum testosterone to low levels in human prostate cancer trials, this paradigm was used in the early agonist trials on suppression of spermatogenesis. The agonists were known to have longer blood half lives than authentic GnRH and were potent in stimulating LH and FSH secretion in the initial stimulatory phase (Bhasin and Swerdloff, 1995). It was also known that GnRH, when given as a constant infusion, suppressed LH and FSH when compared to single or spaced injections of the authentic GnRH peptide (Schürmeyer et al., 1984b; Michel et al., 1985; Pavlou et al., 1986; Bhasin et al., 1987). The GnRH agonist treatment trials of prostate cancer demonstrated that a sufficiently high daily dose of GnRH agonist resulted in suppression of testosterone levels for 24 hours (Rajfer et al., 1986; Handelsman and Swerdloff, 1985). While the sensitivities of the LH and FSH assays may have been marginal in their ability to separate complete from near complete suppression of LH and FSH levels, careful assessment of gonadotropin levels during agonist treatment, suggested that partial LH and testosterone escape may occur (Resko et al., 1982). These observations led to studies in monkey and humans to assess the possibility that constant GnRH agonist infusion might produce more reliable down regulatory effects on the pituitary, and thereby block escape of LH and FSH  from suppression. This was a rational consideration since constant infusion of authentic GnRH had potent paradoxical suppressive effects on LH and FSH secretion and the pharmacodynamic studies of GnRH agonists indicated a time-related maximum effect.

Results in monkeys treated with agonist infusions by minipumps at rates of 3.5-5 ug/kg/day were highly successful with two investigators (Akhtar et al., 1983; Mann et al., 1987) reporting azoospermia in 13/14 monkeys. We and others attempted to demonstrate an enhanced effect of continuous subcutaneous infusions of GnRH agonists (compared to intermittent injections) in  human subjects. The results failed to show major advantage of the continuous over intermittent pattern of administration, although the highest dose of infusion of Nafarelin (400 ug/d) gave better results than historical controls given 200 ug dose of the same drug, once daily (Bhasin et al., 1985; Bhasin et al., 1987). Additional trials comparing continuously infused agonists against historical controls using intermittent injections did not produce greater suppression of spermatogenesis (Michel et al., 1985; Pavlou et al., 1986; Schürmeyer et al., 1984). It should be noted that none of these studies rigorously tested the hypothesis in a multilevel dose response fashion, and small differences in effectiveness between the two methods of drugs administration could not be detected because of the small sample size.

A second explanation for incomplete suppression of spermatogenesis could be partial refractoriness of FSH to the inhibitory effects of GnRH agonist. This possibility was raised over a decade ago by Santen who noted that in men treated with GnRH agonist for prostate cancer, LH levels remained low, while FSH levels initially suppressed and then escaped after protracted treatment (Santen et al., 1984; Huhtaniemi et al., 1985). Since FSH is believed to be a factor in maintenance of spermatogenesis, such escape, even if partial, could result in failure to predictably induce azoospermia.

Another controversy related to incomplete suppression of gonadotropins in GnRH analogue plus testosterone treated men, is whether the androgen component augments or inhibits the effects of the analogue on gonadotropin levels. Early studies from our laboratories on rats clearly demonstrated that testosterone amplified the inhibitory effects of GnRH analogues on suppression of gonadotropins and spermatogenesis (Heber et al., 1982; Heber and Swerdloff, 1980; Heber and Swerdloff, 1981). Most studies in non-human primates and humans failed to show this

# Table 1 CLINICAL TRIALS OF GnRH AGONISTS AS MALE CONTRACEPTIVES

| Trial | Drug | N | Dose | Androgen | Time | Results | Comments |
|---|---|---|---|---|---|---|---|
| Bergquist (1979) | Buserelin | 4 | 5 µg/d sc | None | 17 wk | No in sperm ct. | Initial low-dose trial Gtns & T ! |
| Linde (1981) | D-Trp[6] | 8 | 50 µg/d sc | None | 6-10 wk | Azo 1/8<br>Oligo 6/8 (<6) | Low dose<br>Poor gtn suppression impotence: 5/8 |
| Doelle (1983) | D-trp[6] | 6 | 50 µ/d sc | TE 100 q 2 wk | 20 wk | No azo<br>Oligo 3/6 (≤6.2)<br>LMSC = 12 | T repleted: sexual function OK<br>T blunts agonist effect relative to Linde 1981 |
| Rabin(1984) | D-Trp[6] | 3<br>5 | I. 100 µg sc qd<br>II. 500 µg sc qd | TE 100 q 2 wk | 20 wk | I. azo 1/3<br>II. azo 3/5<br>Overall: oligo-azo 5/8 | Higher dose: azo inconsistent |
| Schurmeyer (1984) | Buserelin | 7<br>4 | I. 118 µg/d sc.<br>II. 230 µg/d sc. (minipumps) | TU 80-120 mg po qd, start w/ Sx's (~5th wk) | 12 wk | No azo<br>I. LMSC 18<br>II. LMSC 10 | First constant infusion |
| Michel (1985) | Buserelin | 7 | 450 µg/d sc (minipumps) | TU 80 mg po qd, start @ wk 5 _ to 120/d by wk 8 | 12 wk | No Δ in sperm ct.<br>LMSC 44 | Higher dose constant infusion<br>Worse results @ 2x max dose of Schurmeyer<br>! b/i LH ratio |
| Bhasin (1985) | Nafarelin | 7 | 200 µg/d sc | TE 200 q 2 wk | 16 wk | No azo<br>Oligo 3/7 (<5)<br>LMSC 17 | Failed because unable to maintain agonist levels by sc injection? |
| Bhasin (1987) | Nafarelin | 7 | 400 µg/d sc constant infusion (mechanical) pump | TE 200 q 2 wk | 16 wk | Azo 3/7<br>Oligo 5/7 (<5)<br>LMSC 6 | Better results than Bhasin 1985 @ 2x dose and constant infusion<br>! b/i LH ratio; LH pulsatility |

| Study | Agonist | n | Regimen | Androgen | Duration | Results | Comments |
|---|---|---|---|---|---|---|---|
| Frick (1986) | Buserelin | 6 | I. 3 x 50 µg/wk | I. None | 5 mo | I. No Δ sperm ct. | Direct Study + or - androgen; T blunts agonist effect |
| | | 4 | II. 3 x 100 µg/wk | II. None | 6 mo | II. "All virtually azo" | |
| | | 4 | III. 3 x 200 µg/wk (intranasal) | III. 5 mg po qd fluoxymesterone | 5 mo | III. No sperm ct. Libido/potency OK | |
| Pavlou (1986) | D-trp[6] | 8 | 500 µg/d constant infusion (sc insulin pump) | TE 100 q 2 wk | 16 wk | No azo Oligo 6/8 ↓ b/i LH | High-dose continuous infusion. Responders vs. non-responders not distinguished by T or LH profile. Continuous infusion no better than daily injection |
| Bouchard (1987) | D-Trp[6] | 5 | I. 100 µg/d (microspheres) | I. TE 125 q mo (low-dose replete) | 15-30 wk | I. Azo 5/5 LMSC~5 | T blunts agonist: Direct study. Additional T inj's given to one of the azo's in I: sperm reappeared. Return to low-dose T -azo |
| | | 5 | II. 100 µg/d (microspheres) | II. TU 120 q day (nrl T repletion) | 4..5-100 wk | II. No azo LMSC~35 | |
| Behre (1992) | Buserelin | 8 | I. Placebo | 19-NT Load:400 Maint:200 q 3 wk | 24 wk | I. Azo 4/8 6 wk to azo | Agonist blunts T suppression of sperm (time to & % of azo), in dose-department fashion. |
| | | 8 | II. 3.3 mf sc depot implant | | | II. Azo 2/8 15 wk to azo | |
| | | 8 | III. 6.6 mg sc depot implant | | | III. Azo 2/8 21 wk to azo | |

AZO, azoospermia; b/i, bioactive:immunoreactive ratio; gtn, gonadotropin; inj, injection; LMSC, lowest mean sperm count; oligo, oligospermia; sc, subcutaneous; SX, symptoms; T, testosterone; w/, with; change.
Table adapted from Cummings and Bremner (1994): "Prospects for new hormonal male contraceptives." Endocrinology and Metabolism Clinics of North America 23:4; 893-922, 94. (Permission granted by W.B. Saunders Co.)

effect and many studies showed antagonistic or interfering effects of testosterone on GnRH analogue suppression of FSH. Studies in monkeys treated with Buserelin (Akhtar et al., 1983) produced azoospermia in 4 of 4 animals; azoospermia was not seen when testosterone was added to the Buserelin regimen in other animals (Akhtar et al., 1983). Men treated with Buserelin alone had a greater degree of sperm suppression than men treated with a higher dose of the agonist combined with an androgen, fluoxymesterone (Frick and Aulitzky, 1986). Bouchard and Garcia produced azoospermia in four of five men treated with D-trp[6] GnRH (100 mg/d by microspheres) and TE 125 mg given intramuscularly once a month (Bouchard and Garcia, 1987). In one azoospermic subject, when the dose of testosterone was increased, sperm reappeared in the semen; decreasing the testosterone levels reproduced azoospermia. When the same investigators, using the same dose of D-trp[6] GnRH formulation, added what is presumed to be higher doses of testosterone (testosterone undecenoate 120 mg/d orally), they failed to induce azoospermia in any subject. FSH escape may be the mechanism for this secondary failure to maintain azoospermia in subjects when testosterone and GnRH agonist are combined. Support for this concept comes from several laboratories (Behre et al., 1992; Bhasin et al., 1994); Using Lupron and testosterone microspheres in normal men, LH and FSH were initially suppressed, but FSH escaped with continued treatment. It is unclear if this effect could be overcome with much higher doses of GnRH agonist. Studies are underway to test this hypothesis.

## GnRH ANTAGONISTS

This second class of GnRH analogues (antagonists) has been shown to be more effective in suppressing sperm counts to azoospermia levels. Antagonists predictably suppress LH and FSH by competitive binding and slow disassociation from the GnRH receptor. Problems with this class include: the relatively low potency of the agents (much larger doses than that for agonists were required for effect); expense due to the incorporation of costly unnatural amino acids at several positions in the back bone of the molecule, and the tendency to stimulate histamine released from mast cells.

Despite these problems, antagonists were pursued as male contraceptives since they were highly effective in rapidly lowering LH, FSH, testosterone and sperm counts, without an initial stimulatory phase.

Five clinical studies have assessed antagonist plus testosterone combinations on spermatogenesis. Overall, 88% became azoospermic. In the first two trials (Pavlou et al., 1991; Tom et al., 1992), 14 of 16 men became azoospermia after treatment with Nal Glu-GnRH plus delayed addition of testosterone; the remaining two men became severely oligospermic. In the third study, a higher dose of testosterone was given coincident with GnRH antagonist; the results were poorer with only 70% of the men becoming azoospermic (Bagatell et al., 1993). In two later studies (Pavlou et al., 1994; Behre et al., 1995b), azoospermia was produced in all subjects (14/14). Testosterone administration was delayed in one study and given simultaneously with analogue in the last one.

In all human studies, recovery was complete with normal sperm densities seen within 10 to 14 weeks. We believe that recovery can be predictably anticipated because GnRH analogue suppression of gonadotropin secretion accelerates normal cell death (apoptosis) of germ cells, rather than producing abnormal degenerative effects on spermatogenic cells (Sinha-Hikim et al., 1995). Apoptosis is a reversible event.

It is unclear whether the function of residual sperm in subjects where spermatogenesis is partially suppressed, is abnormal. Studies in non-human primates (Weinbauer et al., 1988; Weinbauer et al., 1989) and men (Pavlou et al., 1991) have found impaired morphology and/or motility; hamster oocyte penetration testing suggests impaired function in oligospermic monkeys (Mann et al., 1987), but normal function was observed in a relatively small number of oligospermic GnRH antagonist treated human subjects (Tom et al., 1992). Since azoospermia was not predictably produced in all GnRH antagonist plus testosterone treated men, the possibility of impaired sperm function in the oligospermic subjects is of great interest. Unfortunately, it is difficult to answer the question definitively due to the small numbers of tested subjects, the rapid fall to azoospermia, and the limited number of subjects that continue to have chronically low (not absent) sperm counts.

The issue of androgen attenuation of antagonist antifertility effects has been raised. Data from studies on rats consistently showed testosterone blunting of antagonist suppression of FSH (Bhasin et al 1987, 1988; Rhea and Marshall et al., 1986; Rhea and Weinbauer et al., 1986; Rivier et al., 1981). In studies by Bhasin et al. (1987, 1988) and Rivier et al (1981), high doses of testosterone added to GnRH antagonists resulted in rising FSH levels, while lower doses of testosterone maintained mating behavior without increasing serum FSH levels or reversing the antifertility effects (Bhasin et al., 1988; Bhasin et al., 1987; Rivier et al., 1981). Data in non-human primates have given inconsistent results. Bremner and colleagues produced azoospermia in 9 of 10 monkeys treated with Detirelix (antagonist) plus replacement doses of testosterone (Bremner et al., 1991). Weinbauer et al. (1987) found that concurrent testosterone replacement produced less sperm suppression in 4 monkeys than anticipated, compared to earlier studies in which GnRH antagonist was given alone. In additional monkey studies, the same investigators showed that delay in adding testosterone for as little as 2 weeks after beginning GnRH antagonist, gave a much higher degree of azoospermia than concomitant treatment. In a subsequent study, testosterone was shown to produce a dose related blunting of GnRH antagonist suppression of sperm levels. Because of the necessity of maintaining normal sexual function, direct trials of GnRH antagonist alone, compared to combined GnRH antagonist and testosterone have not been performed in humans. Despite the lack of conclusive data, it now appears that GnRH antagonists produce a high degree of azoospermia, independent of whether androgens are delayed or given concomitantly with the analogue.

Even with the above issues incompletely resolved, GnRH antagonists are the gold standard of success in inducing azoospermia in most Caucasian men and producing the most rapid onset of action. The problems with GnRH antagonists are: (1) their high cost; (2) difficulty in loading sufficient amounts of antagonist in a depot form to assure long term suppression of spermatogenesis; and (3) local irritation at the site of injection due to histamine release. Inroads have been made with longer acting depot preparations and the newest generation of antagonists are less irritating to the user. It is hoped that less histaminergic and more potent antagonists will be developed or that non peptide analogues will replace the more expensive and difficult to produce peptide analogues. Recently reported and ongoing studies in several laboratories (Behre, Swerdloff, and Bremner) are testing the possibility that azoospermia induced by GnRH antagonists plus testosterone will be maintained with testosterone alone.

# REFERENCES

Akhtar FB, Marshall GR, Nieschlag E (1983): Testosterone supplementation attenuates the antifertility effects of an LHRH agonist in male rhesus monkeys. Int J Androl 6:461.

Akhtar FB, Marshall GR, Wickings EJ, Nieschlag E. (1983): Reversible induction of azoospermia in rhesus monkeys by constant infusion of a gonadotropin-releasing hormone agonist using osmotic minipumps. J Clin Endocrinol Metab 56:534.

Bagatell CJ, Matsumoto AM, Christensen RB, Rivier JE, Bremner WJ (1993): Comparison of a gonadotropin releasing hormone antagonist plus testosterone (T) versus T alone as potential male contraceptive regimens. J Clin Endocrinol Metab 77:427-432.

Behre HM, Nashan D, Hubert W, Nieschlag E (1992): Depot gonadotropin-releasing hormone agonist blunts the androgen-induced suppression of spermatogenesis in a clinical trial of male contraception. J Clin Endocrinol Metab 74:84.

Behre HM, Sandow J, Nieschlag E (1992): Pharmacokinetics of the gonadotropin-releasing hormone agonist Buserelin after injection of a slow-release preparation in normal men. Arzneim-Forsch 42:80.

Behre HM, Kliesch S, Lemeke B, Nieschlag E (1995): Suppression of spermato-genesis to azoospermia by combined administration of GnRH antagonist and 19-nortestosterone cannot be maintained by 19-nortestosterone alone in normal men. (submitted).

Berquist C, Nillius SJ, Bergh R (1979): Inhibitory effects on gonadotropin secretion and gonadal function in men during chronic treatment with a potent stimulatory luteinizing hormone-releasing hormone analogue. Acta Endocrinol 91:601.

Bhasin S, Steiner B, Swerdloff R (1985): Does constant infusion of gonadotropin-releasing hormone agonist lead to greater suppression of gonadal function in man than its intermittent administration? Fertil Steril 44:96.

Bhasin S, Fielder TJ, Swerdloff RS (1987): Testosterone selectivity increases serum follicle-stimulating hormone (FSH) but not luteinizing hormone (LH) in gonadotropin-releasing hormone antagonist-treated male rats: Evidence for differential regulation of LH and FSH secretion. Biol Reprod 37:55.

Bhasin S, Yuan QX, Steiner BS, Swerdloff RS (1987): Hormonal effects of gonado-tropin-releasing hormone (GnRH) agonist in men. Effects of long term treatment with GnRH agonist infusion and androgens. J Clin Endocrinol Metab 65:568-574.

Bhasin S, Fielder T, Peacock N, Sod-Moriah UA, Swerdloff RS (1988): Dissociating antifertility effects of GnRH-antagonist from its adverse effects on mating behavior in male rats. Am J Physiol 17:E84.

Bhasin S, Berman N, Swerdloff, RS (1994): Follicle-stimulating hormone (FSH) escape during chronic gonadotropin-releasing hormone (GnRH) agonist and testosterone treatment. J Androl, 15: 386.

Bhasin S, Swerdloff RS (1995): Follicle stimulating hormone and luteinizing hormone. In "The Pituitary " Melmeds, (ed), Blackwell Scientific Co., Cambridge, MA.

Bhasin S, Heber D, Steiner BS, Handelsman DJ, Swerdloff RS (1985): Hormonal effects of gonadotropin-releasing hormone (GnRH) agonist in the human male: III. Effects of long term combined treatment with GnRH agonist and androgen. J Clin Endocrinol Metab 60:998.

Bouchard P, Garcia E (1987): Influence of testosterone substitution on sperm suppression by LHRH agonists. Horm Res 28:175.

Bremner WJ, Bagatell CJ, Steiner RA (1991): Gonadotropin-releasing hormone antagonist plus testosterone: A potential male contraceptive. J Clin Endocrinol Metab 73:465-469.

Cunningham GR, Silverman VE, Kohler PO (1986): Clinical evaluation of testosterone enanthate for induction and maintenance of reversible azoospermia in man. In Patanelli DJ (ed): Hormonal Control of Male Fertility. Washington, DC, US Department of Health, Education, and Welfare, p 71.

Frick J Aulitzky W (1986): Effects of a potent LHRH-agonist on the pituitary gonadal axis with and without testosterone substitution. Urol Res 14:261.

Handelsman DJ, Swerdloff RS (1985): Male gonadal dysfunction. Clinics in Endo and Metab. 14: 89-124.

Heber D, Swerdloff RS (1981): Gonadotropin-releasing hormone analog and testosterone synergistically inhibit spermatogenesis. Endocrinology 108:2019.

Heber D, Dodson R, Stoskopf C, Peterson M, Swerdloff RS (1982): Pituitary desensitization and the regulation of pituitary gonadotropin-releasing hormone (GnRH) receptors following chronic administration of a superactive GnRH analog and testosterone. Life Sci 30:2301.

Heber D, Swerdloff RS (1908): Male contraception: Synergism of gonadotropin-releasing hormone analog and testosterone in suppressing gonadotropin. Science 209:936.

Hikim AP, Wang C, Leung A, Swerdloff RS (1995): Involvement of apoptosis in the induction of germ cell degeneration in adult rats after gonadotropin-releasing hormone antagonist treatment. Endocrinology, in press.

Hikim, A, Swerdloff RS (1993): Temporal and stage-specific changes in spermatogenesis of rat following gonadotropin deprivation by a potent gonadotropin-releasing hormone (GnRH) antagonist treatment. Endocrinology 133:2161-2170.

Huhtaniemi I, Nikula H, Rannikko S (1985): Treatment of prostate cancer with a gonadotropin-releasing hormone agonist analog: Acute and long term effects on endocrine functions of testis tissue. J Clin Endocrinol Metab 61:698.

Linde R, Doelle GC, Alexander N, Kirchner F, Vale W, Rivier J, Rabin D (1981): Reversible inhibition of testicular steroido-genesis and spermatogenesis by a potent gonadotropin-releasing hormone agonist in normal men. N Engl J Med 305:663.

Mann DR, Collins DC, Smith MM, Gould KG (1987): Effect of continuous infusion of a low dose of GnRH antagonist on serum LH and testosterone concentrations, spermatogenesis and semen quality in the rhesus monkey (Macaca mulatta). J Reprod Fertil 81:485.

Mann DR, Gould KG, Collins DC (1987): Influence of simultaneous gonadotropin-releasing hormone agonist and testosterone treatment on spermatogenesis and potential fertilizing capacity in male monkeys. J Clin Endocrinol Metab 65:1215.

Michel E, Bents H, Akhtar FB, Hönigl W, Knuth UA, Sandow J, Nieschlag E (1985): Failure of high-dose sustained-release luteinizing hormone agonist (Buserelin) plus oral testosterone to suppress male fertility. Clin Endocrinol 23:663-675.

Paulsen CA, Bremner WJ, Leonard JM (1982): Male contraception: Clinical trials. In Mishell DR (ed): Advances in Fertility Research. New York, Raven Press, p 157.

Pavlou SN, Debold CR, Iland DP, Wakefield G, Rivier J, Vale W, Rabin D (1986): Single subcutaneous doses of a luteinizing hormone-releasing hormone antagonist suppress serum gonadotropin and testosterone levels in normal men. J Clin Endocrinol Metab 63:303-308.

Pavlou SN, Brewer K, Farley MG, Lindner J, Bastias M, Rogers BJ, Swift LL, Rivier JE, Vale WW, Conn PM, Herbert CM (1991): Combined administration of a gonadotropin-releasing hormone antagonist and testosterone in men induces reversible azoospermia without loss of libido. J Clin Endocrinol Metab 73:1360-1369.

Pavlou SN, Interlandi JW, Wakefield G, Rivier J, Vale W, Rabin D (1986): Heterogeneity of sperm density profiles following 16-week therapy with continuous infusion of high-dose LHRH analog plus testosterone. J Androl 7:228.

Rabin D, Evans RM, Alexander AN, (1984): Heterogeneity of sperm density profiles following 20-week therapy with high-dose LHRH analog plus testosterone J Androl 5:176.

Rajfer J, Handelsman D, Hurwitz R, Kaplan H, Vandergast T, Swerdloff RS, Erlich, RM (1986): Hormonal therapy of cryptorchidism: Randomized double blind study comparing hCG and GnRH. N. Engl. Med 314:466-470.

Resko JA, Belanger A, Labrie F (1982): Effects of chronic treatment with a potent luteinizing hormone releasing hormone agonist on serum luteinizing hormone and steroid levels in the male rhesus monkey. Biol Reprod 26:378.

Rivier C, Rivier J, Vale W (1981): Effect of a potent antagonist and testosterone propionate on mating behavior and fertility in the male rat. Endocrinology 108:1998.

Rowley MJ, Heller CG (1977): Summary of studies utilizing androgens in the normal human male. In Patanelli DJ (eds): Hormonal Control of Male Fertility. Washington, DC, US Department of Health, Education, and Welfare, p 145.

Santen RJ, Demers LM, Max DT, (1984): Long term effects of administration of a gonadotropin-releasing hormone superagonist analog in men with prostatic carcinoma. J Clin Endocrinol Metab 58:397.

Schürmeyer T, Knuth UA, Freischem CW, Sandow J, Akhtar FB, Nieschlag E (1984b): Suppression of pituitary and testicular function in normal men by constant gonadotropin-releasing hormone agonist infusion. J Clin Endocrinol Metab 59:19.

Schürmeyer Th, Knuth UA, Freischem CW, Sandow J, Akhtar FB, Nieschlag E (1984): Suppression of pituitary and testicular function in normal men by constant gonadotropin-releasing hormone agonist infusion. J Clin Endocrinol Metab 59:1-6.

Steinberger E, Smith KD (1977): Effect of chronic administration of testosterone enanthate on sperm production and plasma testosterone, FSH, and LH levels: A preliminary evaluation of a possible male contraceptive. Fertil Steril 28:1320.

Swerdloff RS, Campfield LA, Palacios A, McClure RD (1979): Suppression of human spermatogenesis by depot androgen: Potential for male contraception. J Steroid Biochem 11:663.

Tom L, Bhasin S, Salameh W, Steiner B, Pederson M, Sokol R, Bermon N, Rivier J, Vale W, Swerdloff RS (1992): Induction of azoospermia in normal men with combined Nal-Glu gonadotropin-releasing hormone antagonist and testosterone enanthate. J Clin Endocrinol Metab 75:476.

Weinbauer GF, Surmann FJ, Nieschlag E (1987): suppression of spermatogenesis in a non- human primate (Macaca fascicularis) by concomitant gonadotropin-releasing hormone antagonist and testosterone treatment. Acta Endocrinol 114:138.

Weinbauer GF, Gockeler E, Nieschlag E (1988): Testosterone prevents complete suppression of spermatogenesis in the gonadotropin-releasing hormone antagonist-treated non-human primate (Macaca fascicularis). J Clin Endocrinol Metab 67:284.

Weinbauer GF, Khurshid S, Fingscheidt U, Nieschlag E (1989): Sustained inhibition of sperm production and inhibin secretion induced by a gonadotropin releasing hormone antagonist and delayed testosterone substitution in non-human primates (Macaca fasicularis). J Endocrinol 123:303.

# 35

# HORMONAL MALE CONTRACEPTIVE DEVELOPMENT: COMBINED ADMINISTRATION OF ANDROGENS AND PROGESTOGENS

Alvin M. Matsumoto

University of Washington, School of Medicine
Department of Veterans Affairs Medical Center
Seattle, Washington 98108

## INTRODUCTION

The maintenance of quantitatively normal spermatogenesis in man requires the stimulatory action of both pituitary gonadotropins, luteinizing hormone (LH), and follicle-stimulating hormone (FSH) (Matsumoto, 1987). Hormonal approaches to achieve contraception in men have attempted to reversibly suppress sperm production by inhibiting endogenous LH and FSH secretion. Among methods studied so far, the most promising approaches have been androgen (mostly testosterone) administration alone, or in combination with progestogens, or gonadotropin-releasing hormone (GnRH) analogs (Cummings and Bremner, 1994).

## HIGH-DOSE TESTOSTERONE ALONE  REGIMENS

Administration of testosterone alone in high doses has been the major approach used in hormonal male contraceptive development trials. Testosterone inhibits gonadotropin secretion via hypothalamic-pituitary negative feedback mechanisms, resulting in  suppression of spermatogenesis to very low levels. The most extensively tested and effective regimen in suppressing sperm production utilizing testosterone alone has been administration of the parenteral testosterone ester,  testosterone enanthate, at a dose of 200 mg weekly (Cummings and Bremner, 1994 ).

Several studies, including those recently performed by the World Health Organization (WHO, 1990), have demonstrated that azoospermia (zero sperm count) occurs in 50-70% of Caucasian, and greater than 95% of Asian men, and severe oligospermia (sperm count less than 3 million/ml) is achieved in over 90% of all

*Pharmacology, Biology, and Clinical Applications of Androgens*, edited by Shalender Bhasin et al.
ISBN 0-471-13320-5 © 1996 Wiley-Liss, Inc.

men receiving 200 mg of testosterone enanthate weekly. From these studies, it is also clear that testosterone enanthate must be administered at least weekly to be maximally effective in suppressing sperm production; probably because declining serum testosterone levels near the end of longer dosing intervals fail to maintain maximal gonadotropin suppression. High-dose induction regimens (Bajaj and Madan, 1984) and longer term administration of higher doses of testosterone enanthate (up to 300 mg weekly) (Matsumoto, 1990) have not resulted in greater suppression of spermatogenesis.

The WHO studies demonstrated contraceptive efficacy that is comparable to that of female oral contraceptives and greater than that of the condom in men, with azoospermia (WHO, 1990) or sperm counts less than 3 million/ml induced by testosterone enanthate, administered at a dose of 200 mg weekly. This high-dose testosterone enanthate regimen has been tolerated well by normal men; only mild acne and weight gain in some subjects and no significant behavioral effects or other toxicity have occurred. Furthermore, the suppression of sperm production has been completely reversible. Despite this evidence for the relatively good effectiveness, lack of significant adverse effects, and complete reversibility of testosterone administration alone as a male contraceptive agent, concerns have been raised over the use of high doses of testosterone for prolonged periods of time.

Plasma high-density lipoprotein (HDL) cholesterol levels decrease in normal men treated with testosterone enanthate at a dosage of 200 mg weekly, or above (Bagatell et al., 1994). Although the clinical significance of testosterone-induced HDL cholesterol reduction is unclear, epidemiological studies have suggested that lower HDL cholesterol levels are associated with an increased risk of atherosclerotic coronary artery disease. As a result, there has been some concern raised regarding the potential long-term risk of cardiovascular disease in normal men receiving high-dose testosterone enanthate for contraception (Cummings and Bremner, 1994). Another concern with the use of high-dose testosterone is the unknown long-term effect of supraphysiologic testosterone administration on the prostate gland and on development of benign prostatic hyperplasia (Cummings and Bremner, 1994).

Issues of cardiovascular risk, if any, of pharmacologically reducing HDL cholesterol by testosterone administration and the effects of testosterone on the prostate, can only be resolved with long-term observations. However, despite the lack of information on the chronic effects of supraphysiologic testosterone administration in normal men, these issues have raised enough concern that strategies are being tested to reduce the dosage of testosterone in contraceptive regimens to more nearly physiologic levels. In this regard, a major approach has been to combine testosterone with another agent that is known to suppress endogenous gonadotropin secretion, e.g., combined administration of a lower dosage of testosterone enanthate with GnRH analogs or progestogens (Cummings and Bremner, 1994).

# TESTOSTERONE-PROGESTOGEN COMBINATION REGIMENS

## Mechanism of Suppression of Spermatogenesis

Administration of progestogens alone suppresses endogenous LH and FSH secretion in normal men (Meyer et al., 1985) by hypothalamic-pituitary feedback mechanisms that are different from those responsible for gonadotropin inhibition induced by testosterone, acting in large part through progesterone receptors. Thus, combined administration of testosterone and progestogens would be expected to have additive or synergistic effects on the suppression of gonadotropin production. Although this has not been carefully assessed in men, the demonstrated enhanced ovulation suppression achieved by adding a progestogen to estrogen in female oral contraceptives provides a precedent for potential synergistic actions of combining sex steroid hormones on gonadotropin and spermatogenic suppression.

Progestogens may also inhibit spermatogenesis directly (Goldzieher and Castracane, 1984). Since relatively high intratesticular androgen levels are thought to be important for maintenance of quantitatively normal sperm production, progestogens may interfere with sperm production locally by acting as an antiandrogen and competing with testosterone for binding to testicular androgen receptors (Buzek and Sanborn, 1990), and by inhibiting $5\alpha$-reductase activity (Southern et al., 1977) and reducing the conversion of testosterone to the more potent androgen, dihydrotestosterone, within the testis. Thus, the independent mechanisms of gonadotropin inhibition and possible dual sites of action of testosterone-progestogen combinations, at both the hypothalamic-pituitary and testicular levels, could enhance the efficacy of these combined regimens in suppressing sperm production and permit use of more physiologic testosterone dosages.

## Rationale

Combined administration of testosterone and a progestogen has been administered to normal men in previous contraceptive development trials. Some testosterone-progestogen combinations appeared to suppress sperm production to azoospermia and severe oligospermia at least as effectively as testosterone alone regimens. However, in most of these studies, testosterone was given at intervals (usually monthly) that were too infrequent to result in effective suppression of spermatogenesis if administered alone; and no direct comparisons of testosterone-progestogen combinations with the same dose of testosterone alone were performed.

Although a number of androgen-progestogen combinations were studied in the past, the majority of previous studies utilized various combinations of testosterone enanthate and depomedroxyprogesterone acetate (DMPA), both given by intramuscular injections. In combining the results of those studies that administered DMPA at a dosage of 150 to 300 mg monthly (with or without an initial induction dose of 1000 mg), plus testosterone enanthate 250 to 500 mg monthly, completely reversible azoospermia occurred in approximately 70% and severe oligospermia (sperm counts less than 3 million/ml) was induced in approximately 95% of Caucasian men (Alvarez-Sanchez et al., 1979; Faundes et al., 1981; Frick et al., 1977, 1982; Paulsen et al., 1982; Wu and Aitken, 1989). Similar to results with high-dose testosterone, combined administration of testosterone enanthate (100 to 200 mg monthly) and DMPA (100 to 200 mg monthly) in Asian (Indonesian) men uniformly resulted in azoospermia (Pangkahila, 1991).

Thus, the degree of suppression of spermatogenesis achieved with these testosterone-progestogen combinations that utilized lower doses of testosterone was comparable to that achieved by high-dose testosterone administration alone. These results suggest that the addition of a progestogen to a relatively ineffective testosterone dose (e.g. testosterone enanthate 200 mg monthly) greatly increases suppression of sperm production and that combining a progestogen with a more maximally effective testosterone dose might further suppress spermatogenesis.

No significant adverse effects occurred during combined administration of testosterone enanthate and DMPA in normal men. However, as in high-dose testosterone alone regimens, combined administration of testosterone enanthate and DMPA, reduced HDL cholesterol levels (Hedman et al., 1988; Wallace and Wu, 1990). Furthermore, because of the very long half-life of DMPA, although the recovery of sperm counts after discontinuation of this progestogen and testosterone was complete, it was much more prolonged than after high-dose testosterone alone (Cummings and Bremner, 1994).

Compared to GnRH analogs, sex steroid hormones, such as testosterone and progestogens, are relatively inexpensive to synthesize. There is also considerable long-term experience with use of testosterone in men and progestogens in women. Finally, development of long-acting testosterone and progestogen delivery methods are well underway and currently being tested. Thus, if a safe testosterone-progestogen combination is found that effectively and reversibly suppressed sperm production in normal men, the prospects for a relatively inexpensive and practical male contraceptive method would be greatly enhanced.

For these reasons, and based on the encouraging results of earlier trials using testosterone enanthate-DMPA combinations, we embarked on studies to further develop a male contraceptive strategy using a combination of relatively low-dose testosterone and a progestogen that would be more effective in reversibly suppressing sperm production in normal men, than high-dose testosterone alone regimens, without causing significant adverse effects or suppression of HDL cholesterol levels.

## TESTOSTERONE ENANTHATE-LEVONORGESTREL COMBINATIONS

### Rationale

We initially chose to investigate the combination of testosterone enanthate and levonorgestrel. A testosterone enanthate dosage of 100 mg given intramuscularly weekly, was chosen for these studies. This dose is half that used in the majority of male contraceptive development trials.    At steady-state, serum testosterone levels increase to slightly above the normal range, one to two days, following an injection of this dose and are maintained consistently within the normal range thereafter; mean serum testosterone concentrations between weekly injections are in the upper normal range (unpublished observations).  This dosage of testosterone enanthate was chosen because, in contrast to higher doses (e.g. 200 mg weekly), when administered alone to normal men, it does not suppress HDL cholesterol levels (Bagatell et al., 1992).  Furthermore, previous studies suggested that weekly administration of testosterone enanthate at a dosage of 100 mg weekly was very effective in suppressing sperm production (Matsumoto, 1990).

The progestogen chosen for initial studies was levonorgestrel (generously provided by Wyeth-Ayerst Research) because of its potency, ready availability, and ability to achieve steady-state levels rapidly after oral administration.    Levonorgestrel is one of the most potent progestogens in suppressing gonadotropins *in vivo* (Brotherton J, 1976).    There is also extensive clinical experience with this progestogen as a safe contraceptive agent in women, both as an oral and implanted (Norplant®) contraceptive.  Levonorgestrel is well absorbed orally with little first pass metabolism in the liver.  Therefore, oral doses provide serum levels similar to parenteral and implanted preparations releasing the same amount of steroid daily (Orme et al., 1983).    This bioavailability feature and measurements of serum levonorgestrel levels will permit estimation of the release rates required to achieve the same effect by long-acting parenteral or implantable formulations.

## COMPARISON OF TESTOSTERONE ENANTHATE AND LEVONORGESTREL COMBINATION WITH TESTOSTERONE ENANTHATE ALONE

In our initial study, we tested the hypothesis that combined administration of testosterone enanthate and levonorgestrel will suppress gonadotropin secretion and sperm production in normal men more effectively than the same dose of testosterone enanthate alone (Bebb et al., Submitted, 1995).    This study was sponsored by the Contraceptive Research and Development (CONRAD) Program of the United States Agency for International Development.

After a 3 month-control period during which no hormones were administered, 36 normal young men, age 19 to 45 years, were randomly assigned, in a balanced-design, single-blind fashion, to receive either combined administration of testosterone enanthate 100 mg intramuscularly weekly and levonorgestrel 500 μg orally daily for 6 months (18 subjects), or testosterone enanthate 100 mg intramuscular weekly and a placebo capsule orally daily for 6 months (18 subjects). Following the treatment period, all hormones were discontinued and the subjects entered a recovery period, until three successive sperm counts were within their control range. Twice monthly sperm counts, monthly serum LH and FSH levels and clinical evaluations, and serum lipid levels at the end of each study period were performed throughout the study.

Preliminary analysis of the results of this study revealed that compared with testosterone enanthate alone, sperm counts were suppressed more rapidly and effectively by combined administration of testosterone enanthate and levonorgestrel.

The testosterone-levonorgestrel combination resulted in azoospermia in approximately 70% of subjects in 10 weeks and severe oligospermia (sperm counts less than 3 million/ml) in 95% of men in 9 weeks, compared with testosterone alone, which resulted in azoospermia in approximately 30% of subjects in 15 weeks and severe oligospermia in 70% of men in 14 weeks. Both serum LH and FSH levels were also suppressed more rapidly and effectively by combined administration of testosterone enanthate and levonorgestrel.

Both regimens were tolerated well with mild acne and weight gain occurring in both groups. However, total and HDL cholesterol levels were reduced by approximately 6% and 24%, respectively, while low density lipoprotein (LDL) cholesterol and triglyceride levels were unchanged in men who received the combination of testosterone and levonorgestrel; whereas those who received testosterone alone demonstrated no significant changes in blood lipids.

In summary, the combination of testosterone enanthate and levonorgestrel resulted in a greater and more rapid suppression of gonadotropin and sperm production than the testosterone enanthate administration at the same dose alone; however, HDL cholesterol levels were significantly reduced with the combination regimen. These results suggest that combined administration of testosterone and a progestogen is a very promising approach to the development of effective male contraceptives.

Future studies should determine whether reducing the dose of either levonorgestrel or testosterone enanthate will suppress spermatogenesis to the same degree without reducing HDL cholesterol, and whether testosterone combined with newer, less androgenic progestogens, such as desogestrel, norgestimate or gestodene, results in greater suppression sperm production without affecting blood lipids.

## REFERENCES

Alvarez-Sanchez F, Brache V, Leon P, Faundes A (1979): Inhibition of spermatogenesis with monthly injections of medroxyprogesterone acetate and low dose testosterone enanthate. Int J Androl 2:136-149.

Bagatell CJ, Knopp RH, Vale WW, Rivier JE, Bremner WJ (1992): Physiologic testosterone levels in normal men suppress high-density lipoprotein cholesterol levels. Ann Intern Med 116:967-973.

Bagatell CJ, Heiman JR, Matsumoto AM, Rivier JE, Bremner WJ (1994): Metabolic and behavioral effects of high-dose exogenous testosterone in healthy men. J Clin Endocrinol Metab 79:561-567.

Bajaj JS, Madan R (1984): New approaches to male fertility regulation: LHRH analogs, steroidal contraception and inhibin. In Benagiano G, Diczfalusy E (eds): "Endocrine mechanisms in fertility regulation." New York: Raven Press, pp 203-232.

Bebb RA, Anawalt BD, Christensen RB, Paulsen CA, Bremner WJ, Matsumoto AM (1995): Combined administration of levonorgestrel and testosterone induces more rapid and effective suppression of spermatogenesis than testosterone alone: a promising male contraceptive approach. Submitted.

Brotherton J (1976): Animal biological assessment. In Brotherton J (ed): "Sex Hormone Pharmacology." London: Academic Press, pp 43-75.

Buzek SW, Sanborn BM (1990): Nuclear androgen receptor dynamics in testicular peritubular and Sertoli cells. J Androl 11:514-520.

Cummings DE, Bremner WJ (1994): Prospects for new hormonal male contraceptives. Endocrinol Metab Clin North Am 23:893-922.

Faundes A, Brache V, Leon P, Schmidt F, Alvarez-Sanchez F (1981): Sperm suppression with monthly injections of medroxyprogesterone acetate combined with testosterone enanthate at a high dose (500 mg). Int J Androl 4:235-245.

Frick J, Bartsch G, Weiske WH (1977): The effect of monthly depot medroxyprogesterone acetate and testosterone on human spermatogenesis. II. High initial dose. Contraception 15:669-677.

Frick J, Danner C, Kunit G, Joos H, Kohle R (1982): Spermatogenesis in men treated with injections of medroxyprogesterone acetate combined with testosterone enanthate. Int J Androl 5:246-252.

Goldzieher JW, Castracane VD (1984): Antifertility effects of progestational steroids. In Benagiano G, Diczfalusy E (eds): "Endocrine mechanisms in fertility regulation." New York: Raven Press, pp 49-69.

Hedman M Gottlieb C, Svanborg K, Bygdeman M, de la Torre B (1988): Endocrine, seminal and peripheral effects of depot medroxyprogesterone acetate and testosterone enanthate in men. Int J Androl 11:265-276.

Matsumoto AM (1987): Hormonal control of human spermatogenesis. In Burger H, de Kretser D (eds.): "The Testis, Second Edition." New York: Raven Press, pp 181-196.

Matsumoto AM (1990): Effects of chronic testosterone administration in normal men: safety and efficacy of high-dosage testosterone enanthate and parallel dose-dependent suppression of luteinizing hormone, follicle-stimulating hormone and sperm production. J Clin Endocrinol Metab 70:282-287.

Meyer WJ, Walker PA, Emory LA, Smith ER (1985): Physical, metabolic, and hormonal effects on men of long-term therapy with depomedroxyprogesterone acetate. Fertil Steril 43:102-109.

Orme M, Back DJ, Breckenridge AM (1983): Clinical pharmacokinetics of oral contraceptive steroids. Clin Pharmacokinet 8:95-136.

Pangkahila W (1991): Reversible azoospermia induced by an androgen-progestin combination regimen in Indonesian men. Int J Androl 14:248-256.

Paulsen CA, Bremner WJ, Leonard JM (1982): Male contraception: clinical trials. In Mishell D (ed): "Advances in Fertility Research." New York: Raven Press, pp 157-170.

Southern AL, Gordon GG, Vitek J, Altman K (1977): Effect of progesterone on androgen metabolism. In Martini L, Motta M (eds): "Androgens and Antiandrogens." New York: Raven Press, pp 263-279.

Wallace EM, Wu FWC (1990): Effect of depot medroxyprogesterone acetate and testosterone oenanthate on serum lipoproteins in man. Contraception 41:63-71.

World Health Organization Task Force on Methods for the Regulation of Male Fertility (1990): Contraceptive efficacy of testosterone-induced azoospermia in normal men. Lancet 336:955-959.

Wu FWC, Aitken RJ (1989): Suppression of sperm function by depot
    medroxyprogesterone acetate and testosterone enanthate in steroid male
    contraception. Fertil Steril 51:691-698.

# 36

# EFFECT OF TE/DMPA AND 19-NT/DMPA ON SPERMATOGENESIS IN INDONESIAN MEN

**K. M. Arsyad[1], N. Moeloek[2], P. Hadiluwih[3], A. Adimoelja[4], and W. Pangkahila[5]**

[1]Faculties of Medicine, Sriwijaya University
[2]University of Indonesia
[3]Diponegoro University
[4]Airlangga University
[5]Udayana University

## INTRODUCTION

Androgen alone (Patanelli, 1978; Paulsen et al., 1982), or in combination with progestogens (Schearer et al., 1978) have been widely used in the past to suppress spermatogenesis in normal men. Testosterone enanthate (TE), if administered in doses of 50 to 200 mg every 7 - 12 days for 12 weeks, will suppress spermatogenesis to some extent in all men (Paulsen, et al., 1982; Matsumoto, 1988). Another androgen, 19-nortestosterone-hexyloxyphenyl propionate (19-NT), has been used clinically without toxic side effects for many years (Knuth et al., 1986).

Progestogens administered either by implantation or injection also suppress spermatogenesis by inhibition of pituitary gonadotropin secretion (Schearer et al., 1978). Depot-medroxy-progesterone acetate (DMPA) is widely used for female contraception.

The TE and DMPA combination has already been investigated for its effectiveness to suppress spermatogenesis to azoospermia, and between 14% and 70% of men achieved azoospermia (Schearer et al., 1978). Knuth et al. (1978) conducted a study of 19-NT and DMPA combination on 12 German volunteers. Azoospermia was achieved in 6 men; 4 men achieved oligozoospermia with sperm concentration 5 less than $2 \times 10^6$/ml, and the remaining 2 men produced only a single sperm per ejaculate. In contrast, a previous study conducted by Pangkahila (1991) in Indonesia, using TE and DMPA combination, demonstrated higher rates of azoospermia (20/20) than those found in men of European background.

*Pharmacology, Biology, and Clinical Applications of Androgens*, edited by Shalender Bhasin et al.
ISBN 0-471-13320-5 © 1996 Wiley-Liss, Inc.

The aim of this study, adopted from the design of Knuth et al. (1986), was to compare the effect of TE/DMPA with that of 19-NT/DMPA in suppression of spermatogenesis in healthy Indonesian men.

## MATERIALS AND METHODS

The study consisted of pre-treatment, treatment, and recovery phases. Up to 20 healthy male volunteers from each of five Indonesian centers (Palem-bang, Jakarta, Semarang, Surabaya and Denpasar) were randomized, using sealed envelopes, to one of two treatment groups: TE plus DMPA or 19-NT plus DMPA. Seven weekly injections of TE or 19-NT, 200 mg IM followed by injections every 4 weeks to week 24. In both groups 250 DMPA was injected IM at 0, 6, 12 and 18 weeks. Sperm suppression was measured by semen analysis at 3-week intervals and clinical chemistry, hematology, and gonadotrophin hormones were monitored at 6-week intervals. Recovery was assessed monthly until return to normal sperm concentration ($\geq 20 \times 10^6$ mL).

## RESULTS

A total of 96 men were recruited to the study. Their baseline physical characteristics are shown in Table 1. The men from Denpasar were taller and had larger body size and testicular volume, than those from the other centers, but the physical characteristics of the men were similar in the two treatment groups.

Table 1.  Baseline Physical characteristics of subjects by center

| Center | Age* | Height | Weight | BMI | Mean Testis volume |
|---|---|---|---|---|---|
|  | g | cm | kg | kg/m$^2$ | ml |
| All Centers (n=96) | 34.7 ± 5.8 | 162.6 ± 5.1 | 57.6 ± 7.6 | 21.8 ± 2.8 | 22.4 ± 5.3 |
| Denpasar (n=20) | 37.8 ± 4.7 | 165.7 ± 4.8 | 62.9 ± 8.2 | 23.0 ± 3.2 | 27.8 ± 4.1 |
| Jakarta (n=20 | 34.9 ± 6.7 | 161.6± 6.7 | 54.4 ± 8.5 | 20.8 ± 3.0 | 23.8 ± 4.8 |
| Palembang (n=20) | 33.8 ± 6.0 | 161.6 ± 5.3 | 55.3 ± 5.4 | 21.2 ± 2.2 | 21.3 ±  3.3 |
| Semarang (n=20) | 34.1 ± 5.3 | 161.5 ± 4.0 | 59.4 ± 6.3 | 22.8 ± 2.0 | 19.8 ± 4.3 |
| Surabaya (n=16) | 32.8 ± 5.6 | 163.1 ± 5.9 | 55.8 ± 6.5 | 21.1 ± 2.6 | 18.6 ± 4.0 |
| 19-NT (n-47) | 34.7 ± 6.0 | 162.5 ± 4.9 | 55.9 ± 6.8 | 21.2 ± 2.6 | 21.1 ± 5.3 |
| TE (n=49) | 34.7 ± 5.7 | 162.8 ± 5.4 | 59.2 ± 8.1 | 22.3 ± 2.9 | 23.5 ± 5.1 |
| P  value+ | 0..91 | 0.83 | 0.029 | 0.043 | 0.020 |

* Value are mean ± SD
+ P value for differences between drug groups adjusted for center (two-way ANOVA)

The baseline semen characteristics (Table 2) varied from center to center. However these factors were balanced across the two treatment groups, with the exception of sperm concentration, which was slightly higher in the TE group (P=0.05, two-way ANOVA adjusting for between center differences). The median sperm concentrations (5th and 95th percentiles) were 46.3 (22.7,123.2) x $10^6$ /mL in all men and 40.7 (21.8,109.4) and 55.7 (23.0,141.5) x $10^6$ /mL in the 19-NT and TE groups respectively. The mean ± SD levels among all men for hemoglobin, white blood cells, and platelet count were 145 ± 12 g/L, 6.4 ± 1.3 x $10^9$/L, and 241 ± 47x $10^9$/L, respectively, and did not differ between the two treatment groups.

A total of 90 of the 96 men completed the treatment phase. Of these, 87 (96.7%; 95% confidence interval, 90.6% to 99.3%) achieved azoospermia (two or more consecutive azoospermic samples). The rates and degree of suppression were similar in the two treatment groups (Table 1) and in the different centers (data not shown). Once azoospermia in two samples was achieved, a subsequent increase in sperm production occurred in only one man during the treatment phase and then only to 0.4 x $10^6$ /mL. The median time to recovery of normal sperm concentration (>/ 20.0 x $10^6$ /mL) after the last injection was 6.5 months in those men who had achieved azoospermia (Table 1.). Two of the three men who failed to achieve consistent azoospermia had the lowest sperm concentration of 0.1 and .08 x $10^6$

Table 2. Baseline Semen Characteristics of Subjects by Center

| Center | Volume * | Concen-tration++ | Viability* | Motility* | Morphology* |
|---|---|---|---|---|---|
| | ml | x $10^6$/ml | % live | % motile | % normal |
| All centers (n=96) | 2.95 ± 0.87 | 49.2 | 78.8 ± 10.6 | 62.9 ± 12.6 | 71.4 ± 10.1 |
| Denpasar (n=20) | 2.83 ± 1.03 | 43.5 | 74.4 ± 7.6 | 70.5 ± 7.2 | 66.4 ± 7.6 |
| Jakarta (n=20) | 2.72 ± 0.73 | 70.2 | 69.1 ± 9.5 | 63.1 ± 7.6 | 84.1 ± 4.2 |
| Palembang (n=20) | 3.09 ± 0.85 | 39.9 | 84.7 ± 3.3 | 53.4 ± 2.6 | 62.3 ± 8.3 |
| Semarang (n=20) | 3.23 ± 0.73 | 46.5 | 89.2 ± 9.4 | 77.5 ± 5.2 | 73.3 ± 8.1 |
| Surabaya (n=16) | 2.87 ± 1.00 | 51.4 | 76.4 ± 6.9 | 47.0 ± 8.2 | 70.6 ± 5.0 |
| 19-NT (n=47) | 2.85 ± 0.87 | 44.2 | 79.3 ± 9.9 | 62.1 ± 12.4 | 71.3 ± 9.9 |
| TE (n=49 | 3.05 ± 0.87 | 54.6 | 78.4 ± 11.3 | 63.7 ± 12.8 | 71.4 ± 10.5 |
| P value+ | 0.78 | 0.051 | 0.30 | 0.23 | 0.29 |

* Value are mean ± SD
+ P value for differences between drug groups adjusted for center (two-way ANOVA)
++ Geometric mean

/mL, respectively, and the third had a single azoospermic sample. They were similar in anthropometric characteristics to the other men. There was a decrease in testicular volume (mean ± SE) during the period of injections of 12.8% ± 2.5% and 9.9% ± 2.6% and an increase in body weight of 9.2% ± 1.4% and 8.8% ± 1.1% in the 19-NT and TE groups, respectively. Both changes were returning to pre-treatment levels by 6 months after the last injection.

Plasma FSH and LH levels were suppressed during the treatment phase (Table 2) and exhibited a rebound elevation 3 and 5 months after cessation of injections.

## DISCUSSION

A hormonal contraceptive method for men must reduce the number of sperm in the ejaculate to a sufficient degree to induce consistent infertility. This study has demonstrated that Indonesian men can be rendered azoospermic, or near azoo-spermic, by 3-weekly injections of TE or 19-NT, plus DMPA at 6-week intervals for > 6 months. Almost 100% azoospermia was achieved by both combinations in all centers, even though there were inter-center differences in baseline semen quality that may suggest lower fertility potential among some volunteers.

These differences probably reflect poor control of subjective measures despite use of standard semen analysis methods in all centers. It is unlikely that such differences would account for the considerably higher rates of azoospermia compared with those attained in similar studies on men of European background. The TE and DMPA combination has been investigated in men where only 14% to 70% of the subjects achieved azoospermia (Schearer et al., 1978, Knuth et al., 1986, Knuth et al., 1989, Brenner et al., 1977). The only investigation of the 19-NT plus DMPA combination was on 12 healthy German volunteers of whom only 6 achieved azoospermia, whereas two more were suppressed to near azoospermia. As in the WHO multicenter trial involving androgen suppression to azoospermia (WHO, 1990), rebound from established azoospermia was rare, occurring in only one sample in 87. The possible explanation for the differences between Indonesian and Caucasian men may be related to genetic or on pharmacologic differences between ethnic groups. There were no significant changes in liver function tests in this or the German study (Knuth et al., 1978); such changes have only previously been noted with 17 alpha alkylated androgens and not with the compounds used in this study. The variations in sperm suppression could be due to differences in nutritional, metabolic, cultural, or genetic factors, both between and within populations. Similar patterns of sperm suppression were also observed in a multicenter study involving Chinese and non-Chinese men using weekly TE injections (WHO, 1990) and would appear not to depend on the nature of the hormonal regimen used to suppress spermatogenesis. Comparative pharmacologic studies are underway to throw light on these important observations.

Androgen and progestogen combination have been in clinical and experimental clinical use for many decades (Schearer et al., 1978). The low rates of discontinuation for side effects in the present study confirm the acceptability of such combination drug regimens in Indonesian men for ≤6 months duration of exposure. A major limitation of this regimen is the frequency of injections. Weekly intra-muscular injections of androgen on seven occasions, and the continuation with injections of androgen at 3-week intervals, was chosen as the simplest prototype regimen because of its safety, reversibility, and effectiveness in inducing azoospermia. The pharmacokinetic properties of androgen preparations seem to be of critical importance in achieving azoospermia in men. The more frequent complaints of loss of libido during treatment with 19-NT, compared with TE, could reflect differences either in the efficacy of 19-NT and TE as androgens, or in dose equivalence of the two regimens used for androgen replacement. Both androgens act upon the same androgen receptor and exhibit similar androgenic and anabolic effects, as demonstrated by the similarity of their effect on androgen-sensitive variables in this study (body weight, testis size, hemoglobin, LH and FSH). Nevertheless, differences in biological action are possible since 19-NT is nonaromatizable, whereas the aromatization of TE to estradiol is involved in some effects of TE on brain function. It remains controversial whether 19-NT is able to support sexual function only partially (Michael et al., 1984) or fully (Weinbauer et al., 1990) in orchiectomized monkeys. Alternatively, the efficacy of the 19-NT regimen for androgen replacement therapy when administered at 3-week intervals (as during maintenance phase in this study) is less well established than that for TE (Snyder and Lawrence, 1980).

Although very high rates of azoospermia were achieved in this study, a small minority of men (3 of 90, 3.3%) failed to reach consistent azoospermic levels. The very low levels of residual sperm output however, suggest that these men may also be rendered sufficiently infertile to equate with reliable contraception. Indeed, the function of residual sperm during steroid-induced suppression appears to be markedly decreased as judged by their impaired ability to fuse with zona-free hamster oocyte (Wu and Aitken, 1989).

Hormonally induced azoospermia can provide effective reversible contraception with minimal side effects (WHO, 1990). These data also confirm the acceptability and efficacy of such combination drug regimens in Indonesian men. A major limitation of this regimen is the frequency of injections. Effectiveness of a simpler regimen using 6-weekly DMPA and a monthly TE in inducing azoospermia should be tested in Indonesia.

## REFERENCES

Brenner PF, Mishell DR, Bernstein GS, Ortiz A (1977): Study of depot medroxyprogesterone acetate and testosterone enanthate as a male contraceptive. Contraception 15:679-91.

Knuth UA, Behre H, Belkein L, Bents H, Nieschlag E (1986): 19-Nortestosterone for male fertility regulation, in: Zatuchni GI, Goldsmith A, Spieler JM, Sciarra JJ, (eds), Male contraception, advances and future prospects. Philadelphia: Harper and Row 320-8.

Knuth UA, Yeung CH, Nieschlag E (1989): Combination of 19-nortestosterone hexyloxyphenylpropionate (Anadur) and depot-medroxyprogesterone acetate (Clinovir) for male contraception. Fertil Steril 51:1011-8.

Matsumoto AM, (1988): Is high dosage testosterone an effective male contraceptive agent? Fertil Steril 50:324-8.

Micallef JV, Ahsan R, Gandy S, Latif A, Shapton R, Edward PR et al. (1992): Standardization of laboratory performance, In: Developments in radioimmunoassay and related procedures, Vienna, Austria: International Atomic Agency 393-402.

Michael RP, Bonsall RW, Zumpe D (1984): The behavioral thresholds of testosterone in castrated male rhesus monkeys (maccaca mulatta). Horm Behav 18:161-76.

Pangkahila W (1991): Reversible azoospermia induced by an androgen-progestin combination regimen in Indonesian men. Int J Androl 14:248-56.

Patanelli DJ, (1978): editor. Hormonal control of male fertility, Washington (DC): U.S. Department of Health, Education and Welfare, Publication no. (NIH) 78-1097.

Paulsen CA, Bremner WJ, Leonard JM, (1982): Male contraception clinical trials, In: Mishell, D.R., Jr., editor, Advances in fertility research. Raven Press, 157-70.

Schearer SB, Alvarez-Sanchez F, Anselmo J, Brenner PF, Coutinho E, Latham-Faundes A et al. (1978): Hormonal contraception for men. Int J Androl suppl. 2:680-712.

Snyder PJ, Lawrence DA (1980): Treatment of male hypogonadism with testosterone enanthate. J Clin Endocrinol Metab, 51:1335-9.

Sufi SB, Donaldson A, Jeffcoate SL, editors (1992): Programme for the provision of matched assay reagents for the radioimmunoassay of hormones in reproductive physiology. Method Manual, 16th ed., Geneva, Switzerland; World Health Organization.

Weinbauer GF, Jaekwert B, Yoon YD, Behre HM, Yeung CH, Nieschlag E, (1990): Pharmacokinetics and pharmacodynamics of testosterone enanthate and dihydrotestosterone enanthate in non-human primates. Acta Endocrinol (Copenhagen) 122:432-42.

World Health Organization Task Force on Methods for the Regulation of Male Fertility (1990): Contraceptive efficacy of testosterone induced azoospermia in normal men. Lancet 336:955-9.

Wu FCW, Aitken RJ (1989): Suppression of sperm function by depot medroxyprogesterone acetate and testosterone enanthate in steroid male contraception. Fertil Steril 51:691-8.

# 37

# COMPARISON BETWEEN TESTOS-TERONE-INDUCED AZOOSPERMIA (RESPONDERS) AND OLIGOZOO-SPERMIA (NON-RESPONDERS) IN A MALE CONTRACEPTIVE STUDY

**F.C.W. Wu**

**Department of Medicine,**
**University of Manchester,**
**Manchester Royal Infirmary**
**Manchester, England**

## INTRODUCTION

The use of exogenous sex steroids to inhibit pituitary gonadotrophin secretion and, secondarily, to deplete intratesticular testosterone, induces a profound suppression of spermatogenesis which can confer effective contraception in men (WHO, 1990). Since endogenous testosterone secretion is abrogated by this treatment, one of the mandatory requirements of these regimes is the maintenance of extratesticular secondary sexual functions by androgen supplementation. In this respect, androgens alone achieve both the suppression and maintenance functions simultaneously and consequently, testosterone enanthate, as a prototype single agent regime, has been most studied in recent trials of male contraception. A consistent finding in all the studies to date is that azoospermia is not uniformly achieved. Typically, 50-70% became azoospermic (so-called responders) while the rest remained oligozoospermic (non-responders) with mean sperm density of around 2 million/mL. The azoospermic responders also had a significantly faster rate of suppression apparent by the end of the first month (Handelsman et al., 1995). Furthermore, there is a significantly greater rebound rise in plasma FSH during recovery (Wallace et al., 1993). These observations suggest that there may be some intrinsic polymorphism in the hormonal regulation of spermatogenesis in men which could differentiate between these two distinct response patterns. The reason(s) for this apparent polymorphism is unknown but a better understanding of this phenomenon is clearly germane to the overall success of this method of contraception.

*Pharmacology, Biology, and Clinical Applications of Androgens*, edited by Shalender Bhasin et al.
ISBN 0-471-13320-5 © 1996 Wiley-Liss, Inc.

The aim of our investigations is to identify possible differences in the acute (week 1) and steady state (week 16) pharmacokinetics and pharmacodynamics of exogenously administered testosterone between the azoospermic and oligozoospermic responders amongst 33 healthy Caucasian men recruited into a male contraceptive efficacy trial using TE 200 mg im weekly.

## PHARMACOKINETICS OF TOTAL AND FREE T

The total and free T concentrations following the first and the 16th injections, increased in both azoospermic and oligozoospermic groups after 16 weeks. Compared to baseline, pre-injection levels of total T increased 2.5-fold, reaching a steady state around 4 weeks of treatment. Peak concentrations of total testosterone increased by 5-fold, but non-SHBG-bound testosterone was increased by 9-fold and free testosterone by 20-fold after 16 weeks. The plasma levels of estradiol showed similar changes to testosterone. However, neither testosterone (bound or free) nor estradiol were significantly different between azoospermic and oligozoospermic responders in the first or the sixteenth week.

## GONADOTROPHIN SUPPRESSION

TE treatment induced a progressive fall in both LH and FSH to undetectable levels (with Delfia assay sensivities of 0.04 U/L for both LH and FSH) between day 56 to 84 with no difference in either the rate or the degree of suppression between the 18 azoospermic and 15 oligozoospermic responders.

## METABOLIC CLEARANCE RATE (MCR) AND
## CONVERSION RATION (CR$^{T\text{-}DHT}$)

Before treatment, there was no difference in the MCR of T between the azoospermic (1120L/24h) and oligozoospermic (1020L/24h) responders. After 16 weeks of treatment, the MCR in both groups increased significantly to 1300 and 1280 L/24th respectively, but again, there was no difference between the groups.

Although there was no difference in the CR of T to DHT at baseline, after 16 weeks of TE treatment, a significant increase (from 3.2 to 4%) was observed in the oligozoospermic but not the azoospermic group (which remained at 3.4 to 3.1%). This suggested that 5α-reductase activity was higher in the oligozoospermic subjects at 16 weeks but not at baseline.

## DHT & ANDROSTANEDIOL GLUCURONIDE (A'DIOLG)

Mean plasma DHT and A'DiolG concentrations at baseline in the azoospermic and oligozoospermic responders were similar. After 16 weeks of TE treatment, both the free and conjugated 5α-reduced steroid levels increased significantly in all subjects. Consistent with the CR result, the increase in DHT was greater in the oligozoospermic (66% from 2.6 to 4.1 nMol/L) compared to the azoospermic subjects (33% from 2.5 to 3.1 nMol/L). Similarly, the increase in A'DiolG was

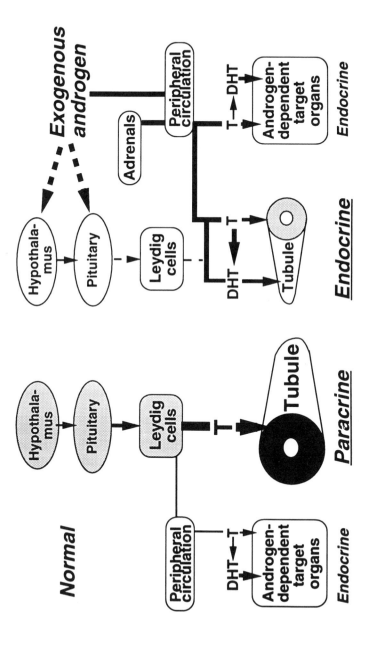

Figure 1. Model of androgen sources and mode of androgen action in the physiological state (left) and during suppression of gonodotropins to deplete intratesticular testosterone (right).

greater in the oligozoospermic (110% from 18 to 40 nMol/L) compared to the azoospermic subjects (69% 20 to 31 nMol/L). Since these subjects have similar bioavailable T and clearance rates, these results would also suggest that there is a significantly higher 5α-reductase activity in the oligozoospermic subjects, but this only becomes apparent following a period of sustained exogenous androgen loading.

## URINARY T AND EPISTESTOSTERONE

Following TE administration, urinary total T increased significantly by 4-5 fold to a similar extent between azoospermic and oligozoospermic responders. Urinary ET decreased from 64 to 5 and 50 to 5 μg/24h in azoospermic and oligozoospermic responders respectively. Since urinary ET is believed to be derived predominately or exclusively from testicular synthesis and secretion, the data suggest that endogenous testosterone production by the testis have been reduced to <10% of pre-treatment levels in both azoospermic and oligozoospermic responders.

## URINARY DEHYDROEPIANDROSTERONE (DHA AND PLASMA DHA-SULFATE (DHAS)

Urinary DHA decreased significantly only in the azoospermic (910 to 370 μg/24h) but not in the oligozoospermic group (850 to 720 μg/24h). This pattern was replicated by plasma DHAS levels with a significant decrease only in the azoospermic group.

## CONCLUSIONS

We conclude that non-suppression of spermatogenesis during TE treatment could not be accounted for by incomplete gonadotrophin inhibition, or differences in testosterone absorption or clearance. Exogenous TE reduces testicular steroid production to less than 10% normal in both azoospermic and non azoospermic responders. An increase in 5α-reductase activity was evident in the oligozoospermic, but not azoospermic responders, during TE suppression. Exogenous TE also appears to inhibit adrenal androgen secretion in the azoospermic, but not the oligozoospermic group. Taking these findings together, it is possible that conversion of circulating T and/or adrenal androgens to more potent 5α-reduced androgens plays a role in sustaining a degree of spermatogenesis in the androgen-depleted testis (Figure 1). In the physiological state, testosterone over-abundance in the testis is such that the tubules, unlike the extratesticular target tissues, respond to the paracrine action of very high intratesticular levels of testosterone and 5α-reductase and DHT are, not surprisingly, redundant. However, during gonadotrophin suppression, Leydig cell steroidogenesis is drastically reduced to create a testosterone-depleted state in the testis. The tubules therefore, now have to function as an endocrine target organ relying largely on peripherally-delivered exogenously-administered androgen. Under these circumstances, the action of 5α-reductase in converting either testosterone or adrenal androgens becomes disproportionately important. Hence, those subjects with evidence of a higher level of 5α-reductase activity and higher (less suppressed) levels of DHEA during TE treatment, are able to maintain a degree of spermatogenesis compatible with oligozoospermia, despite the lack of gonadotrophin stimulation. This hypothesis provides a conceptual model for further investigation and validation.

## ACKNOWLEDGMENTS

This work is supported by the UNDP/UNFPR/WHO/World Bank Special Program of Research, Development and Research Training in Human Reproduction.

## REFERENCES

Handelsman DJ, Farley TMM, Peregoudov A, Waites GMH (1995): Factors in the non-uniform induction of azoospermia by testosterone enanthate in normal men. Fertil & Steril 63: 125-133.

Wallace EM, Gow SM, Wu FCW (1993): Comparison between testosterone enanthate-induced azoospermia and oligozoospermia in a male contraceptive study I: plasma luteinizing hormone, follicle stimulating hormone, testosterone, estradiol and inhibin concentrations. J Clin Endocrinol Metab 77:290-293.

World Health Organization Task Force for the Regulation of Male Fertility (1990): Contraceptive efficacy of testosterone-induced azoospermia in normal men. Lancet 336:955-959.

# 38

# HORMONAL METHODS OF MALE CONTRACEPTION ARE FLAWED AND IMPRACTICAL

Gabriel Bialy

Center for Population Research
National Institute of Child Health and
Human Development
Bethesda, Maryland  20892

## THE HORMONAL APPROACHES

Hormonal approaches to male contraception are all based on the fact that gametogenic function of the testes is dependent on proper functioning of the hypothalamo-pituitary axis.  If the function of this axis can be impaired to the point where gonadotropic support is insufficient to maintain spermatogenesis, we reach the state of infertility and good contraceptive efficacy.

Over the last 25 years, a whole variety of hormonal approaches to male contraception have been attempted (Nieschlag et al., 1992). The word "hormonal" is used very broadly to include both hormones and their synthetic analogs. While important advances, both in basic male reproductive and applied research have been made, we still do not have nor will have in the near future, a male contraceptive based on a hormonal approach.  I must admit that the title of this presentation was not generated by Gabe Bialy nor do I believe with absolute certainty that a hormonal approach will not work.  However, it is incumbent on my part to bring forth certain criteria that must be met before we can make the statement that we have a reasonable prototype approach.  The true task that I have assigned to myself is that of a devil's advocate:  To question and to suggest.

In any product development program it is mandatory to set a number of attributes that we want the product to achieve.  In basic research we have a different orientation in that we are satisfied with a null hypothesis.  What then must be satisfied in order to develop a contraceptive agent and why have the current approaches failed to meet one or more of these attributes/criteria?  I shall try to discuss them, knowing full well that others may disagree or may add to my list.

*Pharmacology, Biology, and Clinical Applications of Androgens*, edited by Shalender Bhasin et al.
ISBN 0-471-13320-5 © 1996 Wiley-Liss, Inc.

## WHAT IS AN ACCEPTABLE LEVEL OF RESPONSE?

The majority of clinical studies aimed at arrest of spermatogenesis as a potential contraceptive method have involved relatively small numbers of volunteers. Under these types of circumstances, it is exceedingly difficult to establish the true percentage of responders and nonresponders. A shift of one or two individuals from one category to another can produce a dramatic shift in the level of response and the degree of enthusiasm for the regimen. This is true for most of the studies conducted with GnRH agonists and antagonists (Weinbauer et al., 1990). The data for the antagonists are suggestive that azoospermia can be achieved in 90% of the volunteers, but even after combining all of the studies, involving different antagonists, we are left with relatively small numbers.

The only comfort that can be drawn comes from the WHO sponsored studies involving testosterone enanthate (TE) alone (WHO Task Force on Methods for the Regulation of Male Fertility, 1990) and the combination of DMPA and an androgen (WHO Task Force on Methods for the Regulation of Male Fertility, 1993). These studies have spotlighted the fact that ethnic differences in level of response may exist. The Chinese men in the TE study and Indonesian men in the combination study responded to the drug treatment at a rate higher than 90%. The Caucasian population in the TE study showed azoospermia rate of only 70% or so (WHO, 1993).

There is a recent combination oral levonorgestrel, together with TE study in the USA, which suggest a response rate of 90%, but once again the number of volunteers is small (Bebb et al., 1995).

What then is the level of response that could make a "hormonal" approach practical? It is my opinion that the response rate must be at least 90% and preferably 95%. The argument that other male controlled methods such as condoms, show a contraceptive failure rate of 10 to 15%, does not in any way justify a similar failure for a hormonal approach. We must keep in mind that a large contributor to the condom failure rate is noncompliance. This element has not been properly evaluated with hormonal methods and may result in lower response rate if injections or pills are not taken on schedule.

Therefore, in summary, the response rates that have been achieved with hormonal-like approaches have not been sufficiently high for practical contraception (Handelsman et al., 1995). The positive high rate responses in Chinese and Indonesian men need to be substantiated in additional clinical studies.

## ACHIEVEMENT OF INFERTILE STATUS

It is important, at least for the present, to think about a successful male contraceptive method as one which achieves azoospermia. There is good and logical evidence that azoospermia results in high contraceptive efficacy and, consequently, this is the therapeutic end point that we must strive for (WHO, 1993). Careful review of clinical data suggests that even with the "successful" experimental methods, there is considerable variation in time required to achieve azoospermia. While in clinical studies there is room for careful monitoring of sperm numbers in the ejaculate, that luxury rapidly disappears when an approach reaches the marketing stage.

We are advised not to worry too much about this problem because even after a vasectomy, there is a delay before functional infertility sets in. I do not believe for a moment, that at the present time, we have any evidence that will allow us to set practical guidelines telling men using a hormonal contraceptive when they can have an unprotected coitus. Very conservative, play it safe, guidelines will make such approaches unattractive to users and a simple do it yourself assessment kit is not on the horizon.

In trying to establish guidelines for a successful hormonal method, one needs to state an acceptable time frame for induction of azoospermia. Obviously, one cycle of spermatogenesis would be a desirable induction period. But, if that is not achieved, then what? In experimental protocols we can set just about any induction period and indeed, in the WHO (1993) studies, induction period of six months was the limit. I do not believe that this is viable under real-use conditions.

The utilization of GnRH antagonists has brought hope that these chemical entities could induce azoospermia in a reliable and predictable fashion. At this time, we have no good answer since the total experience with these drugs is so very limited. In one of the small studies, there were nonresponders at the dose level used and significant increases in dosage had to be utilized in order to achieve a positive response. This experience, together with the experience with other hormonal approaches, suggests considerable variability in the dose-response relationship among different men. We know very little about the responsive/nonresponsive characteristics of individuals, and until such time that we can prospectively identify the responders from nonresponders, the proposed hormonal contraceptive is not likely to be practical. This is especially true if the proportion of nonresponders is high (20%+).

## MAINTENANCE OF INFERTILE STATUS

Success of any approach to male contraception will to a degree be dependent on the uniformity of the inhibitory response. This does not represent a problem with weekly injections of TE or when we look at the response to a single administration of a long-acting drug. But the situation can be critical when one must determine when the next treatment is to be instituted. In the study conducted by Behre and associates (Behre, 1994) in which 1200 mg of testosterone buciclate (TB) were administered to healthy male volunteers, three subjects out of eight became azoospermic. Surprisingly-singly, all three subjects became azoospermic at ten weeks, but one remained azoospermic for two weeks, another for ten and the third for 12 weeks. One then asks when should the second injection be given? We can give valid answers for subjects who are closely monitored. Unfortunately, this is not the case when we are dealing with a product in the field.

Will the variability disappear if we go to higher doses of TB? Not likely, since pharmacokinetics-kinetics of long-acting drugs show high variability among different individuals. Even when testosterone will not be the primary inhibitor of the hypo-thalamic/pituitary/gonadal axis, a similar situation may very well arise.

If we choose a specific interval for the next drug injection, we will be faced with the situation that some individuals will receive an extra burden of the drug. In some cases, this may not be acceptable and will make the hormonal approach a difficult one.

## SAFETY

Recent clinical studies have strict criteria for inclusion and exclusion of subjects from the trial. At the same time, there exists the tendency to minimize the problems that have arisen with some of the hormonal approaches. While there may not have been any life threatening episodes, there may have been some close calls with the GnRH antagonists.

To my knowledge, we have no reliable information on safety of the numerous approaches. The reasons for the lack of this information are numerous. First of all, majority of the studies involve very small numbers of volunteers, thus precluding observation of potential life threatening manifestations. Where the numbers of volunteers have been larger, such as in the WHO multi-center studies, some potential toxicities have emerged. These side effects are generally dismissed by the enthusiastic clinicians, while at the same time, they may be unacceptable to others.

Another potential problem that looms on the horizon involves the transition from carefully conducted clinical trials to the introduction of a method into a general population. We must recognize that any and all problems that were apparent at the stage of clinical studies will be magnified in less selected populations. We can anticipate that unacceptable weight gain or acne will contribute significantly to discontinuation rates (Bardin et al., 1991). What about cardiovascular risks to subjects on androgen alone regimens? Review of the literature dealing with the long-term safety of androgen treatment of hypogonadal men suggests that the risk to benefit ratio is acceptable. But it is also of interest that in the advertisement of their transdermal patch, Testoderm$^T$, Alza makes the following statement: "In clinical studies, the following events occurred rarely: stroke (2/104); deep vein phlebitis (1/104); congestive heart failure (1/104). A casual relationship to Testoderm$^R$ treatment was not always determined" (Alza Corporation, 1994). None of the serious complications mentioned in the Alza advertisement occurred in the WHO trials. This may very well reflect the fact that the health status of men with idiopathic hypogonadism is different from that observed in men with drug-induced hypogonadism.

In summary, it can be stated that the safety of any and all hormonal approaches to male contraception is not well documented. We must proceed with due caution, especially when we consider phase II and III clinical studies.

## COST

Discussion of cost factors is not one of the favorite topics among researchers conducting male contraceptive trials. There exists the apprehension that a frank discussion of costs can jeopardize funding of specific projects. On the other side, to those who are funding development of new methods, consideration of costs is one of the most important decision making points.

The issue of costs is complicated by the fact that there is no current hormonal method of male contraception. Thus, there is no comparison standard. There is also a degree of confusion between research aimed at testing of an hypothesis and actual product development research. The few studies done with GnRH antagonists were critical to our understanding of the pharmacology of these drugs even though there was the general understanding that the current generation of drugs was much too expensive for contraception purposes. Economics of large scale production could not provide a rescue. The cost issue with GnRH antagonists is further complicated by the multiplicity of therapeutic uses. Obviously, we cannot charge for contraception what can be charged for cancer chemotherapy. We only need to look at the current costs of GnRH agonists to realize how the cost situation will dictate utility of a product for a specific therapeutic use.

Moving to a less expensive category of drugs, namely steroids, we must still examine the impact of costs on the development of a hormonal male contraceptive. In the Indonesian study, looking at the combination of DMPA with androgens, the progestin was given at the dose of 250 mg every six weeks and the androgen was given initially at weekly intervals and then spaced at every three weeks. The conservative yearly cost of these drugs in the USA would be around $450. When doctor and clinic costs are added to that figure, we can readily see that costs are not inconsequential. I would, therefore, suggest that when we are attempting to develop a contraceptive approach based on marketed drugs, we should make every effort to calculate potential costs of the proposed regimen. In order to be a viable male contraceptive, what should its cost be relative to a female contraceptive? Or should we even think in those terms?

In order to bring a product to the market, public sector agencies will require a viable industrial partner. Costs are a very important issue in decision making processes and cannot be ignored. We need to be realistic and appreciate the fact that a man suffering from idiopathic hypogonadism is driven by a somewhat different set of values than a normal man looking at the cost of contraception.

## LEGAL ISSUES

Developers of male hormonal contraceptive methods must be aware and consider the legal aspects of androgen replacement therapy. I am addressing the universal problem of the male athlete and the designation in the USA of androgenic/anabolic steroids as controlled substances. Unfortunately, good medical practice takes a back seat to regulations and laws. It is very unlikely that the doses used for contraception can have any impact on athletic performance. But how do we convince athletic associations of this fact? We may take comfort in the fact that the number of competitive male and female athletes is relatively small and we may develop for them alternative methods.

The legal situation in the USA is of importance to those of us who are concerned with the development of methods for the males in the USA How overwhelming will the paperwork become when a practical method is developed and popularized? The answer can be provided by physicians who treat patients with androgens. The Drug Enforcement Agency requires record keeping at every step, going back to the manufacturer and ending with the prescribing physician.

To what degree are the legal issues an impediment to successful male contraceptive development? I do not have an answer, but the problems must be addressed since they are not likely to go away.

## CONCLUSIONS

Development of a male hormonal contraceptive poses a difficult challenge to research. In the field of contraceptive development, that for the male has been the province of public sector agencies. The pharmaceutical industry has been on occasion supportive by providing drugs to the academic researcher, while at the same time, it has been passive in terms of actual involvement. While the position of industry may be influenced by a variety of factors, we need to ask ourselves which of these factors should we worry about as well? At the third European Congress of Endocrinology, our distinguished colleague, Prof. Nieschlag, delivered a plenary lecture titled "Hormonal Contraception in the Male." In conclusion, he stated that "Further development, however, is impeded by the lack of interest on the part of the pharmaceutical industry which persists in withholding its skills in drug development from the field of male contraception" (Nieschlag et al., 1994). Is it possible that the leads we have identified are significant in terms of improving our understanding of testicular function and its control, but are less significant in identifying product development?

Before we can develop a product, we must identify a clear-cut set of criteria/attributes that a drug or a combination of drugs must have before we can proceed on the R & D path. Failure to recognize and consider the factors that are part of a successful drug development continue to plague this field. Progress will continue to be slow. The difficulties are surmountable only if we recognize them and develop reasonable solutions.

## REFERENCES

Alza Corporation 1994: (Advertisement) Alza Transforms Testosterone Delivery. Testoderm.

Bardin WC, Swerdloff RS, Santen RJ (1991): Androgens: Risks and Benefits. J Clin Endocrinol Metab 73:4-7.

Bebb RA, Anawalt BD, Christensen RB, Paulsen CA, Bremner WJ, Matsumoto AM (1995): A Promising Male Contraceptive Approach: Combined Testosterone and Levonorgestrel. Submitted for publication. New Engl J Med.

Behre HM (1994): Private Communication .

Handelsman DJ, Farley TMM, Peregoudov A, Waites GMH (1995): Factors in Nonuniform Induction of Azoospermia by Testosterone Enanthate in Normal Men. Fertil Steril 63:125-133.

Nieschlag E, Behre HM, Weinbauer GF (1992): Hormonal Male Contraception: A Real Chance? In Nieschlag E and Halbernicht UF (eds.), Spermatogenesis-Fertilization-Contraception: Molecular Cellular and Endocrine Events in Male Reproduction. Springer Verlag, Heidelberg, pp. 477-501.

Nieschlag E, Weinbauer GF, Gromoll J, Behre HM (1994): Hormonal
    Contraception in the Male. Eur J Endocrinol 130 (Suppl. 2):11-12.
Weinbauer GF, Behre HM, Nieschlag E (1990): Contraceptive Studies with
    GnRH Analogs in Men and Non-Human Primates. In Bouchard P, Haour F,
    Schatz B (eds.), Recent Progress on GnRh and Gonadal Peptides. Elsevier,
    Paris, pp. 181-194.
WHO Task Force on Methods for the Regulation of Male Fertility (1990):
    Contraceptive Efficacy of Testosterone-Induced Azoospermia in Normal Men.
    Lancet 336:955-959.
WHO Task Force on Methods for the Regulation of Male Fertility (1993):
    Comparison of Two Androgens Plus Depo-Medroxy-Progesterone Acetate for
    Suppression to Azoospermia in Indonesian Men. Fertil Steril 60:1062-1068.

# 39

# ANDROGEN-BASED REGIMENS FOR HORMONAL MALE CONTRACEPTION

David J. Handelsman

Andrology Unit, Royal Prince Alfred Hospital
Departments of Medicine, Obstetrics and Gynecology
University of Sydney
Sydney, NSW, 2006 Australia

## INTRODUCTION

The *fin de siecle* dilemma for wider application of global male contra-contraception is that the reversible male methods are unreliable and the reliable male method is irreversible. Despite this, men continue to take a major share of responsibility for family planning with 160 million couples currently relying on methods requiring active male participation. This represents 35% of all couples using family planning methods world-wide and >55% of couples in developed countries (United Nations, 1989), but their overall failure rates are 3-4 times higher than modern female methods (Handelsman, 1994). The prime task is therefore to develop a reliable and reversible male method of family planning. A male contraceptive must reduce the number of fertile sperm in the ejaculate to levels that reliably prevent fertilization. This can be achieved by the pre-20th Century methods of mechanically diverting sperm by using periodic abstinence, withdrawal, condoms, and vasectomy. A more sophisticated approach, yet to be realized, would be to reduce sperm output and/or function. This would be analogous to the highly effective, convenient and reversible contraceptive methods developed over the last 3 decades for women which aim to inhibit ovulation and/or uterine function. Among various novel approaches in development, hormonal methods are the closest to introducing the first novel male contraceptive method in the last century. Two landmark WHO-sponsored studies of contraceptive efficacy of hormonally-induced azoospermia (WHO, 1990) and oligozoospermia (WHO, 1995) demon-demonstrated that a prototype androgen-alone regimen can suppress sperm output to levels that provide reliable and reversible contraception with acceptable levels of minor side-effects. In setting the cornerstone for development of hormonal male contraceptive regimens, these studies establish that under clinical trial conditions, azoospermia can be regarded as analogous to anovulation for female hormonal contraception; both are sufficient, but not necessary for highly effective contraception (Trussell et

*Pharmacology, Biology, and Clinical Applications of Androgens*, edited by Shalender Bhasin et al.
ISBN 0-471-13320-5 © 1996 Wiley-Liss, Inc.
395

al., 1987). Although universal azoospermia may not be strictly necessary, it is desirable to provide a better tolerance margin for human error and is achievable already in some Asian countries. Thus hormonal male contraception has moved from concept and feasibility studies to product development with field testing still to follow. Presently, the focus must be on better (faster, universal, predictable) suppression of spermatogenesis to give a wider safety margin and on better products to deliver a convenient contraceptive. This review considers the relative merits of regimens likely to best realize this potential, emphasizing androgen-alone methods.

## FEATURES OF HORMONAL REGIMENS

Hormonal male contraceptive methods classically exploit the pivotal role of GnRH in regulating pituitary gonadotropin secretion. They aim to abolish sperm production by withdrawing gonadotropin stimulation of the testes but without diminishing androgen supply to the body. Spermatogenesis is highly dependent upon gonadotropins and their paracrine modulators within the testis (including testosterone) that relay and amplify testicular gonadotropin action. Spermatogenesis is effectively abolished by inhibition of gonadotropin secretion. This inhibition, however, must be sustained and complete in order to deplete fully testicular testosterone from ambient concentrations well above either blood levels, or the threshold required to maintain spermatogenesis, as well as depleting other gonadotropin-dependent paracrine factors (Spiteri-Grech et al., 1993; Sharpe, 1994). Inhibition of GnRH action, whether by negative feedback from sex steroids, synthetic GnRH analogs, or GnRH immunoneutralization, would inevitably lead to androgen deficiency due to the abolition of LH secretion, upon which testicular testosterone production is wholly reliant. Consequently, androgen replacement is essential for all such regimens. Thus, the two fundamental principles of hormonal male contraception are to block gonadotropin action, and replace testosterone. The former can be achieved with androgens, progestins, or GnRH analogs, whereas the latter is usually provided by testosterone itself.

Potential regimens include (1) androgens alone, (2) androgen combined with a second agent, either a GnRH analog, or progestin, and (3) androgen-independent methods. In addition, hybrid regimens, such as induction or intermittent use of a progestin, or GnRH antagonist, with androgen and maintenance by androgen alone, are also possible. Androgen-independent methods have the theoretical advantage of avoiding this need to co-administer an androgen. Among these approaches, antiandrogens alone (Wang et al., 1980) and selective FSH suppression (Nieschlag, 1986) are considered insufficiently effective, whereas paracrine hormonal approaches remain promising future developments when their safety, efficacy and feasibility in humans is established. Thus, the main contenders in the immediate future remain androgen-based regimens, such as androgens alone, or in conjunction with a second agent, such as progestin, or GnRH analog. Although this review will contrast these options, in reality a diversity of choice in contraception is optimal and more than a single hormonal regimen would be used by men if they were available. In evaluating competing directions for product development, various options must be compared against ideal criteria, which broadly include, efficacy, safety, convenience, acceptability (to users, producers and regulators), and affordability.

# EFFICACY

## Androgen-Alone Regimens

Androgen-alone regimens have the unique advantage of providing simultaneously both gonadotropin suppression and androgen replacement in a single agent. This simplicity makes an androgen-alone regimen an obvious first choice for a reversible hormonal male contraceptive. The choice of androgen is governed by safety and efficacy considerations, leaving testosterone as the major natural androgen, the default choice. The most comprehensive experience with androgen-alone regimens derives from the WHO multicentre studies which included over 670 men using a standard protocol of weekly intramuscular injections of 200 mg testosterone enanthate (TE) in an oil vehicle (WHO, 1990 and 1995). Within 6 months of weekly injections of 200 mg, TE-produced azoospermia was produced in 425/620 (69% [65%-72%]) and severe oligozoospermia (<3 M/ml) in 349/357 (98% [96%-99%]). This effectiveness exceeds earlier feasibility studies (Patanelli, 1977) probably due to regular monitoring of compliance with scheduled injections. The identical regimen also renders azoospermic virtually all men living in China (WHO, 1990 and 1995) and Indonesia (Arsyad, 1993). Combining the 2 studies, contraceptive efficacy of azoospermia was high with only 1 (extramarital) pregnancy observed during 354 subject-years (0.3 [0-1.6]), and efficacy virtually equivalent to vasectomy (Trussell et al., 1987), which is itself not perfect (Smith et al., 1994). Nevertheless, 3.3% of non-Asian men were not rendered sufficiently oligozoospermic and contraception would be more reliable if men became consistently azoospermic, as the contraceptive failure rate among the 10% of persistently oligozoospermic men remains 8 per 100 person-years, which is still better than other reversible male methods. While universal azoospermia is no longer strictly essential, it would be desirable to ensure a better tolerance margin for efficacy. This is already achievable in some Asian countries, but second generation hormonal regimens for men are needed and the question is, whether androgens alone can make such improvements, or whether second agents must be added.

The suboptimal pharmacokinetics of TE dictate that dose reduction, or spacing, fail to sustain spermatogenic suppression (Patanelli, 1977; Matsumoto, 1990) illustrating the need for improved depot formulations that provide physiological testosterone levels for prolonged periods. This requires novel depot testosterone preparations as the pharmacokinetics of currently available testosterone esters are no better than TE (Behre et al., 1990). Prolonged physiological testosterone levels can be provided by true long-acting testosterone depots, such as testosterone pellets, lasting for 4-6 months (Handelsman, 1990; Handelsman et al., 1990), and testosterone-loaded biodegradable microspheres (Bhasin et al., 1992), or testosterone buciclate (Behre et al., 1992b), lasting for 2-3 months. Using testosterone pellets as a model depot, benefits deriving from the highly favorable kinetics included equally effective, but faster suppression >50 % dose-sparing (9 vs 21 mg/day), and fewer metabolic side-effects than weekly TE injections; nonetheless, azoospermia was not achieved universally (Handelsman et al., 1992; Behre et al., 1994a). Whether other androgen-alone regimens can induce universal azoospermia, remains to be established.

A practical disadvantage of testosterone is the large mass of steroid that must be delivered to replicate its endogenous production of 3-10 mg daily. Synthetic androgens with sufficient potency (Avery et al, 1990) to substantially reduce the daily dose have unproven safety and the limitation that their spectrum of androgen action across a range of tissues may be incomplete if they lack metabolic activation by 5-alpha reduction and aromatization. On balancing potential advantages and disadvantages, developing improved depot testosterone delivery systems are preferable to seeking novel, more potent, but restricted androgens, at present.

## Androgen/GnRH Analog Regimens

Superactive GnRH analogs, co-administered with androgens have proven ineffective at inhibiting spermatogenesis. In 12 reports (Nieschlag et al., 1992), only 21/106 (20%, [95% CI 13%-29%]) of healthy men were rendered azoospermic, although significant heterogeneity in achieving azoospermia (0-100%; p=0.0001), among these, mostly small studies (n=4-11) presumably indicates inclusion of suboptimal regimens. The failure of superactive GnRH agonists may reflect their persistent, partial, agonist activity, preventing adequate depletion of intratesticular testosterone (Bouchard et al., 1987; Lunn et al., 1990; Behre et al., 1992a), and/or incomplete FSH suppression (Behre et al., 1992a; Bhasin et al., 1994). Pure GnRH antagonists combined with testosterone are more promising as they produce rapid, reversible and virtually complete inhibition of spermatogenesis in monkeys (Weinbauer et al., 1987; Weinbauer et al., 1989; Bremner et al., 1991) and men (Pavlou et al., 1991; Tom et al., 1992; Bagatell et al., 1993; Pavlou et al., 1994). In four small human studies 29/34 (85% [69%-95%]), healthy men were rendered azoospermic which, statistically, barely exceeds that of weekly TE injection (69%, n=620 overall; 65%, n=389 for non-Asian men). These studies were consistent with non-human primate studies indicating that delayed commencement of androgen replacement facilitated suppression of spermatogenesis, presumably by allowing greater depletion of testicular testosterone and/or other paracrine modulators of testicular gonadotropin action; delayed starting of androgen may be circumvented by lowering androgen dosage (Bremner et al., 1991; Pavlou et al., 1994). The efficacy of a GnRH vaccine (Giri et al., 1991) to inhibit testicular function, remains to be established by ongoing pilot studies in men with prostate cancer (Talwar et al., 1989).

## Androgen/Progestin Regimens

The rationale for introducing androgen/progestin regimens is that the combination may have additive effects lowering doses of both agents, and/or that a potent synthetic progestin which suppresses gonadotropin secretion, reduces the dose requirement for testosterone. Such theoretical benefits in efficacy, or safety, have yet to be established empirically, and additive complexities could also arise. Various androgen/progestin combinations used in 16 small studies lasting at least 3 months, attained azoospermia in 147/214 (69% [62%-75%]) healthy European men (Schearer et al., 1978; Nieschlag et al., 1992; Cummings et al., 1994) and virtually all (87/90, 98%) Indonesian men (Pangkahila, 1991; WHO, 1993), with the remainder having severe oligozoospermia and impaired sperm function (Matsumoto, 1988; Wu et al., 1989). Thus, while direct controlled comparisons are lacking, available studies do not support any major benefit in efficacy for the androgen/progestin combination over standard androgen-alone regimens (Patanelli, 1977; Schearer et al., 1978; Nieschlag et al., 1992; Cummings et al., 1994). Rather than adding a synthetic progestin, androgen dose reduction (>50%) is achievable by using true depots which deliver steady-state testosterone levels over prolonged periods (Handelsman et al., 1992; Behre et al., 1994a).

## Population Differences in Susceptibility

Using an androgen-alone regimen, strikingly higher susceptibility to hormonally-induced azoospermia, has been observed among men living in China (WHO, 1990 and 1995) and Indonesia (Pangkahila, 1991; Arsyad, 1993; WHO, 1993), compared with non-Asian men. Although the reasons remain unclear (Handelsman et al., 1995), these findings suggest that induction of azoospermia universally in all men might be feasible by improved androgen-based regimens. These population differences in efficacy were not associated with corresponding differences in safety as indicated by the lack of region- or center-specific differences in safety profile, in the WHO multicentre studies (WHO, 1990 and 1995).

Ultimately, it remains difficult to compare the three main regimens for suppressing spermatogenesis, due to the lack of direct controlled studies and the small size of the available studies. Nevertheless, it is clear that all hormonal regimens have been fully reversible and that steroidal regimens are clearly superior to androgen/GnRH agonist regimens. While androgen/GnRH antagonist regimens may be more effective than steroidal regimens, larger studies are needed to determine directly whether either androgen/2nd agent combination regimens have advantages over androgen-alone studies. Studies are also needed to estimate the tolerance in efficacy for each regimen for human error, including irregular compliance.

## SAFETY

The safety record of testosterone is well established over decades of use in numerous formulations for treating androgen deficiency. Androgen-alone contraceptive regimens, using a higher testosterone dose, also demonstrated satisfactory safety in both earlier feasibility studies (Patanelli, 1977), as well as the large multicentre WHO studies (WHO, 1990 and 1995), amounting to over 800 men. In the WHO studies, using weekly injections of 200 mg TE for up to 18 months, there were few medical discontinuations (<10% per annum) and none for serious adverse effects (Wu et al., 1995). Medical discontinuations (35/401 men) were mostly for acne (8), or for changes in mood (4), behavior (3), or libido (3), while other idiosyncratic or incidental conditions were uncommon (<1%), and there were none for palpable prostatic enlargement. This safety experience sets a benchmark for subsequent comparisons and lower dose regimens, such as standard androgen replacement (e.g. 100 mg TE per week) or optimized depot testosterone regimens (63 mg/week) that can be considered safe in the medium term. In contrast, synthetic androgens, such as 17-alpha alkylated derivatives, are unsuitable for clinical use and their toxicology casts a shadow over the long-term safety profile of newer synthetic androgens (Avery et al., 1990), which has yet to be established.

Wide usage of a hormonal male contraceptive requires consideration of long-term safety of androgen-based regimens on cardiovascular and prostate disease, and psychological function. Ultimately, only long-term surveillance can accurately quantitate or rule out small changes in risks and benefits involving common medical disorders, such as cardiovascular and prostate disease. Androgen-induced lipid changes of uncertain significance, limited to small decreases in HDL-cholesterol in some, but not all studies, do not differentiate between androgen-based regimens (Friedl et al., 1990; WHO, 1990; Handelsman et al., 1992). The major predictors of prostate disease in later life are age, genetics, and exposure to eugonadal testosterone levels in early manhood (Krieg et al., 1990; Schroeder, 1990). The relationship of blood androgen levels to prostatic disease is poorly understood (Nomura et al., 1988; Krieg et al., 1990) and both replacement (Behre et al., 1994b) nor suppressive (Wallace et al., 1993) androgen doses have minimal effects on prostate size. While prevalence of in-situ prostate cancer rises steeply with age in all populations, rates of invasive prostate cancer differ many-fold between populations with similar blood testosterone levels. This suggests androgen exposure in early adult life imprints the risk of prostatic disease, which is then precipitated into invasive form later in life by subsequent androgen-independent environmental factors (Schroeder, 1990). The absence of serious mood or behavioral changes with androgen-alone regimens has been consistent in studies with well over 800 healthy men (Patanelli, 1977; WHO, 1990 and 1995). This contrasts sharply with uncontrolled observations and tabloid self-reports from body-builders, athletes and prisoners where psychological self-selection and placebo responses explain high levels of observed psychopathology, rather than androgen effects (Bahrke et al., 1990; Hubert, 1990). Given the inevitable uncertainties regarding long-term risks at this early stage of development, the soundest approach is to aim to maintain physiological testosterone levels and, within these bounds, it seems unlikely that small variations in testosterone dose would substantially influence risks of cardiovascular or prostate disease, or psychological changes in mood, or behavior, compared with eugonadal testosterone levels.

GnRH analogs, having a highly specific and localized site of action, have proven safe in extensive clinical usage of superactive GnRH agonists, including depot formulations. In contrast, GnRH antagonists have so far only been used in small, short-term studies. The latest generation of GnRH antagonists still has relatively low molar potency and use expensive, highly hydrophobic, and exotic synthetic amino-acids, which cause histamine release and irritation at the injection site, as well as being difficult to formulate into true long-acting (3 month) depots.

Future development of GnRH antagonists must overcome these limitations to develop more potent, affordable, and tractable compounds for depot delivery. Non-peptide GnRH antagonists might improve the applicability of GnRH analogs if they provide long-acting depots, whereas multi-daily oral dosing would be impractical for male contraception. Larger and longer studies with GnRH antagonists are needed to clarify their practicability, as well as safety, for hormonal male contraception, and in particular, whether they are really superior to androgen-alone regimens (Bremner et al., 1991). A GnRH vaccine would entail risks due to the inability to regulate the immune response (autoimmunization, unpredictable titres and duration of effect, uncertain reversibility), which raises safety concerns for application to healthy men.

Although synthetic progestins are well tolerated in the short-term, the long-term safety of 17-alpha alkylated progestins, particularly in combination with an exogenous androgen, has not been established in men. For example, the risk of hepatotoxicity and/or hepatic tumors, compared with 17-alpha alkylated androgens, is unclear. The putative safety advantage of introducing a progestin assumes that replacing part of the daily testosterone dosage by a potent synthetic progestin is beneficial. As testosterone is still required for androgen replacement, the saving in testosterone dosage is the difference between the standard testosterone replacement dosage and the minimum for satisfactory spermatogenic suppression, using depot testosterone regimens. From our ongoing studies, this amounts to about 3 mg/day of testosterone. It is unclear that such reduction in androgen dosage influences safety, or that spermatogenic suppressive doses of synthetic progestins are significantly safer than this amount of testosterone. Nonetheless, progestins in superior long-acting depot formulations, such as levonorgestrel butanoate (HRP002), and non-biodegradable implants of norgestrel, or ketodesogestrel, would be very valuable to determine the benefits, if any, of combination regimens, compared with optimized androgen-alone depot regimens.

Idiosyncratic reactions to androgens, such as polycythemia and worsening obstructive sleep apnea, both occurring in <1% of the target age-group of men, must constitute precautions related to predisposing conditions for androgen-based regimens, much as estrogen-sensitive migraine or epilepsy are for female hormonal contraception. Absolute contraindications to androgens, such as prostate cancer, or breast cancer are rare in reproductivly active men.

A full evaluation of safety must also include consideration of potential non-contraceptive benefits of androgen-based regimens involving androgen-sensitive tissues, such as bone, muscle, bone marrow, and collagen. Nevertheless, while side-benefits must not be ignored, they cannot constitute a realistic development strategy in immediate future for hormonal male contraception. More broadly still, the safety of not having a reliable, reversible male contraceptive method, in terms of unwanted conceptions, abortions, and premature sterilization, as well as in social equity, can only be guessed.

## CONVENIENCE

The ideal contraceptive would be user-friendly with a simple and non-intrusive method of administration that is, (1) non-coital to remove interference with spontaneous pleasurability of sex, (2) infrequent, so reducing demands for compliance by fallible humans, (3) reliable, without monitoring, and (4) rapid in onset and offset. All hormonal regimens satisfy the first criterion. Steroidal regimens potentially also satisfy the second criterion with long-acting form of delivery at 3 month intervals, as exemplified by testosterone pellets (Handelsman, 1990), testosterone buciclate (Behre et al., 1992b; Behre et al., 1994a), and testosterone microspheres (Bhasin et al., 1992). Suitable GnRH antagonist depots lasting a comparable duration are not yet available and shorter-acting ones would defeat the purpose of infrequent administration of a testosterone depot. Short-acting testosterone preparations (e.g., oral, transdermal) requiring daily or more administration, while acceptable to hypogonadal men, would be impractical for male contraception. No available depots are yet ideal as pellets require minor surgery for implantation and can extrude, while the buciclate ester and microsphere formulations require large injection volumes. Using androgen-alone regimen, onset of azoospermia, takes an average of 3 months and a similar period for sperm to reappear after cessation of injections, and similar durations are expected for combination regimens. Relatively slow onset and offset, dictated by the duration of the spermatogenic cycle (>70 days), is likely to be an unavoidable feature of all hormonal methods, however. Suboptimal hormonal regimens may also exhibit slower onset, and high dose steroidal regimens may exhibit slower offset than optimized depot androgen regimens. Future hormonal methods interfering with paracrine hormonal influence on late stages of spermatogenesis (spermiogenesis), or post-testicular approaches, may fill the need for faster acting male contraceptives. Obviating the need to monitor sperm output and enhancing the speed of suppression are high priorities for improved 2nd generation hormonal regimens, even though such delay and monitoring is accepted after vasectomy (Liskin et al., 1992).

## ACCEPTABILITY

Numerous surveys (Gallen, 1986; Cummings et al., 1994), confirmed by the enthusiasm of over 670 volunteers in 16 centers and 10 countries in the WHO studies, indicate that men remain willing to share responsibility for effective family planning. Specific niches for hormonal male methods to lighten women's burden of treatment include, (1) post-partum contraception , (2) delaying sterilization and, (3) intolerance of reliable female methods. In each situation male methods have advantages, and even a small fraction of the 150 million birth per year would constitute a substantial global market. Like any other discretionary-use products in consumerist societies, acceptability of contraceptives is governed largely by subjective factors related more to fashion and marketing than medicine or science. A key factor is peace of mind for users in the form of freedom from baseless scare publicity created by the swelling ranks of self-serving crusading journalists, single-issue political activists, and predatory product-liability lawyers. In the modern equivalent of a gold rush, any of these groups can, in pursuit of a "scalp," effectively derail novel medical products, regardless of, or even unwittingly abetted by, reasoned judgments by dispassionate observers and experts. This potentially lethal political aspect of acceptability is inherently more unpredictable than any other. Undoubtedly, prudent risk-aversive strategies by the pharmaceutical industry will continue to deter contraceptive R&D unless exceptional profit margins, or legislative shielding from opportunistic piracy, can be provided. Finally, the abuse potential of androgens is a new consideration in regulatory acceptability, but should be acceptably low in the setting of appropriate delivery systems.

## AFFORDABILITY

The costs of manufacture and delivery of steroidal products is likely to remain comparable with female hormonal contraception, with the exception that testosterone microspheres are more expensive. GnRH antagonists are likely to remain substantially more costly than steroidal regimens until their market for medical castration grows. Such efficiencies of scale and market size were instrumental in lowering the originally very high costs of contraceptive steroids. Economic factors in the interim may limit hormonal male contraception to steroidal regimens in less affluent countries until costs of potent GnRH antagonists fall substantially.

## SUMMARY

Following the substantial progress in recent years, there is now a need to develop second generation products that are convenient and deliver improved regimens. These should induce universal azoospermia so as to provide a wider tolerance margin in efficacy for users. The present indications are that androgens alone, as well as combination regimens with progestins as the poor man's GnRH antagonist, could form the basis of reliable and reversible male contraceptives. In some Asian countries this is already feasible with existing non-optimized products which remain affordable and have acceptable levels of efficacy and safety, but are suboptimal in convenience. Whether better products will actually emerge on the wider market will largely be determined by political factors, including the funding of R and D in male contraception, as well as, whether governments act to halt the predatory exploitation of product liability laws. This requires recognition by legislators that sustain commercial deterrence of pharmaceutical innovation in male contraception precludes people from enjoying the benefits promised by advances in biomedical science. Meanwhile, developing countries with a sense of urgency to provide a wider range of attractive family planning options may lead the way by introducing the first practical hormonal male contraceptive regimens. Men worldwide are clearly willing to share burdens, as well as benefits of effective family planning, and increase their already substantial share of responsibility, but need more effective options to choose from. By ignoring men's contribution in this generation, we neglect the needs of our children.

## REFERENCES

Arsyad KM (1993): Sperm function in Indonesian men treated with testosterone enanthate. Int. J. Androl. 16: 355-361.

Avery MA, Tanabe M, Crowe DF, Detre G, Peters RH, Chong WKM (1990):
    Synthesis and testing of 17ab-hydroxy-7a methyl-D-homoestra-4,16-dien-3-one; a
    highly potent orally active androgen. Steroids. 55:59-64.

Bagatell CJ, Matsumoto AM, Christensen RB, Rivier JE, Bremner WJ (1993):
    Comparison of a gonadotropin-releasing hormone antagonist plus testosterone (T)
    versus T alone as a potential male contraceptive. J. Clin. Endocrinol. Metab. 77:
    427-32.

Bahrke MS, Yesalis CE, Wright JE (1990): Psychological and behavioural effects of
    endogenous testosterone levels and anabolic-androgenic steroids among male. A
    review. Sports Medicine. 10: 303-337.

Behre HM, Baus S, Kliesch S, Keck C, Nieschlag E (1994a). US Endocrine Society,
    Anaheim, #1312.

Behre HM, Bohmeyer J, Nieschlag E (1994b): Prostate volume in testosterone-
    treated and untreated hypogonadal men in comparison to age-matched normal
    controls. Clin. Endocrinol. 40: 341-9.

Behre HM, Nashan D, Hubert W, Nieschlag E (1992a): Depot gonadotropin-
    releasing hormone agonist blunts the androgen-induced suppression of
    spermatogenesis in a clinical trial of male contraception. J Clin Endocrinol
    Metab. 74: 84-90.

Behre HM, Nieschlag E (1992b): Testosterone buciclate (20 Act-1) in hypogonadal
    men: pharmacokinetics and pharmacodynamics of the new long-acting androgen
    ester. J Clin Endocrinol Metab. 75: 1204-1210.

Behre HM, Oberpenning F, Nieschlag E (1990): Comparative pharmacokinetics of
    androgen preparations: application of computer analysis and simulation. In E.
    Nieschlag & H. M. Behre (eds): "Testosterone: Action Deficiency Substitution"
    Berlin: Springer-Verlag, 115-135.

Bhasin S, Swerdloff RS, Steiner B, Peterson MA, Meridores T, Galmirini M,
    Pandian MR, Goldberg R, Berman N (1994): Follicle-stimulating hormone (FSH)
    escape during chronic gonadotropin-releasing hormone (GnRH) agonist and
    testosterone treatment. J. Androl. 15: 386-91.

Bhasin S et al. (1992): A biodegradable testosterone microcapsule formulation
    provides uniform eugonadal levels of testosterone for 10-11 weeks in hypogonadal
    men. J Clin Endocrinol Metab. 74: 75-83.

Bouchard P, Garcia E (1987): Influence of testosterone substitution on sperm
    suppression by LHRH agonists. Hormone Res. 28: 175-180.

Bremner WJ, WJ, Bagatell CJ, Steiner RA (1991): Gonadotropin-releasing hormone
    antagonist plus testosterone: a potential male contraceptive. J Clin Endocrinol
    Metab. 73: 465-469.

Cummings DE, Bremner WJ (1994): Prospects for new hormonal male
    contraceptives. In W. J. Bremner (eds): "Clinical Andrology" Philadelphia: W B
    Saunders Company, 893-922.

Friedl KE, Hannan CJ, Jones RE, Plymate SR (1990): High-density lipoprotein
    cholesterol is not decreased if an aromatisable androgen is administered.
    Metabolism. 39: 69-74.

Gallen ME (1986): Men - new focus for family planning programs. Population
    Reports. 14: J889-920.

Giri DK, Jayaraman S, Neelaram GS, Jayashankar R, Talwar GP (1991): Prostatic hypoplasia in bonnet monkeys following active immunization with semisynthetic anti-LHRH vaccine. Exp Mol Pathol. 54: 255-264.

Handelsman DJ (1990): Pharmacology of testosterone pellet implants. In E. Nieschlag & H. M. Behre (eds): "Testosterone: Action Deficiency Substitution" Berlin: Springer-Verlag, 136-154.

Handelsman DJ (1994): Contraception in the male. In L. J. DeGroot (ed): "Endocrinology": W B Saunders, 2449-58.

Handelsman DJ, Conway AJ, Boylan LM (1990): Pharmacokinetics and pharmacodynamics of testosterone pellets in man. J Clin Endocrinol Metab. 71: 216-222.

Handelsman DJ, Conway AJ, Boylan LM (1992): Suppression of human spermatogenesis by testosterone implants in man. J Clin Endocrinol Metab. 75: 1326-1332.

Handelsman DJ, Farley TMM, Peregauder A, Waites GMH, WHOMTF (1995): Factors in the nonuniform induction of azoospermia by testosterone enanthate in normal men. Fert. Steril. 63: 125-33.

Hubert W (1990): Psychotropic effects of testosterone. In E. Nieschlag & H. M. Behre (eds): "Testosterone: Action Deficiency substitution" Berlin: Springer-Verlag, 51-71.

Krieg M, Tunn S (1990): Androgens and human benign prostatic hyperplasia. In E. Nieschlag & H. M. Behre (eds): "Testosterone: Action Deficiency substitution" Berlin: Springer-Verlag, 219-244.

Liskin L, Benoit E, Blackburn R (1992): Vasectomy: New Opportunities. Population Information Program, Johns Hopkins University, Baltimore, MD.

Lunn SF, Dixson AF, Sandow J, Fraser HM (1990): Pituitary-testicular function is suppressed by an LHRH antagonist but not by an LHRH agonist in the marmoset monkey. J Endocr 125.

Matsumoto AM (1988): Is high dosage testosterone an effective male contraceptive agent? Fertil Steril 50: 324-328.

Matsumoto AM (1990): Effects of chronic testosterone administration in normal men: safety and efficacy of high dosage testosterone and parallel dose-dependent suppression of luteinizing hormone, follicle-stimulating hormone and sperm production. J Clin Endocrinol Metab. 70: 282-287.

Nieschlag E (1986): Reasons for abandoning immunization against FSH as an approach to male fertility regulation. In G. I. Zatuchni, A. Goldsmith, J. M. Spieler & J. J. Sciarra (eds): "Male Contraception: Advances and Future Prospects" Harper & Row, 395-400.

Nieschlag E et al. (1992): Hormonal male contraception: a real chance? In E. Nieschlag & U. F. Habenicht (eds): "Spermatogenesis, Fertilization, Contraception: Molecular, Cellular and Endocrine Events in Male Reproduction" Berlin: Springer-Verlag, 477-501.

Nomura A, Heilbrun LK, Stemmermann GN, Judd HL (1988): Prediagnostic serum hormones and the risk of prostate cancer. Cancer Res. 48: 3515-3517.

Pangkahila W (1991): Reversible azoospermia induced by an androgen-progestagen combination regimen in Indonesian men. Int J Androl. 44: 248-256.

Patanelli DJ, Ed. (1977). Hormonal control of fertility. Washington, US Department of Health and Welfare.

Pavlou SN, Brewer K, Farley MG, Lindner J, Bastias MC, Rogers BJ, Swift LL, Rivier JE, Vale VW, Conn PM, Herbert CM (1991): Combined administration of a gonadotropin-releasing hormone antagonist and testosterone in men induces reversible azoospermia without loss of libido. J Clin Endocrinol Metab. 73: 1360-1369.

Pavlou SN, Heredotou D, Curtain M, Minaretzis D (1994). US Endocrine Society, Anaheim, #1324.

Schearer SB, Alvarez-Sanchez F, Anselmo J, Brenner P, Coutinho E, Latham-Faundes A, Frick J, Heinild B, Johansson EDB (1978): Hormonal contraception for men. Int J Androl. (suppl 2):680-712.

Schroeder FH (1990): Androgens and carcinoma of the prostate. In E. Nieschlag & H. M. Behre (eds): "Testosterone: Action Deficiency Substitution" Berlin: Springer-Verlag, 245-260.

Sharpe RM (1994): Regulation of spermatogenesis. In E. Knobil & JD Neill (eds): "The Physiology of Reproduction" Raven Press. Smith JC et al. (1994): Lancet. 344: 30.

Smith JC, Cranston D, O'Brien T, Guillebaud J, Hindmarsh J, Turner AG (1994): Fatherhood without apparent spermatozoa after vasectomy. Lancet. 344:30.

Spiteri-Grech J, Nieschlag E (1993): Paracrine control of testicular function: a review. J. Reprod. Fertil. 98: 1-14.

Talwar GP, Raghupathy R (1989): Anti-fertility vaccines. Vaccine. 7: 97-101.

Tom L, Bhasin S, Salameh W, Steiner B, Peterson M, Sokol R, Rivier J, Vale VW, Swerdloff RS (1992): Induction of azoospermia in normal men with combined Nal-Glu GnRH antagonist and testosterone enanthate. J Clin Endocrinol Metab. 75:476-483.

Trussell J, Kost K (1987): Contraceptive failure in the United States. A critical review of the literature. Stud Fam Planning. 18: 237-283.

United Nations (1989): Levels and trends of contraceptive use as assessed in 1988. Department of International Economic and Social Affairs, New York, 1989.

Wallace EM, Pye SD, Wild SR, Wu FCW (1993): Prostate-specific antigen and prostate gland size in men receiving exogenous testosterone for male contraception. Int J Androl. 16: 35-40.

Wang C, Yeung KK (1980): Use of low-dosage oral cyproterone acetate as a male contraceptive. Contraception. 21: 245-272.

Weinbauer GF, Khurshid S, Findscheidt U, Nieschlag E (1989): Sustained inhibition of sperm production and *inhibin* secretion by a gonadotrophin-releasing hormone antagonist and delayed testosterone substitution in non-human primates. (Macaca Fascicularis). Acta Endocr. 123: 303-310.

Weinbauer GF, Surmann FJ, Nieschlag E (1987): Suppression of spermatogenesis in a non-human primate (Macaca Fascicularis) by concomitant gonadotrophin-releasing hormone antagonist and testosterone treatment. Acta Endocr. 114: 138-146.

WHO Task Force on Methods for the Regulation of Male Fertility (1990): Contraceptive efficacy of testosterone-induced azoospermia in normal men. Lancet. 336: 955-959.

WHO Task Force on Methods for the Regulation of Male Fertility (1995): Contraceptive efficacy of testosterone-induced oligozoospermia in normal men (submitted).

WHO Task Force on Methods for the Regulation of Male Fertility (1993): Comparison of two androgens plus depot-medroxyprogesterone acetate for suppression to azoospermia in Indonesian men. Fert. Steril. 60: 1062-8.

Wu FCW, Aitken RJ (1989): Suppression of sperm function by depot medroxyprogesterone acetate and testosterone enanthate in steroid male contraception. Fertil Steril. 51: 691-698.

Wu FCW, Farley TMM, Peregaudon A, Waites GMH, WHOMTF (1995): Biochemical effects of exogenous testosterone in normal men; experiences from a multi-centre contraceptive efficacy study using testosterone enanthate. Fert. Steril. (in press).

# 40

# MALE CONTRACEPTION BASED ON TESTOSTERONE IN COMBINATION WITH OTHER AGENTS

**Eberhard Nieschlag, Gerhard F. Weinbauer and Hermann M. Behre**

**Institute of Reproductive Medicine University of Münster (WHO Collaborating Center for Research in Human Reproduction) D-48149 Münster, Germany**

## INTRODUCTION

This paper is based on the final presentation of a tripartite debate on the feasibility of hormonal contraception in the male. While the first discussant, G. Bialy, questioned the hormonal approach as such, the second, D.J. Handelsman, defended the position that testosterone alone would be sufficient for male contraception. The task of the third debater was to explore whether the combination of testosterone with other agents might have advantages over testosterone alone. Since previous speakers had reviewed individual approaches (Waites: testosterone alone; Swerdloff: GnRH analogs; Matsumoto, and also Arsyad: gestagens), this paper will not provide a complete survey of the field of hormonal male contraception, but will quote specific papers as required for the purpose of this presentation.

## REQUIREMENTS OF A HORMONAL MALE CONTRACEPTIVE

Concerned individuals, pressure groups and health advocates, as well as international conferences, such as the Womens' Conference on Contraception (Mexico, 1992) demand more and more that men play an active role in contraception and family planning. Representative public opinion polls reveal that a large proportion of men would be ready to accept a male contraceptive and to share the burden of birth control with their partners. However, aside from condom and vasectomy, men have little choice; in particular, there is no pharmacological method available for men. Although two large multicenter trials conducted by WHO (the only efficacy studies performed in hormonal male contraception to date), have

*Pharmacology, Biology, and Clinical Applications of Androgens*, edited by Shalender Bhasin et al.
ISBN 0-471-13320-5 © 1996 Wiley-Liss, Inc.

shown that testosterone alone suppresses spermatogenesis to a level compatible with contraceptive protection (WHO, 1990), no pharmaceutical company has adopted this approach and developed a male contraceptive based on testosterone. While representatives of industry assure us that they will remain "the major suppliers of innovative contraceptive methods in the future" (Vemer and Bergink, 1994), none of the companies engaged in the field of contraception is known to be actively involved in the development of hormonal male methods. The risk of unexpected side effects leading to huge damage claims may be particularly discouraging for the industry in the prevailing climate of litigation, but cannot be the only cause for the industry's lethargy towards hormonal male contraception. We may rather ask whether industry considers the approaches which have emerged from research so far insufficient for general application.

Pharmaceutical companies rely heavily on opinion surveys as part of their market analysis before they enter new fields. As mentioned above, opinion polls demonstrate readiness to use a male contraceptive. Nevertheless, they also reveal the major drawbacks of male contraceptives based on testosterone alone as seen by the potential users (Survey Research Associates, 1992): injections as such, and the long-lead time to effect, are considered as major drawbacks; and injections, even at monthly intervals, and the necessary visits to a doctor's office, loom as great deterrants. The negative attitudes describe the needs for a male contraceptive quite precisely: if injections are unavoidable, they should be as infrequent as possible and contraceptive protection should be guaranteed as quickly as possible. Furthermore, in the WHO multicenter trials quoted above testosterone enanthate alone produced azoospermia, which provides the safest contraceptive protection, only in 75% of all volunteers. In the remaining 25% the pregnancy rate was as high as 20 per 100 years of exposure as extrapolated from Table 2 in Waites and Farley (this volume). It appears that a higher rate of suppression and thus azoospermia should be achieved.

If testosterone alone may not achieve this goal, let us explore whether a combination with other agents may be more promising. An overview of the various possibilities and results is shown in Fig. 1.

## EFFECTIVENESS OF TESTOSTERONE PLUS GESTAGENS

When considering "effectiveness" of hormonal male contraception, it should be kept in mind that only two trials have been performed to date analyzing effectiveness of hormonal male contraception in terms of pregnancy rates, i.e. the two WHO multicenter trials (see Waites and Farley, this volume). "Effectiveness" in this chapter refers to the completeness of suppression of spermatogenesis as shown by azoospermia, or severe oligozoospermia, and to the time required to achieve this suppression.

Gestagens are potent inhibitors of LH and FSH secretion and therefore have been tested, in combination with testosterone, for male fertility regulation. Nore-thindrone, medroxyprogesterone acetate (MPA), depot-MPA (DMPA), 17-hydroxy-progesterone capronate and megestrol acetate have been used in clinical trials initiated by the WHO (1972 - 1983) and the Population Council (Schearer et al., 1978). The most favorable combination was the monthly intramuscular injection of 200 mg DMPA plus 200 mg testosterone enanthate or testosterone cypionate; this

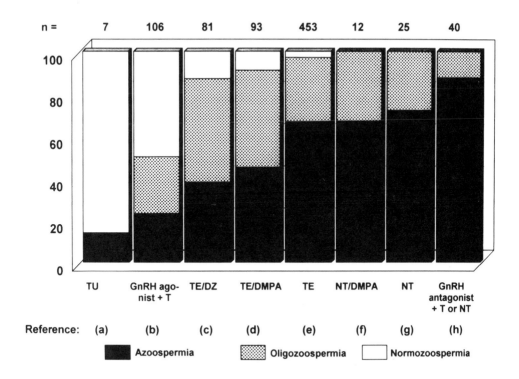

Fig. 1. Effectiveness of androgens alone or in combination with other steroids or GnRH analogs in achieving azoospermia or oligozoospermia in Caucasian men. T = testosterone; TU = testosterone undecaonate; TE = testosterone enanthate; NT = 19 nortestosterone hexyloxyphenylpropionate; DZ = danazol; DMPA = depot medroxyprogesterone acetate. Results from the following publications: a) Nieschlag et al., 1978; b) see Table 1; c) Paulsen et al., 1982; d) Schearer et al., 1978; Wu and Aitken, 1989; e) Waites and Farley, this volume; f) Knuth et al., 1989; g) Schürmeyer et al., 1984a; Knuth et al., 1985; Behre et al., 1992; h) see Table 2.

combination gave the best results in suppressing spermatogenesis and the incidence of untoward side effects was low. No negative effects on libido and potency were observed. However, this combination did not produce azoospermia uniformly; therefore its possible efficacy remained uncertain.

To develop a method that could be self-administered, 20 mg of MPA was given orally, together with 50 to 100 mg of testosterone percutaneously via a cream for one year (Soufir et al., 1983). Sperm counts in the six volunteers were suppressed to less than 5 million/ml for most of the study time, but azoospermia was not achieved. Guerin and Roullet (1988) tried various combinations of oral gestagens and transdermal or oral testosterone preparations. In all 12 volunteers treated with 5 or 10 mg/day 19-norethisterone orally, plus 250 mg (!) percutaneous testosterone daily, azoospermia was achieved within 8 weeks. These favorable results were mitigated by the elevated testosterone levels in the blood of female partners. In a similar study, the wives of five of the twelve men treated developed hirsutism secondary to testosterone being transferred to their skin from their husband's abdomen or buttocks (Delanoe et al., 1984). These untoward side effects made this approach, based on topical androgen application, unattractive, although it demonstrated the potential of a combined regimen.

Animal studies and studies in sexual delinquents have shown that the antiandrogen cyproterone acetate, which can be considered a potent gestagen, suppresses spermatogenesis, an effect exerted through the suppression of pituitary gonadotropin secretion. In clinical trials using 5 to 20 mg cyproterone acetate per day for up to 16 weeks, sperm counts and motility were reduced markedly (Fogh et al., 1979; Moltz et al., 1980; Wang and Yeung, 1980). Thus, cyproterone acetate appeared to be a possibility for male fertility control. However, decreases in serum testosterone levels to below normal were also observed. Some of the volunteers complained of fatigue, lassitude and decrease in libido and potency attributable to the diminished testosterone levels. Thus, although cyproterone acetate produces infertility, clinical trials have not been continued as the lowered testosterone levels were considered intolerable. The consequence would have been to combine it with testosterone. The combination of an androgen with an antiandrogen, however, appeared somewhat illogical and has therefore never been tested.

Danazol, a derivative of ethinyltestosterone, strongly inhibits LH and FSH secretion when given orally, but is devoid of other significant estrogenic or gestagenic activities. Various combinations of daily and oral doses of danazol with monthly injections of testosterone enanthate have been tested (Leonard and Paulsen, 1978). A daily oral dose of 600 - 800 mg danazol, in combination with 200 mg of testosterone enanthate monthly, induced azoospermia, or severe oligozoospermia. However, since the rate of azoospermia was not significantly higher than that achieved with testosterone alone, and since the daily steroid load was quite high and liver toxicity had been reported by female users (for treatment of endometriosis), these studies were not continued.

Since monotherapy with the long-acting androgen ester 19-nortestosterone injected every three weeks resulted in effective suppression of spermatogenesis to azoospermia in about 70% of the volunteers (Schürmeyer et al., 1984a), we tested the combination of 19-nortestosterone with DMPA to see whether it would result in even more complete suppression of spermatogenesis (Knuth et al., 1989). Twelve volunteers were injected weekly with 200 mg 19-nortestosterone hexyloxyphenyl-propionate, followed by injections with the same dose every three weeks up to week 15. In addition, the volunteers were injected with 250 mg DMPA in weeks 0, 6 and 9. Azoospermia was achieved in 9 of 12 volunteers during the study course, while in 3 of the remaining 4 volunteers, spermatogenesis was suppressed to single sperm, and in one volunteer to a sperm concentration of 1,3 mill/ml.

These promising results prompted the WHO Task Force on the Regulation of Male Fertility to launch a large-scale multicenter trial in five centers in Indonesia, comparing the effectiveness of testosterone enanthate, or 19-nortestosterone hexyloxyphenylpropionate in combination with DMPA (WHO, 1993). Surprisingly, 43/45 and 44/45 subjects in the testosterone and the 19-nortestosterone groups respectively suppressed to azoospermia. Unfortunately, this study had failed to include groups treated with the androgens alone, so that it remained unclear whether the azoospermia rates of 97% and 98% were due to the combination treatment, or could also be achieved by the androgens alone. The answer to this question was provided by Arsyad (1993) in an independent study who achieved azoospermia in 7/7 men from Palembang (Indonesia) by weekly injections of 100 mg testosterone enanthate.

The results from Germany and Indonesia quoted above highlight the ethnic differences in response to the same contraceptive agent which is also seen in Chinese men compared to Caucasians. The results reveal that testosterone alone may be a much more effective contraceptive in Asian than in Caucasian men. Notwithstanding these promising results, it should be kept in mind that in the Indonesian as well as in European studies, it took 20 weeks to achieve azoospermia. Therefore, even in the good responders, i.e. Asian men, another agent may be required to suppress spermatogenesis more rapidly. Perhaps such an additional agent may only be required at the beginning of the contraceptive phase. From all published evidence it appears that DMPA may not be the appropriate candidate for faster suppression. However, Wu and Aitken (1989) showed that the remaining sperm in the non-azoospermic men under DMPA, plus testosterone enanthate, may be impaired in their function. Since sperm function can ultimately only be tested *in vivo*, their observation requires confirmation in clinical efficacy studies, taking pregnancy rates, and not sperm counts, as the end point.

## EFFECTIVENESS OF TESTOSTERONE PLUS GnRH AGONISTS

Given in appropriate doses and after transient stimulation of the pituitary, GnRH agonists down regulate the pituitary GnRH receptors and cessation of gonadotropin secretion results. As a consequence, testicular function is suppressed. Exploiting the ensuing decrease of testosterone production, GnRH agonists are widely used clinically for the treatment of hormone-dependent prostate carcinoma. Since spermatogenesis is also suppressed, whether GnRH agonists, in combination with testosterone, may provide a male contraceptive, has been tested.

Between 1979 and 1992, results from 106 healthy men participating in 12 trials for male fertility regulation were published. In these studies the GnRH agonists decapeptyl, buserelin and nafarelin were administered at daily doses of 5 - 500 µg/volunteer for periods of 10 to 30 weeks. In about 30% of men, sperm production could be suppressed below $5 \times 10^6$/ml and in 21 men azoospermia occurred, while in the remaining volunteers, the sperm number was only slightly reduced or remained unaffected.

These results are not as good as those generated by steroid trials for male contraception, and therefore, GnRH agonists are no longer considered useful for male contraception. Two important general findings, however, emerged which were first described in monkeys serving as models in trials for male contraception. These results are important pointers for future investigations.

First, constant infusion of the GnRH agonist is much more effective in suppressing gonadotropins and testicular functions than single injections

Table 1. Overview of twelve clinical trials with GnRH agonists for male contraception involving 106 volunteers (from Nieschlag et al., 1992)

| Reference | Sub-jects (n) | Agonist | Daily dose μg/day | Route of admini-stration | Weeks of admini-stration | Androgen | Effect on sperm counts |
|---|---|---|---|---|---|---|---|
| Berquist et al. (1979) | 4 | buserelin | 5 | sc injection | 17 | none | none |
| Linde et al. (1981) | 8 | D-Trp[6] | 50 | sc injection | 6-10 | none | azoospermia in 1/8 |
| Doelle et al. (1983) | 6 | D-Trp[6] | 50 | sc injection | 20 | TE[a]100 mg biweekly | 12±4[b] |
| Rabin et al. (1984) | 8 | D-Trp[6] | 100 -500 | sc injection | 20 | TE 100 mg biweekly | 5.5[b] |
| Bhasin et al. (1985) | 7 | nafarelin | 200 | sc injection | 16 | TE 200 mg biweekly | 17±6[b] |
| Schürmeyer et al. (1984b) | 7 4 | buserelin buserelin | 118 230 | sc infusion sc infusion | 12 12 | TU daily TU daily | 18±5[b] 10±3[b] |
| Michel et al. (1985) | 7 | buserelin | 440 | sc infusion | 12 | TU daily | 44±14[b] |
| Pavlou et al. (1986) | 8 | D-Trp[6] | 500 | sc infusion | 16 | TE 100 mg biweekly | 4.5±11[b] in 5/8 |

| Study | N | Drug | Dose | Route | | Androgen | Result |
|---|---|---|---|---|---|---|---|
| Frick and Aulitzky (1986) | 6 | buserelin | 3x50 | nasal | 20 | none | none |
| | 4 | buserelin | 3x100 | nasal | 24 | none | azoospermia |
| | 4 | buserelin | 3x200 | nasal | 20 | fluoxymest | none |
| Bouchard and Garcia (1987) | 5 | D-Trp[6] microsperes | 100 | im | 15-60 | TE 125 mg biweekly | azoospermia in 0/5 |
| | 5 | D-Trp[6] | 100 | im | 15-60 | TU daily | azoospermia in 0/5 |
| Bhasin et al. (1987) | 7 | nafarelin | 400 | sc infusion | 16 | TE 200 mg biweekly | $4.5\pm1.1^{b}$ in 5/8 |
| Behre et al. (1992) | 8 | buserelin(3.3 mg) | | implant | 24 | 19NT 200mg | azoospermia in 2/8 |
| | 8 | buserelin(6.6 mg) | | implant | 24 | 19NT 200mg every 3 wk | azoospermia in 2/8 |

[a]Abbreviations: TE: testosterone enanthate; TU: testosterone undecanoate; fluoxymest: fluoxymesterolone; NT: 19-nortestosterone-hexyloxyphenylproprionate. [b]Lowest mean sperm counts.

(Schürmeyer et al., 1984b; Michel et al., 1985; Pavlou et al., 1986; Bhasin et al., 1987). Since this principle is also of advantage for patients with prostatic carcinoma, pharmaceutical companies have been working successfully on the development of slow-release preparations of GnRH agonists. From these, in turn, clinical trials for male contraception also benefited since the various implants developed obviated the cumbersome wearing of extracorporal pumps by the volunteers (Bouchard and Garcia, 1987; Behre et al., 1992b).

Secondly, as in monkeys (Akhtar et al., 1983), testosterone supplementation appeared to attenuate sperm-suppressing effects of GnRH agonists, since lower sperm counts were achieved in men receiving GnRH agonists, without simultaneous testosterone supplementation (Linde et al., 1981; Frick et al., 1986). Since it would be impossible to leave volunteers without testosterone substitution, i.e., with serum levels in the hypogonadal range, we tried to give androgens first and then added buserelin at a later stage. However, it could be shown in this controlled study that the combination of GnRH agonist with androgen is less effective than the androgen alone. An explanation for the ineffectiveness of GnRH agonist plus androgen is the escape of FSH suppression after several weeks of GnRH agonist treatment (Behre et al., 1992), a result that was later confirmed by others (Bhasin et al., 1994).

Altogether, GnRH agonists in combination with testosterone did not prove useful in male contraception and no further clinical studies appear to be under way.

## EFFECTIVENESS OF TESTOSTERONE PLUS GnRH ANTAGONISTS

In contrast to GnRH agonists, GnRH antagonists produce a precipitous and prolonged fall of gonadotropins and testosterone in men (e.g. Pavlou et al., 1989; Behre et al., 1994). However, as it was extremely difficult to develop GnRH antagonists suitable for clinical use (Karten et al., 1990), trials for male contraception using GnRH antagonists started later than those applying agonists. Meanwhile, preclinical studies in monkeys were undertaken and served as models for later trials in humans.

The studies in monkeys indicated that concomitant testosterone replacement using testosterone buciclate prevented the induction of azoospermia (Weinbauer et al., 1988), whereas a delay of androgen substitution permitted the induction of complete and sustained suppression of sperm numbers (Weinbauer, et al., 1989). In contrast, Bremner et al. (1991) reported induction of azoospermia during GnRH antagonist and concomitant testosterone administration using a different mode of androgen substitution and animals characterized by rather low sperm numbers at initiation of the study.

In five clinical trials summarized in Table 2, 35 of 40 volunteers, i.e. 88%, became azoospermic. In comparison to testosterone enanthate alone, which produces azoospermia in only 67% of Caucasian men within 6 months, this is a much better rate of complete suppression. In addition, the mean time to achieve azoospermia with testosterone enanthate alone is as long as 4 months, but appears to be considerably shorter when GnRH antagonists were added. Most of the GnRH antagonist-treated men became azoospermic within 12 weeks of treatment. Although the

Table 2. Overview of five clinical trials with GnRH antagonists and testosterone for male contraception

| Study | Antagonist | Daily dose | Duration of antagonist administration (weeks) | Androgen substitution | Rate of azoospermia (n/n) | Azoospermia reached by week |
|---|---|---|---|---|---|---|
| Pavlou et. al. 1991 | Nal-Glu | 10 mg | 20 | Delayed TE 25 mg/week | 6/6 | 12 |
| | " | 10 mg | 10 | dto. | | 16 |
| | | 20 mg | +10 | | 1/2 | |
| Tom et. al. 1992 | Nal-Glu | 7,5 mg | 16 | Delayed TE 150 mg/2 weeks | 7/8 | 10 |
| Bagatell et. al. 1993 | Nal-Glu | 100 µg/kg | 20 | Simult. TE 200 mg/week | 7/10 | 4-24 |
| Pavlou et. al. 1994 | Nal-Glu | 10 mg | 20 | Simult. TE 100 mg/week | 8/8 | 6-10 |
| Behre et. al. 1995 | Cetrorelix | Loading dose: 10 mg/day Maint. dose 2 mg/day | 12 | Delayed 19NT 400 mg initial 200 mg maint. | 6/6 | 4-12 |
| | | | | | 35/40 | |

TE = Testosterone enanthate; 19NT = 19 nortestosterone hexyloxyphenylproionate clinical investigations with GnRH antagonist are phase-I studies involving few subjects, it seems that in the human delayed testosterone administration (azoospermia in 20/22 men) offers little advantage over concomitant administration (azoospermia in 15/18 men). However, a higher dose of testosterone appears to prolong the time to complete suppression, indicating that testosterone does influence the effectiveness of the antagonist.

Recent studies in monkeys suggested that the suppression of spermatogenesis achieved by GnRH antagonists could be maintained after withdrawal of the antagonist by a testosterone preparation alone (Weinbauer et al., 1994). This finding could not be confirmed in a first human trial since sperm reappeared under continued 19-nortestosterone treatment when the antagonist cetrorelix was withdrawn (Behre et al., 1995b). This study, however, showed that much lower doses of the GnRH antagonist may be required to maintain suppression of spermatogenesis than to reduce it.

While Nal-Glu caused side effects in a few subjects, cetrorelix was well tolerated by all subjects who received it first in single doses, and then up to 12 weeks (Behre et al., 1992, 1994, 1995) or longer (for review: Reissmann et al., 1994). Cetrorelix is also being used for other indications including ovarian suppression for controlled ovulation induction in *in vitro* fertilization (Diedrich et al., 1994) and normal children have been delivered following this treatment. Since a depot preparation of cetrorelix was recently developed (Behre et al., 1995a), this antagonist has further potential for male contraception (and other indications).

In summary, GnRH antagonists, in combination with testosterone, appear to harbor a great potential for successful application in male contraception.

## CONCLUSION

From the above considerations it can be concluded that testosterone, in combination with GnRH antagonists, represents a favorable modality for male contraception. There are strong indications that testosterone depot preparations, such as testosterone buciclate or implants given together with GnRH antagonist depot preparations, may fulfill both requirements for a quick onset of contraceptive protection as well as for long injection intervals. However, these trials have yet to be conducted and the studies performed to date, although promising, provide only leads. From all existing evidence it can be concluded that such a combination (if appropriate antagonists are used) would be free of major side effects and the suppression of spermatogenesis should be fully reversible. Skeptics may argue that the price for GnRH antagonists may preclude them from development as a male contraceptive which should be affordable and in the price range of comparable female methods. If prices for GnRH antagonists would be in the range of those for GnRH agonists prescribed for the treatment of prostate carcinoma, they could never become part of a male contraceptive. However, prices are dictated by many variables and production costs will decrease with greater demand. In addition, based on screening of new compounds by binding to GnRH receptors *in vitro,* a chance exists that a cheap and perhaps orally effective GnRH antagonist may be identified. Therefore, it remains the scientists' task to demonstrate the feasibility of the combined use of testosterone and GnRH antagonist.

## ACKNOWLEDGMENT

The work from the Institute of Reproductive Medicine, University of Münster, summarized in this chapter was supported by the Max Planck Society, the Deutsche Forschungsgemeinschaft, the Federal Ministry of Health (Bonn) and the WHO.

## REFERENCES

Akhtar FB, Marshall GR, Wickings E., Nieschlag E (1983): Reversible induction of azoospermia in rhesus monkeys by constant infusion of a GnRH agonist using osmotic minipumps. J Clin Endocrinol Metab 56:534-540.

Arsyad KM (1993): Sperm function in Indonesian men treated with testosterone enanthate. Int J Androl 16:355-361.

Bagatell CJ, Matsumoto AM, Christensen RB, Rivier JE, Bremner WJ (1993): Comparison of a gonadotropin-releasing hormone antagonist plus testosterone (T) versus T alone as potential male contraceptive regimens. J Clin Endocrinol Metab 77:427-432.

Behre HM, Böckers A, Schlingheider A, Nieschlag E (1994a): Sustained suppression of serum LH, FSH, and testosterone and increase of high-density lipoprotein cholesterol by daily injections of the GnRH antagonist cetrorelix over 8 days in normal men. Clin Endocrinol 40:241-248.

Behre HM, Klein B, Steinmeyer E, McGregor GP, Voigt K, Nieschlag E (1992): Effective suppression of luteinizing hormone and testosterone by single doses of the new gonadotrophin-releasing hormone antagonist cetrorelix (SB-75) in normal men. J Clin Endocrinol Metab 75:393-398.

Behre HM, Kliesch S, Bock W, Hermann R, Reissmann Th, Engel J, Nieschlag E (1995a): Suppression of serum testosterone in normal men by Cetrorelix pamoate, a GnRH antagonist depot preparation. Exp Clin Endocrinol 103, Suppl 1.

Behre HM, Kliesch S, Lemcke B, Nieschlag E (1995b): Suppression of spermatogenesis to azoospermia by combined administration of GnRH antagonist and 19-nortestosterone cannot be maintained by 19-nortestosterone alone in normal men. (submitted).

Behre HM, Nashan D, Hubert W, Nieschlag E (1992): Depot gonadotropin-releasing hormone agonist blunts the androgen-induced suppression of spermatogenesis in a clinical trial of male contraception. J Clin Endocrinol Metab 74:84-90.

Bergquist C., Nillius SG, Bergh T, Skering G, Wide G (1979): Inhibitory effects on gonadotropin secretion and gonadal function in men during chronic treatment with a potent stimulatory luteinizing hormone-releasing hormone analogue. Acta Endocrinol 91:610-618.

Bhasin S, Heber D, Steiner BS, Handelsman DJ, Swerdloff RS (1985): Hormonal effects of gonadotropin-releasing hormone (GnRH) agonist in the human male. III. Effects of long-term combined treatment with GnRH agonist and androgen. J Clin Endocrinol Metab 60:998-1003.

Bhasin S, Berman N, Swerdloff RS (1994): Follicle-stimulating hormone (FSH) escape during chronic gonadotropin-releasing hormone (GnRH) agonist and testosterone treatment. J Androl 15:386-391.

Bhasin S, Yuan QX, Steiner BS, Swerdloff RS (1987): Hormonal effects of gonadotropin-releasing hormone (GnRH) agonist in men. Effects of long-term
treatment with GnRH agonist infusion and androgens. J Clin Endocrinol Metab
65:568-574.

Bouchard P, Garcia E (1987): Influence of testosterone substitution on sperm suppression by LHRH agonists. Horm Res 28:175-180.

Bremner WJ, Bagatell CJ, Steiner RA (1991): Gonadotropin-releasing hormone
antagonist plus testosterone: a potential male contraceptive. J Clin Endocrinol
Metab 73:465-469.

Delanoe D, Fougevrollas B, Meyer L, Thonneau P (1984): Androgenisation of
female partners of men on medroxyprogesterone acetate/percutaneous testosterone
contraception. Lancet 1:276.

Diedrich K, Diedrich C, Santos E, Zoll C, Al-Hasani S, Reissmann T, Krebs D,
Klingmüller D (1994): Suppression of the endogenous luteinizing hormone surge
by the gonadotrophin-releasing hormone antagonist Cetrorelix during ovarian
stimulation. Hum Reprod 9:788-791.

Doelle GC, Alexander AN, Evans RM, Linde R, Rivier J, Vale W, Rabin D (1983):
Combined treatment with an LHRH agonist and testosterone in man. J Androl
4:298:302.

Fogh M, Corcker CS, Hunter WM, McLean H, Philip J, Schon G, Skakkebaek NE
(1979): The effects of low doses of cyproterone acetate on some functions of the
reproductive system in normal men. Acta Endocrinol 91:545.

Frick J, Aulitzky W (1986): Effects of a potent LHRH agonist on the pituitary-
gonadal axis with and without testosterone substitution. Urol Res 14:261-264.

Guerin JF, Rollet J (1988): Inhibition of spermatogenesis in men using various
combinations of oral progestagens and percutaneous or oral androgens. Int J
Androl 11:187-199.

Karten MJ, Hoeger CA, Hook WA, Lindberg MC, Naqvi RH (1990): The development of safer GnRH antagonists: strategy and status. In Bouchard P, Haour F,
Franchimont P, Schatz B (eds): "Recent progress on GnRH and gonadal peptides." Paris: Elsevier, pp 147-158.

Knuth UA, Behre HB, Belkien L, Bents H, Nieschlag E (1985): Clinical trial of 19-
nortestosterone of male fertility regulation. Fertil Steril 44:814-821.

Knuth UA, Yeung CH, Nieschlag E (1989): Combination of 19-nortestosterone-
hexyloxyphenylpropionate (Anadur) and depot-medroxyprogesterone-acetate
(Clinovir) for male contraception. Fertil Steril 51:1011-1018.

Leonard JM, Paulsen Ca (1978): The use of androgens plus synthetic steroids as a
reversible means of regulating male fertility. In Fabbrini A, Steinberger E (eds):
"Recent progress in andrology." New York: Academic Press, p 271.

Linde R, Doelle GC, Alexander N, Kirchner F, Vale W, Rivier J, Rabin D (1981):
Reversible inhibition of testicular steroidogenesis and spermatogenesis by a potent
gonadotropin-releasing hormone agonist in normal men. N Engl J Med 305:663-
667.

Michel E, Bents H, Akhtar FB, Hönigl W, Knuth UA, Sandow J, Nieschlag E
(1985): Failure of high-dose sustained-release luteinizing hormone agonist
(buserelin) plus oral testosterone to suppress male fertility. Clin Endocrinol
23:663-675.

Moltz L, Römmler A., Post K, Schwartz U, Hammerstein J (1980): Medium dose cyproterone acetate (CPA): effects on hormone secretion and on spermatogenesis in man. Contraception 21:393.

Nieschlag E, Behre HM, Weinbauer GF (1992): Hormonal male contraception: a real chance? In Nieschlag E, Habenicht UF (eds): "Spermatogenesis - fertilization - contraception. Molecular, cellular and endocrine events in male reproduction." Heidelberg: Springer, pp 477-501.

Nieschlag E, Hoogen H, Bölk M, Schuster H, Wickings EJ (1978): Clinical trial with testosterone undecanoate for male fertility control. Contraception 18:607-614.

Paulsen CA, Bremner WJ, Leonard JM (1982): Male contraception: Clinical trials. In Mishell DR (ed): "Advances in fertility research." New York: Raven Press, pp 157-170.

Pavlou SN, Debold CR, Island DP, Wakefield G, Rivier J, Vale W, Rabin D (1986): Single subcutaneous doses of a luteinizing hormone-releasing hormone antagonist suppress serum gonadotropin and testosterone levels in normal men. J Clin Endocrinol Metab 63:303-308.

Pavlou SN, Brewer K, Farley MG, Lindner J, Bastias MC, Rogers BJ, Swift LL, Rivier JE, Vale WW, Conn PM, Herbert CM (1991): Combined administration of a gonadotropin-releasing hormone antagonist and testosterone in men induces reversible azoospermia without loss of libido. J Clin Endocrinol Metab 73:1360-1369.

Pavlou SN, Herodotou D, Curtain M, Minaretzis D (1994): Complete suppression of spermatogenesis by co-administration of a GnRH antagonist plus a physiologic dose of testosterone. 76th Meeting, Am Endocr Soc (Abstract) 1324.

Pavlou SN, Wakefield G, Schlechter NL, Lindner J, Souza KH, Kamilaris TC, Konidaris S, Rivier JE, Vale WW, Toglia M (1989): Mode of suppression of pituitary and gonadal function after acute or prolonged administration of a luteinizing hormone-releasing hormone antagonist in normal men. J Clin Endocrinol Metab 68:446-454.

Rabin D, Evans RM, Alexander AN, Doelle GC, Rivier J, Vale W, Liddle G (1984): Heterogeneity of sperm density profiles following 20-week therapy with high-dose LHRH analog plus testosterone. J Androl 5:176-180.

Reissmann T, Engel J, Kutscher B, Bernd M, Hilgard P, Peukert M, Szelenyi I, Reichert S, Gonzales-Barcena D, Nieschlag E, Comaru-Schally A (1994): Cetrorelix. Drugs of the Future 19:228-237.

Schearer SB, Alvarez-Sanchez F, Anselmo G, Brenner P, Coutinho E, Lathen-Faundes A, Frick J, Heinild B, Johansson EDB (1978): Hormonal contraception for men. Int J Androl Suppl 2:680-712.

Schürmeyer Th, Knuth UA, Belkien L, Nieschlag E (1984a): Reversible azoospermia induced by the anabolic steroid 19-nortestosterone. Lancet 1:417-420.

Schürmeyer Th, Knuth UA, Freischem CW, Sandow J, Akhtar FB, Nieschlag E (1984b): Suppression of pituitary and testicular function in normal men by constant gonadotropin-releasing hormone agonist infusion. J Clin Endocrinol Metab 59:1-6.

Nieschlag et al.

Tom L, Bhasin S, Salameh W, Steiner B, Peterson M, Sokol RZ, Rivier J, Vale W, Swerdloff RS (1992): Induction of azoospermia in normal men with combined Nal-Glu gonadotropin-releasing hormone antagonist and testosterone enanthate. Clin Endocrinol Metab 75:476-483.

Vemer H, Bergink W (1994): The role of industry in contraceptive research and development. Hum Reprod 9:376-379.

Wang C, Yeung KK (1980): Use of a low dosage oral cyproterone acetate as a male contraceptive. Contraception 21:245.

Weinbauer, GF, Göckeler E, Nieschlag E (1988): Testosterone prevents complete suppression of spermatogenesis in the gonadotropin-releasing hormone (GnRH) antagonist-treated non-human primate (*Macaca fascicularis*). J Clin Endocrinol Metab 67:284-290.

Weinbauer GF, Khurshid S, Fingscheidt U, Nieschlag E (1989): Sustained inhibition of sperm production and inhibin secretion induced by a gonadotropin-releasing hormone antagonist and delayed testosterone substitution in non-human primates (*Macaca fascicularis*). J Endocrinol 123:303-310.

Weinbauer GF, Limberger A, Behre HM, Nieschlag E (1994): Can testosterone alone maintain the GnRH antagonist-induced suppression of spermatogenesis in the non-human primate? J Endocrinol 142,485-495.

WHO (1972-1983): Special Program of Research Development and Research Training in Human Reproduction: Annual Reports. Geneva.

WHO (1993): Comparison of two androgens plus depot-medroxyprogesterone-acetate for suppression to azoospermia in Indonesian men. Fertil Steril 60:1062-1068.

Wu FCW, Aitken RJ (1989): Suppression of sperm function by depot medroxyprogesterone acetate and testosterone enanthate in steroid male contraception. Fertil Steril 51:691-698.

# DISCUSSION: HORMONAL METHODS FOR MALE CONTRACEPTION
## Chairpersons - Alvin Paulsen, Geoffrey Waites

**C. Alvin Paulsen:** In a stable union, if the wife or significant other becomes pregnant, the male can start the hormonal method (injections or pills) and be "infertile" by the time the wife has delivered and is in a position to resume sexual activity.

**David Handelsman:** I would like to make one point about the delay in achieving satisfactory contraceptive levels of sperm output. In the WHO studies it was always the third specimen that was required for what was called "consistent" azoospermia or "consistent" oligospermia. As the samples were two weeks apart, the first specimens at those levels were obtained a month in advance of those times shown on the slides. Suppression is still slow but it is not quite as slow as it looked.

**Jack Geller:** In the western world, the number one cause of mortality is heart disease. Testosterone enanthate in the dose of 200 mg a week, with its effects on lowering HDL, would be unacceptable if given for any length of time. If you lower the dose of androgen and add DMPA to achieve azoospermia you again create an HDL problem. If you use a GnRH antagonist with testosterone, you are dealing with a practical problem of cost. I wish to make a suggestion. For management of prostate cancer, progestational agents such as Megace, are quite effective, but there is an escape from it. There is tremendous synergism between very low doses of estrogen and other sex steroids whether they be progestational or androgenic. I suggest that in combination with lower doses of testosterone, 0.1 mg daily of DES, which has no effects on serum gonadotropins or testosterone by itself, might allow us to achieve adequate suppression of gonadotropins and the goal of azoospermia. The addition of low dose DES would not lower HDL and it would be cheap. A very mild non-progressive gynecomastia after about four to six months might be a potential concern.

**C. Alvin Paulsen:** The International Contraceptive Research Committee of the Population Council originally used the 19-nor progestational compounds (which are ordinarily found in the oral contraceptive agents), without the added estrogen. But *in vivo*, these 19-nor compounds are converted to estrogen. They noted adverse reactions such as gynecomastia, that caused them to disband that strategy. I believe that the estrogen in combination with androgens was tried by Bernard Robaire and Larry Ewing in monkeys, but this strategy was not found to be very effective in suppressing spermatogenesis, but perhaps this approach should be looked at again.

**Eberhard Nieschlag:** We should not fall into the trap of studying side effects on the nonfinal entity we are going to use in the clinic. We should concentrate on the underlying principles and develop better products. The side effects should be dealt with when we have a viable entity. For example, we now have a depot preparation for cetrorelix with much smaller doses. Now the question arises, how the original effects with the high dose would compare with those with the low dose. Similarly, testosterone enanthate given in these studies is something completely different than testosterone bucciclate or microspheres. Nevertheless, we should keep our eyes open for potential risk areas and identify those topics that require further attention.

**Bernard Robaire:** Testosterone and estradiol given via sustained release capsules were proposed in the late 70's by Ewing and myself as male contraceptives and those rat studies were expanded to monkey studies. The concern about gynecomastia was investigated and in the animal studies, where we can measure increases in breast mass, no increases were found. The doses of estradiol are very low. The basis of the principle for that therapy is that you are getting rid of the pulsatility of the steroid signals and that the hypothalamic pituitary complex responds to pulses, as opposed to flat signals. I believe the time has come for this group to re-examine the possibility of testing testosterone-estradiol combinations given in a sustained-release device as contraceptive in humans. Furthermore, the addition of estradiol should counteract any potential negative effect of testosterone on serum lipids and synergistically augment the action of testosterone on suppression of spermatogenesis.

**David Handelsman:** In studies using testosterone enanthate, the blood estradiol levels are quite high. Another point in reference to Dr. Geller's comment. It is very important not to focus entirely on biochemical markers like HDL cholesterol in isolation. It is one of a whole variety of risk factors for cardiovascular disease in an epidemiological context. We need to be looking at real outcomes, such as cardiovascular events, and not surrogate short-term biochemical markers.

**Gabriel Bialy:** Much of the work that Larry Ewing did, that Dr. Robaire mentioned, took place with NIH support. The primary effect of combined estrogen and testosterone implant in the monkeys was on motility of the spermatozoa; there was not much of an effect on the sperm numbers.

**Bernard Robaire:** There was 100% inhibition of fertility, which was completely reversible. But there was a decrease in both the number of spermatozoa and motility. The biochemistry of the sperm was not analyzed. The suppression was not complete, the doses were limited. We should look at these issues in the human.

**Wayne Meikle:** It seems that for these studies one dose of testosterone fits all, regardless of body size. The question is, whether there are differences in responses of suppression of sperm counts among different ethnic groups?

**David Handelsman:** In female contraception, one dose fits all, not only in one population, but in virtually all populations. In terms of the population differences in susceptibility to suppression, the question of body physique was looked at. There is no convincing evidence that response was related to physique.

**Cristina Meriggiola:** In Italy, we used cyproterone-acetate in combination with testosterone enanthate. Cyproterone-acetate is an antiandrogen but is also a progestin, so it can act both at the central level synergistically with testosterone in suppressing gonadotropins, and at the gonadal level, competing with endogenous or exogenous testosterone. We administered cyproterone-acetate at the dose of 100 mg/day and 50 mg/day together with testosterone enanthate 100 mg/week. We achieved a very quick and consistent suppression of spermatogenesis. All of our subjects became azoospermic. The group had only 10 subjects, but the azoospermia was consistent and very quick. Most importantly, we did not see any metabolic effects like the decrease of HDL that you show is present with testosterone alone, or with testosterone in combination with androgenic progestin, like Matsumoto showed with the combination of testosterone enanthate and levonorgestrol. This combination is very promising.

**Somnath Roy:** We carried out this study with cyproterone-acetate using 20 mg daily dose and testosterone enanthate 150 mg every two weeks. The suppression of gonadotropins was faster and more prolonged. The LH suppression is greater and intratesticular androgen levels are suppressed. Intratesticular testosterone plays an important role in the responders and nonresponders. The intratesticular testosterone levels are suppressed and cyproterone-acetate can counteract even that low level of androgen. We find rapid spermatogenic suppression within six to eight weeks. Simultaneous administration of testosterone prevents changes in libido. Any fear for suppressing the anabolic effect for a long time is also counteracted by this procedure. HDL level is increased by CPA treatment. Lastly, the dosage of both the steroids in the combination are much lower than have ever been used to achieve azoospermia.

**Ronald Swerdloff:** If you could turn off gonadotropins completely, you would have azoospermia. If you do hypophysectomy, the gonadotropins are gone and azoospermia occurs. Is it possible that there are differences between the responders and nonresponders in terms of the degree of LH and FSH suppression, that we cannot yet detect with the hormone assays that are available for LH and FSH?

**F.C. Wu:** Unfortunately, the levels of gonadotropins are so low that they are below the limit of detection of bioassay. But perhaps with the recombinant FSH receptor assays, we will be able to address this question more directly in the future. At present, we do have an *in vivo* index of gonadotropin bioactivity, which I tried to show by measuring the urinary epitestosterone excretion, if we agree that that is an index of endogenous Leydig cell activity, and if we agree that the adrenal does not contribute to epitestosterone secretion. We did not see any difference between the responders versus the nonresponders and, therefore, by deduction, it is unlikely that there will be any differences in the degree or the rates of gonadotropin suppression.

**Hermann Behre:** Some information on this question will be gained from the first study with testosterone bucciclate for male contraception. In this study, 3 out of 8 men became azoospermic after a single injection of 1200 mg testosterone bucciclate. In these 3 men, serum levels of LH and FSH were suppressed to the respective detection limit of the assay. Those 5 men who did not suppress to azoospermia had not clearly suppressed gonadotropin levels.

**F.C. Wu:** It is an interesting observation from Dr. Behre, but the numbers in each group is small. I would like to see a larger number before putting any significance into that.

**Alvin Matsumoto:** We have had experience in approximately 40 men that have either become, or not become, azoospermic on high-dose testosterone. In comparing gonadotropin levels, measured by immunofluorometric assays, most all of these individuals, except for maybe one or two, have detectable levels of immunoreactive LH and FSH. When comparing azoospermic versus nonazoospermic men on testosterone, we do not find a significant difference in the degree of gonadotropin suppression using these sensitive immunoassays. We also determined bioactive LH and FSH levels in men that were treated with high-dose testosterone using heterologous *in vitro* bioassays and found there was no difference in either serum LH or FSH bioactivity in those individuals that suppressed sperm production to azoospermia, compared to those that did not.

**Eberhard Nieschlag:**  The methodology used to measure gonadotropins is extremely important.  Here we are dealing with minute differences and you have to keep your assay under extreme control.  There is now assay technology available with better precision and sensitivity that may be very useful to answer this question.  I do not think that the gonadotropins alone are responsible for the different responses; it is the whole set point of the hypothalamic pituitary gonadal axis in these men.  That is what makes the difference and the gonadotropins are only an indicator for that.

**Stephen Winters:**  Several groups have reported data which suggest that 5 alpha-reductase activity is higher in Caucasians than in Asians.  Ethnic differences in 5 alpha-reductase activity, in part, may explain this ethnic difference in suppression of spermatogenesis by testosterone enanthate.

**Gui-Yuan Zhang:**  In order to answer the question whether there are ethnic differences in 5 alpha-reductase activity in Caucasians and Asians, we performed two studies.  In the first study we determined the overall 5 alpha-reductase activities following constant infusion of 3H-T in Chinese and American men.  No difference was found in the conversion rate of T to DHT in the two ethnic groups.  We further measured the 5 reductase activity in foreskin of normal Chinese men after a circumcision and we did not find any difference in 5 reductase activity between Chinese and American men.  We have found the same activities, particularly for type II isozyme.

I would like to ask Dr. Arsyad about the lipid metabolism in Indonesian men.  Did you find any changes in total cholesterol or HDL cholesterol levels after treatment by testosterone enanthate in combination with progestogens?  If you did, it would be very interesting to compare your results with results reported by Dr. Matsumoto from Seattle.  I want to know whether there was any difference in response between Oriental men and the Caucasian men.

**Kiagus Arsyad:**  Yes, there is an increase in metabolism, but it is still in normal range in Indonesian men.  Total cholesterol increased, HDL cholesterol also increased while receiving treatment, and both returned back to normal levels after injection stopped.

**Gui-yuan Zhang:**  Several pregnancies occurred in Caucasian couples when sperm count decreased to less than 5 mil/ml.  It is well known that testosterone induced oligospermia always caused severe damage to sperm function.  We have found that during the first two months after injection of testosterone, the sperm movement parameters significantly decreased.  I am wondering whether there is any extramarital pregnancy in Caucasian couples?

**Eberhard Nieschlag:**  If this method is so effective in China, why are you not using testosterone alone?

**Gui-yuan Zhang:**  Before WHO multicenter studies, we had no experience using testosterone enanthate alone but we have some experience using testosterone in combination with DMPA.  Overall, our experience has been limited.  We are going to conduct a national multicenter clinical trial using testosterone undecanoate alone, which is a long-acting injectable preparation.

**C. Alvin Paulsen:** Since you have this tremendous experience with testosterone enanthate alone demonstrating efficacy in the field trial, why not put that on the market now in China?

**Gui-yuan Zhang:** Because we have no TE produced in China. We have only imported preparation of TE. In addition, weekly injections of TE would not be acceptable as a male contraceptive in China.

**Christian Wang:** We only observed pregnancies in the Caucasian subjects who were consistently oligospermic (between 0.1 to 3 million). Because most of the Asian men became either completely azoospermic or had sperm count less than 1,000,000, it is anticipated that you will not see any pregnancies in Asians.

**David de Kretser:** It is also raising issues regarding elements of vital exposure. One element in exposure that has not been touched on is the frequency of intercourse, because that influences vital exposure rate. What are the intercourse rates in marital couples in different ethnic communities?

**Geoffrey Waites:** Yes we have some data on that. Menstrual diaries and frequency of intercourse were recorded. The frequency was higher in the non-Asian centers than in the Asian centers.

**Avraam Grinvald:** When the rectal digital exam is done for diagnosis of metastatic cancer, we know that 50% of cancers will be missed. Even if PSA test is done, still about 25% of the early cancers will still be missed. What is the risk that you are missing a patient with early stage prostate cancer? In order to be sure that these patients do not have prostate cancer, you must do a digital exam, PSA, and transrectal ultrasound, and you have to monitor the patients. Also, what is the chance for the patients to develop BPH?

**David Handelsman:** I think these are important considerations for anyone designing such trials and they were considered very carefully in the design and conduct of the WHO studies. First of all the subjects coming into the study were all under the age of 45, an age group in which clinical prostate disease is rare. The subjects had regular rectal examinations throughout the studies. In some centers, PSA measurements were done and there were no significant changes in PSA. The degree of additional monitoring is a question of degree and practicality. In men under the age of 45, no matter what treatment you use, highly invasive investigation for occult prostate cancer is not justifiable because the disease is very rare in that age group.

**F.C. Wu:** I would like to take issue with Professor Nieschlag. I disagree with his statement that we should not document the side effects in the prototype regimen. Testosterone enanthate 200 mg/week is indeed a prototype regimen and that in the very near future we will have much better long-acting androgens. However, we cannot ignore any of the side effects that the volunteers are currently reporting to us. After all, we are hopefully looking at a situation where these men will take testosterone for a very long time in the future and it may be a considerable time before we will be able to document what kind of serious side effects we have to deal with. We need long-term surveillance. When do you suggest we start long-term surveillance, and if so, what kind of monitoring do you think we should be doing?

**Eberhard Nieschlag:** I would fully agree with what you said. We should study the physiology and the pathophysiology of testosterone as much as we can. I did not say we should not monitor these effects, but the question is what to do with detailed observation of side effects of these prototype regimens? We run into problems if we have a study with 27 men and 3 have been found to be aggressive and oversexed on testosterone enanthate. This has far reaching implications if such information is spread widely while enanthate in these high doses will never be used for male contraception. It would be counter-productive to publicize this information widely. Instead, when performing trials with more definite testosterone preparations, we should carefully monitor issues which emerged as sensitive areas from pilot studies.

**Avraam Grinvald:** I would like to ask you why did you not include a Black population in your studies, because we know that in Black population, prostate cancer is a much higher risk than in the white population.

**Geoffrey Waites:** It was hard to recruit centers and principal investigators. We did not have a take-up in Africa, for example. We had only two centers in the United States where there might have been African-American volunteers. But we did not specifically encourage such volunteers to join the study and the end result was that no men of African origin participated. But you have raised an important issue, the variability of risk to prostate cancer between different population groups. While the risk is relatively high in African-Americans, it is currently very low in the Chinese and Indian populations.

**Richard Sharpe:** I would like to touch on a subject of reversibility. Every talker this morning has worked on the presumption that there is complete reversibility after suppression of spermatogenesis, whether that is complete or incomplete. And that is obviously justified by the recovery data from studies up to a year in man and perhaps longer in nonhuman primates. However, when spermatogenesis is suppressed for contraceptive purposes in the long-term, in the real world, five-ten years or longer (it does not really matter what methods you use to suppress it), how confidant can we be that at the end of that period there will be complete recovery, not only of sperm production rates, but of Leydig cell numbers and function?

**C. Alvin Paulsen:** I do not believe at this moment we have anyone who has been exposed continuously to steroids for spermatogenic suppression using testosterone singly or in combination with another agent for longer than a couple of years. We have had volunteers who have participated in about six of our studies at separate times over the last twenty years and they seem to recover each time. But I agree with Dr. Sharpe that we have to keep in mind there are conditions that we may not even think about at present that may occur.

**Geoffrey Waites:** The excellent work of Gerald Lincoln in Edinburgh showing that seasonally breeding animals decline to azoospermia and then recover normal spermatogenesis every season is encouraging, even though the period of intermittent suppression is less than five years.

**Bernard Robaire:** If you suppress spermatogenesis in rats with either testosterone alone or in combination, and you let them come back, is the progeny going to be normal? Have you affected the quality of the genome? This is the other side of your question "are the Leydig cells normal?" In our studies, after reversal, testosterone production was normal and progeny outcome was absolutely the same as in the controls.

**Eberhard Nieschlag:** I would like to remind you that none of the over 2,000 subjects who have participated in clinical trials for hormonal male contraception, have not returned to normal fertility. It gives the clinician a very safe feeling to know that we can always re-stimulate hypogonadotropic male patients even after long periods of azoospermia. The WHO in its wisdom commissioned studies in India where monkeys were exposed to GnRH agonists for two years. After recovery, fertility was tested and they were all as fertile as before. In addition, their testes were dissected and they were perfectly normal.

**Henry Gabelnick:** The clinical study was not done with testosterone and estradiol combination because, based on Larry Ewing's calculations, we were going to need about 20 feet of testosterone silicone tubing in the human. We have much better delivery systems today. In addition, we have more data. So I would suggest that we reconsider this protocol in humans.

**Hermann Behre:** We have recently done the first study with a GnRH antagonist depot preparation in men. One injection of this depot suppresses gonadotropins and testosterone for 3 to 4 weeks. There is no histamine release at all. In addition, the total dose of the depot GnRH antagonist to be given will be much lower and therefore the cost will come down as well.

Dr. Waites presented very encouraging results of the two WHO efficacy trials. You have shown that there was a relatively high rate of, but not complete, azoospermia. David Handelsman has shown in the first WHO efficacy trial that those men who suppressed to azoospermia had initially high FSH levels. Therefore, if we include in future trials unselected men without excluding those men with higher FSH, the rate of azoospermia might be even higher.

**C. Alvin Paulsen:** The issue is whether or not someone who has impaired spermatogenesis will be more sensitive to azoospermia by the injection of testosterone. Testosterone has been used in the United States since 1952 for the treatment of oligospermia and there does not appear, in the majority of individuals, to be increased sensitivity to suppression nor lack of recovery. Also, in our controversial radiation studies there was a consideration, but again, no definitive data to indicate that those individuals with oligospermia were more sensitive to the administration of ionizing radiation. But it is possible that you may encounter some individuals who are more sensitive to suppression of spermatogenesis and who may not fully recover to their original levels.

**David Handelsman:** There was a study from Seattle pointing out that higher FSH levels did predict a higher rate of azoospermia in a non-WHO contraceptive study. That was from Alvin Matsumoto.

**C. Alvin Paulsen:** Well, we have an honest difference of opinion. We analyzed all of our studies. We were unable to confirm that point.

**Amiya Sinha-Hikim:** The basic difference between an azoospermic subject and oligospermic subject is that in the latter case the spermatogenesis is still continuing though in a very slow rate. My question is, what are the driving forces in the oligospermic subjects which are helping to continue this spermatogenesis?

**Eberhard Nieschlag:** I presume it is the remaining testosterone in the testes, because we are not depleting the testes completely of testosterone. At the same time there may be some FSH left in circulation. And these two together guarantee that spermatogenesis continues. This is a very efficient system that can run with very low doses of fuel.

**Amiya Sinha-Hikim:** Is there any data showing that there is a difference in the levels of intratesticular testosterone or FSH between responders and nonresponders?

**Eberhard Nieschlag:** We know from monkey studies that antagonists can suppress gonadotropins very effectively and we can more or less deplete the testes of testosterone. So the antagonists are much more effective than agonists and they are much better for contraception than agonists.

**Amiya Sinha-Hikim:** Our studies on the time course of recovery of spermatogenesis in rats after GnRH-antagonist treatment demonstrate that the spermatogenesis recovers completely after GnRH antagonist treatment is discontinued. Most importantly, it follows the same time schedule as the normal germ cell development. The recovery of spermatogenesis is also accompanied by complete recovery of the Leydig cell morphology, total volume of Leydig cells, and the Leydig cell function.

**Gabriel Bialy:** I believe clinical studies need to be well designed and all the risks be taken into account. But I would also remind people that when Gregory Pincus was trying to introduce the first oral contraceptive, all kinds of fantastic scare scenarios were put forth; that women who took OCs for 20 years would have menopause at the age of 70 rather than 50. Most of these fears were not sustained. That is not to say that careful attention should not be given. NIH requires that if we do clinical studies that minority and gender representation be there. But if you have a group of individuals that is unusually susceptible to whatever disorder may be, you have to handle them very carefully and their representation on certain occasion may not be indicated.

# PART VII: ANDROGEN DELIVERY SYSTEMS

# 41

# ANDROGEN DELIVERY SYSTEMS: OVERVIEW OF EXISTING METHODS AND APPLICATIONS

Christina Wang

Division of Endocrinology
Department of Medicine
Harbor-UCLA Medical Center
1000 West Carson Street
Torrance, California 90509

An ideal androgen delivery system should be effective in correcting the symptoms and signs of hypogonadism; convenient to administer; acceptable to users; have predictable pharmacokinetics; simulate physiological levels of androgen; inexpensive; safe; and with low abuse potential (Wilson, 1988; Wang and Swerdloff, 1992). The currently available methods, as well as the methods under development, are shown in Table 1.

Table 1. Androgen Delivery Systems

| Currently Available | Under Development |
|---|---|
| Oral/Sublingual | Sublingual |
| 17 alkylated oral androgens (fluoxymesterone, methyl T) | T cyclodextrins |
| T undecanoate | |
| Micronized T | |
| Injectable | Long-Acting Injectables |
| T enanthate/cypionate | T buciclate |
| | T microspheres |
| Transdermal systems | Transdermal systems |
| Scrotal | Non-scrotal |
| Implants | |
| Pellets | |

*Pharmacology, Biology, and Clinical Applications of Androgens*, edited by Shalender Bhasin et al.
ISBN 0-471-13320-5 © 1996 Wiley-Liss, Inc.

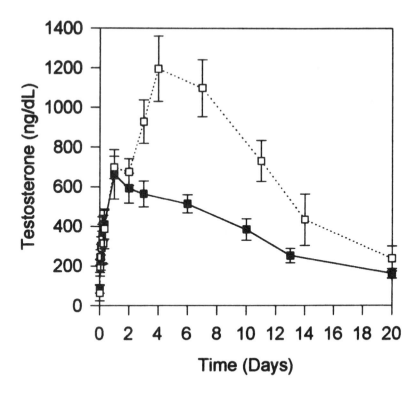

Figure 1. Serum T levels (mean ± SEM) after a single intramuscular dose of TE 200 or 400 mg administered to hypogonadal men at Day 0.

The 17 alkylated oral androgens, such as methyl T and fluoxymesterone, have significant higher risks of hepatoxicity than testosterone and its esters (e.g., testosterone enanthate, cypionate, undecanoate) (de Lorimier et al., 1965; Wilson, 1988). Moreover, the 17 alkylated oral androgens alter lipid profile, resulting in elevations of total and LDL cholesterol and suppression of HDL cholesterol (Friedl et al., 1990).

The most common intermediate-acting T preparation used throughout the world is T enanthate (TE). TE is usually given as an IM injection. Figure 1 shows the pharmacokinetics of TE (Delatestryl, BioTechnology General Corp., Iselin, N.J.) after a single administration of 200 mg IM to hypogonadal men (n=19) in the recent study. After a single IM injection of TE 200 mg, mean serum T levels rose twofold at half to one hour, and three to fourfold at four hours. Thereafter, serum T rose gradually to peak at two-to-four days after the injections. The levels fell, but not to pretreatment level, even at 20 days after injection. The calculated half life was 6.1 ± 0.9 days (range 1.7 to 16.2 days). This pharmacokinetic profile of TE was different from that previously reported by our group (Sokol et al., 1982) in that the peak levels of serum T appeared to be lower (day 1: present study 662 ± 125 ng/dl; Sokol et al., 1233 ± 484 ng/dl). When a single injection of 400 mg IM of TE was administered to another group of hypogonadal men (n=5), the serum T levels plateaued from 3 to 7 days and then decreased gradually to reach below normal adult range by about 3 weeks. From these studies, it could be concluded that increasing the TE dosage did not prolong its duration of action but increased the peak levels achieved during the first ten days after the injection. The usual recommended dosage of TE for replacement therapy is 200 mg once every 2 to 3 weeks. If patients became symptomatic or experienced large fluctuations in mood or sexual function, then TE could be administered as 100 mg IM once every 7 to 10 days.

Since the indications of androgen therapy might be expanded over the next few years to include possibly: male contraception, aging men, wasting diseases (HIV, cachexia) and post menopausal women, it is timely that the advantages and disadvantages of various alternative delivery systems will be reviewed in the following chapters. The questions that we may consider in the development of new androgen delivery systems are:

1. Do we need more potent androgens?
2. Which is the most efficient and acceptable androgen preparation/delivery system?
3. Can we develop "designer" androgens that have minimum side effects without loss of androgenic activity?
4. Do we need more androgen delivery systems than what we have now?

## ACKNOWLEDGMENT

The studies on the pharmacokinetics of TE were supported by a grant from BioTechnology General Corporation. (GYN-91-11) and the studies were performed at the General Clinical Research Center at Harbor-UCLA Medical Center, supported by NIH-NCRR (MO1 RR00425).

## REFERENCES

de Lorimier AA, Gordery GS, Lower RC, Carbone JV (1965): Methyltestosterone, related steroids, and liver function. Arch Intern Med 116:289-294.

Freidl KE, Hannan C, Jones RE, Kettler TM, Plymate SR (1990): High-density lipoprotein is not decreased if an aromatizable androgen is administered. Metabolism 39:69-77.

Sokol RZ, Palacios A, Campfield LA, Saul C, Swerdloff RS (1982): Comparison of the kinetics of injectable testosterone in eugonadal and hypogonadal men. Fertil Steril 37:425-430.

Wang C, Swerdloff RS (1992): Androgens. In: Smith CM, Raynand AM (eds.): "Textbook of Pharmacology." Philadelphia: W.B. Saunders, pp 683-694.

Wilson JD (1988): Androgen abuse by athletes. Endocr Rev 9:181-199.

# 42

# TESTOSTERONE TRANSDERMAL DELIVERY SYSTEM

Glenn R. Cunningham[1], Peter J. Snyder[2], Linda E. Atkinson[3]

[1]Departments of Medicine and Cell Biology
Baylor College of Medicine and
VA Medical Center
Houston, Texas 77030
[2]Department of Medicine
University of Pennsylvania School of Medicine
Philadelphia, PA 19104
[3]ALZA Corporation
Palo Alto, California 94303

## INTRODUCTION

Testoderm® (testosterone transdermal system) represents the first new form of androgen that has been cleared by the United States Food and Drug Administration in more than two decades. Previous efforts to develop a more effective androgen by chemically modifying the chemical structure were either less effective or less safe than the available depot forms of testosterone. The short-acting testosterone propionate, the longer-acting testosterone enanthate, and testosterone cypionate, have been the mainstays of replacement therapy even though their pharmacokinetics are not completely satisfactory. Testosterone undecanoate can be given orally, but its limited duration of action requires multiple large daily doses. For this reason it has never been approved for use in this country, although it is popular in Europe.

In 1983, scientists at ALZA Corporation explored the use of a transdermal system to administer testosterone. They found that the major problem was the quantity of testosterone to be delivered. Testosterone production rates in young adult men were estimated to be 6 to 7 mg/day (Southern et al, 1967). This required delivery of steroid that was 2 orders of magnitude greater than that delivered by the estradiol transdermal system that ALZA developed. The options for increasing delivery included, having very large systems, using enhancers to facilitate transdermal penetration, or finding skin that was more efficient in transporting testosterone. This led to the development of a trans-scrotal delivery system for testosterone.

*Pharmacology, Biology, and Clinical Applications of Androgens,* edited by Shalender Bhasin et al.
ISBN 0-471-13320-5 © 1996 Wiley-Liss, Inc.

Pilot studies conducted by Dr. Korenman proved that it was possible to absorb adequate amounts of testosterone from these systems (Korenman et al., 1987). Furthermore, the efficacy persisted for up to one year, and the systems were not associated with local or systemic side effects. Those studies did note that dihydrotestosterone (DHT) levels were increased above the normal range. Dr. Place and his colleagues at ALZA were sufficiently impressed with these results that they undertook multicenter studies in 1985.

## CLINICAL TRIALS

Two sizes (40 cm$^2$ or 60 cm$^2$) of the delivery system were studied in hypogonadal men at 14 academic centers. These systems contained 10 mg and 15 mg of testosterone. They were worn 22 hours per day, and the estimated testosterone delivery was approximately 2.4 mg and 3.6 mg of testosterone per day. In the initial studies, seventy-nine men in the United States, whose ages ranged from 18 to 77, used the systems on a daily basis. Eighty-five percent previously received an injectable form of testosterone. The major studies consisted of a 5-week pharmacokinetic study, two 12-week studies, and continued use. Several investigators have published the results from their institutions (Bals-Pratch et al., 1986; Findlay et al., 1987; Carey et al., 1988; Ahmed et al., 1988; Findlay et al., 1989; Cunningham et al., 1989), and the entire data has been summarized through two years and published (Place et al., 1990).

## 5-WEEK STUDY

Twenty-six patients completed the 5-week pharmacokinetic study (Figure 1).

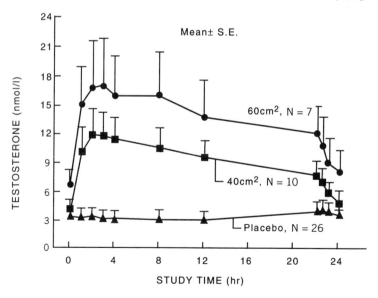

Figure 1. Pharmacokinetics of the 40 cm$^2$ and the 60 cm$^2$ of Testoderm® (testosterone transdermal system) in hypogonadal men (Place et al., 1990).

Patients applied the active Testoderm® system, or the placebo, daily, and the serum level of testosterone was determined on day 7. Peak concentrations of 12 and 17 nmol/L were obtained with the 40 cm² and 60 cm² systems. The maximum serum concentrations of testosterone with both systems occurred between 3 and 5 hours. The mean areas under the curve differed significantly between the two doses and with the placebo. As noted previously, the pharmacokinetic patterns resemble those observed in normal young men (Bremner et al., 1983).

## 12-WEEK STUDY

Fifty-four patients completed a 12-week study (Figure 2). Forty-two patients used the 40 cm² Testoderm systems for 4 weeks, followed by the 60 cm² systems for the next 8 weeks. Some patients who achieved normal blood levels of testosterone with the 40 cm² systems did not use the 60 cm² systems. Blood specimens were obtained 3 to 5 hours after application of the systems. Peak serum testosterone levels increased progressively during the first 3 weeks of the study. No differences were observed between values for week 3 and those for week 4. The mean levels achieved with the 60 cm² systems (weeks 5-12) were greater (p<0.001) than those achieved with the 40 cm² systems on week 4. This study was used to estimate the delivery of 2.4 mg and 3.6 mg of testosterone per day. Later, systems produced by a different and commercial process were re-evaluated and found to deliver 4 mg and 6 mg of testosterone per day.

The fractions of patients achieving normal testosterone and total androgen concentrations during the 12-week study are depicted in Table 1. Mean serum testosterone (T) levels were within the normal range in 61.5%. If the mean T + DHT levels are combined to represent total serum androgen, 80% of the men had values within the normal range.

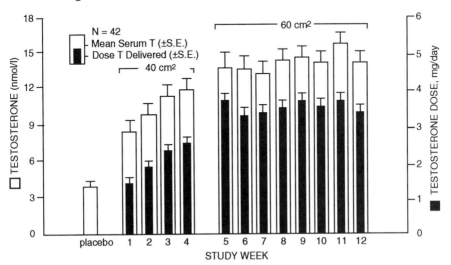

Figure 2. Mean serum testosterone levels and calculated dose of testosterone delivered (Place et al, 1990).

**Table 1: Patients Achieving Normal Testosterone and Total Androgen Concentrations After 12 Weeks of Testoderm® System Use**

| Mean Serum Level (nmol/L) | # Patients/Total | % |
|---|---|---|
| Total Testosterone | | |
| ≥ 12 | 48/78 | 61.5 |
| 10-12 | 7/78 | 9.0 |
| < 10 | 23/78 | 29.5 |
| Total T + Total DHT | | |
| ≥ 13 | 63/78 | 80.8 |
| < 13 | 15/78 | 19.2 |

The observation that serum DHT levels were increased raised the question as to the bioavailability of the circulating levels of androgen. Although not included in the original study design, sufficient serum was available from 28 men to permit measurements of T, bioavailable T, DHT, bioavailable DHT, $3\alpha$-androstanediol glucuronide, and sex hormone binding globulin (Demers et al., 1990). Values for the 40 cm$^2$ systems are from weeks 3 and 4. Values for the 60 cm$^2$ systems are from weeks 11 and 12. The mean values for total T, bioavailable T and sex hormone binding globulin are

**Table 2: Serum Testosterone (T) and Sex Hormone Binding Globulin (SHBG) in Hypogonadal Men Using Testoderm® Systems**

| | Placebo | 40cm$^2$ | 60cm$^2$ | Normal Range |
|---|---|---|---|---|
| Total DHT | 3.1±0.6 | 10.2±1.2 | 14.4±1.4 | 8.7-31.2 |
| (nmol/L) | (0) | (50) | (78) | |
| Bioavailable DHT | 1.0±0.3 | 4.0±0.5 | 6.9±0.8 | 3.8-12.7 |
| (nmol/L) | (0) | (39) | (76) | |
| SHBG | 37±3 | 36±3 | 33±3 | 10-73 |
| (nmol/L) | (100) | (100) | (100) | |
| N=28; Mean ±SE; (% patients above normal range) | | | | |

**Table 3: Serum Dihydrotestosterone (DHT) and $3\alpha$-Androstanediol Glucuronide ($3\alpha$-A-diol-G) in Hypogonadal Men UsingTestoderm® Systems**

| | Placebo | 40cm$^2$ | 60cm$^2$ | Normal Range |
|---|---|---|---|---|
| Total DHT | 0.5±0.1 | 4.9±0.7 | 6.5±0.7 | 1.0-5.2 |
| | | (32) | (50) | |
| Bioavailable DHT | 0.1±0.02 | 1.4±0.2 | 2.1±0.2 | 0.5-2.6 |
| | | (4) | (20) | |
| $3\alpha$-A-diol-G | 45±5 | 119±11 | 141±11 | 42-213 |
| | | (8) | (10) | |
| N=28; Mean ±SE; (% patients above normal range) | | | | |

shown in Table 2. The mean serum levels of total T and bioavailable T were proportional to the size of the system and were within the normal ranges at both doses. Bioavailable DHT and $3\alpha$-androstanediol glucuronide (Table 3) were within the normal ranges at both doses. The mean total DHT levels with the 60 cm$^2$ systems exceeded the normal range.

Subjective reports during the 12-week study have been tabulated. There were increases in mood and energy that were correlated with duration of treatment (Figure 3) and the serum level of testosterone over the range from 5 to 12 nmol/L (not shown). The number of waking erections and spontaneous erections/week were also strongly correlated with duration of treatment (Figure 4) and serum testosterone levels over this range.

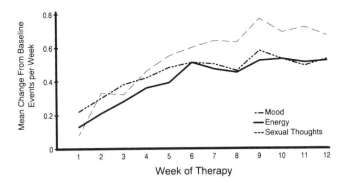

Figure 3. Subjective changes in mood, energy and sexual thoughts following initiation of Testoderm® therapy.

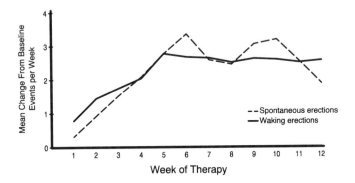

Figure 4. Subjective changes in spontaneous and awakening erections following initiation of Testoderm® therapy.

## CHRONIC USE

Sixty-eight patients used either the 40 cm$^2$ or the 60 cm$^2$ systems for one year or longer (Table 4). Thirty-two men have used the systems for 6 or more years. If one restricts the observations to those 32 men who completed 6 years of treatment, serum levels have remained remarkably stable (Table 5).

**Table 4:  Testosterone, Dihydrotestosterone, and Estradiol Levels During Chronic Testoderm® Therapy**

| Duration (yr) | Pts (#) | T (nmol/L) | DHT (nmol/L) | T/DHT | E$_2$ (nmol/L) | T/E$_2$ |
|---|---|---|---|---|---|---|
| B | 68 | 3.9+3.4 | 0.6+0.5 | 6.5+3.1 | 0.037+0.03 | 108+ 79 |
| 1 | 68 | 16.1+8.0 | 6.5+3.3 | 2.6+0.9 | 0.066+0.04 | 307+166 |
| 2 | 55 | 16.8+8.6 | 5.4+2.6 | 3.4+1.3 | 0.066+0.04 | 320+187 |
| 3 | 46 | 15.2+7.9 | 4.9+2.4 | 3.2+0.9 | 0.055+0.03 | 344+208 |
| 4 | 43 | 15.4+8.2 | 4.5+2.2 | 3.8+1.8 | 0.058+0.03 | 329+192 |
| 5 | 39 | 13.9+7.0 | 5.8+2.6 | 2.6+1.1 | 0.055+0.02 | 286+134 |
| 6 | 36 | 13.4+5.9 | 5.6+2.6 | 2.6+1.0 | 0.060+0.03 | 258+116 |
|  |  | Mean + SD |  |  |  |  |

**Table 5:  Testosterone, Dihydrotestosterone, and Estradiol Levels in 32 Men During Chronic Testoderm® Therapy**

| Duration (yr) | T (nmol/L) | DHT (nmol/L) | T/DHT | E$_2$ (nmol/L) | T/E$_2$ |
|---|---|---|---|---|---|
| B | 3.7+3.4 | 0.5+0.4 | 6.2+3.1 | 0.037+0.02 | 108+ 88 |
| 1 | 17.3+6.7 | 7.0+2.6 | 2.6+0.9 | 0.073+0.04 | 292+138 |
| 2 | 16.6+6.9 | 5.4+2.3 | 3.3+1.1 | 0.065+0.03 | 325+192 |
| 3 | 16.0+6.6 | 5.3+2.4 | 3.2+1.0 | 0.062+0.03 | 314+171 |
| 4 | 15.4+6.3 | 4.7+2.1 | 3.6+1.5 | 0.063+0.03 | 306+153 |
| 5 | 14.1+5.6 | 6.0+2.5 | 2.6+1.0 | 0.057+0.02 | 287+135 |
| 6 | 13.7+5.6 | 5.7+2.4 | 2.6+0.9 | 0.060+0.02 | 263+102 |
| Mean + SD |  |  |  |  |  |

The effects of Testoderm® systems on serum LH levels in 36 men with primary hypogonadism are illustrated in Figure 5.  LH levels became normal (<10 mIU/ml) in 17 men during the first year of treatment.  The mean serum T level in these 17 men was 17 nmol/L.

## HEMATOLOGY AND BLOOD CHEMISTRIES

Mean values for serum electrolytes, prostatic acid phosphatase, hepatic enzymes, and hematological measurements have remained within the normal range throughout the studies.  Longitudinal data for the 32 patients who have used the systems for 6 years are shown in Table 6.  Since patients were not required to be fasting, accurate measurements of serum triglycerides and LDL-cholesterol are not available.  Mean serum concentrations of total and HDL-cholesterol declined during the first year and then stabilized (Table 7).  The total cholesterol/HDL-cholesterol ratio  was increased by treatment, a finding that has been observed in hypogonadal men treated with testosterone esters (Godsland et al., 1987).

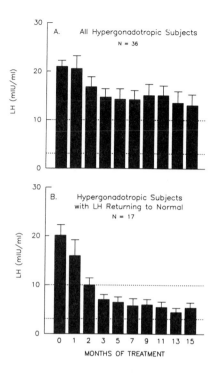

Figure 5. Serum LH levels in men with primary hypogonadism during Testoderm®
therapy (Place et al., 1990).

**Table 6: Hemoglobin, Serum AST and ALT in 32 Men
During Chronic Testoderm® Therapy**

| Duration (yr) | Hemoglobin (g/dL) | AST (7-41u/L) | ALT (0-49 u/L) |
|---|---|---|---|
| B | 15+1 | 27+11 | 34+27 |
| 1 | 15+1 | 24+ 5 | 21+10 |
| 2 | 15+2 | 23+ 9 | 17+10 |
| 3 | 15+2 | 20+10 | 20+12 |
| 4 | 15+1 | 15+ 1 | 18+ 8 |
| 5 | 15+2 | 17+ 5 | 18+11 |
| 6 | 15+2 | 21+ 8 | 28+21 |
|   | Mean + SD |  |  |

## SIDE EFFECTS

Patients using the systems have been remarkably free of local irritative side
effects. Over the initial 90,000 patient-days of wearing the systems, no patient had to stop
using the systems because of local irritative problems. In subsequent use, of 182,500

**Table 7:  Serum Lipids in 32 Men During Chronic Testoderm® Therapy**

| Duration (yr) | Total Cholesterol (nmol/L) | HDL Cholesterol (nmol/L) | TC/HDL |
|---|---|---|---|
| B | 6.3±1.1 | 1.2±0.3 | 5.3 |
| 1 | 6.0±1.1 | 1.1±0.3 | 5.5 |
| 2 | 5.5±1.0 | 1.1±0.2 | 5.2 |
| 3 | 5.5±1.0 | 1.1±0.2 | 5.8 |
| 4 | 5.6±1.0 | 1.1±0.3 | 6.1 |
| 5 | 5.7±1.0 | 1.1±0.3 | 6.2 |
| 6 | 5.9±1.0 | 1.0±0.2 | 6.3 |
| | Mean ± SD | | |

patient days, we are aware of four patients who stopped using the systems because of irritation.

A second study evaluating chronic use of Testoderm® systems examined serum prostate specific antigen (PSA) and prostate changes during treatment of hypogonadal men (Table 8). PSA levels at 6 and 12 months were not increased significantly, even though serum T became normal and serum DHT levels were elevated.

**Table 8:  Prostate Specific Antigen (PSA) Concentrations During Chronic Testoderm® System Use**

| Time (months) | PSA (ng/ml) | T (nmol/L) | DHT (nmol/L) |
|---|---|---|---|
| Baseline | 2.01±0.05 | 5.7±4.2 | 0.6±0.5 |
| 6 | 2.04±0.19 | 14.9±5.4 | 5.8±3.1 |
| 12 | 2.06±0.27 | 16.7±7.5 | 5.6±3.5 |
| p value | B v 6 mo: >0.7<br>B v 12 mo: >0.5 | B v 6 mo: <0.001<br>B v 12 mo: <0.001 | B v 6 mo: <0.001<br>B v 12 mo: <0.001 |

Mean ± SD; N=35

It is essential that patients treated with androgen are assessed for prostatic disease. As of June, 1994, an estimated 330 patients had used the system for approximately 500 patient-years in clinical trials. Five patients were diagnosed as having benign prostatic hyperplasia. Their ages, duration of prior androgen treatment, and duration of Testoderm® therapy are shown in Table 9. For three men, the diagnosis was prostate cancer. One of them is in a blinded study, so it is not known if he is receiving active drugs.

**Table 9:  Prostatic Disease During Androgen Replacement With Testoderm® Therapy**

| Patient (ID#) | Age (yrs) | Condition | Duration of Treatment | |
|---|---|---|---|---|
| | | | Prior (yrs) | Testoderm® (yrs) |
| 913 | 57 | BPH | 9+ | 0.5 |
| 4710 | 57 | BPH | 6+ | 0.5 |
| 26552 | 53 | BPH | 0.5 | 0.8 |
| 28003 | 77 | BPH | 1 | 7.0 |
| 28555 | 73 | BPH | 2 | 6.0 |
| 2113 | 56 | Ca | 3.2 | 0.6 |
| 1601 | 51 | Ca | 2.0 | 0.2 |
| 22 | 86 | Ca | 0 | 1.0(?) |

## COMMENTS

The delivery of testosterone to hypogonadal men by scrotal transdermal delivery systems has provided normal serum levels of testosterone in more than 60% of  patients. The pharmacokinetic pattern resembles that of young normal men.  While serum DHT levels are increased presumably by 5α-reductase in the scrotal skin, it is important to note that mean bioavailable serum DHT levels are not above normal.  Since DHT is an active androgen, this results in normal total androgen (T + DHT) levels in 80% of men. Further, the greater affinity of DHT for sex hormone-binding globulin, results in a bioavailable-T/total-T ratio that is slightly greater than that observed in normal men (0.68 vs 0.56), perhaps making this form of therapy more efficient in delivering testosterone to target tissues.

It is important to note that mean PSA levels are not increased above normal during chronic Testoderm® treatment.  Behre and colleagues (1994), also have shown that serum PSA levels are normal  and prostate volume increase to normal when hypo-gonadal men receive a variety of androgen replacement therapies.   Lack of effect on prostate and/or circulating PSA with other drugs that elevate serum DHT, such as percutaneous DHT gel (de Lignieres, 1995), or testosterone undecanoate (Gooren, 1986), point to the safety of higher-than-normal serum DHT concentrations.

Patients who use the transdermal systems have been remarkably free of local side effects or systemic toxicity.   No patient has had to stop treatment because of polycythemia, or hepatotoxicity.  Because androgen therapy returns prostate size and activity to normal, it is essential that patients treated with androgen be examined periodically for prostatic disease because benign prostatic hyperplasia, or prostate cancer, may occasionally appear.

## ACKNOWLEDGMENTS

The authors wish to recognize the important contribution of Virgil Place, M.D. and Nancy Trunnell, ALZA Corporation, and principal investigators listed below who participated in the multicenter studies.

M. Feingloss, Duke Medical Center; S. Korenman, UCLA; R. Krauss, University of California, Berkeley; A. Manni, Penn State University; J. Melby, Boston University; C.A. Paulson, University of Washington; R. Swerdloff, Harbor-UCLA Medical Center; J. B. Tyrrell, UCSF; M. L. Vance, University of Virginia; S. Winters, University of Pittsburgh; and T. C. Wong, Honolulu, Hawaii.

## REFERENCES

Ahmed SR, Boucher AE, Manni A, Santen RJ, Bartholomew M, Demers LM (1988): Transdermal testosterone therapy in the treatment of male hypogonadism. J Clin Endocrinol Metab 66:546-551.

Bals-Pratsch M, Knuth UA, Yoon Y-D, Nieschlag E (1986): Transdermal testosterone substitution therapy for male hypogonadism. Lancet 2:943-946.

Behre HM, Bohmeyer J, Nieschlag E (1994): Prostate volume in testosterone-treated and untreated hypogonadal men in comparison to age-matched normal controls. Clin Endocrinol 40:341-349.

Bremner WJ, Vitiello MV, Prinz PM (1983): Loss of circadian rhythmicity in blood testosterone levels with aging in normal men. J Clin Endocrinol Metab 56:1278-1281.

Carey PO, Howards SS, Vance ML (1988): Transdermal testosterone treatment of hypogonadal men. J Urol 140:76-79.

Cunningham GR, Cordero E, Thornby JI (1989): Testosterone replacement with transdermal therapeutic systems. JAMA 261:2525-2530.

de Lignieres B (1995): Effect of high dihydrotestosterone plasma levels on prostate of aged men. Second International Androgen Workshop, Long Beach CA, Abstract #27.

Demers LM, Atkinson LE, Place VA, Santen RJ (1990): Circulating androgen levels in hypogonadal men during therapy with TESTODERM® transdermal testosterone. Workshop Conference on Androgen Therapy, Marco Island, Florida. Abstract.

Findlay JC, Place VA, Snyder PJ (1987): Transdermal delivery of testosterone. J Clin Endocrinol Metab 64:266-268.

Findlay JC, Place VA, Snyder PJ (1989): Treatment of primary hypogonadism in men by the transdermal administration of testosterone. J Clin Endocrinol Metab 68:369-373.

Godsland BA, Wynn V, Crook D, Miller NE (1987): Sex, plasma lipoproteins, and atherosclerosis: prevailing assumptions and outstanding questions. Am Heart J 114:1467-1503.

Gooren LG (1986): Long-term safety of the oral androgen testosterone undecanoate. Int J Androl 9:21-26.

Korenman SG, Viosca S, Garza D, Guralnik M, Place V, Campbell P, Davis SS (1987): Androgen therapy of hypogonadal men with transscrotal testosterone systems. Am J Med 83:471-478.

McClure RD, Oses R, Ernest ML (1991): Hypogonadal impotence treated by transdermal testosterone. Urology 37:224-228.

Place VA, Atkinson L, Prather DA, Trunnell N, Yates FE (1990): Transdermal testosterone replacement through genital skin. IN: Nieschlag E, Behre HM (eds): Testosterone: Action, Deficiency, Substitution. Springer-Verlag.

Southern AL, Gordon GG, Tochimoto S, et al (1967): Mean plasma concentration, metabolic clearance and basal plasma production rates of testosterone in normal young men and women using a constant infusion procedure: Effect of time of day and plasma concentration on the metabolic clearance rate of testosterone. J Clin Endocrinol 27:686-694.

# 43

# *ANDRODERM*™: A PERMEATION ENHANCED NON-SCROTAL TESTOSTERONE TRANSDERMAL SYSTEM FOR THE TREATMENT OF MALE HYPOGONADISM

A. Wayne Meikle[1], Stefan Arver[3], Adrian S. Dobs[4], Steven W. Sanders[5], and Norman A. Mazer[2,5]

[1]Department of Medicine and Pathology, and

[2]Pharmaceutics, University of Utah, Salt Lake City, Utah

[3]Karolinska Institute, Stockholm, Sweden,

[4]Johns Hopkins University, Baltimore, Maryland

[5]TheraTech, Inc., Salt Lake City, Utah

## ABSTRACT

*Androderm*™ is a permeation enhanced non-scrotal testosterone transdermal system designed to treat male hypogonadism. This presentation will summarize the key results of four phase III clinical trials conducted in men between 15 and 65 years of age. The objectives of these studies were to evaluate the pharmacokinetics, metabolism, efficacy, and safety of *Androderm*™.

## Methods

A total of 116 hypogonadal men, including 23 previously untreated men, participated in the trials. Three of the studies had open-label treatment periods of 6 to 12 months duration. The fourth study is an ongoing open-label extension protocol. The primary efficacy parameters were morning hormone concentrations and 24 hour profiles of: testosterone (T), bioavailable testosterone (BT), dihydrotestosterone (DHT), estradiol (E2), sex hormone binding globulin (SHBG), luteinizing hormone (LH), and follicle stimulating hormone (FSH). The secondary

*Pharmacology, Biology, and Clinical Applications of Androgens*, edited by Shalender Bhasin et al.
ISBN 0-471-13320-5 ©1996 Wiley-Liss, Inc.

efficacy parameters included hypogonadal symptoms, mood, and sexual function. The sex hormone parameters were measured by Endocrine Sciences (Calabasas Hills, CA).

## Results

A total of 93% of patients used the standard two-patch regimen applied nightly to the back, abdomen, upper arms or thighs. This regimen delivered an average of 5 mg of testosterone per 24 hours, comparable to normal production rates. During chronic treatment (n=94), mean morning serum hormone concentrations (mg/dL) were: T (589±209 (SD)), BT (312±127), DHT (47±18) and E2 (2.7±1.2). Morning T values were within the normal reference range (306-1031 mg/dL) in 92% of patients. The 24 hour T profiles mimicked the morning peak and nighttime nadir observed in healthy young men. LH values became normal in 48% of patients with primary hypogonadism. In comparison to the untreated hypogonadal state (or androgen withdrawal period), *Androderm*™ treatment produced significant reductions in hypogonadal symptoms, improved mood and improved sexual function (see abstract by S. Arver et al.). Safety evaluations showed comparable results to injectable testosterone-enanthate treatment with regard to prostate, lipid profiles, and systemic laboratory parameters. *Androderm*™ was well tolerated by the majority of patients, with only transient erythema noted at some time during treatment. A total of 9% of patients stopped treatment due to chronic skin irritation (5%) or local allergic contact dermatitis to the system (4%).

## Abstract Conclusion

*Androderm*™ promises to be a more physiological, convenient and "patient-friendly" modality for testosterone replacement therapy than other currently available products.

## INTRODUCTION

Male hypogonadism (testosterone deficiency) may result from a variety of testicular, pituitary or hypothalamic disorders (Nieschlag 1990). Its symptoms include, sexual dysfunction, fatigue, depressed mood, and the absence or regression of secondary sexual characteristics. Testosterone replacement therapy should aim to produce physiological concentrations and mimic normal circadian patterns of testosterone and its active metabolites, dihydrotestosterone, and estradiol, (Behre 1990, Bhasin 1992).

*Androderm*™ is a permeation enhanced non-scrotal testosterone transdermal system, designed for the treatment of male hypogonadism (Mazer, 1992, Meikle, 1992). The *Androderm*™ system has six components as shown in figure 1. The drug reservoir (component 2) contains 12.2 mg of testosterone in a proprietary, permeation enhancing vehicle composed of water, ethyl alcohol, glycerin, glycerol monooleate, methyl laurate, and pharmaceutical gelling agents.

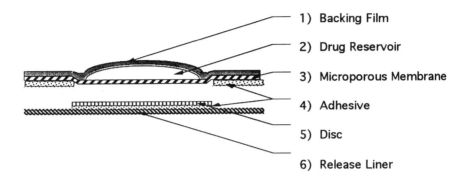

Figure 1. Cross-sectional schematic diagram of the *Androderm*™ Testosterone Transdermal system. The disc/release liner are removed prior to application of the system.

When applied to non-scrotal skin, the system is designed to deliver approximately 2.5 mg of testosterone over a 24 hour period, with approximately 60% of this amount absorbed during the first 12 hours. For adult hypogonadal men, the standard *Androderm*™ dosing regimen is two systems (patches) applied nightly to the abdomen, back, thighs or upper arms. This regimen delivers an average of 5 mg testosterone per 24 hours, comparable to the daily testosterone production rate of eugonadal men (Southren, 1968, Vermulen, 1972, Meikle, 1988).

This presentation will summarize the key results of four Phase III clinical trials involving *Androderm*™ therapy of hypogonadal men. The overall objectives were to evaluate the pharmacokinetics, metabolism, efficacy and safety during *Androderm*™ treatment.

## METHODS

### Clinical Trials

Information on the design and results of the individual clinical trials has appeared in abstract form (Meikle, 1993; Dobs, 1993, 1994; Arver, 1994). In brief, all four studies were multi-center phase III trials in hypogonadal men. Three of the studies had open-label *Androderm*™ treatment periods of 6 to 12 months duration. The fourth study is an ongoing open-label extension protocol.

### Patients

A total of 116 hypogonadal men (ranging in age from 15 to 65 years) participated in the four studies. Twenty-three had received no previous androgen replacement therapy. The study population included men with a variety of testicular, pituitary and hypothalamic causes of hypogonadism. Hypogonadism was defined by a morning serum testosterone of less than 306 mg/dL. All but four patients had developed secondary sexual characteristics before entering the studies.

## Efficacy Parameters

The primary efficacy parameters were morning hormone concentrations and 24-hour profiles of: testosterone (T), bioavailable testosterone (BT), dihydrotestosterone (DHT), estradiol (E2), sex hormone binding globulin (SHBG), luteinizing hormone (LH), and follicle stimulating hormone (FSH). The secondary efficacy parameters included, hypogonadal symptoms, mood, and sexual function (see abstract by S. Arver et al.). The sex hormone parameters were measured by Endocrine Sciences (Calabasas Hills, CA).

## Safety Parameters

The safety parameters included a blood chemistry panel, complete blood counts, urinalysis, prostate size, and appearance measured by transrectal ultrasound (TRUS), prostate specific antigen (PSA), coronary lipid risk profile and local skin tolerability.

## RESULTS

## Pharmacokinetics and Metabolism

Nightly application of two *Androderm*™ systems at approximately 10:00 p.m. results in a profile of serum testosterone concentration that mimics the normal circadian variation observed in healthy young men (Fig. 2). Maximum concentrations occur in the early morning hours with minimum concentrations in the evening. Bioavailable (non-SHBG bound) testosterone concentrations (BT) measured during *Androderm*™ treatment paralleled the total serum testosterone concentration and remained within the normal reference range (92-420 mg/dL).

Morning serum testosterone concentrations reach the normal range during the first day of dosing. There is no accumulation of testosterone during continuous treatment. Upon removal of the Androderm systems, serum testosterone concentrations decrease with an apparent half-life of approximately 70 minutes. Hypogonadal baseline concentrations are reached within 24 hours after removal of the system. During chronic treatment, these baseline concentrations decrease via feedback suppression of the pituitary-gonadal axis.

Single dose pharmacokinetic studies in a group of 34 hypogonadal men (Meikle, 1993), showed that application of two *Androderm*™ systems to the back, abdomen, thighs, or upper arms resulted in average testosterone absorption of 4 to 5 mg over 24 hours. Applications to the chest and shins resulted in greater inter individual variability and a lower mean 24 hour absorption (3 to 4 mg) than other sites used. The serum testosterone concentration profiles during application were

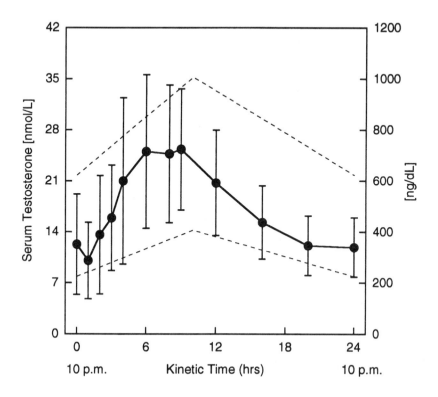

Figure 2. Mean (SD) serum testosterone concentrations derived from steady-state pharmacokinetic studies in hypogonadal patients (n=52). Two *Androderm*™ systems were applied to the back of each patient at approximately 10:00 p.m. Dashed lines represent 95% confidence interval for the circadian variation observed in healthy young men (Mazer, 1993).

similar for all sites.

In both single dose and steady-state pharmacokinetic studies, DHT and E2 levels remained within the normal reference ranges, and the DHT/T and E2/T ratios were comparable to those in eugonadal men, approximately 1:10 and 1:200, respectively (Meikle, 1979, 1989). These findings indicate that the 5α-reductase and aromatase activities of non-scrotal skin do not produce any significant pre-systemic metabolism of testosterone during *Androderm*™ treatment (Mazer, 1992, 1993).

## Normalization Of Hormone Levels

The hormonal effects of *Androderm*™ were demonstrated in 94 hypogonadal men. In this population, 93% of patients were treated with two *Androderm*™ systems daily, 6% used three systems daily, and 1% used one system

Table 1.  Individual morning serum hormone concentrations (mg/dL) and percentage of patients with mean concentrations within the normal range during continuous *Androderm*™ treatment (n=94).

|              | T           | BT         | DHT      | E2         |
|--------------|-------------|------------|----------|------------|
| Normal Range | (306-1031)  | (93-420)   | (28-85)  | (0.9-3.6)  |
| Mean         | 589         | 312        | 47       | 2.7        |
| SD           | 209         | 127        | 18       | 1.2        |
| % Normal     | 92          | 88         | 85       | 77         |
| % High       | 1           | 12         | 2        | 22         |
| % Low        | 7           | 0          | 13       | 1          |

daily.  On these dosing regimens *Androderm*™ produced mean morning serum concentrations of testosterone within the normal reference range in 92% of patients. The mean (SD) serum hormone concentrations of T, BT, DHT and E2 and percentage of patients who achieved average concentrations within the normal reference ranges are shown in Table 1.

A physiological suppression of the pituitary-gonadal axis occurs during continuous *Androderm*™ treatment leading to reduced serum LH concentrations.  In the combined clinical trials, 10 of 21 (48%) men with primary (hypergonadotrophic) hypogonadism achieved normal range LH concentrations within six to 12 months of treatment.  LH concentrations were observed to remain elevated in some patients despite serum testosterone concentrations within the normal range.

## Effects on Hypogonadal Symptoms, Mood, and Sexual Function

In one of the clinical trials, twenty-nine patients, previously treated with testosterone, completed 12 months of *Androderm*™ treatment .  Following an 8-week androgen withdrawal period, *Androderm*™ treatment produced positive effects on fatigue, mood and sexual function.  The percentage of patients complaining of fatigue decreased from 79% to 10% during treatment ($p<0.001$).  The average patient depression score (Beck Depression Inventory)  decreased from 6.9 to 3.9 ($p<0.001$).  Nocturnal penile tumescence and rigidity monitoring showed an increase in mean duration of erections from 0.23 to 0.39 hours per night ($p=0.01$) and an increase in penile tip rigidity from 18% to 50% ($p<0.001$).  The total number of self-reported erections reported increased from 2.3 to 7.8 per week ($p<0.001$) (see abstract by S. Arver et al.).

## Comparison with Intramuscular Testosterone

In another of the trials, sixty-six patients, previously treated with testosterone injections, received *Androderm*™ or intramuscular testosterone enanthate (200 mg every 2 weeks) treatment for 6 months.  The percentage of time that serum concentrations measured throughout the dosing interval remained within the normal range were as follows:

Table 2.

| | *Androderm*™ | IM | *p* value |
|---|---|---|---|
| T | 82% | 72% | 0.05 |
| BT | 87% | 39% | <0.001 |
| DHT | 76% | 70% | 0.06 |
| E2 | 81% | 35% | <0.001 |

Sexual function was comparable between the two groups.

## Effect on Plasma Lipids

In patients who were treated for 6 to 12 months (n=67), the averages (SE) serum total cholesterol and HDL concentrations were 199 (7.6) mg/dL and 46 (2.3) mg/dL.

Compared with a hypogonadal state achieved during eight weeks of androgen withdrawal in 29 patients, the following changes in lipids were observed during one year of *Androderm*™ treatment: Cholesterol decreased 1.2%; HDL decreased 8%; Cholesterol/HDL ratios increased 9%. In these patients, lipids measured during *Androderm*™ treatment were not significantly different from those measured during treatment with IM injection of testosterone.

## Effects on the Prostate

Prostate size and serum prostate specific antigen (PSA) concentrations during treatment were comparable to values reported for eugonadal men. One case of a prostate carcinoma occurred during *Androderm*™ treatment; two cases were detected during IM treatment.

## Skin Tolerability

*Androderm*™ is generally well tolerated with the majority of treated patients having only occasional and/or transient erythema at the application site. Of all patients exposed to *Androderm*™ in the clinical trials (including phase II studies (Meikle, 1992)), only 9% discontinued treatment due to skin reactions, of whom 5% had chronic irritation and 4% had allergic contact dermatitis. The later occurred after 3 to 8 weeks of use. Based on these findings the local tolerability of *Androderm*™ appears comparable to other transdermal products on the market (Hogan, 1990).

## CONCLUSION

*Androderm*™ delivers physiological amounts of testosterone, produces normal range concentrations of testosterone and its metabolites which mimic the circadian rhythms of healthy young men, and improves hypogonadal symptoms, mood and sexual function. In comparison to other currently available products, *Androderm*™ promises to be a more physiological, convenient and "patient-friendly" method for androgen replacement therapy.

## ACKNOWLEDGMENT

Support for these studies was provided by USPHS grants M01 RR-00064, DK-45760, DK-43344 and TheraTech, Inc. AWM, SA, and ASD were independent from TheraTech and contributed in experimental design and data analysis of the investigation.

## REFERENCES

Arver S, Dobs AS, Meikle AW, Sanders SW, Caramelli KE, Laskshminarayan R, Mazer NA (1994): Hormone levels, endocrine responses and sexual function in hypogonadal men treated for one year with a non-scrotal testosterone transdermal delivery system (T-TDS). Program of Endocrine Society 1308 (Abstract).

Behre HM, Oberpenning F, Nieschlag E (1990): Comparative pharmacokinetics of androgen preparations: Application of computer analysis and simulation. in Nieschlag E & Behre HM, eds., Testosterone: Action, Deficiency, Substitution, Springer-Verlag, Berlin, p. 115-135.

Bhasin S (1992): Clinical Review 34: Androgen treatment of hypogonadal men. J Clin Endocrinol Metab 74:1221-1225.

Dobs AS, Rajaram L, Arver S, Meikle AW, Sanders SW, Mazer NA (1993): Pharmacokinetics of non-scrotal testosterone (T) transdermal delivery system (T-TDS) after three months of use in hypogonadal men. Program of Endocrine Society 384 (Abstract).

Dobs AS, Bachorik PS, Arver S, Meikle AW, Sanders SW, Caramelli KE, Lakshminarayan R (1994): Interrelationships between lipoprotein levels, sex hormones and anthropometric parameters in hypogonadal men treated with a non-scrotal testosterone transdermal delivery system (T-TDS). Program of Endocrine Society 1307 (Abstract).

Hogan DJ, Maibach HI (1990): Adverse dermatologic reactions to transdermal drug delivery systems. J Am Acad Dermatol 22:811-814.

Mazer NA, Heiber WE, Moellmer JF, Meikle AW, Stringham JD (1992): Enhanced transdermal delivery of testosterone: A new physiological approach for androgen replacement in hypogonadal men. J Controlled Release 19:347-362.

Mazer NA, Sanders SW, Ebert CD, Meikle AW (1993): Mimicking the circadian pattern of testosterone and metabolite levels with an enhanced transdermal delivery system. In Gurney, Junginger, Peppas, (eds) Pulsatile Drug Delivery: Current Applications and Future Trends. Wiss, Verl, Gess, Stuttgart, pp. 73-97.

Meikle AW, Stringham JD, Wilson DE, Dolman LI (1979): Plasma 5α-reduced androgens in men and hirsute women: Role of adrenals and gonads. J Clin Endocrinol Metab 48:969-975.

Meikle AW, Stringham, JD, Bishop DT, West DW (1988): Quantitating genetic and nongenetic factors influencingandrogen production and clearance rates in men. J Clin Endocrinol Metab 67:014-109.

Meikle AW, Smith JA, Stringham JD (1989): Estradiol and testosterone metabolism and production in men with prostatic cancer. J Steroid Biochem 33:19-24.

Meikle AW, Mazer NA, Moellmer JF, Stringham JD, Tolman KG, Sancers SW Odel WD (1992): Enhanced transdermal delivery of testosterone across non-scrotal skin produces physiological concentrations of testosterone and its metabolites in hypogonadal men. J Clin Endocrinol Metab 74:623-628.

Meikle AW, Arver S, Hoover DR, Sanders SW, Mazer NA (1993): Application site influences on the enhanced transdermal delivery of testosterone to hypogonadal men. Program of Endocrine Society 383(Abstract).

Nieschlag E, Behre HM (1990): Pharmacology and clinical uses of testosterone. In Nieschlag E, Behre HM, eds., Testosterone: Action, Deficiency, Substitution Springer-Verlag, Berlin, p. 92-114.

Southren AL, Gordon GG, Tochimoto S (1968): Further study of factors affecting the metabolic clearance rate of testosterone in man. J Clin Endocrinol 28:1105-1112.

Vermuelen A, Rubens R, Verdonck L (1972): Testosterone secretion and metabolism in male senescence. J Clin Endocrinol 34:730-735.

# 44

# ANDROGEN DELIVERY SYSTEMS: TESTOSTERONE PELLET IMPLANTS

David J. Handelsman

Andrology Unit
Royal Prince Alfred Hospital
Departments of Medicine,
Obstetrics and Gynecology
University of Sydney
Sydney, NSW, 2006 Australia

## INTRODUCTION

Androgen treatment can be considered in three categories: (1) physiological, (2) pharmacological, and (3) androgen misuse/abuse. Pharmacological applications of androgens as second-line therapy in non-androgen deficient individuals (e.g., osteoporosis, anemia, breast cancer, angioedema) as well as the therapeutic irrationality of androgen abuse are outside the scope of this review which focuses on testosterone pellet implants as an androgen delivery system in physiological settings. These include androgen replacement therapy (ART) in hypogonadism, or aging, and for hormonal male contraception, all of which have in common the use of androgens intended at levels for physiological replacement therapy for spontaneous, partial, or induced androgen deficiency, respectively.

## GOALS OF AN ANDROGEN DELIVERY SYSTEM

A physiological androgen delivery system must overcome the basic pharmacological limitations of testosterone which were recognized soon after the first clinical use of androgens (Hamilton, 1937). These features include a very low oral bioavailability (Foss, 1939) and brief duration of action parenterally (Parkes, 1938), due to rapid hepatic metabolism (Frey et al., 1979; Hellman et al., 1956; Nieschlag et al., 1977; Nieschlag et al., 1975) which dictate that achieving durable androgynic effects, requires depot, sustained-release testosterone formulations (Foss, 1939; Parkes, 1938). The goal of ART is pharmacological replication of physiological effects of endogenous testosterone, which, in effect, requires imitating blood testosterone levels. This requires approximating average endogenous, total and free, testosterone levels. Attempts at slavish recreation of other aspects of androgen physiology without known physiological importance (e.g. diurnal or ultradian rhythms; concentrations of other androgens, precursors or metabolites) merely creates unjustified complexity. The practical intent of ART is thus to maintain stable, physiological testosterone levels for prolonged periods. The ideal androgen preparation for long-term ART would be safe, effective, inexpensive, convenient, already marketed, and would be long-acting with reproducible, zero-order dissolution profile. Not surprisingly, even after 5 decades of clinical use of androgens, this requirement is not yet met fully. Testosterone remains the preferred androgen for safety and efficacy reasons, as synthetic androgens may have unpredictable toxicological risk (e.g. hepatotoxicity of 17-$\alpha$ alkylated androgens), and/or an incomplete spectrum of androgynic effects if their metabolic activation (5$\alpha$ reduction, aromatization) is restricted.

## HISTORY

Subdermal implants of crystalline testosterone were among the earliest depot modalities employed for androgen therapy (Deansley et al., 1937; Deansley et al., 1938; Howard et al., 1939; Vest et al., 1939) following experimental observations that they provide the most potent and durable effects of any steroid formulation (Biskind et al., 1941; Deansley and Parkes, 1937; Deansley and Parkes, 1938; Dorfman et al., 1941; Hamilton et al., 1939). Similar depots were reported for most bioactive steroids (Eidelsberg et al., 1940; Emmens, 1941; Forbes, 1941; Foss, 1942; Loeser, 1940), including desoxycorticosterone acetate (DOCA) depots lasting up to 1 year for treatment of Addisons disease (Thorn et al., 1940). Despite long availability, there have been few clinical (Reiter, 1963; Swyer, 1953) or pharmacological (Bishop et al., 1951) studies. Furthermore, clinical applications have dwindled and there were no pharmacological development of implants in the postwar era presumably due to their off-patent status. Recently, interest has been rekindled in the UK (Cantrill et al., 1984) and Australia (Conway et al., 1988) and, particularly after pharmacological studies, showing their near-ideal depot properties and prolonged duration of action (Handelsman, 1990; Handelsman, 1991; Handelsman et al., 1990), have led to a 10-fold increase in the utilization of testosterone pellet implants in Australia over a decade.

## FORMULATION AND PHYSICAL FEATURES

The original testosterone implants were manufactured by high pressure compression of crystalline steroid, mixed with an excipient (usually cholesterol), into discoid or cylindrical shapes with convex ends (Bishop and Folley, 1951). These compressed implants were brittle, difficult to sterilize, provoked fibrotic reactions and had erratic absorption rates late in pellet life (Bishop and Folley, 1951; Emmens, 1941). Consequently, the modern fused, fully biodegradable implants were developed in the early 1950's. Fused pellets are made without excipients by melting testosterone (MP 154-155$^0$ C) and casting the steroid in a suitably shaped mold. Fused implants are more uniform in composition, less brittle or irritating, and provide stable dissolution patterns. Sterilization is ensured by heating during manufacture and terminal gamma-irradiation. Testosterone pellet implants are manufactured as cylinders in 200 and 100 mg sizes; only the 200 mg implants (length 12 mm, diameter 4.5 mm, surface area 202 mm$^2$) are used for ART. Smaller implants (25, 50 & 100mg) have been used for adolescents and in gynecology.

## IMPLANT PROCEDURE

Pellets are implanted under sterile conditions for routine minor office surgery. The procedure takes about 15 minutes and is easily learned by doctors or nurses with experience of minor surgery. The preferred puncture site is the lower abdominal wall in the periumbilical region; but other possible sites used include the deltoid, gluteal, and upper thigh. Under local anesthesia, a small (1 cm) incision about 5 cm from the mid-line at umbilical level to allow introduction of the trocar (7.5 French gauge, 5mm ID, 7 cm length). Pellets are expelled from the trocar by an obturator in individual tracks, 5-10 cm away from the puncture site in a fan-shaped distribution. The puncture is closed without suture by adhesive strips and covered with a water-resistant dressing for a week. Antibiotics are not routinely required.

## ABSORPTION

### Mechanism of Absorption

Testosterone is absorbed from the pellets into the extracellular fluid via a uniform erosion of the pellet's surface. Thus absorption rate is dictated by the exposed surface area from which steroid dissolves. Pellets retain their cylindrical shape for up to 3 months after implantation and a mathematical model incorporating a uniform rate of surface erosion (Forbes, 1941) fits well to data available from direct measurements of release rate (Bishop and Folley, 1951). Direct evidence for pellet surface area-limited dissolution rate in-vivo is provided by higher free testosterone concentrations and greater gonadotropin suppression provided by the 16% higher initial surface area of a 600 mg dose, consisting of six 100 mg implants, compared with three 200 mg implants during the first 3 months (but not later) after implantation (Handelsman, 1990; Handelsman, Conway et al., 1990). Deviations from the simple surface erosion model might occur when the absorbing area enlarges unpredictably due to surface irregularities, pellet fragmentation or if the absorption mechanism changes as the pellet size diminishes (e.g. to matrix-diffusion controlled or encasing by fibrosis); but there have been no human studies examining the influence of pellet geometry, absorption mechanism, or site of implantation.

### Absorption Kinetics

Effective testosterone release rate from pellets calculated directly from measurement of residue in extruded pellets and indirectly from the near-linear, percent absorbed-time plots, are in agreement. The direct estimate of absorption rate

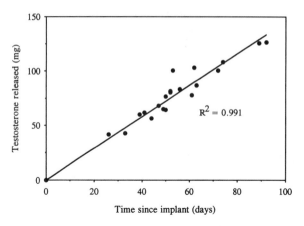

Figure 1.   Testosterone release rate from twenty 200 mg implants collected at various times after spontaneous extrusion.

of 1.5 (95% C.L. 1.4-1.7) mg/day for 200mg pellets was derived from remnants of 20 extruded pellets which exhibit linear dissolution rate in vivo for at least 92 days (figure 1). Additionally, estimates of effective half-time for absorption of 2.5 months and testosterone release rate of 0.65 mg/day/100 mg pellet were derived from the absorption isotherms. The relatively lower dissolution estimates of 1.1 mg/day for 100mg pellets removed at intervals after implantation in the antecubital or subscapular region (Bishop and Folley, 1951) may reflect differences according to implant site. Comparable, but less accurate quantitative estimates, are also derived from increments in blood testosterone following implantation of single 100 mg and 200 mg pellets in women (Dewis et al., 1986; Thom et al., 1981) after correction for gender differences in testosterone clearance rates (Southren et al., 1968).

## Bioavailability

The bioavailability of testosterone from subdermal pellet implants is virtually 100% by 6 months as estimated from the time-course of blood testosterone levels. Net testosterone release is closely correlated with pellet dose so that a 6x200 mg dose regimen gives twice that of either 6x100 mg or 3x200 mg regimen, which were equivalent. This high bioavailability is predictable for a steroid administered parenterally to reach the systemic circulation without first-pass hepatic inactivation.

# PHARMACOLOGY

## Pharmacokinetics

The pharmacokinetics of testosterone pellet implants were studied in 43 hypogonadal men (22 hyper-, 21 hypo-gonadotropic) previously treated with intramuscular testosterone ester injections who underwent 3 testosterone pellet regimens (6x100 mg, 3x200 mg, 6x200 mg; total of 111 implants) in a random

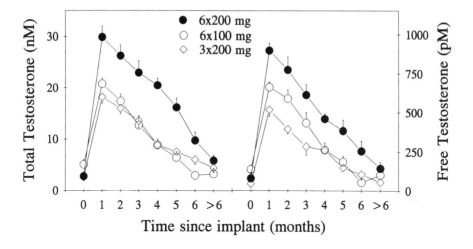

Figure 2. Plasma total (left) and free (right) testosterone following a single implantation in 43 hypgonadal men.

sequence at intervals of [3]6 months with monthly blood sampling for testosterone and gonadotropin assays (Handelsman et al., 1990). Total and free testosterone levels were highly reproducible and dose-dependent. Peak testosterone levels are achieved 2-4 weeks after implantation and initial accelerated ("burst") release (Burris et al., 1988; Diaz-Sanchez et al., 1989) is observed only during the first 24 hours (Jockenhovel et al., 1993) but not in daily (Handelsman et al., 1990) or weekly (Conway et al., 1988) sampling after implantation. Plasma testosterone levels gradually return to baseline by 6 months after 600 mg regimens, but remain elevated after 6 months following the 1200 mg dose. Plasma-free testosterone gave virtually an identical time-course to total testosterone (r=0.90), except that free testosterone levels were significantly higher in the first 3 months after the 600 mg regimen with greater initial surface area, consistent with an effect of initial pellet surface area on early testosterone release rates.

## Pharmacodynamics

The pharmacodynamics of testosterone pellet implants were studied by the effects of implantation on clinical state (well-being, sexual function), gonadotropin suppression (in men with hypergonadotropic hypogonadism), SHBG levels, and biochemistry. Generally, suppression of elevated gonadotropins in men with primary hypogonadism mirrored closely both the clinical androgynic effects, and maintenance of physiological testosterone levels. Thus, clinical monitoring is readily augmented by blood testosterone levels, as well as gonadotropin suppression in men with hypergonadotropic hypogonadism.

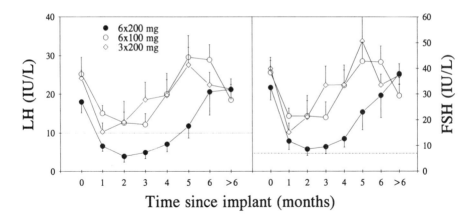

Figure 3. Plasma LH (left) and FSH (right) following a single implantation in 22 men with hypergonadotropic hypogonadism. The horizontal line represents the upper limit of eugonadal reference range.

The clinical effects on sexual function and well-being were consistent between all 3 regimens with adequate replacement for 4-5 months on either 600 mg regimen, or for 6 months on the 1200 mg dose combination. Gonadotropin suppression was studied in 22 hypergonadotropic men. Plasma LH and FSH were markedly suppressed in parallel by all 3 regimens in a dose- and time-dependent fashion. The 1200 mg regimen produced greater and more sustained suppression than either 600 mg regimens. Nadir LH and FSH was between 1-3 months with 600 mg and 1-4 months with the 1200 mg regimen, the latter reaching eugonadal levels. LH levels returned to baseline at 5 (600 mg) and 6 (1200 mg) months. Nadir FSH levels remained elevated above eugonadal levels in all 3 treatment regimens. Plasma SHBG levels are unaffected following implantation of up to 1200 mg testosterone pellets, contrasting with parenteral testosterone esters and oral testosterone undecanoate (Conway et al., 1988). This supports the interpretation (Conway et al., 1988) that reduced SHBG levels should be interpreted as a manifestation of excessive hepatic androgen effects comparable with estrogens (von Schoultz et al., 1989). Routine biochemical variables demonstrated androgynic effects in increasing hemoglobin levels while plasma iron and urea fell reciprocally in a time-course consistent with testosterone and gonadotropin levels. These changes reflect the anabolic effects of androgens (Gardner et al., 1983; Kochakian, 1976; Mooradian et al., 1987). There were no significant or consistent changes in liver function tests, lipids or other routine toxicological, biochemical or hematological variables following pellet implantation (Cantrill et al., 1984; Conway et al., 1988; Handelsman, 1990; Handelsman, 1991; Conway et al., 1990).

## Comparison with Other ART Modalities

Direct comparison of 3 widely used testosterone formulation (intramuscular testosterone ester injections, testosterone pellet implants, oral testosterone undecanoate) in a random-sequence, cross-over clinical trial demonstrated the clear superiority of testosterone pellet implants in clinical and biochemical effects, as well as patient preference (Conway et al., 1988). After experience of all 3 modalities, patients equally preferred pellets (6/14,43%) or im testosterone ester injections (6/14,43%) but one year later most (12/14,86%) had switched to pellet implants and none used oral testosterone. Similarly after the larger pharmacological study (Conway et al., 1990), most (30/43,70%) preferred to continue using testosterone pellets rather than returning to intramuscular injections. The principal reasons for preferring implants were, dislike of wide swings in androgen effects, and need for frequent medical visits with injections.

## ADVERSE EFFECTS

Pellet implantation has few minor and no major side-effects observed in >650 implant procedures over 10 years. Minor discomfort at the puncture site rarely lasts for more than a few hours or requires analgesia. Infection and bleeding are rare (<1%). Minor bleeding from the incision site is readily controlled by topical pressure. The only regular side-effect is pellet extrusion which occurs after ≈7% of implant procedures; the rate depending on operator skill and yet unidentified individual-specific factors. Most extrusions involve the loss of only a single pellet and require no specific treatment. Fibrosis at prior implant sites is uncommon in contrast with older compressed, cholesterol-containing implants (Bishop and Folley, 1951), such as those available in the USA.

## CLINICAL USE

### Indications, Contra-indications & Precautions

Androgen deficiency of any type sufficient to warrant ART is an indication for testosterone pellet implants. Pellets are particularly suitable for hypogonadal men who dislike, or cannot have, regular im injections (e.g. adolescents, travelers, anticoagulants or bleeding disorder). Precautions include using pellets only after tolerance of androgen replacement is established with shorter-acting testosterone preparations. Implantation may be more difficult in very thin or keloid-prone individuals. The only absolute contra-indications are those relating to androgen therapy itself, such as prostate or breast cancer or those relating to minor surgery, such as bleeding disorders, or allergy to local anesthetics. In the rare circumstance requiring rapid termination of testosterone therapy (e.g. diagnosis of prostate cancer), removal could be achieved with minor surgery if necessary, although no removals have been required in >650 implantations over 10 years.

### Dosage and Monitoring

The pellet testosterone release rate of 1.5mg/day for a 200 mg pellet allows a highly flexible dosing schedule to replicate the physiological testosterone production rate (3-9 mg/day; (Southren et al., 1968)) by implantation of two to six

200 mg pellets (400-1200 mg, release rates 3-9 mg/day) lasting for 4-6 months. The standard initial ART dosage is 4x200 mg implants. Using 100 mg pellets as well, it is theoretically possible to span the physiological range in 0.75 mg/day increments. Individual monitoring of adequacy of androgen replacement is monitored by observing clinical effects, testosterone levels and, in men with primary hypogonadism, suppression of gonadotropin levels. A patient's first implant is monitored with monthly blood samples, but, due to the reproducibility of effects within individuals, after subsequent uncomplicated implants, patients are only reviewed after the 4th month to determine need for the next implantation.

## Costs

The average daily retail costs of ART (drug+doctor+overhead costs, $AUD) are comparable between pellet implants ($1.39) and im testosterone esters ($1.28) with both lower than oral testosterone undecanoate ($5.50); relativities differ in UK where pellets are the least expensive (Cantrill et al., 1984). Partitioning the costs for implants and injections, the raw ingredients costs are <2 and ≈20 cents/day, and medical costs 30 cents and 82 cents/day.

## Extended Applications

Beyond the classical indication of ART, testosterone pellet implants might be useful in treating partial androgen deficiency in aging men and for the induced androgen deficiency of hormonal male contraceptive regimens.

Hormonal regimens including androgens alone, or with progestins or GnRH antagonists, are being tested to reversibly suppress spermatogenesis sufficiently to provide a reliable male contraceptive. Testosterone pellet implants (1200 mg) suppress human spermatogenesis as effectively as weekly testosterone enanthate injections but requiring less than half the daily testosterone dosage (9 vs 21 mg/day), thereby eliminating dose-dependent side-effects, including acne (Handelsman et al., 1992). Further downward dose-ranging studies using implants alone or with a depot progestin are underway (Handelsman, unpublished). The popularity of Norplant, which requires implantation as well as removal of six non-biodegradable rods under local anesthesia (McCauley et al., 1992), suggests that testosterone pellet implants might form part of a hormonal male contraceptive regimen acceptable to at least some subpopulation of men.

Recent small, short-term studies have examined the role of androgen therapy to reverse the deleterious effects of declining testosterone levels in aging men, particularly among those with chronic medical illnesses in whom the age-related fall is accentuated (Handelsman et al., 1985; Nieschlag et al., 1982; Vermeulen, 1990). Larger and longer studies are required to establish the safety, efficacy and specific indications for ART in elderly men. Testosterone pellet implants, by virtue of their long-acting properties, convenience and efficacy, together with avoiding supraphysiological testosterone levels, could facilitate such critical studies.

# CONCLUSION

Testosterone pellet implants have many of the ideal features of a long-acting androgen depot, including being safe, highly effective with stable clinical and biochemical effects,  economical, providing flexible dosing, and excellent long-acting properties due to a near-zero-order dissolution. A single biodegradable implant of 600-1200 mg provides stable, effective and well-tolerated androgen replacement for 4-6 months and pellets can provide excellent androgen replacement in most physiological settings. The only limitations are the requirement for minor surgery for implantation and extrusions which occur  after ≈7% of procedures by an experienced operator.

# REFERENCES

Bishop PMF, Folley SJ (1951): Absorption of hormone implants. Lancet. ii: 229-32.

Biskind GR, Escamilla RF, Lisser H (1941): Implantation of testosterone compounds in cases of male eunuchoidism. J Clin Endocrinol Metab 1: 38-49.

Burris AS, Ewing LL, Sherins RJ (1988): Initial trial of slow-release testosterone microspheres in hypogonadal men. Fertil Steril 50: 493-497.

Cantrill JA, Dewis P, Large DM, Newman M, Anderson DC (1984): Which testosterone replacement therapy? Clin Endocrinol 24: 97-107.

Conway AJ, Boylan LM, Howe C, Ross G, Handelsman DJ (1988): A randomised clinical trial of testosterone replacement therapy in hypogonadal men.  Int J Androl 11: 247-264.

Deansley R, Parkes AS (1937): Factors influencing effectiveness of administered hormones. Proceeding of the Royal Society London series B. 124: 279-98.

Deansley R, Parkes AS (1938): Further experiments on the administration of hormones by the subcutaneous implantation of tablets. Lancet. ii: 606-608.

Dewis P, Newman M, Ratcliffe WA, Anderson DC (1986): Does testosterone affect the normal menstrual cycle? Clin Endocrinol 24: 515-21.

Diaz-Sanchez V, Garza-Flores J, Larrea F, Richards E, Ulloa-Aguirre A, Veayra F (1989): Absorption of dihydrotestosterone (DHT) after its intramuscular administration. Fert Steril 51:493-7.

Dorfman RI, Hamilton JB (1941): Rate of excretion of urinary androgens after administration of testosterone by various routes. J Clin Endocrinol Metab 1: 352-8.

Eidelsberg J, Ornstein EA (1940): Observations on the continued use of male sex hormone over long periods of time. Endocrinology 26: 46-53.

Emmens W (1941): Rate of absorption of androgens and estrogens in free and esterified form from subcutaneously implanted pellets. Endocrinology 28: 633-42.

Forbes TR (1941): Absorption of pellets of crystalline testosterone, testosterone propionate, methyl testosterone, progesterone, desoxycorticosterone and stilbestrol implanted in the rat. Endocrinology 32: 70-6.

Foss GL (1939): Clinical administration of androgens. Lancet. i: 502-504.

Foss GL (1942): Implantation of sex hormone tablets in man. J Endocr 3: 107-17.

Frey H, Aakvag A, Saanum D, Falch J (1979): Bioavailability of testosterone in males. Eur J Clin Pharmacol 16: 345-349.

Gardner FH, Besa EC (1983): Physiologic mechanisms and the hematopoetic effects of the androstanes and their derivatives. Curr Top Hematol 4: 123-195.

Hamilton JB (1937): Treatment of sexual underdevelopment with synthetic male hormone substance. Endocrinology 21: 649-654.

Hamilton JB, Dorfman RI (1939): Influence of the vehicle upon the length and strength of the action of male hormone substance, testosterone propionate. Endocrinology 24: 711-9.

Handelsman DJ (1990): Pharmacology of testosterone pellet implants. In E. Nieschlag and H. M. Behre (eds): "Testosterone: Action Deficiency Substitution" Berlin:Springer-Verlag, 136-154.

Handelsman DJ (1991): Testosterone Implants: A Manual of Scientific and Clinical Information. Stredder Print, Auckland.

Handelsman DJ, Conway AJ, Boylan LM (1990): Pharmacokinetics and pharmacodynamics of testosterone pellets in man. J Clin Endocrinol Metab 71: 216-222.

Handelsman DJ, Conway AJ, Boylan LM (1992): Suppression of human spermatogenesis by testosterone implants in man. J Clin Endocrinol Metab 75: 1326-1332.

Handelsman DJ, Staraj S (1985): Testicular size: the effects of aging, malnutrition and illness. J androl 6: 144-151.

Hellman L, Bradlow HL, Frazell EL, Gallagher TF (1956): Tracer studies of the absorption and fate of steroid hormones in man. J Clin Invest 35: 1033-44.

Howard JE, Vest SA (1939): Clinical experiments with male sex hormones. II Further observations on testosterone propionate in adult hypogonadism, and preliminary report on the implantation of testosterone. American Journal of Medical Science. 198: 823-37.

Jockenhovel F, Kreutzer M, Vogel E, Lederbogen S, Wagner R, Olbricht T, Reinwein D (1993): Pharmacokinetics of testosterone subcutaneously implanted in hypogonadal men. Experimental and Clinical Endocrinology 101: 38.

Kochakian CD, Ed. (1976). Anabolic-Androgynic Steroids. Handbook of Experimental Pharmacology. Berlin, Springer-Verlag.

Loeser AA (1940): Subcutaneous implantation of female and male hormone in tablet form in women. Br J Med : 479-82.

McCauley AP, Geller JS (1992): Decisions for Norplant programs. Population Reports 20: 1-32.

Mooradian AD, Morley JE, Korenman SG (1987): Biological actions of androgens. Endocr Rev 8:1-28.

Nieschlag E, Cuppers HJ, Wickings EJ (1977): Influence of sex, testicular development and liver function on the bioavailability of oral testosterone. Eur J Clin Invest 7: 145-147.

Nieschlag E, Lammers U, Freischem CW, Langer K, Wickings EJ (1982): Reproductive function in young fathers and grandfathers. J Clin Endocrinol Metab 55: 676-681.

Nieschlag E, Mauss J, Coert A, Kicovic P (1975): Plasma androgen levels in men after oral administration of testosterone or testosterone undecanoate. Acta Endocrinol 79:

Parkes AS (1938): Effective absorption of hormones. Br Med J : 371-373.

Reiter T (1963): Testosterone implantation: a clinical study of 240 implantations in aging males. Journal of the American Geriatric Society. 11: 54-50.

Southren AL, Gordon GG, Tochimoto S (1968): Further studies of factors affecting metabolic clearance rate of testosterone in man. J Clin Endocrinol Metab 28: 1105-1112.

Swyer GIM (1953): Effects of testosterone implants in men with defective spermatogenesis. Br J Med : 1080-1.

Thom MH, Collins WP, Studd JWW (1981): Hormonal profiles in postmenopausal women after therapy with subcutaneous implants. British Journal of Obstetrics and Gynecology. 88: 426-33.

Thorn GW, Firor WM (1940): Desoxycorticosterone acetate therapy in Addisons disease. J Am Med Assoc 114: 2517-25.

Vermeulen A (1990): Androgens and male senescence. In E. Nieschlag and H. M. Behre (eds): "Testosterone:Action Deficiency Substitution" Berlin: Springer-Verlag 261-276

Vest SA, Howard JE (1939): Clinical experiments with androgens IV a method of implantation of crystalline testosterone. J Am Med Assoc 113: 1869-72.

von Schoultz B, Carlstrom K (1989): On the regulation of sex-hormone-binding globulin. A challenge of an old dogma and outlines of an alternative mechanism. J Steroid Biochem 32: 327-334.

# 45

# TESTOSTERONE BUCICLATE

Hermann M. Behre, Gerhard F. Weinbauer, and
Eberhard Nieschlag

Institute of Reproductive Medicine
University of Münster (WHO Collaborating Center
for Research in Human Reproduction)
D-48149 Münster, Germany

## INTRODUCTION

In view of the shortcomings of the existing testosterone preparations for treatment of male hypogonadism and for male contraception, the WHO Special Programme of Research, Development and Research Training in Human Reproduction (WHO/HRP), in collaboration with the Contraceptive Development Branch of the National Institute of Child Health and Human Development (NICHD), initiated a steroid synthesis program of new testosterone esters, according to a chemical strategy defined during a consultation of leading steroid chemists in 1982. The compound selection criterion used was a long-lasting increase after one injection of the substances in the ventral prostate volume in castrated rats. After initial screening of different esters, testosterone buciclate appeared most promising and was further developed. This chapter provides some information on the pharmacokinetics and pharmacodynamics of this testosterone ester obtained from preclinical and clinical studies.

## CHEMISTRY AND METABOLISM

Testosterone buciclate (testosterone 17ß-trans-4-n-butylcyclohexylcarboxylate) is also known as 20 Aet-1 (HRP code) or CDB 1781 (NIH code). The substance has the empirical formula: $C_{30}H_{48}O_3$ and a molecular weight of 454. It is soluble in acetone, the solubility in ethanol or methanol is low, the solubility in water is very low. Testosterone buciclate is applied intramuscularly as a microcrystalline aqueous suspension. For the preclinical studies described below the substance was provided by the Contraceptive Development Branch, NICHD, Bethesda, or the WHO Special Programme of Research, Development and Research Training in Human Reproduction (WHO/HRP), Geneva. The formulation used in the clinical studies performed under WHO/HRP auspices was prepared by Palmer Research (Holywell, Great Britain) under Good Manufacturing Practice (GMP) conditions. After air milling (Micron Mills Ltd, Orpington, UK) of crystalline testosterone buciclate to a particle size of at least 75% in the range of 10 - 50 μm, the drug was sterilized by gamma radiation (Isotron Ltd, Bradford, UK) and suspended in sterile, aqueous suspension vehicle (Medevale Pharmaservices Ltd, Ashton Under Lyne, UK). The formulation vehicle consisted of benzyl alcohol (1.00 g), sodium carboxymethyl cellulose "50" (0.50 g), sodium hydrogen phosphate dihydrate (0.376 g), sodium dihydrogen phosphate dihydrate (1.495 g) and polysorbate 80 (0.20 g) per 100 ml of aqueous solution, sterilized by filtration. The content uniformity and long-term chemical stability of the steroid formulation were confirmed by analysis (Prof. S.A. Matlin, Chemistry Department, Warwick University, UK).

Studies in rats showed the pharmacokinetic superiority of an aqueous microcrystalline suspension of testosterone buciclate over a solution in ethyl oleate which appeared similar to testosterone enanthate. However, no clear relationship between particle size and prolonged activity could be established (Bialy and Blye, 1994). It was demonstrated *in vitro* studies that testosterone buciclate can be hydrolysed by blood sera of guinea pig, rabbit and rat, but not of horse or man. It is slowly hydrolysed by rat or cynomolgus monkey liver (Monder et al., 1994b). After intravenous administration of testosterone buciclate to cynomolgus monkeys, about 5% of the radioactivity of a dose of doubly labelled ester ($^{14}$C, $^3$H) was excreted via the gastrointestinal tract and most of the radioactivity was excreted in the urine within 5 days. No intact testosterone buciclate was recovered. The buciclic acid and its metabolites were excreted rapidly, while testosterone and its metabolites were excreted over 4 days (Monder et al., 1994a). It can be concluded from these studies that metabolism of testosterone buciclate starts in cynomolgus monkeys *in vivo* by hydrolysis of the ester to testosterone and buciclic acid. The buciclic side chain is rapidly cleared while testosterone is retained in the circulation.

## PRECLINICAL STUDIES

## Pharmacokinetics and Pharmacodynamics of Testosterone Buciclate in Castrated Monkeys

In view of favourable results obtained after injection of testosterone buciclate into female monkeys (Bialy and Blye, 1994), a first study on the pharma-cokinetics of testosterone buciclate was performed in two groups of four long-term orchiectomized cynomolgus monkeys, *Macaca fascicularis*, weighing 2.8 - 4.6 kg (Weinbauer et al., 1986). One group received a single intramuscular injection of 40 mg testosterone buciclate in aqueous suspension or 32.8 mg testosterone enanthate dissolved in sesame oil. Both preparations contained equal amounts of testosterone, namely 23.6 mg. Testosterone enanthate injections resulted in supraphysiological serum levels of testosterone for eight days, followed by a rapid decline with levels lower than the physiological limit after three weeks. In contrast, testosterone buciclate produced a moderate increase of serum testosterone levels into the physiological range with a peak level of 29.9 ± 5.9 nmol/l on day 14. Serum levels of testosterone remained in the physiological range for a period of 4 months. The levels never exceeded the physiological range of testosterone. Serum levels of DHT followed that of testosterone in both groups.

These favorable results on the pharmacokinetics of testosterone buciclate were confirmed in castrated rhesus monkeys. After a single intramuscular injection of 40 mg testosterone buciclate in 1 ml to nine monkeys, serum levels of testosterone remained in the normal physiological range for 80 - 136 days (Rajalakshmi and Ramakrishnan, 1989). Whereas a single intramuscular injection of 40 mg testosterone enanthate to a control group of 9 monkeys suppressed LH from day 1 - 7 post injection, serum levels of LH were suppressed by testosterone buciclate injections from day 5 to 115, but the suppression was of a lower degree than that after testosterone enanthate injection. Similar results were obtained for serum levels of FSH. It could be demonstrated that a single injection of 40 mg testosterone buciclate stimulated accessory gland function as judged by semen weight, fructose content of the ejaculate, seminal alkaline and acid phosphatase activity and seminal glycerylphosphoryl cholin levels to levels lower than in the pre-treatment period. However, the effect was similar to a single injection of 40 mg testosterone enanthate (Rajalakshmi et al., 1991). In addition, it could be demonstrated in castrated rhesus monkeys that significantly higher testosterone levels can be achieved when the intramuscular injection of 80 mg testosterone buciclate is given as four injections of 0.5 ml at four different sites compared to a single injection of 2 ml (Rajalakshmi and Ramakrishnan, 1989).

## Testosterone Buciclate for Suppression of Spermatogenesis in Intact Monkeys

A single intramuscular injection of 40 mg testosterone buciclate to 4 adult male bonnet monkeys did not cause any significant change in sperm concentration or sperm motility while serum levels of testosterone remained unchanged (Sharma and Das, 1992). When the same single dose of testosterone buciclate was combined with intramuscular daily injections of 12 mg of the gestagen STS-557 for 12 weeks, spermatogenesis was suppressed to levels near azoospermia. However, in this study the dose of 40 mg testosterone buciclate given to adult male bonnet monkeys did not maintain serum levels of testosterone in the pre-treatment range.

Testosterone buciclate was also used for androgen substitution in normal adult cynomolgus monkeys (body weight between 4.1 and 8.6 kg) in studies with GnRH antagonists for suppression of spermatogenesis. In a first study, daily subcutaneous injections of 420 - 460 µg/kg of the GnRH antagonist Nal-Glu for 15 weeks suppressed serum levels of testosterone and spermatogenesis to azoospermia in all of 5 monkeys. When an additional single injection of 40 mg testosterone buciclate, or 200 mg testosterone buciclate, was given on the first day of the GnRH antagonist administration, serum levels of testosterone could be maintained in the 40 mg group in the upper normal range during the whole treatment period, while a single injection of 200 mg testosterone buciclate maintained serum levels of testosterone about 1.5-fold above normal. However, no consistent azoospermia could be achieved in these two combination groups (Weinbauer et al., 1988). In a follow-up study, 40 mg of testosterone buciclate was given 6 weeks after the first injection of 450 or 900 µg/kg of the GnRH antagonist antide. Here, serum levels of testosterone

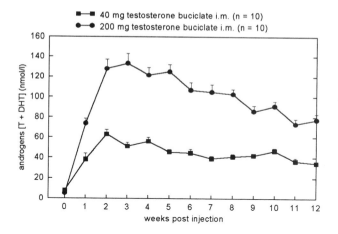

Figure 1. Serum concentrations (mean ± SEM) of androgens after single injection of testosterone buciclate in adult cynomolgous monkeys with suppressed endogenous testosterone by administration of GnRH antagonists (modified from Weinbauer et al., 1992; Weinbauer et al., 1994).

increased to levels in the normal range and complete azoospermia could be achieved in all of 10 monkeys (Weinbauer et al., 1989).

In a third study in adult cynomolgus monkeys, daily injections of 450 µg/kg body weight of the GnRH antagonist cetrorelix for 18 weeks given in combination with a single injection of 200 mg testosterone buciclate during week 6 did not result in consistent azoospermia, whereas serum levels of testosterone were increased to the supraphysiological range (Figure 1) (Weinbauer et al., 1994). However, it could be demonstrated that this supraphysiological dose of 200 mg testosterone buciclate given at study week 6 was able to maintain the suppression of spermatogenesis achieved by administration of the GnRH antagonist when its administration was stopped at week 7.

An interesting observation with practical significance emerging from the monkey studies is the absence of a proportionate increase of maximal serum levels of testosterone with higher doses of testosterone buciclate injected (Weinbauer et al., 1992; Weinbauer et al., 1994; Bialy and Blye, 1994) (Figure 1). Higher doses of testosterone buciclate, however, lead to a substantially increased duration of action and allow even more prolonged injection intervals (Bialy and Blye, 1994).

# CLINICAL STUDIES

## Testosterone Buciclate for Substitution Therapy of Hypogonadal Men

To assess the pharmacokinetics and pharmacodynamics of testosterone buciclate in men, a first clinical study was performed in 8 men with primary hypogonadism under the auspices of the WHO Male Task Force on Methods for the Regulation of Male Fertility (Behre and Nieschlag, 1992). The men were randomly assigned to 2 study groups and were given either 200 (group I) or 600 mg (group II) testosterone buciclate intramuscularly. Whereas in group I serum androgen levels did not rise to normal values, in group II androgens increased significantly and were

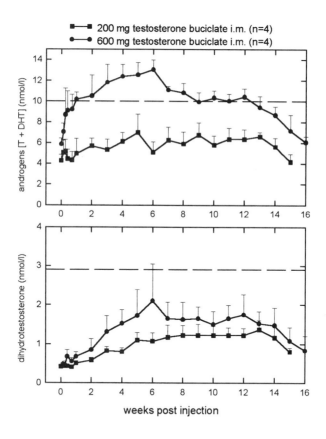

Figure 2. Serum concentrations (mean ± SEM) of androgens (sum of testosterone and DHT measured after HPLC separation) (upper panel) and DHT (lower panel) after single dose injections of 200 mg or 600 mg testosterone buciclate to hypogonadal men. Broken lines indicate the lower normal limit for androgens and the upper normal limit for DHT, respectively (modified from Behre and Nieschlag, 1992).

maintained in the normal range up to 12 weeks with maximal serum levels of 13.1 ± 0.9 nmol/l (mean ± SEM) in study week 6 (Figure 2). No initial burst release of testosterone was observed in either study group.

Pharmacokinetic analysis revealed a terminal elimination half-life of 29.5 ± 3.9 days. This long half-life reflects the more favorable pharmacokinetic profile of testosterone buciclate, compared to testosterone propionate with a terminal half-life of 0.8 days, or testosterone enanthate with 4.5 days (Behre et al., 1990). Serum levels of DHT increased significantly in both study groups with maximal levels in group II of 2.1 ± 0.95 nmol/l in week 6 (Figure 2).

Whereas in the lower dose group, no change was observed in the serum levels of LH or FSH, gonadotropins were significantly suppressed by the single 600

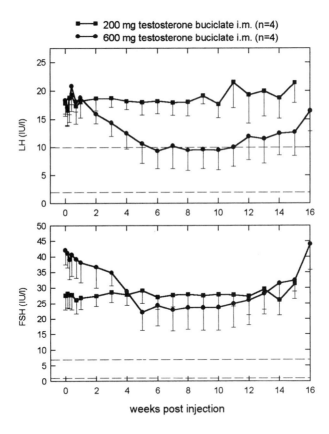

Figure 3. Serum concentrations (mean ± SEM) of LH (upper panel) and FSH (lower panel) after single dose injections of 200 mg or 600 mg testosterone buciclate to hypogonadal men. Broken lines indicate the normal range for LH and FSH, respectively (modified from Behre and Nieschlag, 1992).

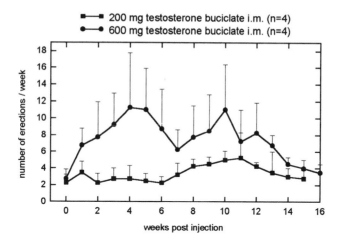

Figure 4. Self-reported number (mean ± SEM) of erections per week after single dose injections of 200 mg or 600 mg testosterone buciclate to hypogonadal men (modified from Behre and Nieschlag, 1992).

mg injection (Figure 3). No significant change was seen in serum levels of SHBG during the study course. Serum levels of estrogens increased slightly in group II without achieving statistical significance.

A significant increase in body weight, hematological parameters, and libido/potency as judged by the number of self-reported erections per week was reported after testosterone buciclate injections, effects that were more pronounced in the higher dose group (Figure 4). No significant change was seen in uroflow, prostate volume as measured by transrectal ultrasonography, or prostate specific antigen. No adverse side-effects including changes in clinical chemistry were observed during the study course.

## Testosterone Buciclate for Hormonal Male Contraception

In view of the favorable results on testosterone buciclate in hypogonadal men, the WHO Task Force on Methods for the Regulation of Male Fertility initiated a clinical trial with testosterone buciclate for suppression of spermatogenesis in normal men. Twelve normal men were enrolled in the first clinical study (Behre et al., 1994a). After 2 control examinations, 4 men were given a single intramuscular injection of 600 mg testosterone buciclate and another group of 8 men was injected with 1200 mg testosterone buciclate. In both groups, serum levels of testosterone remained in the normal physiological range during the study course. Serum levels of DHT increased significantly and reached maximal levels of $3.8 \pm 0.5$ nmol/l in week 6, values that were at this time-point slightly above the normal range for DHT. No suppression of gonadotropins and spermatogenesis was observed after injection of 600 mg testosterone buciclate. However, in the 1200 mg dose group, serum levels of LH and FSH were significantly suppressed; in 3 of 8 volunteers, gonadotropins were lowered to the detection limit of the respective assays for several weeks. In these 3 men, azoospermia that persisted for several weeks was achieved in week 10. No significant change in serum levels of SHBG was seen after injection of testosterone buciclate. However, when the 1200 mg dose group was subdivided into those 3 men who achieved azoospermia (responder) and those who did not (non-responder) a significant and consistent difference in SHBG serum levels was detected between both subgroups. Whether different SHBG levels might be an indicator of or causative for the different suppression of spermatogenesis after testosterone buciclate injections will be subject of further investigations.

## SUMMARY AND CONCLUSION

Of the existing testosterone esters, testosterone buciclate has the most promising pharmacokinetic profile. As demonstrated in non-human primates and men, a single intramuscular injection of testosterone buciclate can maintain serum levels of testosterone in the normal range for several weeks without initial burst release. A significant increase of DHT is observed in the human studies; however, as with other testosterone preparations, e.g. transdermal scrotal testosterone patches, this did not increase prostate volume to levels higher than normal (Behre et al., 1994b). Biological effects of testosterone buciclate on suppression of gonadotropins, erythropoiesis, or libido/potency were demonstrated. No significant adverse side-effects after testosterone buciclate injections were seen in the non-human primate studies, or in hypogonadal or normal men. In conclusion, testosterone buciclate is a new testosterone ester with favourable properties for substitution therapy of male hypogonadism and, possibly with slightly higher doses and repeated injections, or in combination with progestins or GnRH antagonists, for male contraception.

## ACKNOWLEDGMENT

The work from the Institute of Reproductive Medicine of the University of Münster summarized in this chapter was supported by the Max/Planck/Society, the Deutsche Forschungsgemeinschaft, the German Federal Ministry of Health and the WHO Special Programme of Research, Development and Research Training in Human Reproduction.

## REFERENCES

Behre HM, Baus S, Kliesch S, Nieschlag E (1994a): Single injection of the new androgen ester testosterone buciclate leads to azoospermia in normal men: lower SHBG serum levels in responders compared to non-responders (abstract No. 1312). Proceedings of the 76th Annual Meeting of the Endocrine Society, Anaheim.

Behre HM, Bohmeyer J, Nieschlag E (1994b): Prostate volume in testosterone-treated and untreated hypogonadal men in comparison to age-matched controls. Clin Endocrinol 40:341-349.

Behre HM, Nieschlag E (1992): Testosterone buciclate (20 Aet-1) in hypogonadal men: pharmacokinetics and pharmacodynamics of the new long-acting androgen ester. J Clin Endocrinol Metab 75:1204-1210.

Behre HM, Oberpenning F, Nieschlag E (1990): Comparative pharmacokinetics of testosterone preparations: application of computer analysis and simulation. In Nieschlag E, Behre HM (eds.): "Testosterone - action, deficiency, substitution." Berlin, Heidelberg, New York: Springer-Verlag, pp 115-135.

Bialy G, Blye RP (1994): Role of pharmacokinetics in the development of long-acting contraceptive drugs. In Puri CP, van Look PFA (eds.): "Current concepts in fertility regulation and reproduction." New Delhi, Bangalore, Bombay: Wiley Eastern Limited, pp 43-59.

Monder C, Marshall DE, Laughlin LS, Blye RP (1994a): Studies on the metabolism of testosterone trans-4-n-butylcyclohexanoic acid in the cynomolgus monkey, Macaca fascicularis. J Steroid Biochem Mol Biol 50:305-311.

Monder C, Vincze I, Blye RP, Iohan F (1994b): Metabolism of testosterone trans-4-n-butylcyclohexyl carboxylate, a high potency androgen, in rodents and primates: *in vitro* studies. J Endocrinol 140:465-73.

Rajalakshmi M, Ramakrishnan PR (1989): Pharmacokinetics and pharmacodynamics of a new long-acting androgen ester: maintenance of physiological androgen levels for 4 months after a single injection. Contraception 40:399-412.

Rajalakshmi M, Ramakrishnan PR, Kaur J, Sharma DN, Pruthi JS (1991): Evaluation of the ability of a new long-acting androgen ester to maintain accessory gland function in castrated rhesus monkey. Contraception 43:83-90.

Sharma RK, Das RP (1992): Effects of STS-557 and 20 Aet-1 on sperm functions and serum level of testosterone in bonnet monkey (Macaca radiata). Contraception 45:483-491.

Weinbauer GF, Behre HM, Nieschlag E (1992): Concomitant but not delayed androgen supplementation prevents complete testicular involution in GnRH antagonist-treated nonhuman primates (abstract No. 1075). Proceedings of the 74th Annual Meeting of the Endocrine Society, San Antonio.

Weinbauer GF, Göckeler E, Nieschlag E (1988): Testosterone prevents complete suppression of spermatogenesis in the gonadotropin-releasing hormone antagonist-treated nonhuman primate (Macaca fascicularis). J Clin Endocrinol Metab 67:284-290.

Weinbauer GF, Khurshid S, Fingscheidt U, Nieschlag E (1989): Sustained inhibition of sperm production and inhibin secretion induced by a gonadotrophin-releasing hormone antagonist and delayed testosterone substitution in non-human primates (Macaca fascicularis). J Endocrinol 123:303-310.

Weinbauer GF, Limberger A, Behre HM, Nieschlag E (1994): Can testosterone alone maintain the gonadotrophin-releasing hormone antagonist-induced suppression of spermatogenesis in the non-human primate? J Endocrinol 142:485-495.

Weinbauer GF, Marshall GR, Nieschlag E (1986): New injectable testosterone ester maintains serum testosterone of castrated monkeys in the normal range for four months. Acta Endocrinol 113:128-132.

# 46

# SUSTAINED DELIVERY OF TESTOSTERONE BY A LONG ACTING, BIODEGRADABLE TESTOSTERONE MICROSPHERE FORMULATION IN HYPOGONADAL MEN

Shalender Bhasin[1] and Ronald S. Swerdloff

Department of Medicine, UCLA School of Medicine
Harbor-UCLA Medical Center and
[1]Drew University of Science and Medicine
Los Angeles, California

## THE WIDENING APPLICATIONS OF TESTOSTERONE

The main indication for testosterone replacement therapy has been the treatment of male hypogonadism (Bhasin, 1993; Snyder, 1985; Sokol and Swerdloff, 1986). Other legitimate indications include, angioneurotic edema, and delayed sexual development (only in carefully selected patients). However, the spectrum of hypogonadal disorders is expanding; it is now widely recognized that systemic illnesses, such as HIV infection and cancer, are associated with a high prevalence of hypogonadism as defined by low serum testosterone levels. Testosterone use as an anabolic agent is being explored in a number of wasting states characterized by a high prevalence of hypogonadism and loss of lean body mass and frailty, such as aging and HIV Wasting Syndrome. In addition, the application of testosterone alone, or in combination with other gonadotropin-inhibitors, such as GnRH analogs, or progestational agents for male contraception, has led to a resurgence of interest in developing more physiological methods of androgen replacement.

## Desirability of a Long-Acting Testosterone Delivery System

Testosterone esters are quite effective in producing and maintaining normal virilization but have a number of undesirable features, such as widely fluctuating serum testosterone levels, and the need for frequent injections (Sokol and Swerdloff, 1986; Nieschlag, 1982; Nankin, 1987; Snyder and Lawrence, 1980; Sokol et al., 1982; Schulte-Beerbuhl et al., 1980). Because of these limitations, a number of new

*Pharmacology, Biology, and Clinical Applications of Androgens*, edited by Shalender Bhasin et al.
ISBN 0-471-13320-5 © 1996 Wiley-Liss, Inc.

androgen delivery systems are under development. A scrotal transdermal system for testosterone was recently approved by the FDA (Korenman et al., 1987; Cunningham et al., 1989). In addition, a non genital transdermal system, a cyclodextrin-complexed sublingual formulation, and several long-acting formulations, are currently being studied (Handelsman et al., 1990; Behre and Nieschlag, 1992).

Longer acting androgen formulations would be particularly attractive for contraceptive use because they would minimize problems related to user compliance. A long acting biodegradable testosterone microsphere formulation, based on the polylactide-polyglycolide microencapsulation technology, that is currently under development, appears particularly attractive. While the first formulation had suboptimal pharmacokinetic profile (Burris, et al., 1988), second generation microcapsule formulation provides reasonably uniform eugonadal levels of serum testosterone for 10-11 weeks in hypogonadal men (Bhasin et al., 1992).

## Composition of the Testosterone Microsphere Formulation

The injectable testosterone formulation was developed and manufactured by the Stolle Research and Development Corporation, Cincinnati, Ohio. Testosterone is microencapsulated in a biodegradable matrix, Medisorb 85/15 lactide/glycolide copolymer, Medisorb Technologies International, L.P., Cincinnati, Ohio, which is completely biodegraded over a period of about 150 days. Testosterone is released from the microspheres by a mechanism of diffusion/leaching and erosion of the polymeric matrix during the remaining treatment period. The release kinetics are determined by the microsphere diameter, testosterone: polymer ratio, and the polymer characteristics, including co-monomer ratio and molecular weight. The microspheres are sterilized by gamma irradiation in the finished package. Biodegradation occurs by simple hydrolysis of the ester linkages and is determined in part by crystallinity and water uptake (Lewis, 1990). The lactide/glycolide polymer chains are cleaved by hydrolysis to the monomeric acids and are cleared through the Krebs cycle, primarily as carbon dioxide, and in urine. A large body of toxicologic data on the safety of these copolymers has emerged from the studies done in relation to the biodegradable sutures (Lewis, 1990; Brady et al., 1973).

Testosterone microspheres were provided in prepackaged syringes, each containing 315 mg of testosterone and designed to release 3 mg of testosterone each day. The microspheres were suspended in approximately 2.5 ml of dextran solution and injected into the gluteal region by deep IM injection. Each subject received two injections, one in each gluteal region. The 6 mg per day dose was selected to approximate the daily production rate of testosterone in normal men.

## Subjects

Hypogonadal men, 18-49 years of age, who were otherwise in good health, were entered into these studies. Subjects who were greater than 15% over their ideal body weight were excluded. Data on 10 subjects who completed all phases of the study are reported here.    Four of these 10 subjects had hypogonadotropic hypogonadism and the other 6 had hypergonadotropic hypogonadism.

## Study Protocol

Any previous testosterone therapy was discontinued for 4-6 weeks before entry into this study.  The study period was divided into a 2 week control period and a 16 week treatment period.  During the control period, the subjects were asked to come to the Clinical Study Center on three occasions for 40 minutes and three, 5 ml blood samples were drawn 20 min. apart and pooled for measurements of hormones and blood chemistries.  Testosterone microsphere formulation was injected on day 1 of treatment period.  The subjects were then followed for up to a minimum of 16 weeks, or until they experienced symptoms attributable to hypogonadism.  Serum LH, FSH, total and free testosterone, estradiol 17 beta (E2), sex hormone binding globulin (SHBG), and dihydrotestosterone (DHT), were measured on multiple occasions.    Sexual function was assessed by means of a specially designed questionnaire on days 0, 28, 56, and 84.

## RESULTS

No adverse local reactions, apart from pain at the site of injection, were noted.  Two subjects reported breast tenderness in the first 2 weeks after injection, but no breast enlargement was noted.  Sexual function was maintained throughout the treatment period, as assessed by patient interviews and sexual questionnaires.

Pre-treatment serum testosterone levels were very low, consistent with hypogonadism.  After injection, serum total testosterone levels rose quickly into the mid-normal range and stayed uniformly in the eugonadal range for about 70-77 days.  After day 77, serum T levels declined gradually into the hypogonadal range. By day 98, all subjects were in the hypogonadal range.

Free testosterone levels measured by equilibrium dialysis method, followed a pattern very similar to that of total testosterone (Bhasin et al., 1992).    Free testosterone levels rose quickly after the microcapsule injection into the normal range, remained in the eugonadal range for about 70-77 days, and then gradually declined into the hypogonadal range.    Serum testosterone to dihydrotestosterone ratios were in the normal male range throughout treatment ($12.2 \pm 1.9$ on day 28 and $13.7 \pm 3.4$ on day 56).  Serum estradiol levels remained in the normal male range for about 70-77 days.  After day 70, serum estradiol levels gradually decreased towards pretreatment levels.

Serum sex-hormone binding globulin levels significantly decreased during treatment ($p<0.01$) thus providing another marker of biological effectiveness of this androgen formulation.

Serum LH and FSH levels decreased significantly in the 6 hypergona-dotropic subjects.  The nadir for LH and FSH was 45.7% and 48.8% respectively of pretreatment baseline levels at day 70.

Total cholesterol, triglycerides, VLDLC, and LDLC levels, did not change significantly during treatment. However, plasma HDLC levels significantly decreased (p<0.03).

## Pharmacokinetic Parameters

The bioavailability of testosterone from the testosterone microspheres, described as area under the curve (AUC), using the Legrange Polynomial Approximation, was quite uniform among the different subjects. The log linear model estimated the onset of terminal phase on day 56 . Slope of the terminal phase was also quite uniform among these 10 subjects (0.0443 $\pm$ 0.0061). The plasma clearance of testosterone estimated by this model independent method was 1268 $\pm$ 109 L/day, which is strikingly close to that calculated by testosterone tracer infusion methods (980 $\pm$ 54 L/day, mean $\pm$ SEM).

In order to assess if the testosterone release from the microspheres was uniform, the areas under the testosterone curve were calculated for 2 week segments. The testosterone release over the 2 week segments, as assessed by comparing the AUC, was not significantly different in any 2 week segment from days 0-84, consistent with uniform release during this period.

## Demonstration of Dose Dependence

Serum testosterone levels are in general, linearly related to testosterone release rates from the microspheres.

In the castrated rat model, testosterone microsphere systems designed to release 25, 75, and 225 ng of testosterone/day, produced dose-dependent increases in serum testosterone levels (Bhasin et al., 1993). In human studies, systems designed to release 6 mg testosterone/day produced mean serum testosterone of approximately 550 ng/dL (Bhasin et al, 1992). In eugonadal men in whom endogenous testosterone secretion had been suppressed by GnRH agonist administration, systems designed to release 4 mg and 8 mg testosterone/day, produced serum testosterone levels of approximately 280 ng/dL, and 800 ng/dL respectively, providing further evidence of dose-dependent release (Byerley et al.)

## Stability Issues

Formal stability studies have not been performed. However, testosterone release profiles from the formulation were identical in hypogonadal men studied sequentially over a period of 30-36 months indicating stability over this period of time.

## Effect of Testosterone Loading on Testosterone Release Rates

It is important to recognize that changes in the composition of solvents, testosterone loading, and particle size, can affect the performance of the systems. Decreasing the testosterone loading to 37% in a subsequent formulation, considerably reduced testosterone release rates and increased the duration of the release.

## SYNOPSIS

These data indicate that testosterone microsphere formulation can provide sustained and uniform release of testosterone for extended periods. Its long duration and uniform drug delivery make it attractive for use in male contraceptive regimens and for androgen replacement in hypogonadal states.

## REFERENCES

Behre HM, Nieschlag E (1992): Testosterone buciclate (20 Aet-1) in hypogonadal men: Pharmacokinetics and pharmacodynamics of the new long-acting androgen ester. J Clin Endocrinol Metab 75:1204-1210.

Bhasin S, Swerdloff RS, Steiner BS et al. (1992): A biodegradable testosterone microcapsule formulation provides uniform eugonadal levels of serum testosterone in hypogonadal men. J Clin Endocrinol Metab 74:75-83.

Bhasin S (1992): Testosterone treatment of hypogonadal men. J Clin Endocrinol Metab 74221.

Brady JM, Cytright DE, Miller RA, Battistone GC )1973): Resorption rate, route of elimination, and ultrastructure of the implant site of polylactic acid in the abdominal wall of the rat. J. Biomed Mater Res 7:155-163.

Burris AS, Ewing LL, Sherins RJ (1988): Initial trial of slow-release testosterone. microspheres in hypogonadal men. Fertil Steril 50:493-497.

Byerley LO, Lee WP, Swerdloff RS, Buena F, Nair SK, Buchnan T, Goldberg R, Bhasin S (1993): Changes in protein, carbohydrate and lipid metabolism when serum testosterone levels are pharmacologically varied within the normal male range. Fertil Steril 59:118.

Cantrill J, Dewis P, Large DM, Newmain M and Anderson DC (1984): Which testosterone replacement therapy? Clin Endocrinol 21:97-107.

Cunningham GR, Cordero E, Thornby JI (1989): Testosterone replacement with transdermal therapeutic systems. JAMA 261:2525-30.

Handelsman DJ, Conway AJ, Boylan LM (1990): Pharmacokinetics and pharmacodynamics of testosterone pellets in man. J Clin Endocrinol Metab 71:216-222.

Korenman SG, Viosca S, Garza D, Guralnik M, Place V, Campbell P, Davis SS (1987): Androgen therapy of hypogondal men with trans-scrotal testosterone systems. Am J Med 83:471-478.

Lewis DH (1990): Controlled release of bioactive agents from lactide/glycolide polymers. In Chasin M, Langer R (eds): Biodegradable Polymers as Drug Delivery Systems. Marcel Dekker, Inc. New York, 1-41.

Nankin HR (1987): Hormone kinetics after intramuscular testosterone cypionate. Fertil Steril 47:1004-1009.

Nieschlag E (1982): Current status of testosterone substitution therapy. Int J Androl 5:225-226.

Peacock NR, Swerdloff RS, Berman N, Gilley RM, Tice TR, Bhasin S (1993): Pharmacokinetics and pharmacodynamics of a testosterone microcapsule formulation in the male rat. Demonstration of dose-dependence and controlled release. J Androl 14:45-52.

Schulte-Beerbuhl M, Nieschlag E (1985): Comparison of testosterone, dihydrotestosterone, luteinizing hormone and follicle-stimulating hormone in serum after injection of testosterone enanthate or testosterone cypionate. Fertil Steril 33:201-203.

Snyder PJ (1985): Clinical use of androgens. Ann Rev Med 35:207-217.

Snyder PJ, Lawrence DA (1980): Treatment of male hypogonadism with testosterone enanthate. J Clin Endocrinol Metab 51:1335-1339.

Sokol RZ, Swerdloff RS (1986): Practical considerations in the use of androgen therapy: In: Santen RJ, Swerdloff RS, (eds.) Male Reproductive Dysfunction, New York: Marcel Dekker 211-225.

# 47

# TESTOSTERONE UNDECANOATE AND TESTOSTERONE CYCLODEXTRIN

**Christina Wang and Ronald S. Swerdloff**

**Division of Endocrinology, Department of Medicine**
**Harbor-UCLA Medical Center**
**1000 West Carson Street**
**Torrance, California, 90509-2910**

## INTRODUCTION

Replacement androgen therapy through oral route of administration has a number of problems. Oral administration of natural or micronized testosterone (T) results in over 98% inactivation by the liver with the remaining 0.5 to 2% appearing in circulation (Nieschlag et al., 1975). Thus, very large doses are required to reach physiological concentration. Moreover, continued administration induces androgen metabolizing liver enzymes and increasing doses are required over time to maintain serum T levels within the normal, physiological range (Nieschlag et al., 1977). Introduction of an alkyl group in the 17 $\alpha$ position (e.g., methyltestosterone, fluoxymestrone) improved oral bioavailability but increased hepatotoxicity (de Lorimier et al., 1965; Wilson 1988). Moreover, because of the first pass hepatic metabolism, these agents increase serum LDL-cholesterol, and lower HDL-cholesterol levels (Friedl et al., 1990). For these reasons, 17$\alpha$-alkylated oral androgens are not recommended for use as androgen replacement therapy.

## TESTOSTERONE UNDECANOATE

Testosterone undecanoate is a T ester with a long fatty acid side chain. It is absorbed in the lymphatics and partially escapes first pass hepatic metabolism. After a single oral dose of T undecanoate, maximal T levels are attained in about 5 hours which fall gradually to baseline by 8 hours (Nieschlag et al., 1975; Coert et al., 1975; Cantrill et al., 1984). The total daily dosage varies between 120 to 240 mg per day administered in three divided doses. There is a large intra- and inter-individual variability in the time of maximum response as well as the maximal serum T levels attained. The causes for this variability are not known but may reflect differences in the rate of absorption of T undecanoate. Despite the short duration of action with peaks and troughs occurring within a day, and the mean T levels which are generally at the lower normal adult male range, clinical effects and

*Pharmacology, Biology, and Clinical Applications of Androgens*, edited by Shalender Bhasin et al.
ISBN 0-471-13320-5 © 1996 Wiley-Liss, Inc.

restoration of sexual function are reported to be satisfactory (Skakkeback et al., 1981; Gooren, 1987).

After T undecanoate administration, serum DHT levels increase dispro- portionately to serum T levels. Although elevated serum DHT levels, in theory, might stimulate prostatic enlargement, long term treatment with T undecanoate has been shown to be safe. Gooren (1994) monitored 33 men treated with standard doses of T undecanoate for a minimum of 10 years. Serum T and DHT levels remained constant and liver function tests were normal over the 10 years. This suggests that hepatic metabolism of this androgen was not altered over time and there was no long term hepatotoxicity. In another study in middle-aged eugonadal men, T undecanoate increased mean prostate volume by 12%, but serum prostate specific antigen levels and peak urine flow remained unchanged (Holmang, 1993). Thus testosterone undecanoate is a safe oral androgen. In a study of the effects of long term T replacement on bone density in patients with Klinefelter's syndrome, it was demonstrated that the patients treated with T undecanoate had similar bone mineral density measurements, as those treated with T enanthate (Wong et al., 1993).

Recent studies in boys with delayed puberty showed that T undecanoate was effective in increasing sexual development, fat free mass and height velocity without compromising final adult height (Bulter et al., 1992; Gregory et al., 1992). These studies indicate that orally active, short-acting androgens are well accepted, effective, and safe treatment for the initiation of male puberty without disproportionate skeletal maturation. Although very popular in Europe and Asia, T undecanoate is not available in the United States.

## TESTOSTERONE CYCLODEXTRIN

Testosterone cyclodextrin utilizes natural T surrounded by a carbohydrate ring (2-hydroxypropyl-beta cyclodextrin) which facilitates the absorption of T through the oral mucosa (Uekama et al., 1987). This sublingual T cyclodextrin preparation (SLT, BioTechnology General Corp., Iselin, NJ) has the advantage of absorption by oral mucosa and avoids the first pass hepatic metabolism. A preliminary study on a small number of hypogonadal men for 7 days established that 2.5 mg, or 5.0 mg tid, appeared to be the appropriate dosages for androgen replacement (Stuenkel et al., 1993). We studied 40 hypogonadal men (age range 22 to 60 years) with basal serum T levels of less than 250 ng/dl. Other than their hypogonadism, they had no other significant medical problems. After enrollment, the 40 subjects were randomized in a double-blind manner to receive SLT 2.5 mg (n=22), or SLT 5.0 mg (n=18), three times per day. Serum T levels rose rapidly after a single dose of either 2.5 mg (data not shown), or 5.0 mg of SLT, and peaked at 20 minutes. Serum T levels then fell and reached baseline levels by 360 minutes (Fig. 1). The calculated half-life was $60.3 \pm 7.5$ minutes (range 19 to 115 minutes) after the first dose of 2.5 mg SLT and $68.8 \pm 5.0$ minutes (range 35 to 102 minutes) after the first dose of 5.0 mg SLT, with no significant difference between the two doses. Similar serum T profile was observed after repeated administration at 21, 41, and 60 days of treatment (Fig. 1) (Salehian et al., 1995). The mean area

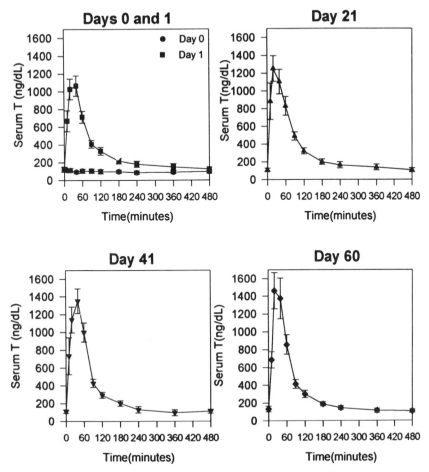

Figure 1. Mean (± SEM) serum T levels before (Day 0) and after administration of SLT 5.0 mg at time 0 minutes on days 1, 21, 41 and 60 in hypogonadal men (n=18).

under the curve (AUC) described by serum T levels was about twofold higher after administration of the 5 mg dose SLT, compared with the 2.5 mg dose. Serum estradiol ($E_2$) and DHT levels paralleled those of serum T. Unlike T undecanoate, the ratios of serum DHT to T were not altered by SLT replacement therapy. Serum sex hormone binding globulin was significantly suppressed in the SLT 5.0 mg, but not in the SLT 2.5 mg group. Serum LH and FSH levels were not significantly lowered by the SLT 2.5 mg group; serum FSH, but not LH, was significantly suppressed in the SLT 5.0 mg group. Administration of T cyclodextrin had no effects on body weight, blood pressure, gynecomastia or testis size. Hematocrit did not significantly rise after SLT treatment. Liver enzymes, renal function, and electrolytes did not change, but serum HDL-cholesterol showed a small but significant decrease after SLT treatment. In both groups of men there were improvements in sexual motivation, including increased frequencies of sexual day dreams, number of days anticipating sexual activity, and increased levels of sexual desire. There were also increases in sexual intercourse, erections, percentage of full erections, and satisfaction with erections after the first three weeks of SLT administration. This improvement was maintained throughout the treatment period (Salehian et al., 1995).

These data showed that T cyclodextrin administration was a safe and effective androgen replacement when improvement in sexual function was used as a marker of efficacy. Because of the ease of administration, lack of significant side effects and achievement of apparently adequate levels of serum T (based on AUC), this preparation can be considered for androgen replacement in hypogonadal men. SLT may be especially useful in constitutional delayed puberty and in elderly men with low androgen levels. The sublingual route of administration and the lower AUC of serum T levels achieved (compared with T enanthate injections) may make SLT more acceptable to pubertal boys. Since SLT lasts only 6 hours after administration, this short off-time may be helpful, should older men develop signs and symptoms of urinary obstruction during androgen replacement. The efficacy of SLT in maintaining bone and muscle mass must be demonstrated before this preparation can be recommended for long-term maintenance therapy. Long term studies on the effect of SLT on the maintenance of bone density, muscle mass and strength, are currently on-going at our center. Thus, SLT may be a useful addition to the limited androgen delivery systems currently available for androgen substitution therapy.

## SUMMARY

In conclusion, orally or sublingually administered T preparations, such as T undecanoate, and T cyclodextrin, are not hepatotoxic and have no significant adverse effects. Because of the ease of administration and short duration of action, such preparations may be especially suitable for treatment of boys with delayed puberty and elderly men with androgen deficiency. However, the long-term effects of these short-acting androgens on maintenance of bone density and muscle strength should be ascertained before these androgen preparations can be universally recommended for chronic long-term maintenance therapy.

## ACKNOWLEDGMENTS

The study on cyclodextrin was supported by a grant from BioTechnology General Corporation (GYN-91-71), and the General Clinical Research Center at Harbor-UCLA Medical Center (NIH grant No. MO1 RR00425). We are grateful for the help of B. Salahian, T. Davidson, V. McDonald, N. Berman, G. Alexander, R. Dudley, F. Ziel and L. Hall, in the T cyclodextrin study.

## REFERENCES

Bulter GE, Sellar RE, Walker RF, Hendry M, Kelnar CJ, Wu FC (1992): Oral testosterone undecanoate in the management of delayed puberty in boys: pharmacokinetics and effects on sexual maturation and growth. J Clin Endocrinol Metab 75:37-44.

Cantrill JA, Davis P, Laya DM, Newman M, Anderson DC (1984): Which testosterone replacement therapy? Clin Endocrinol (Oxf) 21: 97-107.

Coert A, Geelen J, De Vieser J, Van der Vies J (1975): The pharmacology and metabolism of testosterone undecanoate (TU), a new orally active androgen. Acta Endocrinol (Copenh) 79:789-800.

de Lorimier AA, Gorday GS, Lower RC, Carbone JV (1965): Methyltestosterone, related steroids, and liver function. Arch Intern Med 116:289-94.

Friedl KE, Hannan CJ, Jones RE, Plymate SR (1990): High-density lipoprotein cholesterol is not decreased if an aromatizable androgen is administered. Metabolism 39:69-74.

Gooren LJG (1987): Androgen levels and sex functions in testosterone-treated hypogonadal men. Arch Sex Behav 16:463-73.

Gooren LJG (1994): A ten-year safety study of the oral androgen testosterone undecanoate. J Androl 15:212-215.

Gregory JW, Greene SA, Thompson J, Scrimgeour CM, Rennie MJ (1992): Effects of oral testosterone undecanoate on growth, body composition, strength and energy expenditure of adolescent boys. Clin Endocrinol (Oxf) 37:207-13.

Holmang S, Marin P, Lindstedt G, Hedelin H (1993): Effect of long-term and testosterone undecanoate treatment or prostate volume, serum prostate-specific antigen concentration in eugonadal middle aged men. Prostate 23:99-106.

Nieschlag E, Clippers HJ, Wickings EJ (1977): Influence of sex, testicular development and liver function on the bioavailability of oral testosterone. Eur J Clin Invest 7:145-147.

Nieschlag E, Mauss J, Coert A, Kicovic PM (1975): Plasma androgen levels in men after oral administration of testosterone or testosterone undecanoate. Acta Endocrinol (Copenh) 79:366-374.

Salehian B, Wang C, Alexander G, Davidson T, McDonald V, Berman N, Dudley RE, Ziel F, Swerdloff RS (1995): Pharmacokinetics, bioefficacy and safety of sublingual testosterone cyclodextrin in hypogonadal men: Comparison to testosterone enanthate. J Clin Endocrinol Metab (submitted).

Skakkeback NE, Bancroft J, Davidson DW, Warner P (1981): Androgen replacement with oral testosterone undecanoate in hypogonadal men: A double blind controlled study. Clin Endocrinol (Oxf) 14:49-61.

Stuenkel CA, Dudley RE, Yen SS (1991): Sublingual administration of testosterone-hydroxypropyl-b-cyclodextrin inclusion complex simulates episodic androgen release in hypogonadal men. J Clin Endocrinol Metab 72:1054-59.

Uekama K, Otagiri M (1987): Cyclodextrin in drug carrier systems. Cur Rev Ther Drug Carrier Syst 3:1-40.

Wong FH, Pun KK, Wang C (1993): Loss of bone mass in patients with Klinefelter's syndrome despite sufficient testosterone replacement. Osteoporosis Int 3:3-7.

# 48

# 7α-METHYL-19-NORTESTOSTERONE (MENT): AN IDEAL ANDROGEN FOR REPLACEMENT THERAPY

**Kalyan Sundaram, Narender Kumar, and C. Wayne Bardin**

**Center for Biomedical Research**
**The Population Council,**
**1230 York Avenue**
**New York, New York 10021**

## INTRODUCTION

The androgens most commonly used clinically, and others under development, are testosterone (T) and it esters (Behre et al., 1990). The preceding chapters have covered the wide range of uses as well as the various products that are currently available and those under development. Testosterone and its esters have certain limitations (Sundaram et al., 1993). Assuming a normal production rate of 5 mg/day, T replacement has required either frequent im injections (T enanthate and T cypionate) or im injections of large bulk at less frequent intervals e.g., T buciclate and T microcapsules (Bhasin et al., 1992). These considerations led us to investigate the possibility of using a synthetic androgen, 7α-methyl-19-nortestosterone (MENT) whose biopotency has been reported to be 10 times greater than that of T (Segaloff, 1963; Kumar et al., 1992). Because of its higher potency, the dose of MENT for replacement therapy is estimated to be 500 μg/day. It is feasible to administer this dose of MENT via sustained release subdermal implants that will last for a year or longer. This report compares the biological properties and metabolism of MENT and T and discusses the advantages of using MENT as a replacement androgen.

### Androgenic and Anabolic Actions

The biopotency of MENT and T were compared in castrated male rats. The dose related increase in the weight of ventral prostate (VP) was used as an index of androgenic potency, while that in the levator ani (muscle) was used as an index of anabolic activity. An estimate of the pituitary suppressive activity (anti-

*Pharmacology, Biology, and Clinical Applications of Androgens,* edited by Shalender Bhasin et al.
ISBN 0-471-13320-5 © 1996 Wiley-Liss, Inc.

gonadotropic) was based on the suppression of the post-castration rise in serum LH levels. Compared to T, MENT was found to be 4 times more androgenic and 10 times more anabolic. The antigonadotropic potency was also 10-fold greater than that of T. An explanation for the dissociation of the androgenic potency from the anabolic and antigonadotropic potency can be found in the differences in the metabolism of T and MENT. In the prostate, T is enzymatically 5α-reduced to DHT, which has a higher affinity for androgen receptors (AR) and is more potent than T (Mooradian et al., 1987). This leads to a 2-3 fold amplification of T action on the prostate. In contrast, due to the almost total lack of 5α-reductase in muscle, the action of T is not amplified in this tissue. *In vitro* studies have suggested that MENT does not undergo 5α-reduction due to steric hindrance from the 7α-methyl group (Agarwal and Monder, 1988). Hence, the action of MENT is not amplified in the prostate. Further support for this hypothesis is provided by the use of 5α-reductase inhibitor (5αRI) (Table 1). When castrated rats were treated with T and MENT, with or without the 5αRI, the stimulatory action of T on the prostate was decreased by 35%. In contrast, 5αRI did not alter the action of MENT on the prostate since 5α-reduction of T does not play a significant role in the anabolic action of T, 5αRI had no effect on the muscle weight.

Table 1. Effect of 5α-reductase inhibitor (5αRI) on the androgenic and anabolic actions of T, MENT and NT.

|              | Prostate | Muscle |
| ------------ | -------- | ------ |
| T            | 100      | 100    |
| T +5αRI      | 64       | 92     |
|              |          |        |
| MENT         | 100      | 100    |
| MENT +5αRI   | 102      | 112    |
|              |          |        |
| NT           | 100      | 100    |
| NT +5αRI     | 159      | 96     |

The androgen stimulated response is designated 100%.

Based on the above findings, it is concluded that the anabolic properties of MENT derive from the fact that, unlike testosterone, it cannot be 5α-reduced. The role of 5α-reductase as a determinant of the anabolic property of an androgen is further illustrated by the action of 19-nortestosterone (NT), another anabolic androgen. Compared to T, NT has higher binding affinity for AR and exhibits greater stimulatory effect on muscle. However, in contrast to the situation with T, 5α-reduction of NT in the prostate leads to a reduction in its binding affinity for AR, leading to a decrease in its androgenic activity (Celotti et al., 1992). A clear explanation for this mechanism of action is illustrated by the use of 5αRI (Table 1). Blocking 5α-reduction causes a decrease in the androgenic action of T, an increase in the androgenic action of NT and no change in the androgenic action of MENT.

Part of the physiological action of T is mediated by its enzymatic aromatization to estradiol ($E_2$). Hence, the estrogenic activity of T and MENT was compared in immature ovariectomized rats. Both T and MENT caused a dose related increase in uterine weight. MENT was 50 times more uterotropic than T. Further studies showed that the increase in uterine weight was a result of, at least in part, the anabolic properties of T and MENT. For example, the uterotropic action of the androgens could not be blocked by tamoxifen and other specific antiestrogens. However, it was partially blocked by flutamide, an antiandrogen.

## Gonadotropin Suppression

The antigonadotropic potential of MENT was compared with that of T by their ability to inhibit post-castration rise in serum LH levels. In this regard, MENT was at least 12 times as potent as T. Indeed, when the potency comparison was based on the serum levels of T and MENT, the antigonadotropic potency of MENT was 30 times greater than that of T (Kumar et al., 1992). Administration of 5αRI did not affect the antigonadotropic activity of T and NT, indicating that the regulation of pituitary gonadotropin secretion by T does not depend upon its 5α-reduction to DHT (Kumar et al., 1995).

## Aromatization

Whether or not MENT can undergo aromatization to androgenic products was investigated *in vitro* using human placental aromatase (LaMorte et al., 1994). Products isolated following incubation of MENT with placental microsomes behaved like 7α-methyl-estradiol on thin layer chromatography. Furthermore, the metabolite exhibited specific binding to rat uterine estrogen receptors.

## Support of Libido and Mating Behavior

The ability of MENT to restore ejaculatory response after blocking pituitary and testicular function with an LHRH agonist was investigated in rhesus monkeys. Administration of MENT subdermally, via sustained release implants, was able to restore ejaculatory response to electrical stimulation while maintaining azoospermia in 3 of 4 animals (Sundaram et al., 1987). In castrated rats, MENT was 10 times more potent than T in restoring mating behavior (Morali et al., 1993). Similar results were obtained in hamsters and mice.

## Pharmacokinetics

Studies in rats, rabbits and monkeys showed that the metabolic clearance rate (MCR) of MENT was much faster than that of T. Pharmacokinetic studies in men also gave similar results. Following iv injection, MENT was cleared with a terminal half-life of approximately 30 min. which is approximately half of that reported for T. MCR of MENT was approximately 2,000 L per day, which is twice the rate reported for T. This could be partly related to the finding that MENT did not bind to TEBG.

## SUMMARY

The advantage of using MENT as a replacement androgen for male contraception and for other clinical conditions requiring long-time androgen therapy can be summarized as follows:

1.     Because of its high potency, the doses required are much lower.

2.     It is feasible to administer it continuously over a long period via subdermal implants.

3.     Unlike testosterone, its stimulatory action is not amplified in the prostate. Hence, it could have health benefits.

4.     Its high potency in blocking gonadotropin secretion may have additional advantage when used as a male contraceptive.

5.     MENT can support libido at low doses.

## REFERENCES

Agarwal AK, Monder C (1988): *In vitro* metabolism of 7α-methyl-19 nortestosterone by rat liver, prostate, and epididymis: Comparison with testosterone and 19-nortestosterone. Endocrinology 123:2187-2193.

Behre HM, Oberpenning F, Nieschlag E (1990): Comparative pharmacokinetics of androgen preparations: Application of computer analysis and simulation. In E. Nieschlag & H.M. Behre (eds.): "Testosterone: Action, Deficiency, Substitution," Berlin: Springer-Verlag pp. 115-135.

Bhasin S, Swerdloff RS Steiner B, Peterson MA, Meridores T, Galmirini M, Pandian MR Goldberg R, Berman N (1992): A biodegradable testosterone microcapsule formulation provides uniform eugonadal levels of testosterone for 10-11 weeks in hypogonadal men. J Clin Endocrinol Metab 74:75-83.

Celotti F, Negri CP (1992): Anabolic steroids: A review of their effects on the muscles, of their possible mechanisms of action and of their use in rabbits. J Steroid Biochem Molec Biol 43-469-477.

Kumar N, Didolkar A, Monder C, Bardin CW, Sundaram K (1992): The biological activity of 7α-methyl-19-nortestosterone is not amplified in male reproductive tract as is that of testosterone. Endocrinology 130:3677-3683.

Kumar N, Sundaram K, Bardin CW (1995): Feedback regulation of gonadotropins by androgens in rats: Is 5α-reductase involved? J Steroid Biochem Mol Biol 52:105-112.

LaMorte A, Kumar N, Bardin CW, Sundaram K (1994): Aromatization of 7α-methyl-19-nortestosterone by human placental microsomes *in vitro*. J Steroid Biochem Mol Biol 48:297-303.

Mooradian AD, Morley JE, Korenman SG (1987): Biological actions of androgens. Endocrine Review 8:1-27.

Morali G, Lemus AE, Munguia R, Arteaga M, Perez-Palacios G, Sundaram K, Kumar N, Bardin CW (1993): Induction of male sexual behavior in the rat by 7α-methyl-19-nortestosterone, of an androgen that does not undergo 5α-reduction. Biol Reprod 49:577-581.

Segaloff A (1963): The enhanced local androgenic activity of 19-nor steroids and stabilization of their structure by 7α-and 17α-methyl substituents to highly potent androgens by any route of administration. Steroids 1:299-315.

Sundaram K, Keizer-Zucker A, Thau R, Bardin CW (1987): Reversal of testicular function after prolonged suppression with an LHRH agonist in rhesus monkeys. J Androl 8:103-107.

Sundaram K, Kumar N, Bardin CW (1993): 7α-methyl-nortestosterone (MENT): The optimal androgen for male contraception. Ann Med 25:199-205.

# DISCUSSION: ANDROGEN DELIVERY SYSTEMS
## Chairpersons: Christina Wang and Kiagus Arsyad

**Gus Fried:** I would like to make a brief comment on the paper of testosterone bucciclate (TB). Dr. Behre inadvertently omitted mentioning that The International Organization for Chemistry in Development (IOCD), which I represent, collaborated with WHO and NIH on the development of TB. IOCD is a group of international chemists mainly from developing countries like China and Brazil. Testosterone bucciclate was synthesized by a chemist from Tehran. The reason I mentioned this is because this collaboration was initiated because industry in the western countries was not willing to undertake such a study.

**David Handelsman:** I would like to respond to your invitation to discuss the best delivery systems and suggest that we ask the patients rather than make our own decisions. I think that oral agents are preferable to intramuscular injections. I think anyone who has had experience with patients having intramuscular injections knows that they will choose anything than to have those injections every two or three weeks. In that context, oral androgens are preferred, but in our experience, the patches would probably be equally attractive.

**Shalender Bhasin:** We need multiple choices. We have hundreds of models of cars, and there is no ideal model of a car for everybody. There are individuals who would prefer a long-acting injectable delivery system while there are others who would take anything but an injection. Although we have a number of very attractive formulations, it is premature to compare these formulations because they are at different stages of development; a formulation that looks very attractive in early stages may look very different in its final form.

**Wayne Meikle:** I think the androgen patch offers a lot of opportunities for physiologic replacement, especially in prepubertal adolescent individuals. As adolescents go through puberty, hormone levels are not sustained and the testosterone patch duplicates early as well as late puberty; it has this flexibility in dosing.

**Hermann Behre:** For different indications, for example, treatment of male hypogonadism or contraception, different androgen preparations are needed. For male contraception, questions of the frequency of injection or whether you have to have some surgical procedure might be very important, but this might not be so important if you treat hypogonadal patients.

**Norm Mazer:** Although I am not unbiased, I would like to make two comments. It would behoove us to try to compare the number of products being developed on a similar foundation, even from the hormone measurement perspective. We use a time average testosterone level based on the dosing interval, and the area under the curve, to make it possible for endocrinologists to readily appreciate the differences between these formulations. When we express the AUC, people are unfamiliar with the values. The majority of studies that have looked at testosterone enanthate show that one is really delivering a very high average testosterone level to patients. It averages approximately 700-800 ng/dL when it is averaged over a two-week interval with the 200 mg dose. An alternative, and an equally useful way to compare products, is by their delivery rates. This is something that is readily done for the transdermal systems and pellets. When you give 200 mg of testosterone enanthate every two weeks, and if you assume and most studies would support that you have a complete absorption of that product, you are actually delivering a little more than 10 mg of testosterone a day for the patient. If you give 300 mg every three weeks or 100 mg every week, you are still delivering 10 of testosterone per day. This is above the normal range of daily production for most healthy men and we have to keep that in mind.

**Christina Wang:**     Testosterone enanthate includes testosterone and the enanthate side chain.

**Norm Mazer:**   I have converted it to the amount of testosterone. The last comment that I would like to make is that in our experience of looking at the non-scrotal testosterone patch, and in conversations with patients to help us understand what they feel about the product, there is certainly a substantial number of individuals who feel that by doing something everyday they feel that they are taking an active step in the treatment of their condition. There may be some men who would rather forget about the fact that they have hypogonadism, but those that have been using our product actually get an additional feeling of doing something for themselves that they appreciate.

**Ronald Swerdloff:**   It strikes me that when you are asking, even for an indication like hypogonadism, what is the best type of preparation, that there are a number of factors that come to mind and most of these have not really been carefully analyzed in a comparison-type study. We have heard about the issue of compliance, of subject or patient satisfaction, and a little bit about the issues of marketing. It looks as though most of these agents that have been talked about seem to have positive effects on sexual function, libido, and mood. If they are all equal in that regard, then it is a matter of what seems to satisfy the client. However, there are lots of other indications for androgen treatment in patients with hypogonadism. For instance, there are the issues of effects on muscle and on bone. We also can see from the data that were presented with these different preparations that not all the metabolic profiles seems to be identical. We see different ratios of DHT to T, we have seen different effects on aromatization and we really have little insight on what the relative comparative impacts of these would be on some of these metabolic functions. There is a lot that we do not know about these preparations.

**Somnath Roy:**   For the time being, I am not considering the efficacy part of various types of administration, but let us talk from the aspect of patient compliance and motivation. If you take oral preparations for hypogonadal man, motivation is of one type. But if you are using that for contraceptive purposes, the motivation is completely different. I would also like to ask a question, when you gave testosterone undecanoate by oral administration, how much patient compliance did you get?

**Christina Wang:**  If they like the drug, they will take it, if they do not think it is working, they will not take it.   Similarly for testosterone cyclodextran.   So, compliance is good in patients who think that the drug is working. It varies from patient to patient.

**Somnath Roy:**  Did you monitor what proportion of medication your clients had taken regularly?

**Christina Wang:** We had a drug chart and we collected pills. Because this was a very closely monitored clinical trial, we had the same physician and nurses looking after them all the time. I think the compliance was higher than you would get in field trials.

**David Handelsman:** Our experience in a closely controlled trial of testosterone undecanoate orally is that it causes substantial amount of gastrointestinal intolerance. In terms of whether it works for the patient or not, sometimes it works on some days and not on the others in the same patient. So it is not a great preparation.

**Somnath Roy:** The injectables have the attraction that you can administer them at longer intervals. In India, as a physician, if you give something orally, the people in general will not really like it as much as an injection which they think is more effective.

**William Bremner:** I am somewhat dubious about the androgens used in terms of the speed of the induction of suppressed sperm counts and, perhaps, the completeness of suppression as well. There are the other potential combination agents. Either a progestin or a GnRH analogue with a lower dose testosterone preparation is preferable to an androgen alone. What we are trying to aim at is the greatest suppression possible of both gonadotropins and sperm production while at that same time as low as possible intratesticular levels of steroids that stimulate spermatogenesis while maintaining circulating T levels that approximate the mid end of the normal range. I think if we aim at those three criteria, we will probably do a fairly reasonable job. It is hard for me to see a regimen that will do that with an androgen alone.

**Carlos Callegari:** I got the impression from one of the speakers that it was very clear the lipids (HDL) were going down with testosterone treatment in patients with hypogonadism. But today, looking at the studies that were presented, it seems that some of the preparations did not have any changes on HDL. I was also concerned about the SHBG and hematocrit changes. To what extent does this relate to the selection of patients, whether they are hypogonadal and for how long? Is it necessary to standardize the methods and population so that we can compare different preparations?

**Shalender Bhasin:** Let me respond to your second question first. The issue of changes in sex hormone binding globulin with testosterone treatment has been debated between many of us here. The effects of testosterone on SHBG depend on a number of variables including the duration of the washout in the studies and the assay that is used to determine SHBG. The results may not be the same using the immunoradiometric assay which measures the mass of SHBG versus the tritiated-DHT binding assay that measures the binding capacity of SHBG. My assessment of the literature is that the older literature where people used tritiated binding assay as we have done, showed a modest decrease in SHBG concentrations with testosterone treatment. We use a fairly long washout period. Some of the discrepancies may be related to the types of assays used. Testosterone may have some post translational effects. The other point related to the effects on lipids. In hypogonadal men in our studies, the basal HDLC concentrations are about 10-15% higher and with testosterone replacement, they fall about 10-15%. Total cholesterol concentrations do not change. Dr. Bremner's data in normal men using suppression with GnRH antagonist provided similar data.

**Wayne Meikle:** We have looked at SHBG with binding assays as well immunoassays and we really do not see a change with androgen therapy. Concerning your question about standardization of men and washout protocols, part of that is very difficult. You accept the men who come along and some of them have primary gonadal disease and some of them have secondary or tertiary disease. But washing these men out for longer periods than eight weeks may be unusually cruel. That is why we have selected eight weeks rather than a longer interval.

**F.C. Wu:** I have a question for David Handelsman regarding the cost of the testosterone implant. I think he is correct in calculating the doctors time in his assessment of the cost of implants versus injections. But I wonder whether you have costed the equipment such as the sterilizer, the packaging, and also the use of a room for insertions, and any required assistance. I have had to do that exercise recently, and the hospital actually made us curtail the number of implants that we had to do because of the overall cost of the implant.

**David Handelsman:** These are very good points. The calculation I showed you was done for a specific purpose of the national pharmaceutical benefits gain which considered only those particular categories of cost. I think you are quite right about that those other overhead costs. I would say though that there is now a disposable trocar which would probably reduce the sterilization cost, but the room cost and the nurse costs are additional.

**F.C. Wu:** My other question to you is how do you know whether there is less fibrosis after the new implant versus the previous version of the implants?

**David Handelsman:** What I meant to say was that fibrosis has never interfered with the ability to put implants in the same site. Occasionally you do get individuals who seem to be more prone to fibrosis and you can sometimes feel where the implants were in the past, but that is unusual and it has never interfered with the ability to put implants in again, and the patients themselves do not notice it.

**Avraam Grinvald:** My question is to Dr. Handelsman. When you insert those pellets subcutaneously, do you close the wound?

**David Handelsman:** No sutures are needed.

**Avraam Grinvald:** When you have an extrusion, it is because of infection?

**David Handelsman:** The mean time to extrusions is about 60 days. It occurs because the pellet migrates down. It seems to be aseptic. We have cultured virtually all of the 40 or so episodes in ten years and we have had two of them that became infected. We never see infections outside the circumstance of an extrusion, but infection seems to follow the extrusion if it is not kept clean.

**Avraam Grinvald:** My second question is to Dr. Cunningham. You are using those scrotal patches to maintain a normal level of testosterone. Do you have to change the patch everyday?

**Glenn Cunningham:** Correct.

**Avraam Grinvald:** How long do you have to wear those patches in order to maintain a normal level of testosterone? How comfortable is the patch on the patient's scrotum? What is the temperature of the scrotum?

**Glenn Cunningham:** Obviously the patch will deliver testosterone as long as it is adherent to the scrotum. One of the issues that we faced initially was trying to maintain adherence, but what we learned quickly was that you had to shave the scrotum once every four to five days in order to maintain the best adherence. Once the patch is removed, testosterone levels begin to fall very quickly. At this point, we have data through six years, so presumably patients can wear these for a long period of time without any untoward effects. As far as temperature is concerned, there is no evidence that there is any increase in scrotal temperature as a result of wearing these.

**Avraam Grinvald:** What happens if you wear the patches on other parts of the body, not on the scrotum?

**Glenn Cunningham:** These patches do not have an enhancer and when attempts were made to apply them to the torso and other areas, less testosterone was absorbed.

**Ronald Swerdloff:** My question is for David Handelsman. I would suggest that it would be worthwhile for us to look at the data on AUCs for multiple delivery systems to get a much better idea about this issue of effect on suppression of gonadotropins. There is a fair bit of variability in the ability to suppress gonadotropins with different preparations and routes of administration. The second point that I wanted to make is that the TE, which is being delivered here in the United States, may give somewhat of a different pattern of delivery than what the original Schering preparation does in Europe and other parts of the world.

**C. Alvin Paulsen:** Dr. Swerdloff, we heard about your observations and so I checked this out on a couple of patients with Klinefelter's Syndrome, and indeed the peak was one day, two to three like we had always seen before. Maybe we are using a different preparation, but it is the testosterone enanthate, not the generic.

**Alvin Matsumoto:** My suspicion is that there is something different about the preparation within the United States and that it has changed over time.

**Christina Wang:** We studied the 400 mg dose of TE and we didn't get a very high peak. The same preparation was sent to Dr. Bailey to be put into castrated monkeys and he sent me data that looked exactly the same profile as men. We also have data from Dr. Bhasin's group using 100 mg in hypogonadal men and the peaks were not high.

**Richard Clark:** As we develop these new modes of testosterone replacement systems, it is very important to capture populations of men that are carried through, not only the initial clinical trials, but maintained on therapy after approval has been given and after the product has been marketed to monitor for effects that we are not really aware of.

## DISCUSSION: CRITICAL ISSUES FOR THE FUTURE
## Chairpersons: Eberhard Nieschlag, Jean Wilson, Terry Brown, and Ronald Swerdloff

**Eberhard Nieschlag:** The ultimate study in assessing the effects of testosterone on the male body is castrating prepubertal boys and following them through life. Over the centuries, as you know, lots of boys with good voices have been castrated to preserve their voices as sopranos. We investigated the life expectancy of these individuals and compared them with intact singers who had their full testicles in place and had voices - bassos, baritones, and tenors. There were 50 singers who were castrated between 1580 and 1859 and we matched them with 50 intact singers born on the same years when these castrated singers were born. The life expectancy of the castrates was an average of 65 years. The intact singers had exactly the same life expectancy. So what we can say from this study is that obviously the presence of testes and of testosterone does not shorten your life, neither does the removal lengthen your life. With this notion, we would like to discuss the question whether supraphysiologic levels of testosterone may be toxic to your health. I would like to ask Dr. Wilson to address this topic first.

**Jean Wilson:** A recurring theme of this workshop is the question of whether androgen excess will have pathological consequences. In the field of endocrinology, for every other hormonal system that I can think of, the excess secretion or excess administration clearly causes a toxic effect. It is also true that androgen excess in women, in children of both sexes, and in female embryos, causes pathological virilization. But there is simply no natural state of androgen excess in adult men. Consequently, we do not have guidelines for assessing the long-term consequences of supraphysiological doses of androgen in men. Nor is it intuitively obvious how to study this issue. My personal prejudice is that androgen excess is probably safe, because most of the androgen receptors appear to be saturated at plasma. At any rate, in simplistic terms, there are at least two ways that toxic or unwanted side effects might arise. One, is that the effects are consistent, predictable, and statistically measurable. For example, a decrease in HDL, or a rise in LDL cholesterol, is measurable and could either occur or not occur and could be dose-related or nondose-related. Likewise, evidence was presented at this meeting that a significant increase in plasma testosterone may cause consistent and predictable increases in lean body mass. The other possibility is that androgens could cause inconsistent effects as the result of genetic polymorphisms in the population among normal men. For example, profound hypercholesterolemia has been reported in the literature to occur occasionally in people who take androgens and patients have been reported to develop odd tumors while abusing androgens. At present we do not know whether these rare occurrences are coincidental or whether there are a variety of polymorphisms that predispose occasional people to unusual effects. We do know that underlying medical problems predispose to certain complications. Liver disease, for example, is said to increase the feminizing complications of androgen therapy. There may also be ethnic differences in the incidence of side effects. One can only conclude that valid assessment of androgen safety may require long-term studies of large numbers of individuals. It should also be pointed out that the literature on androgen abuse is not a useful guide for this problem because it involves the use of various dosages, various schedules of administration, and multiple drug formulations, each of which has different turnovers, different metabolites, and toxicities. Some, for example, can be aromatized and some cannot. Some have not been studied in detail in humans. For example, those drugs that are only approved for veterinary use may have totally unexpected effects in athletes. All studies of this subject were poorly controlled and poorly designed. Everyone must be concerned about potential cardiovascular complications. Another issue that was raised by Dr. Schroder has to do with whether or not raising plasma androgen levels will have pathological consequences for the prostate; either increasing the progression of benign prostatic hyperplasia, or possibly predispose to prostate cancer. Once again, this is not going to be an easy question to answer, but it may be possible to design prospective studies that might provide guidance as to how to design such studies. It would be very interesting to determine, for example, whether raising plasma testosterone levels above the physiological range influences prostate androgen levels. Once again, my prejudice is that it will not because if one administers increasing doses of androgens to dogs, a plateau level is noted in the prostate. I think it would also be interesting to know whether over a relatively long-term increasing the plasma testosterone influences prostate size. Negative findings with either of these studies would not necessarily mean that such therapy is safe as far as prostatic hyperplasia is concerned, but if a progressive dose-related increase in size or in intraprostatic testosterone concentration occurred, one would be very worried about the long-term use of such dosages.

**Eberhard Nieschlag:** Thank you very much for these very lucid thoughts on things that should be done. I am not so sure that I understood you correctly concerning the anabolic steroid users. Although these are not very well designed studies, I think they provide an opportunity to look at long-term effects.

**Ronald Swerdloff:** I wanted to add a comment to what Dr. Wilson had to say. We heard earlier in this workshop from Dr. Coffey who was not concerned at all about the effects of testosterone on the prostate but felt obliged to comment about other areas, including potential adverse effects of testosterone on behavior, including the so-called rage reaction. Unfortunately, we have much to learn about androgen effects on human cognitive and behavioral activities. Despite supportive data from studies in animals including subhuman primates, evidence demonstrating that androgens are responsible for aggressiveness in humans is limited. Furthermore, Dr. Wilson I know of no data to support the notion that testosterone will induce rage reactions in humans.

**Eberhard Nieschlag:** In this context I think it was very important to hear that we should look at other psychological and social parameters rather than so-called aggression. Dr. Dabbs clearly said that dominance and sociability may be important parameters.

**Gabriel Bialy:** When we do toxicological studies we try to estimate the potential human level and then use some multiple, let us say 25 times. We do not go up to 100 times. A number of years ago Peter Ramwell at Georgetown gave very high doses of testosterone to male rats and was able to show excess mortality in these animals. Now it seems to me that if, indeed, we are going to use testosterone preparations quite extensively, both for replacement therapy or androgen alone contraception, we should see if in rats, or some other animal, whether these excessive doses of androgens are leading to excess morbidity and maybe mortality.

**Eberhard Nieschlag:** This is a valuable comment and we may consider just which animal model is the proper one. However, for contraception we are seeking normal physiological levels to get away from the supraphysiological ones. Perhaps we should touch upon another point which came up on the first day. In the 1950s and 1960s, steroid pharmacologists had "a dream" that they would find steroids that would mimic one specific function of testosterone only, be it hematopoietic or be it anabolic. In the end they did not really succeed. But now with knowledge about targeting organs and about receptors and modulators, the question comes up whether it is possible to have organ-specific androgen actions. Dr. Terry Brown might be willing to address this point.

**Terry Brown:** One of the approaches that we have taken in identifying mutations in the androgen receptor is to learn something about the structure-function relationships that affect binding of the ligand to the receptor protein and the functional effects that result. As I pointed out in my presentation during this meeting, we have identified quite a few different mutations in the androgen receptor that occur naturally and, of course, you can always produce additional mutations by site-specific mutagenesis and then study the structure-function relationships. The unfortunate part of these studies is that they have not really told us what we had expected. As you may recall, I pointed out a large number of heterogeneous mutations, affecting both the ligand binding and DNA binding properties of the receptor but we probably now understand less from those mutations than we expected going into it naively several years ago. The benefit of such studies, however, is that now we know some of the structural properties of the receptor and hopefully can prepare sufficient quantities of purified receptors to perform some crystallographic analysis and computer modeling that will then allow us to better understand the protein structure. The goal is to design appropriate ligands to bind the protein that will then allow the specific responses that we are looking for, whether we are looking for responses in bone, muscle, or specifically in the prostate, from the perspective of agonist activity, or antagonist activity. Hopefully, we can model some compounds that will fulfill our desire for so-called designer drugs. One drawback that has been mentioned today is that many of the pharmaceutical companies are really not interested in synthesizing the compounds that would be necessary to do these kinds of studies. Maybe it is the individual chemists that will be able to devote time, effort, and resources to developing some of those compounds. The positive way of looking at it is that once we know the appropriate protein structural information and the computer modeling can be done, then maybe new interest will resurface within the pharmaceutical industry to pursue the design of compounds that are necessary to create the effects that we are interested in defining.

**David Handelsman:** I just want to raise the issue when we say we aim for physiological testosterone levels, the range that we call physiological is quite wide in normal men and the tissue effects are probably very diverse. We have reasonably good evidence that the threshold for restoration of sexual function in men is actually quite low while it may be higher for other tissues. While we are aiming for physiological replacement and yet not knowing the thresholds for those tissues, it makes it very difficult to target more finely what we are doing. I wonder if people have ideas about how to go about trying to understand what the androgen requirements of different tissues are?

**Eberhard Nieschlag:** Who could answer that, Dr. Wilson?

**Jean Wilson:** That is a question that only Dr. Nieschlag can answer.

**Eberhard Nieschlag:** I do not think so. You mean because it is unanswerable?

**Jean Wilson:** I do not know how to answer this.

**Eberhard Nieschlag:** Ron, can you answer?

**Ronald Swerdloff:** No, but I can certainly acknowledge that it is a very important question. Let me comment upon another point which may stimulate better response from our panel. We have talked about the normal range of serum testosterone levels of a normal population; it was correctly noted that this range is fairly wide. Presumably the individual's serum testosterone is determined by a testosterone Sensor that reflects the set point within the hypothalamic-pituitary axis. I have always wondered whether the hypothalamic-pituitary set point reflected the total body set point and that the body has wisdom to know that serum testosterone should be 800 ng/dl in one person in order to have the appropriate biological effects on all the tissues. An alternate possibility is that the serum level of testosterone is really the slave to the hypothalamus and pituitary and the other organs are either starved or overfed.

**Bernard Robaire:** I would like to try and get at Dr. Handelsman's question from another angle. Since we know that spermatogenesis takes a lot more testosterone than say maintaining prostate weight, which seems to require more testosterone than sexual behavior so, in fact, we have within the body different systems that respond to different amounts of testosterone. What we have to do is figure out the cellular and molecular biology of why those different systems need different amounts of testosterone. That is the gap in our knowledge. My impression is that the androgen receptor is going to be very much the same throughout the body so that if you have a tissue-specific defect in the structure of a receptor, that defect is going to be in all tissues and will have occurred in the gene from conception on. Thus, if we want to target androgen action I think we have to target the gene action within the cell where androgen receptors are working. Trying to determine the androgen responsive genes in different cell types and seeing how we can interfere at that level should provide more specific tools than trying to interfere with the receptor itself.

**Terry Brown:** Well I would agree with Bernard. I was trying to approach it from the perspective that conformational changes which occur in the receptor can be modified by the design of the ligands. I mean, we know that antiandrogens as well as androgens bind to the receptor. Obviously the receptor conformation is different because one activates and the other one does not activate, or in some instances other compounds act as partial agonists. So in each case, the receptor binds to the ligand, but as you said, the other tissue-specific or cell-specific factors may interact with the receptor and ultimately determine the target gene expression.

**Glenn Cunningham:** Perhaps one other approach would be to use another agent which might affect the response of an androgen in a given tissue. For instance, 5 alpha-reductase inhibitors might have a greater effect on the prostate than they would on other tissues. There is a great deal of interest at this time in looking at the effects of retinoic acid analogues and vitamin D analogues in certain tissues. These compounds may prevent neoplastic changes in the prostate.

**Eberhard Nieschlag:** I think the great outcome from the first Androgen Workshop in Marco Island in 1990 was the consensus that whatever we try to do in substituting testosterone levels, it should be as close to physiological as possible. Now I would like to ask the panel and maybe the audience, is that still the dogma we are following, or do we have modified dogmas?

**Ronald Swerdloff:** That certainly is a sound principle in terms of safety. To a certain extent it depends upon what you are trying to do. And if it requires a pharmacologic dose in order to accomplish your goal, then you have to give a pharmacologic dose. Nevertheless, care should be given to administer the lowest pharmacologic dose that is consistent with the desired effect in order to minimize the chances of dose-related adverse actions. That, I think, remains a reasonable principle.

**Kalyan Sundaram:** We still have not identified what is the adverse effect we are trying to avoid with androgens. For example, are you trying to protect the prostate, or are we concerned about lipid levels? Is there a specific concern that you are trying to address? Do we know what harm is the high level of testosterone doing that we want to avoid? I mentioned that MENT can spare the prostate.

**Eberhard Nieschlag:** This discussion clarifies the needs for future studies.

**David Handelsman:** The safety record of synthetic androgens is unenviable. It would take a lot of work to persuade people that a synthetic androgen's potential benefits in being selective really are justifying its introduction.

**Stephen Winters:** I was intrigued with Dr. Sundaram's approach of identifying an androgen which is metabolized differently than testosterone in various tissues. If we are concerned about the proliferative effects of testosterone treatment on the prostate, the identification of an androgen which is 5 alpha-reduced to a less biologically active compound would be further advantageous.

**Eberhard Nieschlag:** This is a valid and important statement. We have not seen clinical studies of MENT yet. And I presume that the Population Council has not done any clinical studies. The great problem here is that we are not getting the pharmaceutical industry involved. So maybe we could ask members of the audience whether they could help us in identifying the problems of why the pharmaceutical industry is not interested in this area and does not help us. Dr. Fried, would you be able to comment on this question or other representatives from the pharmaceutical industry, or Henry Gabelnick?

**Henry Gabelnick:** I do not want to respond on behalf of the pharmaceutical industry, but I did want to respond to David Handelsman's remark a moment ago. Just because there have been problems in the past, and I assume you are talking about methyl-testosterone for one, I do not understand why one extrapolates from that to saying that all synthetic androgens are damned. We have to keep an open mind that there are certain advantages to the synthetic androgens. I do not think we should rule them out. As far as your question about the pharmaceutical industry, it is clearly one that has been repeated over and over again in this workshop and in many others. The issue is the cost-to-benefit ratio and what drugs are in wide use and will lead to large profits compared to the risks associated with small volume drugs and high liability.

**Eberhard Nieschlag:** That is a good explanation. Dr. Fried, please.

**G. Fried:** I can only subscribe to Dr. Gabelnick's comment. The pharmaceutical industry, as any industry, is profit-driven and no project whose promise for an adequate return is too small compared with the risks involved, including liability problems, will gain approval. This is particularly true for drug developments that would benefit poorer populations as would be the case with testosterone bucciclate.

**Eberhard Nieschlag:** The question arises whether this is an area in which the public sector might step in, in particular, in developing countries.

**Norm Mazer:** As a representative of the pharmaceutical industry, I find the discussion interesting although I do not want to get into the profit motives. I think, in general, the androgen field was considered to be a small market years ago but that may all be changing because of the science and research that has been going on. What I would like to acknowledge is that rather than synthesizing a "better" androgen than testosterone, the pharmaceutical industry recognized that the real problem was drug delivery. We have had the testosterone molecule for 50 years and not had a good way to administer it. The work presented in today's session shows how hard people have tried with new technologies to make as physiological a replacement delivery system for testosterone as possible. And it is soon going to be in your hands to utilize one that mimics circadian rhythms, has normal metabolism, and can be dosed to achieve low, middle, and high levels. I would like to encourage this group to do as much as they can with systems like that and find out what we can learn about testosterone itself before we head off on the other pathways of trying to do better than the grand synthesizer "herself".

**Eberhard Nieschlag:** Thank you for these comments. It is comforting to know that we have not been left completely alone and that there are colleagues in the industry who are going to help us.

# PART VIII: WORKSHOP PARTICIPANTS

**William Abernathy**
Solvay Pharm.
901 Sawyer Rd
Marietta, GA 30062

**Dimitrios A. Adamopoulos, MD**
Elena's Hos.-Dept of Endo.
2 E. Venizelou Sq.
Athens, 115 21 Greece

**F.X. Arif Adimoelja, MD, PhD**
Airlangga Univ. J1 Dharmahusada
Indah A-5
Surabaya, 60285 Indonesia

**Gerianne M. Alexander, PhD**
University of New Orleans
Lake Front
New Orleans, LA 70148

**Nancy J. Alexander, PhD**
Contraceptive Devlp Branch
Ctr for Popula.
6100 Executive Blvd. -Rm 8B13
Rockville, MD 20892-7510

**Susan S. Allen, MD, MPH**
CONRAD Program
1611 N. Kent St Ste 806
Arlington, VA 22209

**K.M. Arsyad, MD**
Sriwisaya University
Dept. Med. Bio
Palembang, 30126 Indonesia

**Stefan Arver, MD**
Karolinska Hospital
Reproductive Medical Center
Stockholm, S-17176 Sweden

**Linda Atkinson, PhD**
Alza Corp.
950 Page Mill Rd PO Box 10950
Palo Alto, CA 94303-0802

**Carrie Bagatell**
VA Medical Ctr/Univ. Washington
1660 S. Columbia Way
Seattle, WA 98108

**Michael Bailey**
SmithKline Beecham/US Marketing
One Franklin Plz, 200 N. 16th St.
Philadelphia, PA 19102

**Jerald Bain**
Mt Sinai Hospital/Div of Endo.
600 University Ave Ste 781
Toronto, M5G 1X5 Ontario, Canada

**Lisa Banaag, MD**
Harbor-UCLA Res & Ed Inst.
1124 W. Carson St
Torrance, CA 90502

**Elizabeth Barrett-Connor, MD**
Univ. of Calif. San Diego
Dp of Fm and Prev. Med., 0628
9500 Gilman Drive
La Jolla, CA 92093-0628

**Rosemary Basson, MD-BS**
Univ. Hosp/Sexual Med. Un
4500 Oak Street
Vancouver, V6H 3N1 B.C. Canada

**Hermann M. Behre, MD**
Inst. of Rep. Med. Univ. of Munster
Steinfurter Str 107
Muenster, D-48149 Germany

**Shalender Bhasin, MD**
Harbor-UCLA Res & Ed Inst.
1124 W. Carson Street
Torrance, CA 90502

**Gabriel Bialy, PhD**
Ctr for Popul. Res. -NICHD/NIH
6100 Executive Blvd. Rm 8B 07
Bethesda, MD 20892

**Christian Bieglmayer, MD**
A.K. der Stadt Wein-Leitstel-51
Wahringer Gurtel 18-20
Vienna, A-1090 Austria

**Joyce Bierman**
Stolle Research & Develp Corp.
6954 Cornell Rd
Cincinnati, OH 45176

**Juan Bonavera, PhD**
Harbor-UCLA Res & Ed Inst.
1124 W. Carson St
Torrance, CA 90502

**Jo Anne Brasel, MD**
Harbor-UCLA Medical Center
Clinical Study Center
1000 W. Carson St
Torrance, CA 90509

**William J. Bremner, MD, PhD**
University of Washington
VA Med Ctr/Dept. of Med
1660 South Columbian Way
Seattle, WA 98108

**Terry R. Brown, PhD**
John Hopkins Univ. Schl. of Hyg.
615 N. Wolfe Street, Rm 3606
Baltimore, MD 21205

**Carlos Callegari, MD**
Harbor-UCLA Res & Ed Inst.
1124 W. Carson Street
Torrance, CA 90502

**Richard Casaburi, PhD, MD**
Harbor-UCLA Medical Center
1000 W. Carson, St. Box 24
Torrance, CA 90509

**Don H. Catlin, MD**
UCLA Sch of Med/Dept Medicine
2122 Granville Avenue
Los Angeles, CA 90025

**Chawnshang Chang, PhD**
Univ. of WI- Madi., Dept. Ono.
600 Highland Ave.
Madison, WI 53792

**Richard V. Clark, MD, PhD**
Duke Univ. Medical Center
Dept of Medicine Box 3027 DUMC
Durham, NC 27710

**Lee E. Claypool, PhD**
CONRAD Program
1611 N. Kent St. Suite 806
Arlington, VA 22209

**Brenda Clevenger**
Harbor-UCLA Res & Ed Inst.
1124 W. Carson St.
Torrance, CA 90502

**Donald Coffey, PhD**
John Hopkins University
Dept. of Urology
615 N. Wolfe Street
Baltimore, MD 21205

**Douglas S. Colvard, PhD**
CONRAD Program
1611 N. Kent St. Suite 806
Arlington, VA 22209

**M. James Cosentino**
Millersville University
PO Box 1002/Dept of Biology
Millersville, PA 17551

**Patricia S. Cuasnicu, MD**
Inst. de Biologia y Med. Exper.
Obligado 2490
Buenos Aires, 1428 Argentina

**Glenn R. Cunningham, MD**
VA Med Ctr. ACOS-Resch & Dev
2002 Holcombe Blvd.
Houston, TX 77030

**James M. Dabbs Jr., PhD**
College of Arts and Sciences
Georgia State University
Atlanta, GA 30303

**Tina Davidson, RN**
Harbor-UCLA Res & Ed Inst.
1124 W. Carson St
Torrance, CA 90502

**David M. deKretser, MD**
Monash University
Lev 3, Blk E Monash Med. Ctr.
246 Clayton Road
Clayton, Victoria, 3168 Australia

**Bruno DeLignieres, MD**
Service d'Endo et Med dela
Hospital NECKER 149 de Sevres
Paris, 75015 France

**Chuck Dexter**
Torre Renta Lazur Inc.
20 Waterview Blvd.
Parsippany, NJ 07054-1295

**Miguel Diaz, MD**
Mexican Inst. Social Security
AV La Paz 2544
Guadalajara, 44130 Mexico

**Adrian S. Dobs, MD**
John Hopkins Hospital
600 N. Wolfe St.
Baltimore, MD 21287-4906

**Robert E. Dudley, PhD**
Unimed Pharmaceuticals
Buffalo Grove, IL

**Stacy L. Elliot, MD**
Sexual Med. Un, Vancouver Hosp.
G389 4500 Oak St.
Vancouver, V6U 3N1 B.C.

**Mostafa S. Fahim**
Univ. of Missouri, Schl. of Med.
111 Allton Bldg-(DC113)
Columbia, MO 65212

**Gary S. Ferenchick, MD**
Michigan State University
B-338, Clinical center
East Lansing, MI 48824

**Joel S. Finkelstein, MD**
Endocrine Unit, Bulfinch 327
Mass. Gen. Hosp.
32 Fruit Street
Boston, MA 02114

**Charles Fisher, MD**
Harbor-UCLA Medical Center
Clinical Study Center
1000 W. Carson St.
Torrance, CA 90509

**Jean L. Fourcroy, MD, PhD**
Food and Drug Admin.
6310 Swords Way
Bethesda, MD 20817

**Daniel R. Franken**
University of Stellenbosch
Tygerberg Hosp Dept. of OB/GYN
PO Box 19063
Cape Town, 7505 South Africa

**Henry L. Gabelnick, PhD**
CONRAD
1611 North Kent Street Suite 806
Arlington, VA 22209

**Jack Geller, MD**
Mercy Hosp Med Center-Int Med
4077 Fifth Avenue
San Diego, CA 92103

**Joel Gelman, MD**
Harbor-UCLA Res & Ed Inst.
1124 W. Carson Street
Torrance, CA 90502

**Victor Goh, MD**
Hrp/World Health Organization
Avenue Appia
Geneva, CH27 1211 Switzerland

**Erwin Goldberg**
Northwestern Univ/Biochem.
2756 Central Park
Evanston, IL 60201

**Larry S. Goldenberg, MD**
UBC Prostate Clinic
D-9, 2733 Heather St.
Vancouver, V5Z 3J5 B.C. Canada

**Nestor F. Gonzalez-Cadavid, PhD**
Harbor-UCLA Med Ctr/Surgery
1000 W. Carson St.
Torrance, CA 90509

**Louis J. Gooren, MD, PhD**
Free Univ Hosp/Div of Endo
PO Box 7057
Netherlands, 1007 MB Amsterdam

**Roger Gorski, PhD**
UCLA Sch of Med-Biology
Dept of Anatomy and Cell Biology
Los Angeles, CA 90024

**David P. Griffin**
World Health Organization
Avenue Appia CH-1211
Geneva, 27 Switzerland

**Avraam Grinvald, PhD**
Harbor-UCLA Medical Center
Clinical Study Center
1000 W. Carson St.
Torrance, CA 90509

**Michael D. Griswold, PhD**
Washington State University
Prog. in Biochem.
Synthesis Bldg Rm 675
Pullman, WA 99164-4660

**Ralph R. Hall, MD**
University of Missouri
Saint Luke's Hospital
Wornall Road at 44th
Kansas City, MO 64111

**Sang W. Han, MD, PhD**
Dpt of Ur, Yonsei
Univ. College of Med
134 Shinchon-Dong, Seodaemun-Gu
Seoul, 120-752 Korea

**David J. Handelsman, MD, PhD**
University of Sydney
Dept. of OB/GYN
Sydney NSW, 2006 Australia

**John C. Herr, PhD**
Univ. of Virginia Hlth Sci. Ctr.
Dept of Cell Biology
Box 439
Charlottesville, VA 22901

**Walter Heyns**
Katholieke Universiteit Leuven
Legendo, Onderwijs en Navorsing
Gasthuisberg, Herestreat 49
Leuven, B-3000 Belgium

**Yasmin I. Hillmi**
Univ. of Khartoum/Chemistry
PO Box 598
Khartoum, Sudan

**Melissa Hines, PhD**
Goldsmiths College-Dpt of Psych
New Cross
London, UK SE146NW

**Richard Horton, MD**
USC School of Medicine
2025 Zonal Ave, Un I, Rm 18632
Los Angeles, CA 90033

**Hansen M. Hsiung, MD**
Lilly Resch Lab/Dept of Endo
DCO424 Lilly Corp Center
Indianapolis, IN 46285

**Ilpo T. Huhtaniemi, MD, PhD**
University of Turku
Kiinamy 11yukatu 10
Turku, 20520 Finland

**John Isaacs, PhD**
John Hopkins University
Onco. Ctr, Breast Cancer Lab
422 N. Bond St. Rm 201
Baltimore, MD 21231

**Louisa Jenkin**
Univ of Bristol, Dpt of Anatomy
Southwell Street
Bristol, UK BS2 8EJ

**Friedrich Jockenhovel, MD**
Univ Essen/Ablt. Endo
Hufelandstr.55, 45122
Essen, 2980199 Germany

**Frick Julian**
Salsburry, 50201 Australia

**Anu Kapali PhD**
Harbor-UCLA Res & Ed Inst.
1124 W. Carson St
Torrance, CA 90502

**Nadim Y. Kassem, MD**
Bio-Tech General Corp.
70 Wood Avenue South
Iselin, NJ 08830

**Gunter Kaufmann**
Jenapharm GMBH/Medical Resch
Otto-Schott-Strabe 15
Jena, 07745 Germany

**Howard M. Landa, MD**
Loma Linda University/Urology
11370 Anderson St., Ste 1100
Loma Linda, CA 92354

**Gregory Lee**
Univ. of British Columbia-OB/GYN
F107, UBC Hosp 2211 Wesbrook Mall
Vancouver, V67 2B5 BC, Canada

**Andrew Leung**
Harbor-UCLA Res & Ed Inst.
1124 W. Carson St
Torrance, CA 90502

**Tehming Liang, MD, PhD**
Wright St. Univ Sch of Med.
PO Box 927
Dayton, OH 45401-0927

**Gerhard F. Lunglmayr, MD**
Mistelbach Gen Hosp Dpt of Ur
Liechtensteinerstrasse 67
Mistelbach/Zaya, Ak-2130 Austria

**Robert H. Lustig, MD**
Univ of Tenn, Dept of Ped.
50 North Dunlap/Child Med Ctr
Memphis, TN 38103

**Helen Maclean**
Royal Child's Hospital
Dept of Endo.-Flemington Rd
Parkville, 3052 Vic, Australia

**Mary C. Mahony, PhD**
Jones Inst. for Repd Med/OB-GYN
601 Colley Avenue
Norfolk, VA 23507

**Diana Marquez, MD**
Harbor-UCLA Res & Ed Inst.
1124 W. Carson St.
Torrance, CA 90502

**Stephen A. Matlin**
Warwick University
Chemistry Dept.
Coventry, UK CV4 7AL

**Alvin M. Matsumoto, MD**
VA Medical Center-GRECC(182B)
1660 Columbian Way
Seattle, WA 98108

**Norm Mazer, MD, PhD**
Thera Tech Inc.
417 Wakara Way
Salt Lake City, UT 84108

**Dave McCready**
Organon Canada LTD.
200 Consilium Place, Ste 700
Scarborough, M1H 3E4 Ontario

**Veronica McDonald, RN**
Harbor-UCLA Res & Ed Inst.
1124 W. Carson St.
Torrance, CA 90502

**Robert I. McLachlan, MD, PhD**
Prince Henry's Inst. of Med Rech
PO Box 5152
Clayton, 3168 VIC Australia

**Wayne A. Meikle, MD**
University of Utah Sch of Med
Salt Lake City, UT 84132

**Sunny Melendez, MD**
20911 Earl Str. #220
Torrance, CA 90503

**Aprile Melton, RNC**
Augusta Reprod Biology Assoc.
812 Chafee Ave
Augusta, GA 30904

**M. Cristina Meriggiola, MD**
Universita'Degli Studi Di Bologna
Clinica Ostetrica e Ginecologica
Ospedale S. Orsola V. Massarenti 13
Bologna, 40138 Italy

**Abraham Morgentaler, MD**
Beth Israel Hosp-Dept of Orol
330 Brookline Ave
Boston, MA 02215

**Hossein Najmabadi, PhD**
Harbor-UCLA Res & Ed Inst.
1124 Carson St
Torrance, CA 90502

**Anita Nelson, MD**
Harbor-UCLA Medical Center
1000 W. Carson St
Torrance, CA 90509

**Blake Lee Neubauer, PhD**
Lilly Corp Ctr
CNS/CI/GU Resrch Mail#0510
Indianapolis, IN 56285

**Chris Ng**
Harbor-UCLA Res & Ed Inst.
1124 W. Carson St
Torrance, CA 90502

**Helen Nicholson**
Univer of Bristol, Dpt of Anatomy
Southwell Street
Bristol, UK BS2 8EJ

**Eberhardt Nieschlag, MD**
Max-Planck Clin Res Unit
Steinfurter Strabe 107
Munster, D-48149 Germany

**Todd B. Nippoldt, MD**
Alza Corp
950 Page Mill Rd, PO Box 10950
Palo Alto, CA 94043-0802

**Arlene Noodleman, MD**
Alza Corp
950 Page Mill Rd, PO Box 10950
Palo Alto, CA 94043-0802

**Marie-Claire Orgebin-Crist, PhD**
Vanderbilt University
Dept OB/GYN Rm D-23-3 MCN
Nashville, TN 37232-2633

**Eric Orwoll, MD**
Portland Veterans Admin Med Ctr
Portland, OR

**J. Alfonoso Osuna-Ceballos, MD**
University of the Andes
Apartado #156
Merida, 5101-A Venezuela

**Delores J. Patanelli, MD**
8324 Raymond Lane
Potomac, MD 20954

**C. Alvin Paulsen, MD**
Univ of WA Sch of Med
1200 12th Avenue South
Seattle, WA 98144

**Mark Pavao**
SmithKline Beecham/US Marketing
One Franklin Plz, 200 N. 16th St
Philadelphia, PA 19102

**David Penson, MD**
Harbor-UCLA Res & Ed Inst.
1124 W. Carson St
Torrance, CA 90502

**Dorothy A. Pfeffer**
Mediphacs, Inc.
580 Howard Avenue
Somerset, NY 08873

**Mark Phillipson**
Merck Health Science Service
818 Hastings,
Claremont, CA 91711

**Angelo Poletti**
Univ of Milano, Dept of Endo
Via Balzaretti 9
Milano, 20133 Italy

**Ake Pousette, MD, PhD**
Karolinska Hospital
Karolinska Institutet
Stockholm, S-171 76 Sweden

**Jon L. Pryor, MD**
Univ of Minn/Urologic Sug
420 Delaware St Box 394 UMHC
Minneapolis, MN 55455

**Michael Ramstack, PhD**
Medisorb Technologies
6j954 Cornell Rd
Cincinnati, OH 45242

**Elizabeth Rappaport, MD**
SmithKline Beecham Pharm
Four Falls Corp Ctr Ret
23 & Woodmont Ave.
King of Prussia, PA 19406

**Geoffrey P. Redmond, DM**
Founda for Devlp Endo, Inc.
23200 Chagrin Blvd Ste 325 #5
Cleveland, OH 44122

**Karin Ringheim**
USAID Off of Popul Res Div
G/PHN/R Room 820-SA-18
Washington, DC 20523-1819

**Gail P. Rishbridger**
Inst of Reprod & Devlp, Monash
Blk E, Lev 3, 246 Clayton Rd
Melbourne, 3168 Vic, Australia

**Mark Rispler**
Harbor-UCLA Res & Ed Inst
1124 W. Carson St
Torrance, CA 90502

**Alan D. Rogol, MD, PhD**
Univ of VA Health Sciences Ctr
Lane Road, MR4-Room 3037
Charlottesville, VA 22908

**Somnath Roy, MD**
Reprod Health Foundation
410 Nilgiri Apts, Alaknanda
New Delhi, 110019 India

**Bernard Ruedi, MD**
Hosp des Cadolles
Dept of Int Medicine
Neuchatel, CH-2000 Switzerland

**H. Ruedi-Bettex**
Hosp des Cadolles
Dept of Intern. Medicine
Neuchatel, Ch-2000 Switzerland

**F. H. Schroder, MD**
Erasmus Univ Rotterdam
Prostbus 1738
Rotterdam, 3000 Netherlands

**HCA Schwietert**
N.V. Organon
Molenstraat 110 PO Box 20
Amsterdam 534OBH Oss Netherlands

**Edouard J. Servy, MD**
Augusta Reprod Biology Assoc
812 Chafee Ave
Augusta, GA 30904

**Laurie Shaker-Irwin, PhD**
Pac Oaks Med Gp, Dept of Resch
4940 Van Nuys Blvd 2nd Fl
Sherman Oaks, CA 91403

**Tsang C. Shao, PhD**
VA Med Ctr., Endo Resrch (151B)
2002 Holcombe Blvd.
Houston, TX 77030

**Richard M. Sharpe, PhD**
Centre for Reprod Biology
37 Chalmers Street
Edinburgh EH 393W, UK

**Ruo-King Shen, MD**
Harbor-UCLA Res & Ed Inst
1124 W. Carson St
Torrance, CA 90502

**Barbara Sherwin, PhD**
McGill Univ-Bio Sc Bldg
1205 Dr. Penfield Avenue
Montreal, H3 a 1B1 QC, Canada

**Amiya P. Sinha-Hikim**
Harbor-UCLA Res & Ed Inst
1124 W. Carson St
Torrance, CA 90502

**Indrani Sinha-Hikim PhD**
Harbor-UCLA Res & Ed Inst
1124 W. Carson St
Torrance, CA 90502

**Peter J. Snyder, MD**
Univ of Pennsylvania Sch of Medicine
611 Clinic Research Bldg
422 Curie Blvd.
Philadelphia, PA 19104-6149

**Richard F. Spark, MD**
Beth Israel Hospital
330 Brookline Avenue
Boston, MA 02215

**Jeff Spieler**
Agency for International Development
Research Division
Office of Population
Washington, DC 20523

**Barbara Steiner, RN**
Harbor-UCLA Res & Ed Inst
1124 W. Carson St
Torrance, CA 90502

**Tom Storer, PhD**
Harbor-UCLA Medical Center
1000 W. Carson St
Torrance, CA 90509

**Gerhard Struhal**
Mullnergasse 26
Vienna, A-1090 Austria

**Makam Subbarao, PhD**
Harbor-UCLA Res & Ed Inst
1124 W. Carson St
Torrance, CA 90502

**Kalyan Sundaram, PhD**
The Population Council-Res Ctr
1230 York Avenue
New York, NY 10021

**Laura Superlano, MD**
Harbor-UCLA Res & Ed Inst
1224 W. Carson St
Torrance, CA 90502

**Ronald S. Swerdloff, MD**
Harbor-UCLA Res & Ed Inst
1124 W. Carson St
Torrance, CA 90502

**Lewis S. Sydenstricker, MD**
PO Box 903
Groverland, CA 95321

**Wayne Taylor**
Harbor-UCLA Res & Ed Inst
1124 W. Carson St
Torrance, CA 90502

**Lisa J. Tenover, MD, PhD**
Emory Univ/Wesley Woods Hlth Ctr
1841 Clifton Road NE
Atlanta, GA 30329-5102

**Laurie K.S. Tom, MD**
Queens Physician Office Bldg 1
1380 Lusitand St #806
Honolulu, HI 96813

**Ray Tricker, PhD**
Oregon State University
Walph Hall 311
Corvallys, OR 97331

**Philip Troen, MD**
Montefiore Univ Hosp/Medicine
200 Lothrop Street
Pittsburgh, PA 15213

**Richard J. Udry**
Univ of North Carolina
Carolina Popul Ctr-Univ. Sq
CB #8120, 123 W. Franklin St.
Chapel Hill, NC 27516-3997

**Dirk Vanderschueren, MD, PhD**
U.Z. Gasthuisberg, Dept of Endo
Herestraat 49
Leuven, B-3000 Belgium

**Dolores Vernet, PhD**
Harbor-UCLA Res & Ed Inst
1124 W. Carson St
Torrance, CA 90502

**Geoffrey M.H. Waites, PhD**
Univ Hosp Gena-Dept of OB/GYN
01630 Saint Jean de Gonville
Geneva, 1211 Switzerland

**Christina Wang, MD**
Harbor-UCLA Medical Center
Clinical Study Center Box 16
1000 W. Carson St
Torrance, CA 90509

**Min Wang**
Univ of Missouri, Sch of Med
111 Allton Bldg, (DC113)
Columbia, MO 65212

**Jon E. Wergedal, PhD**
Pettis Veteran Hosp Resch
11201 Benton St
Loma Linda, CA 92357

**Margaret E. Wierman**
Univ of Colorado-Dept of Endo
111H Endo VAMC, 1055 Clermont
Denver, CO 80220

**Cynthia Williams, MD**
Harbor-UCLA Res & Ed Inst
1124 W. Carson St
Torrance, CA 90502

**Jean Wilson, MD**
University of TX Southwestern
Dept of Internal Medicine
5323 Harry Hines Blvd.
Dallas, TX 75235-8857

**Stephen J. Winters, MD**
Univ of Pitts. Sch/Med
UPMC/Montefiore
200 Lothrop Street/9 West
Pittsburgh, PA 15213

**F.C.W. Wu, MD**
Univ of Manchester
Hope Hosp., Eccles Old Road
Salfor M6 8HD
England, UK

**Yining Xie, MD**
Harbor-UCLA Medical Center
Clinical Study Center
1000 W. Carson St
Torrance, CA 90509

**Tatsuhiro Yoshiki**
Univ Hosp/UBC Andrology Lab
2211 Wesbrook Mall
Vancouver, BC N V6T 2B5 Canada

**Gui-yuan Zhang, MD**
Natl Resech Inst for Fm Plan
Dp of Endo #12 Da Hui Si, Haidian
Beijing, 100081 P.R. China

# INDEX